An Introduction to Melanoma

An Introduction to Melanoma

Edited by **Frederick Nash**

FOSTER ACADEMICS

New Jersey

Published by Foster Academics,
61 Van Reypen Street,
Jersey City, NJ 07306, USA
www.fosteracademics.com

An Introduction to Melanoma
Edited by Frederick Nash

International Standard Book Number: 978-1-63242-045-9 (Hardback)

Printed in China.

Contents

Preface

Every book is initially just a concept; it takes months of research and hard work to give it the final shape in which the readers receive it. In its early stages, this book also went through rigorous reviewing. The notable contributions made by experts from across the globe were first molded into patterned chapters and then arranged in a sensibly sequential manner to bring out the best results.

This book intends to present data and knowledge from most experienced experts in the field. The book encompasses important topics related to the fundamental aspects of melanoma biology. It provides a global perspective concerning one of the most frequent types of cancer, which a large number of people come across at some point of time in their life. This book is an invaluable source of reference for those interested in melanoma.

It has been my immense pleasure to be a part of this project and to contribute my years of learning in such a meaningful form. I would like to take this opportunity to thank all the people who have been associated with the completion of this book at any step.

Editor

Section 1

Fundamental Aspects of the Melanoma Biology

Chapter 1

Overcoming Resistance to BRAF and MEK Inhibitors by Simultaneous Suppression of CDK4

Jianli Dong

Additional information is available at the end of the chapter

1. Introduction

Melanoma is one of the most prevalent malignancies and has a very poor prognosis. Mutations in v-raf murine sarcoma viral oncogene homolog B1 (*BRAF*) occur in approximately 50% of melanomas [4]. While the response to selective BRAF inhibitors (BRAFi) in *BRAF*-mutant melanoma is encouraging, virtually all patients rapidly develop secondary resistance [6, 7]. Based on the finding that the mitogen activated protein kinase/ERK kinase (MEK)-extracellular signal regulated kinase (ERK) pathway is frequently reactivated by various BRAFi resistance mechanisms, a combination trial of a selective mutant BRAF inhibitor (dabrafenib, GSK2118436) with a MEK inhibitor (trametinib, GSK1120212) is underway and has achieved clinical responses in 17% and disease control in 67% in patients who failed prior single-agent treatment with a BRAF inhibitor [9]. While these results are promising, there is a critical need to overcome resistance to BRAF and MEK inhibitors. The clinical efficacy of BRAFi and MEKi therapy is believed to rely on a functional retinoblastoma (RB) axis to inhibit cell proliferation. The inhibitor of cyclin-dependent kinase 4A (*INK4A*) gene encode the p16 protein, a critical cell cycle regulator that interacts with cyclin dependent kinase (CDK) 4, inhibiting its ability to phosphorylate and inactivate RB [12, 13]. Genetic disruption of *INK4A* occurs in approximately 50% of melanomas irrespective of *BRAF* mutation and has been detected in melanoma cells that developed resistance to BRAFi. Of note, cyclin D is still expressed even in the setting of maximum tolerance dosing of BRAF inhibitor [7]. We have reported that combination of BRAFi or MEKi with the expression of wild-type *INK4A* or a CDK4 inhibitor (CDK4i) significantly suppresses growth and enhances apoptosis in melanoma cells [1-3]. Currently, CDK4 inhibitors are in active clinical development (http://clinicaltrials.gov/). Based on our previous work and recent insights into molecular mechanisms of resistance to BRAF and MEK inhibitors, we hypothesize that simultaneous suppression of

CDK4 is an effective strategy to overcome resistance to BRAF and MEK inhibitors. BRAF mutation assays have been used to guide treatment with BRAF and MEK inhibitors, development of sensitive and specific INK4A/p16 assays may serve as predictive biomarkers for treatment with CDK4 inhibitors.

2. Body

Constitutive activation of RAS-RAF-MEK-ERK signaling pathway in melanomas.*NRAS* and *BRAF* mutations were found respectively in 10-20% and 60-80% melanomas [4]. NRAS and BRAF are components of the RAS-RAF-mitogen activated protein kinase/ERK kinase (MEK)-extracellular signal regulated kinase (ERK) signaling pathway (Fig. 1) [5]. This signaling pathway plays an essential role in cell proliferation, differentiation and survival [5, 14, 15]. Constitutive activation of the ERK pathway has been shown to mediate the transforming activity of mutant BRAF in melanoma cells [16-18]. Suppression of mutant *BRAF* expression has been shown to inhibit ERK pathway activation and subsequent suppression of melanoma cell proliferation and survival *in vitro* and *in vivo* [19-21]. Our previous data revealed that the inhibition of mutant BRAF decreased levels of phospho-ERK (p-ERK), a marker of ERK pathway activation in melanoma cells [5, 14, 15].

The high frequency of *BRAF* mutation in melanomas makes it an ideal target for therapy. Because normal cells require wild-type *BRAF* for survival [22], specifically inhibiting mutant, but not wild-type *BRAF* in tumor cells could avoid toxic side effects generated by targeting normal cells. The finding that mutations in v-raf murine sarcoma viral oncogene homolog B1 (*BRAF*) occur in approximately 50% of melanomas led to extensive investigation of targeting BRAF for melanoma treatment, resulting in the first approved mutant specific BRAF inhibitor for treatment of advanced melanoma.

Combine BRAF and MEK inhibitors with chemotherapeutic agents. Intrinsic therapy resistance is a major limitation in the treatment of malignant melanomas. The mechanisms involved in the resistance of melanomas are largely unknown [23, 24]. It is believed that apoptosis and cytostasis (growth arrest/differentiation) are two of the main cellular responses to anticancer agents and loss of either process promotes treatment failure [25-27]. Activating *BRAF* mutations could drive cell proliferation and increase the cell death threshold through ERK pathway or alternative mechanisms [28-30], resulting in the blockage of both cytotoxic and cytostatic effects of therapeutic drugs [14, 31, 32]. It has been shown that inhibition of ERK pathway sensitizes melanoma cells to apoptosis induced by DNA damaging agents including cisplatin and ultra-violate (UV) irradiation [32, 33]. Rational combination of BRAF and MEK inhibitors with selective chemotherapeutic agents, for example, dacarbazine (DTIC), may generate additive/synergistic therapeutic effects.

ERK pathway activation and p16 in melanocytic lesions. Melanocytic lesions can be grouped into two main categories: nevi and melanomas. Nevi are divided into several different types based on histology. These include acquired melanocytic nevi, congenital melanocytic nevi, blue nevi, Spitz nevi, and dysplastic nevi. Melanoma can be further divided based on clinical and traditional histological methods as superficial spreading melanoma, lentigo maligna melanoma, acral lentiginous melanoma, and nodular melanoma. In early stages of melanomas, neoplastic cells are confined to the epidermis or with microinvasion into the dermis. In advanced melanomas, cancer cells expand in the dermis and generate tumor nodules and have a high potential for metastatic spread. In the metastatic phase, cancer cells disseminate to lymph nodes or distant organs [34, 35]. For the early diagnosed and localized melanomas, surgery is the choice of treatment. But there is currently no effective treatment for invasive and metastatic melanomas. Patients with late stage melanomas have a high mortality rate and life expectancy averages approximately 6-8 months after diagnosis.

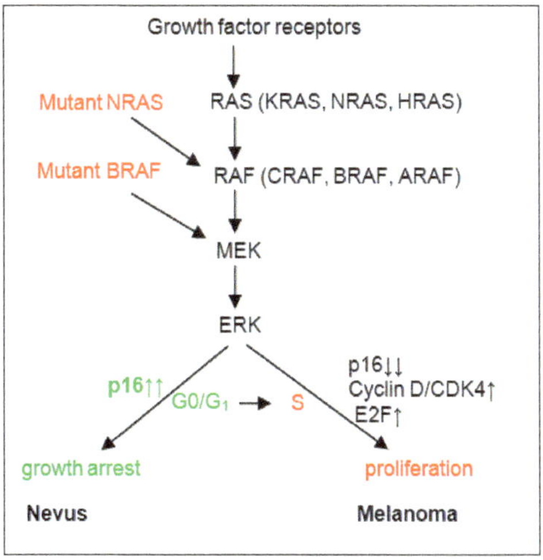

Figure 1. p16-cyclin D/CDK4 modifies the outcome of RAS/RAF/MEK/ERK signaling activation. RAF relays RAS signals through MEK to ERK. The activation of this pathway has multiple effects on cell proliferation, differentiation, and survival depending on the cellular contexts [5]. Constitutive activation of growth factor signaling pathways or NRAS and BRAF activating mutations can trigger over-expression of p16 leading to proliferative senescence, which manifest as benign nevus [10, 11]. Loss of p16 by genetic and epigenetic changes allows activation of cyclin D/CDK4 and inactivation of RB, leading to E2F activation, cell cycle progression from G1 to S phase, cell proliferation and tumor formation [12, 13]. Further genetic changes cause tumor progression to malignant melanoma. Of the three *RAS* and three *RAF* genes, *NRAS* and *BRAF* are mutated in melanoma [4].

Of note, in addition to melanomas, *BRAF* mutations are found at high frequencies (70-80%) in benign melanocytic nevi [36, 37]. There are a large numbers of melanocytic nevi in the general population compared to the relatively low incidence of melanomas [34, 35]. Clinically, it is known that nevi often regress over time. This suggests that BRAF mutations alone are insufficient to induce malignant transformation in nevus cells. The growth arrest of nevi is believed to result from oncogene-induced senescence, which is known as a protective mechanism against unlimited proliferation that could result from *BRAF* mutations and activation of the ERK signaling pathway (nevus in Fig. 1) [10, 11]. Tumor suppressor genes have been found to be involved in senescence process. For example, p16 is one tumor suppressor found to be induced by ERK activation and telomere attrition involving cell senescence [8, 10, 11, 38]. The tumor suppressor p16 is encoded by *INK4A* (Fig. 2) and is often inactivated in a variety of human cancers, including 30-70% in melanomas [39, 40]. Most melanomas, but not nevi, have lost the expression of wild-type *INK4A,* either through DNA deletion/ mutation or promoter hypermethylation [41-45]. It is possible that the loss-of-function of p16 in melanomas may make it possible to bypass the cellular senescence mechanism and function as an anti-tumor mechanism against ERK signal activation triggered by *NRAS* and *BRAF* oncogenic mutation (Fig. 1) [11, 46, 47].

Indirect evidence from cultured cells and animal models reveal that there may be a cooperative role between the constitutive activation of ERK pathway and the loss of p16 in tumor progression. Daniotti et al. [48] reported the co-existence of *BRAF* mutations and *INK4A* mutations/deletions/loss-of-expression in 26 of 41 (63%) short-term cell lines obtained from melanoma biopsies. Recent evidence suggests that growth arrest in benign nevi is due to cell senescence and that p16 at least partially contributes to the process of senescence in nevi [11, 46, 47].

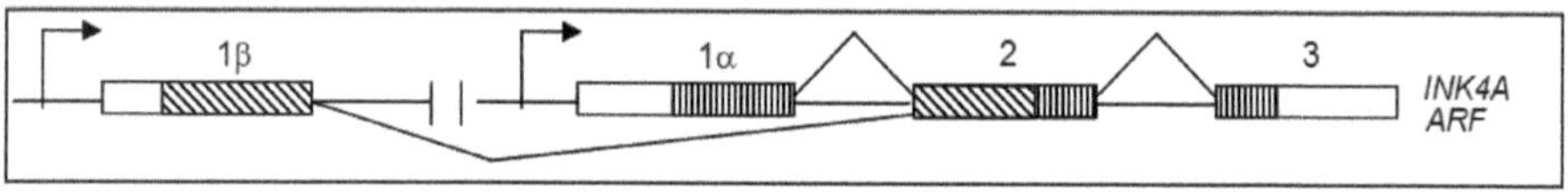

Figure 2. *INK4A* and *ARF* share sequences in the *CDKN2A* locus. Exons are shown as rectangles. Alternative first exons (1α and 1β) are transcribed from different promoters (arrows). Exons 1α and 1β are spliced to the same splicing acceptor site in exon 2 but are translated in alternative reading frames. *INK4A* coding sequences in exons 1α, 2, and 3 and *ARF* coding sequences in exons 1β and 2 are indicated by different shading patterns. Adopted from Sherr [8]. *INK4A* lesions detected by FISH and Sanger sequencing may also affect *ARF*.

Resistance of melanoma to BRAF and MEK inhibitors. The finding that mutations in *BRAF* occur in melanomas led to extensive investigation of targeting BRAF for melanoma treatment. While the response to selective mutant BRAF inhibitors (BRAFi) in *BRAF*-mutant melanoma is encouraging, virtually all patients rapidly develop secondary resistance. Based on the finding that the mitogen activated protein kinase/ERK kinase (MEK)-extracellular signal regulated kinase (ERK) pathway is frequently reactivated by various BRAFi resistance mechanisms, the first combination trial of a selective BRAF inhibitor (dabrafenib, GSK2118436) with a MEK inhibitor (trametinib, GSK1120212) is underway and has achieved clinical responses in 17% and disease control in 67% in patients who failed prior single-agent treatment with a BRAF inhibitor [9]. While these results are promising, again, the treatment response is short-lived; there is a critical need for additional strategies to overcome this deadly disease [49, 50].

There is evidence that treatment response to BRAFi and MEKi relies on a functional p16-cyclin D-CDK4-retinoblastoma (RB) axis. *INK4A* mutations/deletions occur in most of the melanoma cells that demonstrated resistance to BRAFi (e.g.; 451Lu, Mel1617, WM983, WM902, A375, M238, SKMEL28, and A2058) [51-57]. Over-expression of cyclin D and deletion of *RB* confer treatment resistance to BRAFi [56, 58]. Unlike other components of the p16-cyclin D-CDK4-RB axis that harbor genetic changes at low frequency in melanomas (e.g., *CDK4* and *RB* each approximately 3%) [59], and may not overlap with *BRAF* mutation (e.g., amplification of cyclin D1 gene *CCND1* and *CDK4*) [60], *INK4A* lesions are frequently detected in melanomas (~50%) irrespective of *BRAF* mutation [59-61]; therefore, abnormal p16 is a major mechanism of RB-axis attenuation in *BRAF*-mutant melanoma cells. p16 binds to and inhibits the catalytic activity of CDK4, representing a crucial gatekeeper at the G1>S checkpoint [62, 63]. The relative abundance of CDK4-cyclin D and p16 can determine the activity of the CDK4 kinase, thus regulate RB and cell-cycle progression [62, 63]. BRAF-MEK-ERK signaling pathway upregulates/activates the cyclin D-CDK4 enzyme, which phosphorylates and inactivates RB leading to cell cycle progression in melanoma cells; such an effect can be blocked by tumor suppressor p16 [2, 3, 61]. Several pathways that confer BRAFi resistance, including COT, RAF splicing variants, RAF dimerization, NRAS, IGF-1R, and RTK can reactivate cyclin D-CDK4 through signaling pathways including MEK-ERK as well as PI3K-AKT [51-53, 55, 56, 64]. Although the addition of MEKi to BRAFi may suppress reactivation of MEK-ERK-cyclin D-CDK4, alternative resistance mechanisms, including growth factor receptors and PI3K-AKT pathway can activate cyclin D-CDK4 [52, 55, 64-66] *in the absence of a functional p16,* adding CDK4 inhibitor may help overcoming resistance to BRAFi and MEKi (Fig. 3). *BRAF* mutation assays have been used to direct BRAFi treatment. There is significant genotypic heterogeneity of *INK4A* including bi- and mono-allelic deletions, nonsense and missense mutations, and also different levels of epigenetic modification by promoter hyper-methylation. Characterization of whether these *INK4A* changes correlate with different treatment resistance to BRAFi/MEKi/CDK4i may lead to companion molecular tests to better manage melanoma patients under BRAFi, MEKi, and CDK4i therapy.

As shown in Fig. 4, in addition to BRAF and MEK inhibitors, several drugs designed to inhibit the activity of CDK4 are in active clinical trials for melanoma and other cancers including LEE011 (Novartis Pharmaceuticals), LY2835219 (Eli Lilly and Company), PD-0332991 (Pfizer) (http://clinicaltrials.gov/).

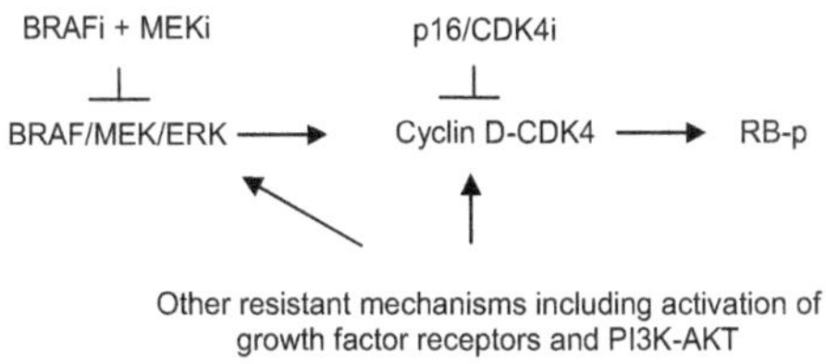

Figure 3. The presence of functional p16 may offset resistance mechanisms that lead to activation of cyclin D-CDK4 in melanomas that progressed under BRAFi/MEKi treatment, whereas abnormal p16 may predict treatment failure in melanomas that develop resistance mechanisms un-opposed by BRAFi + MEKi treatment.

Combined inhibition of CDK4 potentiate the effect of MEKi. In order to design better strategies for the treatment of this devastating disease a better understanding of melanoma biology is necessary. Multiple genetic and environmental factors have been linked to the development and aggressive behavior of melanomas [49, 50]. *BRAF* mutations have been identified in approximately 60–80% of human melanomas, while *NRAS* mutations occur in about 10% of melanomas [4, 67]. Both NRAS and BRAF are components of the RAS-RAF-mitogen activated protein kinase/ERK kinase (MEK)-extracellular signal regulated kinase (ERK) signaling pathway. Apart from *NRAS* and *BRAF* mutation, other factors have been identified leading to constitutive activation of the ERK signaling, for example, amplification and somatic mutations of KIT and constitutive expression of hepatocyte growth factor (HGF) and fibroblast growth factor (FGF) [49, 50]. ERK signaling pathway controls cell proliferation, differentiation, and survival, and has been shown to be a targetable pathway in melanoma treatment [5, 14, 15, 68].

Deregulation of the p16-cyclin D:cyclin-dependent kinases (CDK) 4/6-retinoblastoma (RB) pathway is a common paradigm in malignancy including melanoma [12, 13, 39] and represents another attractive target in melanoma treatment. The great majority of melanoma cells have lost or reduced expression of wild-type *INK4A* caused by genetic and epigenetic changes including mutation, deletion, and promoter hypermethylation [69, 70]. Loss of p16 leaves cyclin D:CDK4 unoppressed to phosphorylate and inactivate RB and cell cycle progression [8, 13, 49, 50, 69, 70]. Amplification of cyclin D1 and CDK4 genes have also been identified, mostly in melanomas that harbor wild-type *NRAS* and *BRAF* [58]. A germ-line Arg24Cys (R24C) mutation in CDK4 was identified in familial melanoma patients [40, 58]. This mutation abolishes CDK4 inhibition by p16 and thus is believed to be a functional equivalent to p16 loss. Both ERK signaling and CDK4 kinase have been shown to regulate RB protein and cell cycle progression [58, 61]. Activation of BRAF-MEK-ERK signaling pathway can cause upregulation of cyclin D resulting in the activation of CDK4 [61]. Activated CDK4 phosphorylates and inactivated RB proteins result in the liberation of E2F transcription factors and cell cycle progression. It has been shown that in advanced melanoma cells, RB is highly phosphorylated and inactive, and E2F transcriptional activity is constitutively high ([5, 12].

Various resistance mechanisms have been identified that contribute to treatment failure of melanoma patients to BRAFi and MEKi therapy. Loss of p16 may represent a common gateway permitting the phenotypic expression of several resistance mechanisms to BRAFi and MEKi (Figs. 1 and 3), a hypothesis that has not been and is waiting to be tested in clinical trials. We reported that simultaneous expression of *BRAF* siRNA and *INK4A* cDNA in melanoma cells leads to dramatically increased apoptosis (17), suggesting that correcting the two most common genetic lesions could be effective in melanoma treatment. It is unclear whether the effect is specific to *BRAF* and *INK4A* or can be generalized to other components of the ERK and RB pathways. It has been shown that *BRAF* and *INK4A* may have activities independent of the corresponding canonical ERK and RB pathways, and the two pathways also mediate cellular signals independent of aberrant *BRAF* and *INK4A*. For example, RAF can act through apoptosis signal-regulating kinase-1 (ASK1)/c-Jun-NH2-kinase or mammalian sterile 20- like-kinase 2 (MST2) pathways ([71]; cyclin D:CDK4 can be activated by enhanced phosphatidylinositol 3-kinase (PI3K) and wingless (WNT) signaling pathways in melanomas [27, 72]. Therefore, we tested PD98059 and 219476, commercially available inhibitors of MEK and CDK4, respectively, in human melanoma cells.

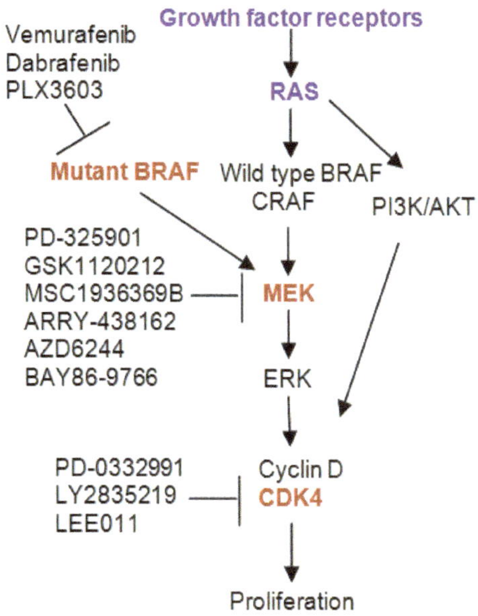

Figure 4. BRAF, MEK and CDK4 inhibitors are in active clinical development and may be used in combination to increase treatment efficacy. Melanoma cells acquire resistance to BRAF and MEK inhibitors by mechanisms including activation of growth factor receptors and RAS signaling pathways. Activation of growth factor receptors and RAS pathways can cause overexpression of cyclin D and activation CDK4 kinase, leading to cell cycle proliferation, which is believed to play major roles in the emergence of treatment resistance. Adding CDK4 inhibitors may overcome resistance to treatment targeting BRAF and MEK. Apart from Vemurafenib (PLX4032, RO5185426) (Hoffmann-La Roche) that has been U.S. Food and Drug Administration (FDA) approved for treatment of melanoma, other mutant BRAF inhibitors including PLX3603 (RO5212054) (Hoffmann-La Roche) and GSK2118436 (dabrafenib) (GlaxoSmithKline) are in active clinical trials. There are clinical trials of MEK inhibitors PD-325901 (Pfizer), GSK1120212 (GlaxoSmithKline), MSC1936369B (EMD Serono), ARRY-438162 (MEK162) (Array BioPharma), AZD6244 (AstraZeneca), and BAY86-9766 (Bayer). Several drugs designed to inhibit the activity of CDK4 are also in active clinical trials for melanoma and other cancers including PD-0332991 (Pfizer), LY2835219 (Eli Lilly and Company), LEE011 (Novartis Pharmaceuticals) (http://clinicaltrials.gov/).

MEK inhibitor PD98059 (Calbiochem, San Diego, CA) was dissolved in dimethyl sulfoxide (DMSO) as a 50 mM stock solution, aliquoted and stored at -20C. CDK4 inhibitor 219476 (Cat. # 219476, Calbiochem, San Diego, CA) was dissolved in DMSO as a 2 mM stock solution and stored at 4C. Human melanoma cell lines 624Mel, A101D, and OM431 were kindly provided by Dr. Stuart Aaronson (Mount Sinai School of Medicine, New York, NY). Cells were maintained in Dulbecco's modified Eagle medium (DMEM) (Mediatech, Herndon, VA) supplemented with 10% fetal bovine serum (FBS; Sigma, St. Louis, MO) and 50 units/mL penicillin–streptomycin (Invitrogen, Carlsbad, CA) in a humidified incubator at 37C with 5% CO2. CellTiter 96® R AQueous One Solution Cell Proliferation Assay (MTS) kit (Promega Corporation, Madison, WI) was used to measure dehydrogenase enzyme activity found in metabolically active cells. Melanoma cells were seeded in a 96 well plate at a density of 2 $\times 10^4$ cells/well in DMEM with 5% FBS. On the second day, the culture medium in each well was changed to 150 μL DMEM without phenol red and supplemented with 0.5% FBS. Cells were treated in triplicate for 24 and 48 hr with either vehicle solvent (control), 25 μM PD98059, 1 μM 219476, or their combination for 624Mel; control solvent, 50 μM PD98059, 1 μM 219476, or their combination for A101D; and control solvent, 50 μM PD98059, 2 μM 219476, or their combination for OM431 cells. CellTiter 96® AQueous One Solution Reagent (30 μL) was then added per well and cell cultures were returned to the incubator for another 4 hr. Subsequently, the absorbance of each well was measured at 450 nm with a Vmax Kinetic Microplate Reader (Molecular Devices, Sunnyvale, CA). The absorbance of the well with only medium and CellTiter 96® AQueous One Solution Regent was background and subtracted from each sample well. The average and standard deviation of three wells with the same treatment were calculated.

Apoptosis was assessed by terminal deoxynucleotidyl transferase-mediated dUTP-biotin nick end labeling of DNA fragments (TUNEL) method using *in situ* Cell Death Detection Kit, Fluorescein (Roche Applied Science, Indianapolis, IN). Melanoma cells were seeded in triplicate in a 6 well plate at a density of 2 $\times$ 10^5 cells/well in DMEM with 5% FBS and antibiotics. On the second day, cells were treated with PD98059 and 219476 under the same conditions as the MTS assay. After treatment with the respective chemicals for 48 hr, cells were harvested to detect apoptotic cells using the TUNEL assay according to the manufacturer's instructions (Roche Applied Science, Indianapolis, IN). Using a cytospin, cells were placed onto Polysine glass slides (Fisher Scientific, Fair lawn, NJ), fixed in 4% paraformaldehyde (Fisher Scientific, Fair lawn, NJ) at room temperature for 1 hr, then permeabilized with a fresh prepared mixture of 0.1% Triton X-100 (MP Biomedicals, Inc. Solon, OH) and 0.1% sodium citrate (Fisher Scientific, Fair lawn, NJ) for 5 min at room temperature. Slides were rinsed with phosphate buffered saline (PBS), air dried, and incubated with 50 μL of TUNEL reaction mixture, containing terminal deoxynucleotidyl transferase (TdT)- and fluorescein isothiocyanate (FITC)-labeled dUTP, in a dark humidified atmosphere at 37C for 2 hr. For nuclei counterstaining, slides were cover-slipped with Vectashield mounting medium containing DAPI (Vector Laboratories, Burlingame, CA). Fluoresce positive cells were viewed with a Nikon Eclipse TE 2000-U inverted microscope (Nikon Corp., Tokyo, Japan) equipped with a FITC filter and a DAPI filter. The percentage of apoptotic cells was determined for each sample in a blind fashion by counting the number of green fluorescent nuclei (TUNEL positive) among a total of 300 or more 4'-6-diamidino-2-phenylindole (DAPI)-stained blue nuclei in three random fields at magnification of 20/0.5 (objective) as described previously [1-3].

For Western blotting, 1 $\times$ 10^6 melanoma cells were seeded in a cell culture dish (10 cm) in DMEM containing 5% FBS and antibiotics. On the second day, cells were treated with PD98059 and 219476 at the same concentration as described in the MTS assay. For cell cycle regulators cyclin-dependent kinase inhibitor p27 kinase interacting protein 1 (KIP1) and RB, cells were treated with the chemicals in medium with 5% FBS for 24 hr and then harvested. For apoptosis-related protein B-cell chronic lymphocytic leukemia (CLL)/lymphoma 2 (BCL2), BCL2-like 1 (BCL2L1 or bcl-xL), inhibitor of apoptosis family (IAP) protein baculoviral IAP repeat-containing 5 (BIRC5 or survivin), apoptosis facilitator BCL2 interacting mediator (BIM), cysteine-aspartic acid protease (caspase) 3, and poly (ADP-ribose) polymerase (PARP), cells were treated with the various chemicals in DMEM with 5% FBS for 48 hr and then harvested. For phospho- and total-ERK, cells were treated with the chemicals in medium with 0.5% FBS for 18 hr and then harvested. Western blots were performed as described [1-3]. Briefly, harvested cells were lysed in Lysis Solution (Cell Signaling, Danvers, MA) supplemented with Complete Mini Protease Inhibitor Cocktail Tablets (Roche Diagnostics Corporation, Indianapolis, IN). Protein concentration of lysates was determined using the Quick Start Bradford 1 × Dye Reagent (Bio-Rad, Hercules, CA). Lysates were separated in either 12 or 15% SDS-polyacrylamide gel, electrophoretically transferred to Immobilon-P membrane (Millipore Corp, Billerica, MA), and probed with primary antibodies followed by incubation with horseradish peroxidase-conjugated secondary antibodies. The following antibodies were used: BCL2 and tubulin, beta (Sigma-Aldrich, St. Louis, MO); BCL2L1 and BIRC5 (Santa Cruz Biotechnology, Santa Cruz, CA); phosphor-ERK, total ERK, Caspase 3, PARP, and PhosphoPlus(R) RB (Ser780, Ser795, Ser807/811) Antibody Kit (Cell Signaling, Boston, MA); p27KIP1 (BD Biosciences, San Jose, CA); and peroxidase-conjugated antimouse and antirabbit secondary antibodies (Calbiochem, San Diego, CA). Immunoreactive bands were visualized with SuperSignal chemiluminescence substrate (Pierce, Rockford, IL). The blots were exposed to blue sensitive blue X-ray film (Phenix Research, Candler, NC) [1-3].

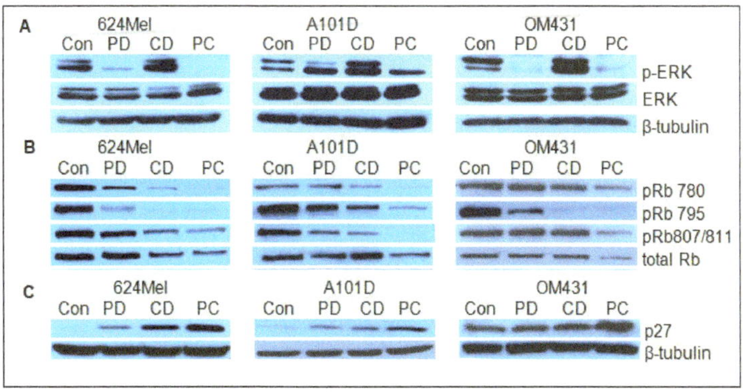

Figure 5. Regulation of ERK phosphorylation, RB phosphorylation, and p27KIP1 expression by PD98059 and 219476, alone and in combination. Human melanoma cell lines 624Mel, A101D, and OM431 were treated with either vehicle solvent (Con), PD98059 (PD), 219476 (CD), or PD98059 plus 219476 (PC) as described in Materials and methods. Western blot was performed using 20 μg total cell lysates, tubulin was used as loading control, as described previously [1-3].

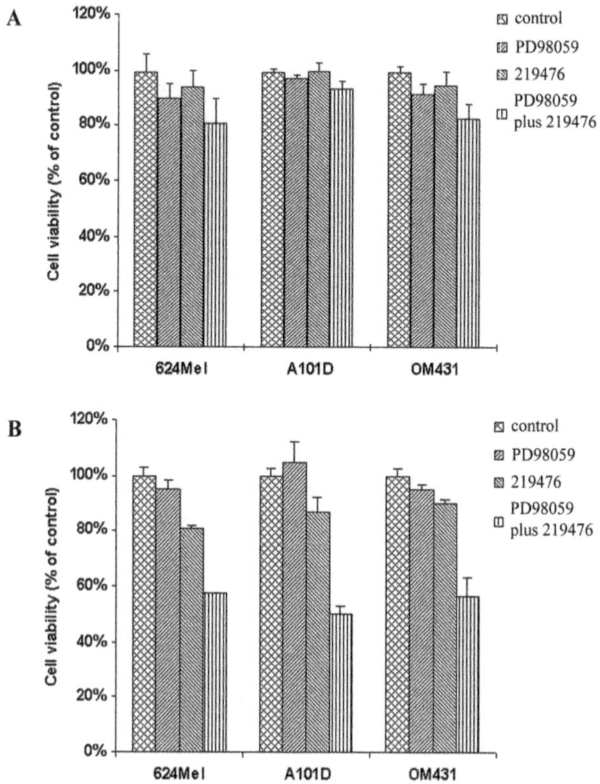

Figure 6. Cytotoxicity by PD98059, 219476, and combinatorial treatment. MTS cytotoxicity assay was performed in 624Mel, A101D, and OM431 cells after (A) 24-hr and (B) 48-hr treatment in medium supplemented with 0.5% FBS. The results are given as means ± SD from three independent tests, as described previously [1-3].

We have shown previously that human melanoma cell lines 624Mel, A101D, and OM431 cell lines harbor heterozygous *BRAF* T1799A mutation and loss of wild-type *INK4A* [1, 61]. Cells were treated, alone or in combination, with MEK inhibitor PD98059 (22) and CDK4 inhibitor 219476 (23). As anticipated, ERK phosphorylation was reduced in cells treated with PD98059, and PD98059 plus 219476 (Fig. 4A). Phosphorylation of S780, S795, and S807/811 of RB, known cyclin D:CDK4 and cyclin E:cyclin dependent kinase 2 (CDK2) targets (7),was decreased in cells treated with either PD98059 or 219476 (except S780 and S807/811 in OM431 cells), and further reduced in cells with combinatorial treatment (Fig. 4B). Of note, total RB was decreased under combinatorial treatment with PD98059 and 219476 in all three melanoma cells (Fig. 4B). Levels of p27KIP1, a negative regulator of cyclin E:CDK2, were increased in cells treated with either PD98059 or 219476, and further increased in cells with combinatorial treatment (Fig. 4C).

PD98059 and 219476 inhibit tumor cell growth in a dose dependent manner [1, 2]. In order to make it possible to monitor the additional therapeutic effects of the combinatorial treatment, both chemicals were used at dosages lower than that which would lead to maximal effect by either agent. The cytotoxicity of PD98059 and 219476 was examined 24 and 48 hr after treatment using the MTS assay that measures the dehydrogenase enzyme activity found in metabolically active cells. After 24-hr treatment, there was no significant difference in cell viability between control, single, and combined treatment groups of 624Mel cells (p = . 05, R-square 0.57320, ANOVA). Small but significant differences were observed in A101D and OM431 cells ($p = .05$, R-square 0.7136 and 0.8091 in A101D and OM431 cells, respectively, ANOVA); the differences were between the combined treatment vs. control and PD98059 in A101D cells, and between the combined treatment vs. control and single treatment of either PD98059 or 219476 in OM431 cells (Figure 2(a), HSD Test at 0.05 significance level). After 48-hr treatment, a significant difference in MTS counts existed for the control, PD98059, 219476, and PD98059 plus 219476 groups in all the three cell lines ($p < .0001$, R-square 0.981444, 0.956956, and 0.991102 in 624Mel, A101D, and OM431, respectively, ANOVA). Further analysis showed that simultaneous treatment with PD98059 and 219476 after 48-hr treatment resulted in significantly reduced numbers of cell survival than control-treatment or monotreatment as measured by MTS in all the three cell lines (Fig. 6B, HSD Test at 0.05 significance level).

Next, we performed the TUNEL DNA fragmentation assay to identify loss of viability due to programmed cell death after 48-hr treatment. As shown in Figure 3, at the drug concentrations used, significantly different levels of apoptosis exist among control for PD98059, 219476, and combinatorial treatment groups ($p < .0001$, R-square 0.973862, 0.990697, and 0.987900 in 624Mel, A101D, and OM431, respectively, ANOVA). Treatment with PD98059 alone resulted in no difference in apoptosis over controls in all three cell lines; 219476 enhanced apoptosis in OM431 but not in the other two cell lines; However, combined treatment dramatically increased apoptosis over that seen for the control-treatment and monotreatment (Fig. 7. HSD Test at 0.05 significance level).

As apoptosis was the major effect observed when melanoma cells were exposed simultaneously to MEK and CDK4 inhibitors, we examined the expression of several pro-apoptotic and anti-apoptotic proteins. Mono-treatment with PD98059 or 219476 caused a decreased or no change in the expression of anti-apoptotic proteins BCL2, BCL2L1, and BIRC5. While there were variations in the patterns of expression of BCL2, BCL2L1, and BIRC5 among the different cell lines (Fig. 8), combinatorial treatment caused a comprehensive down-regulation of the proteins in all three cell lines (Fig. 8). In addition, apoptosis facilitator BIM-EL was increased following treatment with PD98059 and PD98059 plus 219476 in all three cell lines. It was also increased in OM431 cells following treatment with 219476. Consistent with increased apoptosis, caspase 3 was activated by simultaneous treatment with PD98059 plus 219476 in all three cell lines, as shown by decreased procaspase 3, increased levels of the active form of caspase 3 (cleaved caspase 3), and degradation of PARP, a direct substrate of active caspase 3 (Fig. 8).

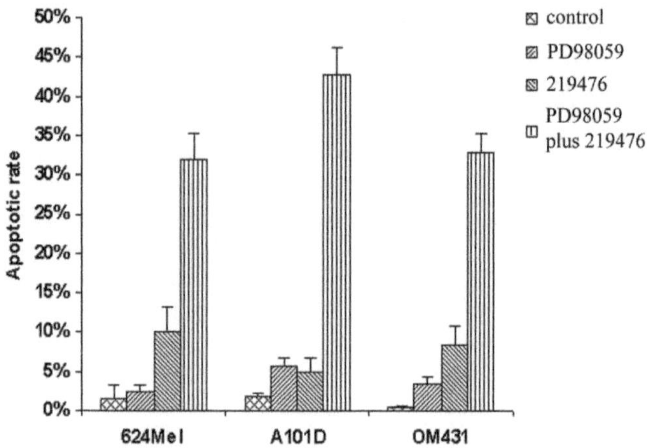

Figure 7. MEK and CDK4 inhibitors induce apoptosis of melanoma cells. TUNEL Assay was performed in 624Mel, A101D and OM431 cells after 48h treatment with vehicle solvent, PD98059, 219476, or PD98059 plus 219476 in medium with 0.5% FBS. The results were given as means ± SD from three independent assays, as described previously [1, 2].

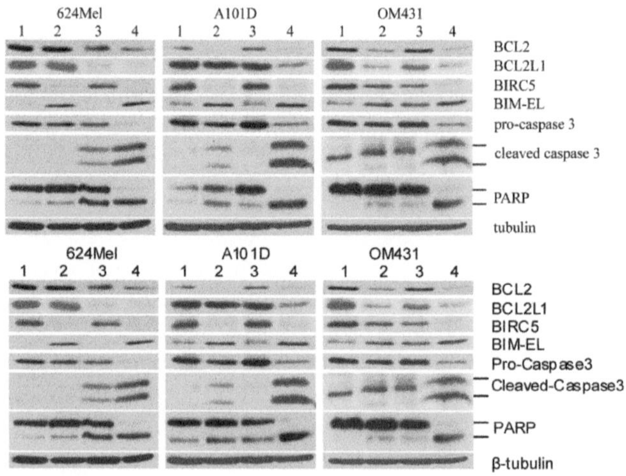

Figure 8. Changes in the expression of pro-survival and pro-apoptotic proteins. Cells were treated with solvent vehicle control (1), PD98059 (2), 219476 (3), and PD98059 plus 219476 (4) for 48 h in medium containing 5% FBS. Western blotting of 20 µg total cell extracts from 624Mel, A101D and OM431 cells using BCL2, BCL2L1, BIRC5, BIM, caspase-3, and PARP antibodies; tubulin was used as loading control, as described previously [1, 2].

In this study, we simultaneously inhibited MEK and CDK4 kinases using pharmacological inhibitors PD98059 and 219476 and observed significantly increased apoptosis compared to control and single agent treatment. This is consistent with our previous report that simultaneous knockdown of BRAF using small interfering RNA (siRNA) and expression of *INK4A* cDNA in melanoma cells leads to a significant increase in apoptosis [1, 3]. These results demonstrate that an increase in apoptosis can be achieved through combinatorial targeting of ERK and RB pathways. It has been well established that constitutive activation of the ERK signaling induces the expression of cyclin D [1, 2, 61], which binds to and activates CDK4 leading to the phosphorylation of RB protein facilitating cell cycle entry [1, 2, 61]. Consistent with an epistatic regulation between ERK pathway and cyclin D:CDK4, amplification of cyclin D1, and CDK4 genes have been identified mainly in melanomas that harbor wild-type *NRAS* and *BRAF* [58, 60]. Additionally, cyclin D:CDK4 mediates resistance to inhibitors of the ERK signaling pathway [58]. Therefore, the enhanced apoptosis and decreased proliferation by simultaneously inhibiting ERK and RB pathways could result from the double hitting of ERK-cyclin D:CDK4-RB that regulate cell cycle progression and cell survival. Alternatively, in support of our previous results that *BRAF* and *INK4A* have a nonlinear functional interaction [1, 61], additional cellular processes could be affected when cells are exposed to both PD98059 and 219476. ERK pathway has pleiopotent activities that regulate cell proliferation, survival, and differentiation through both cyclin D:CDK4 dependent and independent routes [5, 61]. Likewise, cyclin D:CDK4 can be regulated and converges multiple cellular signals. For example, while PI3K signaling can activate CDK4 through downregulation of *INK4A* and upregulation of cyclin D [73], WNT signaling can turn on CDK4 through suppression of *INK4A* transcription [72], It is conceivable that inhibition of MEK and CDK4 not only affects ERK and RB pathways, but also PI3K, WNT, and other ERK signaling activities not mediated through the RB pathway. Therefore, simultaneous targeting of both ERK and RB pathways can generate enhanced effects by targeting both linear and non-overlapping activities.

Apoptosis resistance is a critical factor for therapy failure in melanoma patients. Encouragingly, combined treatment with PD98059 and 219476 leads to significant apoptosis in all the three melanoma cell lines studied (Fig. 7). The apoptotic rate caused by the combined treatment is higher than the combined apoptosis by monotreatment, suggesting that MEK and CDK4 kinases mediate each other's pro-survival effect. The apoptotic effect is associated with changes of apoptosis-related proteins (Fig. 8). PD98059 and 219476 combined treatment leads to significant down-regulation of the pro-survival proteins BCL2, BCL2L1, and BIRC5, and up-regulation of the pro-apoptotic protein BIM. We showed previously that BCL2 and BIM were regulated by *BRAF* and *INK4A* [1, 61]. BCL2L1 and BIRC5 are highly expressed in melanoma cells, and increased expression correlates with tumor progression [74, 75]. A straightforward explanation for the observed apoptosis is that the changes in the pro-apoptotic and anti-apoptotic factors offset the balance and lead to apoptosis [1]. Sequencing analysis of TP53 cDNA [1, 3] showed that 624Mel and OM431cells respectively harbor a T1076G (Cys275Trp) and a G1048A (Gly266Glu) mutations in the DNA binding domain that is likely to compromise the transcription and apoptosis function of p53 [76]. No TP53 mutation has been detected in A101D cells. Although apoptosis is enhanced in all the three cell lines, it is more pronounced in A101D than 624Mel and OM431 cells (Fig. 7), suggesting that TP53 status may influence the magnitude of apoptosis. Combinatorial-treated cells have further inhibited phosphorylation of ERK and RB, reduced total RB, and increased expression of p27KIP1 (Fig. 5). We observed similar effects on ERK and p27KIP1 in a previous report of simultaneous expression of *BRAF* siRNA, and *INK4A* cDNA in melanoma cells [1, 3]. Yu et al. demonstrated that loss of Rb causes apoptosis without effect on cell proliferation [77], and Wang et al. found that overexpression of p27KIP1 leads to apoptosis in melanoma cells [78]. The mechanisms of these changes in relationship to each other and to the observed cooperative effects need to be further investigated. To our knowledge, this study is the first to demonstrate that combined inhibition of MEK and CDK4 using pharmacological inhibitors can cooperate to trigger significant apoptosis in melanoma cells. Deregulation of the RAS-RAF-MEK-ERK and p16-cycylin D:CDK4-RB pathways are common in human malignancies and appears to be important for melanoma development. There has been significant effort to target components of these pathways in cancer treatment. Pharmacologic agents targeting components of the ERK and RB pathways have been developed. However, clinical studies as monotherapy showed that the clinical responses have failed expectations and maximum tolerated doses are often reached before reaching clinical efficacy. Our current study further reinforces the notion that combination targeting of ERK and RB pathways is a promising strategy for melanoma treatment and should encourage further in-depth investigations.

Development of biomarkers to predict treatment response to BRAF, MEK, and CDK4 inhibitors. Apart from *BRAF* mutation, there is no other validated molecular assay to direct BRAFi and MEKi treatment. Comprehensive and standardized *INK4A* molecular assays have not been established in the context of BRAFi and MEKi treatment. Technical and clinical validation of *INK4A* molecular assays may lead to the clinical use of new molecular companion biomarkers to accurately predict clinical response to BRAF and MEK inhibitors, and may also direct future combination treatment that includes CDK4 inhibitors for metastatic melanoma. Because CDK4 is important in both normal and cancerous cells, CDK4 inhibitors are expected to decrease the ability of the bone marrow to make white blood cells, platelets, and red blood cells. Although these effects are expected to be reversible, they can increase the risk of infection, bleeding and fatigue. Like BRAF inhibitors, these drugs are also expected to be expensive. Therefore, development of predictive molecular markers, as in the case of *BRAF* mutation assay for BRAFi, should help selecting patients that are likely to response to the treatment, therefore to maximize efficacy and avoid unnecessary side-effect and treatment cost [79, 80].

Genetic and epigenetic changes of *INK4A* have been identified in 30-70% of melanomas irrespective of *BRAF* mutation [59, 70, 81]. Bi-allelic deletion of *INK4A* (p16 null) occurs in 10-27% of melanomas [60, 82]. Other changes include mono-allelic deletion, point mutation, or promoter hypermethylation, resulting in various levels of p16 expression/activity (Table 1) [57, 60, 81-83]. It is believed that the acquisition of p16 lesions allows melanoma cells to bypass senescence/growth arrest during melanoma development [84]. Although preliminary results with combination therapy of BRAFi and MEKi are encouraging with better clinical response over single agent BRAFi treatment [9], levels of treatment responses vary under the combination treatment [9]. We hypothesize that clinical response to combination therapy of BRAFi and MEKi correlates with status of *INK4A*/p16 (Table 2). The development of clinically useful *INK4A* assays requires an understanding of the underlying biology and access to technology that allows high quality assay performance. Recent advances in molecular technology enable accurate, rapid, and cost-effective *INK4A* molecular testing that can be performed routinely on tumor specimens. However, validation of the technical performance characteristics of *INK4A* assays and understanding of assay limitations are necessary for the accurate interpretation of test results.

***INK4A* status**	**p16 protein sequence and expression**
Wild-type	Normal sequence
Various mutations	Heterogeneous sequence changes
Bi-allelic deletion	Protein null
Promoter hypermethylation	Lower levels of p16

Table 1. Heterogeneity of *INK4A* and p16 in melanoma specimens

As examples, Table 2 is a list of molecular assays to comprehensively examine *INK4A*/p16 lesions in melanoma specimens. Technical and clinical validation studies are necessary before the routine use of these assays in the clinic.

Test	Method	Reference
INK4A deletion	fluorescent *in situ* hybridization (FISH) (p16 SpectrumOrange/ chromosome 9 centromeric probe (CEP9) SpectrumGreen Probe, Abbott Molecular, Des Plaines, IL)	[85, 86]
INK4A mutation	Sanger sequencing	[86, 87]
INK4A promoter methylation	Pyrosequencing (PyroMark Q24 CpG p16 Kit, Qiagen, Valencia, CA)	[82, 88, 89]
p16 expression	Immunohistochemical staining (IHC)	[90, 91]

Table 2. Summary of molecular assays

These assays need to be validated both technically and clinically with defined cut-off values. There should be correlation of results among assay methods; for example, cells with bi-allelic *INK4A* deletion show negative p16 IHC staining and cells with mono-allelic *INK4A* deletion show mutations with loss of heterozygosity (LOH), and p16 expression inversely correlates with levels of *INK4A* promoter methylation. The major obstacles in testing tumor specimens are the presence of non-tumor cells in the samples, the cellular heterogeneity within tumor specimens, and degradation/damage of nucleic acid and protein during sample processing. To ensure accurate testing results, SOPs need to be established with clearly defined instructions on the selection and handling of tumor specimens. For example, FISH assay requires fixation time between 6-48 hrs [92]. Alterations in *INK4A* may also affect the overlapping *ARF* gene (Fig. 2). Although the proposed study focuses on *INK4A*, changes in *INK4A* may also affect *ARF*, which may also be analyzed. Assay clinical sensitivity, clinical specificity, positive predictive value, and negative predictive value of *INK4A* biomarkers for a given treatment response can be calculated as described in Table 4.

INK4A result	**Treatment resistant case**	**Treatment sensitive case**	
Lesion +ve	A	B	Positive predictive value = A / (A + B)
Lesion -ve	C	D	Negative predictive value = D / (C + D)
	Sensitivity = A / (A + C)	Specificity = D / (B + D)	

Table 3. Calculation of clinical sensitivity, clinical specificity and predictive values

3. Conclusion

Patients with metastatic melanoma have a median survival of 6-8 months [93]. Recently, ipilimumab (Yervoy, Bristol-Myers Squibb), an inhibitor of cytotoxic T-lymphocyte antigen 4 (CTLA-4) and vemurafenib (PLX4032, Zelboraf, Plexxikon/Roche), an inhibitor of mutant BRAF, gained FDA approval to treat patients with metastatic melanoma. Although both drugs offer new approaches to the treatment of advanced melanoma, their therapeutic efficacy is limited. Both drugs typically lengthen life by only several months in patients that initially responded to the treatment [94, 95]. There is mounting evidence that acquired resistance to BRAFi frequently correlates with reactivation of the RAS-RAF-MEK-ERK signaling pathway [52, 53, 64]. This finding led to clinical trials combining BRAFi and MEKi in patients with *BRAF*-mutant metastatic melanoma who progressed on a prior BRAFi treatment regimen [94]. Dabrafenib (GSK2118436, GlaxoSmithKline) is a potent and selective inhibitor of mutant BRAF and is comparable in safety and efficacy to vemurafenib. In phase I testing, it achieved a 67% response rate in metastatic melanoma patients with BRAF V600 mutations [96]. Trametinib (GSK1120212, GlaxoSmithKline) is a potent and selective inhibitor of MEK1/2, achieved a clinical response of 40% in patients with an activating *BRAF* mutation in phase I study [97]. A multicenter phase I/II trial of combined treatment with dabrafenib and trametinib demonstrated a disease control rate of 67% (12/18) in patients who failed prior single-agent treatment with a BRAFi [9]. We hypothesize that although reactivation of MEK-ERK-cyclin D-CDK4 in tumors previously treatment with BRAFi may be suppressed by the combination of dabrafenib and trametinib, cyclin D-CDK4 can also be reactivated by alternative resistance mechanisms that cannot be suppressed by the addition of MEKi (e.g.; activation of growth factor receptor and PI3K-AKT pathway) [51-53, 55, 56, 65, 66], if unopposed by p16, can lead to resistance to the BRAFi and MEKi combination therapy (Fig. 1). It has been shown that melanoma cells that harbor abnormal *INK4A* are more sensitive than *INK4A* wild-type cells to the growth inhibitory effect of a p16-mimicking peptide [98] or of flavopiridol, a pan-CDK inhibitor [99], and combination of BRAFi or MEKi with the expression of wild-type *INK4A* or a CDK4 inhibitor significantly suppresses growth and enhances apoptosis in melanoma cells [2, 3]. Therefore, melanoma combination treatments that include CDK4 inhibitors may overcome treatment resistance and enhance efficacy. There is a critical need to identify predictive markers for therapies not only to improve treatment outcomes, but to help avoid ineffective toxic therapies, also because of the likely high cost of combination regimens. Like *BRAF* mutation assay, testing of *INK4A*-p16 may predict which patients will response to BRAF, MEK, and CDK4 inhibitors. Therefore, *INK4A* biomarkers may also have great potential to guide future melanoma combination treatments that include CDK4 inhibitors.

Nomenclature

ASK1: apoptosis signal-regulating kinase-1

ARF: alternative open reading frame

BCL2: B-cell chronic lymphocytic leukemia/lymphoma 2

BCL2L1: BCL2-like 1

BIM: BCL2 interacting mediator

BIRC5: baculoviral IAP repeat-containing 5, also known as survivin

BRAF: v-raf murine sarcoma viral oncogene homolog B1

BRAFi: BRAF inhibitor

Caspase: cysteine-aspartic acid protease

CDK2: cyclin-dependent kinase 2

CDK4: cyclin-dependent kinase 4

CDK4i: CDK4 inhibitor

CEP9: chromosome 9 centromeric probe

CLL: chronic lymphocytic leukemia

DAPI: 4'-6-diamidino-2-phenylindole

DMEM: Dulbecco's modified Eagle medium

DMSO: dimethyl sulfoxide

DTIC: dacarbazine

ERK: extracellular-signal-regulated kinase

FBS: fetal bovine serum

FDA: Food and Drug Administration

FGF: fibroblast growth factor

FISH: fluorescent *in situ* hybridization

FITC: fluorescein isothiocyanate

HGF: hepatocyte growth factor

IAP: inhibitor of apoptosis family

IHC: immunohistochemical staining

INK4A: inhibitor of cyclin-dependent kinase 4A; part of cyclin-dependent kinase inhibitor 2A gene (*CDKN2A*), also known as multiple tumor suppressor 1 (*MTS1*)

KIP1: kinase interacting protein 1

LOH: loss of heterozygosity

MEK: mitogen-activated protein kinase/ERK kinase

MEKi: MEK inhibitor

MST2: sterile 20- like-kinase 2

PAGE: polyacrylamide gel electrophoresis

PARP: poly (ADP-ribose) polymerase

PBS: phosphate buffered saline

PI3K: phosphatidylinositol 3-kinase

p-ERK: phopho-ERK

RAF: v-raf murine sarcoma viral oncogene homolog. Human has three RAF: CRAF, BRAF, and ARAF

RAS: rat sarcoma viral oncogene homolog. Human has three RAS: HRAS, NRAS, and KRAS (KRAS4A and KRAS4B proteins arise from alternative splicing)

RB: retinoblastoma proteins including pRB, p107, and p103

SDS: sodium dodecyl sulfate

siRNA: small interfering RNA

TdT: terminal deoxynucleotidyl transferase

TUNEL: terminal deoxynucleotidyl transferase-mediated dUTP nick end labeling

UV: ultra violate

WNT: wingless

Acknowledgments

We thank Dr. Stuart Aaronson for human melanoma cell lines. This work was supported by Bill Walter III Melanoma Research Fund, Harry J. Lloyd Charitable Trust, and Cancer and Leukemia Group B Foundation (to J.D.).

Author details

Jianli Dong*

Address all correspondence to: jidong@utmb.edu

Molecular Diagnostics Laboratory, University of Texas Medical Branch at Galveston, Galveston, USA

References

[1] Dong, J. and C.L. Schwab, Simultaneous knockdown of mutant BRAF and expression of INK4A in melanoma cells leads to potent growth inhibition and apoptosis. Treatment of Metastatic Melanoma, ed. R.M. R. 2011: InTech. 149-182.

[2] Li, J., et al., Simultaneous inhibition of MEK and CDK4 leads to potent apoptosis in human melanoma cells. Cancer Invest, 2010. 28(4): p. 350-6.

[3] Zhao, Y., et al., Simultaneous knockdown of BRAF and expression of INK4A in melanoma cells leads to potent growth inhibition and apoptosis. Biochem Biophys Res Commun, 2008. 370(3): p. 509-13.

[4] Davies, H., et al., Mutations of the BRAF gene in human cancer. Nature, 2002. 417(6892): p. 949-54.

[5] Peyssonnaux, C. and A. Eychene, The Raf/MEK/ERK pathway: new concepts of activation. Biol Cell, 2001. 93: p. 53-62.

[6] Flaherty, K.T., Next generation therapies change the landscape in melanoma. F1000 Med Rep, 2011. 3: p. 8.

[7] Flaherty, K.T., et al., Inhibition of mutated, activated BRAF in metastatic melanoma. N Engl J Med, 2010. 363(9): p. 809-19.

[8] Sherr, C.J., The INK4a/ARF network in tumour suppression. Nat Rev Mol Cell Biol, 2001. 2: p. 731-7.

[9] Flaherty, K., et al., Phase I/II expansion cohort of BRAF inhibitor GSK2118436 + MEK inhibitor GSK1120212 in patients with BRAF mutant metastatic melanoma who pro-

gressed on a prior BRAF inhibitor [abstract]. In: 8th International Congress of the Society for Melanoma Research. Tampa, FL, November 9–13, 2011. Abstract LBA 1-4. 2011.

[10] Bennett, D.C. and E.E. Medrano, Molecular regulation of melanocyte senescence. Pigment Cell Res, 2002. 15: p. 242-50.

[11] Kuilman, T., et al., The essence of senescence. Genes Dev, 2010. 24(22): p. 2463-79.

[12] Halaban, R., Melanoma cell autonomous growth: the Rb/E2F pathway. Cancer Metastasis Rev, 1999. 18(3): p. 333-43.

[13] Halaban, R., Rb/E2F: a two-edged sword in the melanocytic system. Cancer Metastasis Rev, 2005. 24(2): p. 339-56.

[14] Dent, P. and S. Grant, Pharmacologic interruption of the mitogen-activated extracellular-regulated kinase/mitogen-activated protein kinase signal transduction pathway: potential role in promoting cytotoxic drug action. Clin Cancer Res, 2001. 7: p. 775-83.

[15] English, J.M. and M.H. Cobb, Pharmacological inhibitors of MAPK pathways. Trends Pharmacol Sci, 2002. 23: p. 40-5.

[16] Halaban, R., The regulation of normal melanocyte proliferation. Pigment Cell Res, 2000. 13: p. 4-14.

[17] Busca, R., et al., Ras mediates the cAMP-dependent activation of extracellular signal-regulated kinases (ERKs) in melanocytes. Embo J, 2000. 19: p. 2900-10.

[18] Smalley, K.S., A pivotal role for ERK in the oncogenic behaviour of malignant melanoma? Int J Cancer, 2003. 104(5): p. 527-32.

[19] Hingorani, S.R., et al., Suppression of BRAF(V599E) in human melanoma abrogates transformation. Cancer Res, 2003. 63: p. 5198-202.

[20] Karasarides, M., et al., B-RAF is a therapeutic target in melanoma. Oncogene, 2004.

[21] Sumimoto, H., et al., Inhibition of growth and invasive ability of melanoma by inactivation of mutated BRAF with lentivirus-mediated RNA interference. Oncogene, 2004.

[22] Wojnowski, L., et al., Endothelial apoptosis in Braf-deficient mice. Nat Genet, 1997. 16: p. 293-7.

[23] Ivanov, V.N., A. Bhoumik, and Z. Ronai, Death receptors and melanoma resistance to apoptosis. Oncogene, 2003. 22(20): p. 3152-61.

[24] Soengas, M.S. and S.W. Lowe, Apoptosis and melanoma chemoresistance. Oncogene, 2003. 22: p. 3138-51.

[25] Johnstone, R.W., A.A. Ruefli, and S.W. Lowe, Apoptosis: a link between cancer genetics and chemotherapy. Cell, 2002. 108: p. 153-64.

[26] Schmitt, C.A., Senescence, apoptosis and therapy--cutting the lifelines of cancer. Nat Rev Cancer, 2003. 3: p. 286-95.

[27] Schmitt, C.A., et al., A senescence program controlled by p53 and p16INK4a contributes to the outcome of cancer therapy. Cell, 2002. 109: p. 335-46.

[28] Alavi, A., et al., Role of Raf in vascular protection from distinct apoptotic stimuli. Science, 2003. 301: p. 94-6.

[29] Erhardt, P., E.J. Schremser, and G.M. Cooper, B-Raf inhibits programmed cell death downstream of cytochrome c release from mitochondria by activating the MEK/Erk pathway. Mol Cell Biol, 1999. 19(8): p. 5308-15.

[30] Satyamoorthy, K., et al., Constitutive mitogen-activated protein kinase activation in melanoma is mediated by both BRAF mutations and autocrine growth factor stimulation. Cancer Res, 2003. 63(4): p. 756-9.

[31] Fan, M. and T.C. Chambers, Role of mitogen-activated protein kinases in the response of tumor cells to chemotherapy. Drug Resist Updat, 2001. 4: p. 253-67.

[32] Mandic, A., et al., The MEK1 inhibitor PD98059 sensitizes C8161 melanoma cells to cisplatin-induced apoptosis. Melanoma Res, 2001. 11: p. 11-9.

[33] Halaschek-Wiener, J., et al., Farnesyl thiosalicylic acid chemosensitizes human melanoma in vivo. J Invest Dermatol, 2003. 120: p. 109-15.

[34] Clark, W.H., Jr. and M.A. Tucker, Problems with lesions related to the development of malignant melanoma: common nevi, dysplastic nevi, malignant melanoma in situ, and radial growth phase malignant melanoma. Hum Pathol, 1998. 29: p. 8-14.

[35] Elder, D., Tumor progression, early diagnosis and prognosis of melanoma. Acta Oncol, 1999. 38: p. 535-47.

[36] Pollock, P.M., et al., High frequency of BRAF mutations in nevi. Nat Genet, 2003. 33: p. 19-20.

[37] Dong, J., et al., BRAF oncogenic mutations correlate with progression rather than initiation of human melanoma. Cancer Res, 2003. 63: p. 3883-5.

[38] Sherr, C.J. and F. McCormick, The RB and p53 pathways in cancer. Cancer Cell, 2002. 2: p. 103-12.

[39] Flores, J.F., et al., Loss of the p16INK4a and p15INK4b genes, as well as neighboring 9p21 markers, in sporadic melanoma. Cancer Res, 1996. 56(21): p. 5023-32.

[40] Tsao, H., et al., Melanoma: from mutations to medicine. Genes Dev, 2012. 26(11): p. 1131-55.

[41] Castellano, M., et al., CDKN2A/p16 is inactivated in most melanoma cell lines. Cancer Res, 1997. 57: p. 4868-75.

[42] Funk, J.O., et al., p16INK4a expression is frequently decreased and associated with 9p21 loss of heterozygosity in sporadic melanoma. J Cutan Pathol, 1998. 25: p. 291-6.

[43] von, E.F., et al., Analysis of the tumor suppressor gene p16(INK4A) in microdissected melanoma metastases by sequencing, and microsatellite and methylation screening. Arch Dermatol Res, 1999. 291: p. 474-7.

[44] Welch, J., et al., Lack of genetic and epigenetic changes in CDKN2A in melanocytic nevi. J Invest Dermatol, 2001. 117: p. 383-4.

[45] Zhang, H., J. Schneider, and I. Rosdahl, Expression of p16, p27, p53, p73 and Nup88 proteins in matched primary and metastatic melanoma cells. Int J Oncol, 2002. 21: p. 43-8.

[46] Bannert, N. and R. Kurth, The evolutionary dynamics of human endogenous retroviral families. Annu Rev Genomics Hum Genet, 2006. 7: p. 149-73.

[47] Bandyopadhyay, D., et al., Dynamic assembly of chromatin complexes during cellular senescence: implications for the growth arrest of human melanocytic nevi. Aging Cell, 2007. 6(4): p. 577-91.

[48] Daniotti, M., et al., BRAF alterations are associated with complex mutational profiles in malignant melanoma. Oncogene, 2004. 23(35): p. 5968-77.

[49] Chin, L., L.A. Garraway, and D.E. Fisher, Malignant melanoma: genetics and therapeutics in the genomic era. Genes Dev, 2006. 20(16): p. 2149-82.

[50] Flaherty, K.T., F.S. Hodi, and D.E. Fisher, From genes to drugs: targeted strategies for melanoma. Nat Rev Cancer, 2012. 12(5): p. 349-61.

[51] Johannessen, C.M., et al., COT drives resistance to RAF inhibition through MAP kinase pathway reactivation. Nature, 2011. 468(7326): p. 968-72.

[52] Nazarian, R., et al., Melanomas acquire resistance to B-RAF(V600E) inhibition by RTK or N-RAS upregulation. Nature, 2010. 468(7326): p. 973-7.

[53] Poulikakos, P.I., et al., RAF inhibitor resistance is mediated by dimerization of aberrantly spliced BRAF(V600E). Nature, 2011.

[54] Sondergaard, J.N., et al., Differential sensitivity of melanoma cell lines with BRAFV600E mutation to the specific Raf inhibitor PLX4032. J Transl Med, 2010. 8: p. 39.

[55] Villanueva, J., et al., Acquired resistance to BRAF inhibitors mediated by a RAF kinase switch in melanoma can be overcome by cotargeting MEK and IGF-1R/PI3K. Cancer Cell, 2010. 18(6): p. 683-95.

[56] Xing, F., et al., Concurrent loss of the PTEN and RB1 tumor suppressors attenuates RAF dependence in melanomas harboring (V600E)BRAF. Oncogene, 2011.

[57] Yang, G., A. Rajadurai, and H. Tsao, Recurrent patterns of dual RB and p53 pathway inactivation in melanoma. J Invest Dermatol, 2005. 125(6): p. 1242-51.

[58] Smalley, K.S., et al., Increased cyclin D1 expression can mediate BRAF inhibitor resistance in BRAF V600E-mutated melanomas. Mol Cancer Ther, 2008. 7(9): p. 2876-83.

[59] Dutton-Regester, K. and N.K. Hayward, Reviewing the somatic genetics of melanoma: from current to future analytical approaches. Pigment Cell Melanoma Res, 2012.

[60] Curtin, J.A., et al., Distinct sets of genetic alterations in melanoma. N Engl J Med, 2005. 353(20): p. 2135-47.

[61] Rotolo, S., et al., Effects on proliferation and melanogenesis by inhibition of mutant BRAF and expression of wild-type INK4A in melanoma cells. Int J Cancer, 2005. 115(1): p. 164-9.

[62] Serrano, M., G.J. Hannon, and D. Beach, A new regulatory motif in cell-cycle control causing specific inhibition of cyclin D/CDK4. Nature, 1993. 366(6456): p. 704-7.

[63] Lowe, S.W. and C.J. Sherr, Tumor suppression by Ink4a-Arf: progress and puzzles. Curr Opin Genet Dev, 2003. 13: p. 77-83.

[64] Su, F., et al., Resistance to Selective BRAF Inhibition Can Be Mediated by Modest Upstream Pathway Activation. Cancer Res, 2012.

[65] Recio, J.A. and G. Merlino, Hepatocyte growth factor/scatter factor activates proliferation in melanoma cells through p38 MAPK, ATF-2 and cyclin D1. Oncogene, 2002. 21(7): p. 1000-8.

[66] Spofford, L.S., et al., Cyclin D3 expression in melanoma cells is regulated by adhesion-dependent phosphatidylinositol 3-kinase signaling and contributes to G1-S progression. J Biol Chem, 2006. 281(35): p. 25644-51.

[67] Dong, J., et al., BRAF oncogenic mutations correlate with progression rather than initiation of human melanoma. Cancer Res, 2003. 63(14): p. 3883-5.

[68] Englaro, W., et al., Inhibition of the mitogen-activated protein kinase pathway triggers B16 melanoma cell differentiation. J Biol Chem, 1998. 273: p. 9966-70.

[69] Chin, L., et al., Cooperative effects of INK4a and ras in melanoma susceptibility in vivo. Genes Dev, 1997. 11: p. 2822-34.

[70] Sharpless, E. and L. Chin, The INK4a/ARF locus and melanoma. Oncogene, 2003. 22(20): p. 3092-8.

[71] O'Neill, E.E., D. Matallanas, and W. Kolch, Mammalian sterile 20-like kinases in tumor suppression: an emerging pathway. Cancer Res, 2005. 65(13): p. 5485-7.

[72] Delmas, V., et al., Beta-catenin induces immortalization of melanocytes by suppressing p16INK4a expression and cooperates with N-Ras in melanoma development. Genes Dev, 2007. 21(22): p. 2923-35.

[73] Schmidt, M., et al., Cell cycle inhibition by FoxO forkhead transcription factors involves downregulation of cyclin D. Mol Cell Biol, 2002. 22(22): p. 7842-52.

[74] Piras, F., et al., Nuclear survivin is associated with disease recurrence and poor survival in patients with cutaneous malignant melanoma. Histopathology, 2007. 50(7): p. 835-42.

[75] Zhuang, L., et al., Mcl-1, Bcl-XL and Stat3 expression are associated with progression of melanoma whereas Bcl-2, AP-2 and MITF levels decrease during progression of melanoma. Mod Pathol, 2007. 20(4): p. 416-26.

[76] Petitjean, A., et al., Impact of mutant p53 functional properties on TP53 mutation patterns and tumor phenotype: lessons from recent developments in the IARC TP53 database. Hum Mutat, 2007. 28(6): p. 622-9.

[77] Yu, B.D., et al., Distinct and nonoverlapping roles for pRB and cyclin D:cyclin-dependent kinases 4/6 activity in melanocyte survival. Proc Natl Acad Sci U S A, 2003. 100(25): p. 14881-6.

[78] Wang, X., et al., p27Kip1 overexpression causes apoptotic death of mammalian cells. Oncogene, 1997. 15(24): p. 2991-7.

[79] Engstrom, P.F., et al., NCCN molecular testing white paper: effectiveness, efficiency, and reimbursement. J Natl Compr Canc Netw, 2011. 9 Suppl 6: p. S1-16.

[80] Ong, F.S., et al., Personalized medicine and pharmacogenetic biomarkers: progress in molecular oncology testing. Expert Rev Mol Diagn, 2012. 12(6): p. 593-602.

[81] Grafstrom, E., et al., Biallelic deletions in INK4 in cutaneous melanoma are common and associated with decreased survival. Clin Cancer Res, 2005. 11(8): p. 2991-7.

[82] Jonsson, A., et al., High frequency of p16(INK4A) promoter methylation in NRAS-mutated cutaneous melanoma. J Invest Dermatol, 2010. 130(12): p. 2809-17.

[83] Miller, P.J., et al., Classifying variants of CDKN2A using computational and laboratory studies. Hum Mutat, 2011. 32(8): p. 900-11.

[84] Bennett, D.C., How to make a melanoma: what do we know of the primary clonal events? Pigment Cell Melanoma Res, 2008. 21: p. 27-38.

[85] Chung, C.T., et al., FISH assay development for the detection of p16/CDKN2A deletion in malignant pleural mesothelioma. J Clin Pathol, 2010. 63(7): p. 630-4.

[86] Gerami, P., et al., Fluorescence in situ hybridization (FISH) as an ancillary diagnostic tool in the diagnosis of melanoma. Am J Surg Pathol, 2009. 33(8): p. 1146-56.

[87] Straume, O., et al., Significant impact of promoter hypermethylation and the 540 C>T polymorphism of CDKN2A in cutaneous melanoma of the vertical growth phase. Am J Pathol, 2002. 161(1): p. 229-37.

[88] Tellez, C.S., et al., CpG island methylation profiling in human melanoma cell lines. Melanoma Res, 2009. 19(3): p. 146-55.

[89] Zainuddin, N., et al., Quantitative evaluation of p16(INK4a) promoter methylation using pyrosequencing in de novo diffuse large B-cell lymphoma. Leuk Res, 2011. 35(4): p. 438-43.

[90] Li, Z., et al., Expression of HERV-K correlates with status of MEK-ERK and p16INK4A-CDK4 pathways in melanoma cells. Cancer Invest, 2010. 28(10): p. 1031-7.

[91] Schlosshauer, P.W., et al., Loss of p16INK4A expression in low-grade ovarian serous carcinomas. Int J Gynecol Pathol, 2011. 30(1): p. 22-9.

[92] Middleton, L.P., et al., Implementation of American Society of Clinical Oncology/ College of American Pathologists HER2 Guideline Recommendations in a tertiary care facility increases HER2 immunohistochemistry and fluorescence in situ hybridization concordance and decreases the number of inconclusive cases. Arch Pathol Lab Med, 2009. 133(5): p. 775-80.

[93] Balch, C.M., et al., Final version of 2009 AJCC melanoma staging and classification. J Clin Oncol, 2009. 27(36): p. 6199-206.

[94] Alcala, A.M. and K.T. Flaherty, BRAF Inhibitors for the Treatment of Metastatic Melanoma: Clinical Trials and Mechanisms of Resistance. Clin Cancer Res, 2012. 18(1): p. 33-9.

[95] Patel, S.P. and S.E. Woodman, Profile of ipilimumab and its role in the treatment of metastatic melanoma. Drug Des Devel Ther, 2011. 5: p. 489-95.

[96] Ribas, A. and K.T. Flaherty, BRAF targeted therapy changes the treatment paradigm in melanoma. Nat Rev Clin Oncol, 2011. 8(7): p. 426-33.

[97] Jing, J., et al., Comprehensive predictive biomarker analysis for MEK inhibitor GSK1120212. Mol Cancer Ther, 2011. 11(3): p. 720-9.

[98] Noonan, D.M., et al., In vitro and in vivo tumor growth inhibition by a p16-mimicking peptide in p16INK4A-defective, pRb-positive human melanoma cells. J Cell Physiol, 2005. 202(3): p. 922-8.

[99] Robinson, W.A., et al., The effect of flavopiridol on the growth of p16+ and p16- melanoma cell lines. Melanoma Res, 2003. 13: p. 231-8.

Chapter 2

Targeted Therapies in Melanoma: Successes and Pitfalls

Giuseppe Palmieri, Maria Colombino,
Maria Cristina Sini, Paolo Antonio Ascierto,
Amelia Lissia and Antonio Cossu

Additional information is available at the end of the chapter

1. Introduction

Incidence of melanoma is steadily rising worldwide [1]. Lifetime risk of developing melanoma in Caucasians is estimated as 1 in 50 individuals [2-3]. The incidence of melanoma varies according to the geographical origins of the population and the extent of sun exposure. In Australia and United States, an incidence of melanoma higher than observed in the European countries (with the notable exception of Sweden) has been reported [4-5]. There is a gradient of melanoma incidence from north to south in Europe, with highest frequencies in the northern counties. This suggests that initiation and development of melanoma is due to a combination of the damaging effects of UV and a predisposing genetic background [5].

Melanoma arises from melanocytes, neural crest-derived cells that are located in the basal layer of the epidermis and skin appendages in humans. Melanocytes, by synthesizing melanin pigments and exporting them to adjacent keratonocytes play a key role in protecting the skin from the damaging effects of ultraviolet (UV) and other solar radiation [6]. Melanocytes can proliferate to form nevi (common moles), initially in the basal epidermis (junctional nevus) and later by limited local dermal infiltration (compound nevus). Nevi develop during embryonic life (congenital nevus) and in children and adults, (acquired nevus) partly as a result of solar exposure in the latter two populations. Further progression of melanocytic tumors relates to factors that include intermittent exposure to UV radiation (though a direct relationship between risk of melanoma and UV exposure remains somehow unclear), a history of sunburn and endogenous factors such as skin type and elevated numbers of nevi (especially dysplastic nevi, also known as atypical moles) [7-8].

Considering the growth patterns, four histological types of melanoma have been historically recognized: superficial spreading melanoma (SSM), lentigo maligna melanoma (LMM), nodular melanoma (NM), and acral lentiginous melanoma (ALM) [9]. Comparative genomic hybridization revealed that several genomic regions (mostly, 11q13, 22q11-13, and 5p15) were abnormally amplified in ALM [10]; such regions were different from those found altered in superficial SSM or NM (mainly, 9p21 and 1p22) [11]. Recently, a new classification of melanoma including the site of primary tumour and the degree of chronic sun-induced damage of the surrounding skin has been introduced [12]. Based on these criteria, melanomas are classified into four groups; melanoma on skin with chronic sun-damage (CSD melanoma), melanoma on skin without chronic sun-damage (non-CSD melanoma), melanoma on palms, soles and nail bed (acral melanoma), and melanoma on mucous membrane (mucosal melanoma) [12]. Non-CSD melanomas are characterized by high frequency of BRAF or NRAS mutations (which are mutually exclusive), while CSD, acral, and mucosal melanomas show a low frequency of BRAF/NRAS mutations but a high incidence of alterations in additional genes, such as mutations of receptor tyrosine kinase KIT gene, amplifications of cyclin D1 (CCND1) and cyclin-dependent kinase 4 (CDK4) genes [7, 12-13]. All genes affected into the different types of melanoma are involved in regulating cell-cycle progression and cell survival [12-13]. On the other hand, such a difference of genetic alterations indicates distinct genetic pathways in the pathogenesis of melanoma depending on the anatomical site of the primary lesion. Trying to merge the two classifications, it could be affirmed that non-CSD melanoma roughly corresponds to SSM, CSD melanoma to LMM, and acral melanoma to ALM. Since NM may arise at any anatomical site, this histological type can not be included in any of the subgroups of the latter classification (indeed, no distinct genetic pathway has been so far correlated with NM).

During recent past years, melanocytic transformation is being demonstrated to occur as a sequential accumulation of genetic and molecular alterations [13-14]. In this sense, it is becoming an unquestionable certainty that molecular classification of melanoma patients could be achieved through the assessment of the molecular profile of primary tumors and/or the correspondent metastases, by unveiling which gene or pathway is truly affected. Although pathogenetic mechanisms underlying melanoma development are still largely unknown, several genes and metabolic pathways have been shown to carry molecular alterations in melanoma.

2. Main genes and related pathways

2.1. *BRAF* and MAPK pathway

The *mitogen-activated protein kinase* (MAPK) signal transduction pathway regulates cell growth, survival, and invasion. MAPK signaling is initiated at the cell membrane, either by receptor tyrosine kinases (RTKs) binding ligand or integrin adhesion to extracellular matrix, which transmits activation signals via RAS on the cell membrane inner surface (Figure 1).

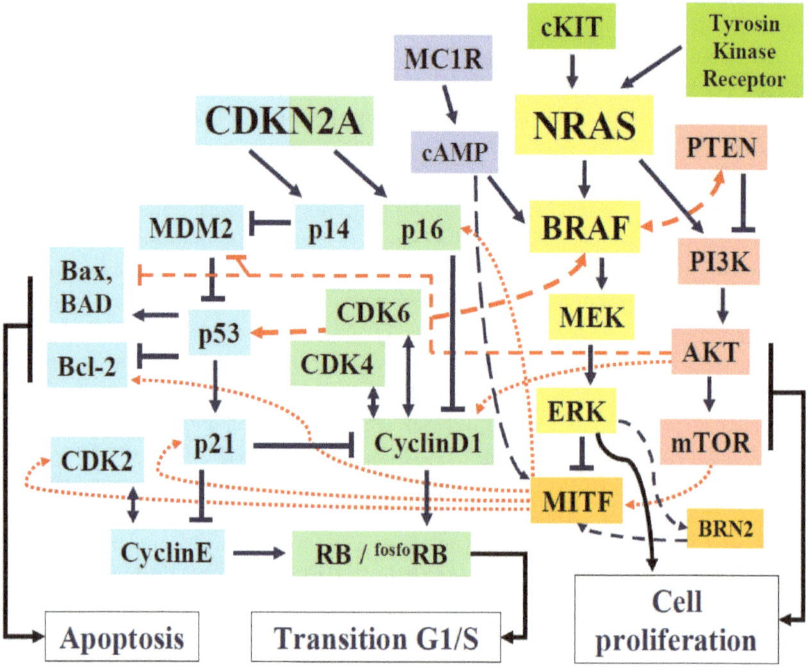

Figure 1. Main pathways involved in melanomagenesis. Arrows, activation signals. Interrupted lines, inhibition signals.

RAS proteins are small GTPases thatare activated by extracellular stimuli and regulate signal transduction of the BRAF-MEK1/2-ERK1/2 and AKT/PI3K pathways, controlling crucial cellular processes such as proliferation, differentiation, cell adhesion, apoptosis, and cell migration [14-16]. RAS gene is mutated in an estimated 20-30% of all cancers [17]. RAS proteins are constituted by three main isoforms - NRAS, KRAS, and HRAS, which present a similar function but a different specificity for tissue distribution [18]. On this regard, KRAS alterations mostly occur in gastrointestinal cancer [17-18], HRAS alterations are frequently observed in bladder cancer, and NRAS is mutated in 15-25% of melanomas [17-18]. Despite the huge amount of knowledge implicating RAS in tumour initiation and promotion, RAS itself has not become a successful target of therapy.

The RAF kinase family consists of three members - ARAF, BRAF, and CRAF, all of which can activate a series of protein kinases; such a signaling cascade culminate in the phosphorylation and activation of the extracellular signal-regulated kinase (ERK) downstream protein [19]. In melanoma, the most commonly mutated component of this pathway is the *BRAF* gene; the prevalent *BRAF* mutation (in nearly, 90% of cases) being a substitution of valine with glutamic acid at position 600 (V600E) [20]. Mutated *BRAF* induces constitutive ERK activation; activated ERK then translocates to the nucleus and initiates the transcription of a variety of growth-related genes, stimulating cell proliferation and survival [20]. Indeed, the increased activity of ERK seems to be implicated in rapid melanoma cell growth, enhanced cell survival and resistance to apoptosis [21]. High levels of activated ERK may further induce the metastatic potential of melanoma by increasing the expression of invasion-promoting integrins [22-23]. Presence of *BRAF* mutations in benign and dysplastic nevi supports the hypothesis that activation of the RAF/MEK/ERK pathway is an early event in melanoma progression [24-25]. In other words, *BRAF* activation is necessary but not sufficient for the development of melanoma and additional co-operating genetic events are required to achieve full malignancy.

In a study aimed to better define the role of BRAF in melanomagenesis, a transgenic zebra fish expressing ^{V600E}BRAF showed dramatic development of patches of ectopic melanocytes (designated as fish-nevi) [26]. Remarkably, activated *BRAF* in p53-deficient zebra fish induced the formation of melanocytic lesions that rapidly developed into invasive melanomas that resembled human melanomas in terms of their histology and biological behaviors [26]. These data provide direct evidence that the p53 and BRAF pathways interact functionally during melanomagenesis.

The *BRAF* gene also cooperates with the cyclin-dependent kinase inhibitor p16^{CDKN2A} (see below). Activating *BRAF* mutations have been reported to constitutively induce up-regulation of *p16*^{CDKN2A} and cell cycle arrest (this phenomenon appears to be a protective response to an inappropriate mitogenic signal). In particular, mutant BRAF protein induces cell senescence by increasing the expression levels of the p16^{CDKN2A} protein, which, in turn, may limit hyperplastic growth caused by *BRAF* mutations [25]. Therefore, inactivation of *p16*^{CDKN2A} gene may promote the melanocytic proliferation depending on oncogenic *BRAF*. In this sense, several factors seem to be able to induce the arrest of the cell cycle and cell senescence caused by *BRAF* activation [27-28].

Finally, it has been showed that primary melanomas arising from chronically sun-damages skin and from mucosal sites, which typically do not harbour *BRAF* and *NRAS* mutations, have increased copy number of the *CCND1/Cyclin D1* gene [12]. In contrast to primary melanomas, a subset (>15%) of metastatic melanoma samples with *BRAF* mutations also exhibit amplification of *CCND1/Cyclin D1*. These melanomas are resistant to BRAF inhibitors highlighting the need for combination therapy [29-30].

2.2. *CDKN2A* and senescence/apoptosis pathways

The cyclin-dependent kinase inhibitor 2 (*CDKN2A*; at chromosome 9p21) gene encodes two proteins, p16^{CDKN2A} and p14^{CDKN2A} (a product of an alternative splicing), that are known to function as tumor suppressors [31-33]. The cyclin proteins are regulatory effectors able to bind and activate the cyclin-dependent kinases (CDKs) that bear catalytic kinase activity. Several distinct cyclin/CDK complexes have been identified and functionally assigned to specific phases of the cell cycle: Cyclin D/CDK4 complex leads the passage from the pre-replicative (G1) to the DNA duplication (S) phase; the Cyclin E/CDK2 complex promotes the progression through the S phase and the Cyclin B/CDK1 complex induces cells to enter mitosis [31-32]. In such a functional network, proteins like p16^{CDKN2A} and p14^{CDKN2A} act as inhibitors of the cell cycle, negatively interfering with the activity of the cyclin/CDK complexes and, in this way, ensuring the control of the cell replication [33]. In particular, p16^{CDKN2A} is part of the G1–S cell cycle checkpoint mechanism that involves the retinoblastoma-susceptibility tumor suppressor protein (pRb). The p16^{CDKN2A} inhibits the Cyclin D/CDK4 complex, which, in turn, phosphorylates pRb and allows progression through the G1–S checkpoint (Figure 1) [33]. The *Cyclin D* (*CCND1*) and *CDK4* genes are found altered in less than 5% of total melanomas [12], though with an heterogeneous prevalence according to the distinct types of melanoma (see above). Somatic *CDK4* amplification is relatively common in acral and mucosal melanomas [12], whereas germline *CDK4* mutations are observed in a limited fraction of melanoma-prone families [34]. The *CCND1* gene amplifications is primarily found in ALM lesions (more than one third of cases) and to a lesser degree in other types (11% for LMM and 6% for SSM) [35]. Regarding the alternative *CDKN2A* gene product, p14^{CDKN2A} is an antagonist of the murine double minute 2 (MDM2) protein, which targets p53 to degradation by ubiquitination and proteasome processing, thus abrogating p53 control of cell growth (Figure 1) [32-33]. In particular, the p14^{CDKN2A} protein exerts a tumor suppressor effect by inhibiting the oncogenic actions of the downstream MDM2 protein, whose direct interaction with p53 blocks any p53-mediated activity and targets the p53 protein for rapid degradation [32-33]. The p53 is a transcription factor that functions as a major negative regulator of cell proliferation and survival, being activated by different adverse signals (i.e. growth factors withdrawal, DNA damage, oncogenic aberrations, hypoxia, etc.) and driving cells to either interrupt progression into the cell-cycle or enter apoptosis program, in order to avoid reproduction of altered cells [33, 36]. In normal conditions, expression levels of p53 within cells are low. In response to DNA damage, p53 accumulates and prevents cell division. Therefore, inactivation of the *TP53* gene results in an intracellular accumulation of genetic damage which promotes tumor formation [36]. In melanoma, such an inactivation is mostly due to functional gene silencing since the frequency of *TP53* mutations is low (less than 10% of cases) [37]. Impairment of the p14^{CDKN2A}-MDM2-p53 cascade, whose final effectors are the Bax/Bcl-2 proteins, has been implicated in defective apoptotic responses to genotoxic damage and, thus, to anticancer agents (in most cases, high expression levels of Bcl-2 protein have been demonstrated to reduce apoptosis and sensitivity of melanoma cells to proapoptotic stimuli, contributing to further increase tumor aggressiveness and refractoriness to therapy) [33].

More in general, genetic loss or rearrangement in the CDKN2A locus may result in impairing or silencing p16^{CDKN2A}, p14^{CDKN2A} or both genes, with the consequence of losing the mechanisms controlling cell proliferation and/or survival. In melanoma, the *CDKN2A* gene is somatically inactivated by genomic deletions (approximately 50% of cases) or point mutations (about 10% of cases); in addition, this gene is often transcriptionally silenced by promoter hypermethylation [38]. A reduced expression of the p16^{CDKN2A} protein seems to be strictly associated with malignant tumor invasion, varying from 5% to about 15% in benign melanocytic lesions, from 10% to about 50% in primary melanomas, and from 50% to about 60% in melanoma metastases [39]. The *CDKN2A* gene is frequently mutated at germline level in patients with a strong familial history of melanoma (three or more affected family members), indicating that it represents a key susceptibility gene for familial melanoma [40]. In melanoma, CDKN2A mutations typically occur in the p16^{CDKN2A} gene, either alone or in combination with p14^{CDKN2A} gene (some families harbor however mutations only in this latter gene) [33, 40].

A recent meta-analysis of studies conducted in independent populations indicated that multiple variants of the melanocortin-1 receptor (*MC1R*) gene increase the melanoma risk in *CDKN2A* mutation carriers [41]. The *MC1R* gene encodes a G-protein coupled receptor. In the skin, two types of melanin pigment, dark-protective eumelanin and red-photo reactive pheomelanin, are present [42]. MC1R plays an important role in determining the ratio of eumelanin and pheomelanin production. After stimulation by UV, keratinocytes produce alpha melanocyte stimulating hormone (MSH) that binds to the MC1R on melanocytes and shifts the balance of these two pigments in the direction of eumelanin [42]. In particular, stimulation of MC1R by MSH mediates activation of adenylate cyclase, subsequent elevation of cAMP levels, and activation of the microphthalmia transcription factor (MITF; see below). Activated MITF binds to a conserved region found in the promoters of the *tyrosinase* (*TYR*), *tyrosinase-related protein 1* (*TYRP1*), and *DOPAchrome tautomerase* (*DCT*) genes, stimulating the transcriptional up-regulation of these proteins and inducing maturation of the melanosomes [43]. This ultimately results in increased eumelanin production and darkening of the skin or hair.

New findings have shed light on the mechanisms by which MC1R contributes to melanoma risk. In vitro studies showed that acute UV irradiation of melanocytes with impaired MC1R results in an increased production of free radicals [44]. Melanomas that arise on body sites only intermittently exposed to sun, and which therefore lack marked signs of chronic solar damage, were found to have a high frequency of *BRAF* mutations [12]. One could speculate that induction of *BRAF* mutations may occur only when solar exposure is not sufficiently prolonged to induce the striking tissue changes that generate the hallmark signs of solar damage. Several *MC1R* variants, that impairing relevant protein function, have been associated with *BRAF* mutation in melanoma arising in Caucasian populations from United States and Europe [45-48]. On the basis of such indications, it is possible that increased production of free radicals following UV exposure is combination with impairment of *MC1R* may induce mutations in the *BRAF* gene.

Additional mechanisms promoting susceptibility to pathogenetic mutations of the *BRAF* gene may however exist since there is no demonstrable association between germ line *MC1R* status and the prevalence of somatic *BRAF* mutations in melanomas from Australian population, even after classifying the melanomas by their location relative to intermittent and chronic sun-exposure [49].

2.3. *PTEN* and mTORC pathways

Phosphatase and tensin homolog deleted in chromosome ten (PTEN) has a key role in cellular signal transduction by decreasing intracellular phosphatidylinositol [3,4-bisphosphate (PIP2) and 3,4,5-triphosphate (PIP3)] that are produced by the activation of phoshoinosite 3-kinase (PI3K) [50]. In the absence of extracellular growth stimuli mediated by cell surface receptors and G-proteins, PTEN dephosphorylates PIP3 generating the PIP2 phospholipid, unable to stimulate phosphorylation of the PI3K protein; this in turn maintains suppression of cell cycle progression and cell growth. In other words, there is a balance between PIP2 and PIP3 which is maintained by the opposite activities of PTEN and PI3K, which instead converts PIP2 into PIP3 [50]. Upon growth stimulation, mainly obtained by triggering the RAS kinase, PI3K is constitutively activated (Figure 1), resulting in an increase of intracellular levels of PIP3 and a consequent activation of AKT by phosphorylation [50-51]. Activated AKT in turn phosphorylates its substrate, the serine/threonine kinase mTOR, leading to increased synthesis of target proteins that promote cell division and survival as well as apoptotic escape [51]. The mechanisms associated with the ability of AKT to suppress apoptosis include the phosphorylation and inactivation of many pro-apoptotic proteins, such as BAD (Bcl-2 antagonist of cell death) and MDM2, as well as the activation of NF-kB [52] (Figure 1).

Three *AKT* genes have been described in humans: *AKT1*, which is involved in apoptosis and protein synthesis; *AKT2*, which is involved in controlling the glucose metabolism; and *AKT3*, whose increased activity (often associated with the amplification of the *AKT3* locus at chromosome 1q43-44) is mainly involved in stimulating cell growth and has been implicated in many cancers including melanoma [51-52]. More than two thirds of primary and metastatic melanomas exhibit higher levels of phosphorylated AKT [52], suggesting that such an alteration might be considered as an early event in melanoma pathogenesis.

Overall, PI3K expression is higher in malignant melanomas, as compared to nevi, and seems to correlate with a worse prognosis [53]. In primary melanomas, since activating mutations of PI3K are quite rare (about 1%), and comparative genomic hybridization did not reveal amplification at this gene locus [12, 37], activation of the PI3K pathway is mostly due to functional silencing of the tumour suppressor gene PTEN. Inactivation of *PTEN* gene is mainly due to hypermethylation-based epigenetic mechanisms, with a low incidence (less than 10%) of somatic mutations and/or allelic deletions; loss of (or reduced) PTEN protein is observed by immunohistochemistry in 20-40% of melanoma tissues [54-55]. Consistent with its role in the PI3K-AKT pathway, vast majority (more than 80%) of melanoma samples with loss of PTEN protein presents a significant increase in expression of phosphorylated AKT [37].

PTEN inactivation has been mostly observed as a late event in melanoma, although a dose-dependent down-regulation of PTEN expression has been implicated in early stages of tumorigenesis, often occurring in conjunction with mutations in *BRAF* gene (which have been demonstrated to indeed play a role in induction of the melanocytic proliferation and early steps of melanoma development) [50]. PTEN downregulation In addition, alterations of the BRAF-MAPK pathway are frequently associated with PTEN-AKT impairment [7, 56]. In summary, the combined effects of the inactivation of *PTEN* gene and activation of the PI3K-AKT effectors may result in aberrant cell growth, apoptosis escape, and abnormal cell spreading and migration [33, 50].

2.4. *MITF* and melanocytic differentiation

The microphthalmia-associated transcription factor (MITF) is a transcription factor that is involved in differentiation and maintenance of melanocytes, playing a role in melanoma development and pathogenesis [43, 57]. MITF is activated by the MAPK pathway as well as by the cAMP pathway (Figure 1), and leads to transcription of genes involved in pigmentation (TYR, TYRP1, and DCT; see above) as well as cell cycle progression and survival [43]. The *MITF* gene is amplified in melanoma (about 20% of cases); *MITF* amplification correlated with increased resistance to chemotherapy and decreased overall survival [57].

The connection between MITF and melanoma development is complex because it plays a double role of inducer/repressor of cellular proliferation. High levels of MITF expression lead to G1 cell-cycle arrest and differentiation, through induction of the cell cycle inhibitors $p16^{CDKN2A}$ and p21 [58-59] (Figure 1). Very low or null MITF expression levels predispose to apoptosis whereas inter-mediate MITF expression levels promote cell proliferation [57-59]. Therefore, it is thought that melanoma cells have developed strategies to maintain MITF levels in the range compatible with tumorigenesis. It has been shown that constitutive ERK activity, stimulated by ^{V600E}BRAF in melanoma cells, is associated with MITF ubiquitin-dependent degradation [60]. Nevertheless, continued expression of MITF is necessary for proliferation and survival of melanoma cells, because it also regulates CDK2 and Bcl-2 genes [61-62]. It has been recently shown that oncogenic BRAF may control intracellular levels of the MITF protein through a fine balance of two opposite mechanisms: a direct reduction of MITF levels, by inducing protein degradation, and an indirect increase of MITF levels, by stimulating transcription factors which increase protein expression levels [63]. Oncogenic *BRAF* mutations are associated with *MITF* amplification in a low fraction (10-15%) of melanomas [63], suggesting that other mechanisms are likely to be involved in ERK-dependent degradation of MITF.

2.5. *iNOS* and *NF-kB* pathways

Human melanoma cells are known to express the inducible nitric oxide synthase (iNOS) enzyme, which is responsible for synthesis of nitric oxide (NO), a free radical involved in several physiological processes such as neurotransmission, vasodilation, and regulation of immune responses [64]. The iNOS enzyme has been found to be frequently expressed in melanoma [65-66] and the subsequent increased concentrations of NO have been demonstrated to contribute to melanomagenesis through a sustained protection of the tumour from apoptosis [67]. However, the role of iNOS in melanoma progression remains controversial. Higher levels of iNOS have been found in subcutaneous and lymph node metastases of non-progressive melanoma as compared to metastases of progressive melanoma [68], however, iNOS was found to be expressed to a lesser extent in metastases as compared with nevi and primary melanomas [69]. Nevertheless, the expression of iNOS in patients with lymph nodes and in-transit metastases (stage III disease) has been proposed as an indicator of poor prognosis [70].

Recently, it has been reported that the constitutive iNOS expression in melanoma cells might be induced by activation of the MAPK pathway through stimulation of the activity of the Nuclear Factor-kB (NF-kB) [71-72]. NF-kB is a protein complex that acts as a transcriptional factor and regulates the transcription of several genes involved in many critical pathways [73]. In a quiescent status, proteins of the NF-kB complex are localized into the cytoplasm. NF-κB exists as cytoplasmic hetero- or homodimers associated with members of the inhibitor-of-kB (IkB) proteins (IkB*a*, IkB*b* and IkB*e*), which form complexes sequestering NF-kB into the cytoplasm [74]. Upon appropriate stimulation, the phosphorylation of IkB proteins is promoted, triggering their ubiquitination and degradation in the proteasome [74]. As a consequence, NF-kB may translocate to the nucleus where it binds to target DNA loci and induces transcription of several genes - including *iNOS* - associated with immune and inflammatory response, angiogenesis, cell proliferation, tumor promotion, and apoptosis [73-74].

Regarding the role of NF-kB in tumorigenesis, there are compelling evidence that activation of NF-kB controls multiple cellular processes in cancer due to its ability to promote cell proliferation, suppress apoptosis, promote cell migration, and suppress cell differentiation, opening the way for new therapeutic approaches against such a target [75-76]. In melanoma, NF-kB is constitutively activated since expression of the IkB proteins seems to be significantly reduced in comparison to nevi [77].

2.6. *cKIT* and tyrosinase kinase receptors

cKIT is a member of the transmenbrane receptor tyrosine kinase family that comprised five immunoglobin-like motifs, a single transmembrane region, an inhibitory cytoplasmic juxtamenbrane domain, and a split cytoplasmic kinase domain separated by a kinase insert segment [78]. Under physiological conditions, binding of the cKIT ligand stem-cell factor (SCF) to the extracellular domain of the receptor leads its dimerization, activation of the intracellular tyrosine kinase domain through autophosporylation of specific tyrosine residue [78]. The intracellular signaling through cKIT plays a critical role in the development of several mammalian cells, including growth, differentiation, migration, and proliferation of melanocytes [79]. It has been defined that cKIT recruits and activates a number of intracellular signaling pathways implicated in tumor progression, such as MAPK, PI3K/AKT, Src, activators of transcription (STAT), and phospholipase-C (PLC) [79-80].

Although the role of cKIT in melanomagenesis is still controversial, several studies have reported its downregulation during melanoma growth and invasion (in vertical growth phase of melanoma and metastatic lesions) [81-83]. Indeed, the majority of highly metastatic human melanomas do not express detectable levels of the cKIT receptor [83]. As a confirmation of this, over-expression of cKIT in metastatic melanoma cell lines led to important reduction in tumor growth, while cKIT activation through exposure to cKIT ligands induced apoptosis [83].

Specific mutations within the cKIT gene cause constitutive phosphorylation and activation of the kinase domain resulting in uncontrolled cell proliferation. [84]. Although such mutations seem to be more rare than *BRAF* and *NRAS* mutations, these may reflect the important role of cKIT tyrosine kinase in melanocyte development [84]. Sequencing of cKIT exons 11, 13, 17, and 18 revealed the most prevalent mutation to be K642, L576P, D816H-V, V559A [84]. The cKIT mutations are more common in mucosal and acral melanomas compared with cutaneous melanomas and are in most cases accompanied by an increase in gene copy number (40% mucosal or acral melanomas - frequently, associated with amplification of *cy-*

clin D1 - as well as 30% of melanomas on skin with chronic sun-induced damage) [84]. High expression levels of cKIT and CDK4 proteins have been identified in another subset of melanomas lacking *BRAF* mutations [85].

2.7. CTLA-4 and T-cell activation

The above-mentioned main intracellular molecular pathways are thus involved in tumor growth and survival, actively participating to the different phases of development and progression of melanoma. Additional extracellular factors, mainly represented by different components of the tumor microenvironment, have been implied to play a role in melanoma tissue invasion and metastatic dissemination. As an example, changes in the expression of adhesion molecules such as MCAM/MUC18, E-cadherin, and integrins occur in the transition from the radial growth phase (RGP) to the vertical growth phase (VGP) of melanoma; they are induced by both intracellular modifications [i.e., activation of the focal adhesion kinase (FAK) and integrin linked kinase (ILK) patways or high levels of activated ERK (phospoERK$_{1-2}$)] and biological signals directly generated by the extracellular matrix (ECM), which is composed of proteins, glycoproteins, proteoglycans, and glycosaminoglycans in complex arrangements [22-23].

Among others, a block of the anti-tumor immune response induced by changes in pericellular microenvironment has been demonstrated to contribute to melanoma progression [86]. In recent past years, research has tried to better define the molecular mechanisms underlying the downregulation of the immune system by such pericellular components, in order to develop new therapeutic targets [87]. Actually, two immunomodulant antibodies, such as anti-CTLA4 and anti-PD1, have been demonstrated to be effective in inhibiting some down-regulators of the anti-tumor immune response [30, 88]. Moreover, drugs able to interfere with the differentiation of the myeloid-derived suppressor cells (MDSC) and T regulatory cells (Treg), which are both physiologically involved in controlling an abnormal immune response during the inflammatory processes and pathologically favoring tumor progression through suppression of T-cell activation, represent additional therapeutic strategies to be exploited [89].

For T-cell activation, melanoma antigens that are bound to the major histocompatibility complex (MHC) on antigen-presenting cells (APCs) require the costimulation of CD28 receptor on T-cells by CD80 or CD86 ligands on APCs [90]. The cytotoxic T-lymphocyte antigen-4 (CTLA-4) can bind with greater affinity to CD80 and CD86, and thus disrupt the necessary costimulatory signal provided by APCs [88, 90]. This led to the hypothesis that blockade of CTLA-4 function may allow for optimal costimulation of CD28 receptors on T-cells by APC CD80/86, and enhanced T-cell activation [88, 90]. Ipilimumab (Yervoy™ Bristol-Myers Squibb, New York, NY) blocks the costimulatory signal required for T-cell activation [30, 88]. In particular, Ipilimumab is a recombinant human IgG1 monoclonal antibody that binds to CTLA-4 and blocks binding to CD80 or CD86 on APCs, thus increasing activation and proliferation of T cells [88]. Two randomized phase III trials have indicated a significant advantage in disease-free survival (DFS) and overall survival (OS) in either monotherapy or combination therapy [91-92]. The first trial compared monotherapy with Ipilimumab 3 mg/kg, combination of Ipilimumab with gp100 vaccine, and gp100 vaccine alone; the study demonstrated a significant advantage in OS for patients treated with Ipilimumab (regardless the addition off gp100) in comparison to those receiving the gp100 vaccine alone [median OS 10.0 vs 6.4 mesi; Hazard Ratio (HR) for death, 0.68; p<0,001) [91]. In the second study, Dacarbazine was administered as standard chemotherapeutic drug for melanoma patients, in association with Ipilimumab or placebo; the OS rate was significantly higher in the group of patients treated with Ipilimumab + Dacarbazine (11.2 *vs.* 9.1 months), with even more significant percentages of survival for such an association after one year (47.3% *vs.* 36.3%), two years (28.5% *vs.* 17.9%), or three years (20.8% *vs.* 12.2%) of follow-up [92]. The DFS and OS curves from the two studies have been indicated as largely overlapping, strongly demonstrating, for the first time in the history of medical treatments for the advanced disease, a clear survival benefit in metastatic (disease stage IV) melanoma. For these reasons, Ipilimumab has been recently approved by FDA and EMEA for the treatment of metastatic melanoma.

3. Melanoma subtypes and targeted therapeutic options

The different molecular *pathways* involved into the pathogenesis of melanoma are functionally linked each other (Figure 1). There is thus a need to consider such biological cascades as part of a functional web, and the alterations detected in distinct components of the various pathways must be globally considered for the effects determining in such a functional web. This new vision helps in clarifying the reasons by which some alterations may coexist or not in specific melanoma subtypes. As an example, *BRAF* mutations may be observed in conjunction with *PI3K* alterations, but none of them may coexist with *NRAS* mutations; since BRAF and PI3K kinases act downstream NRAS protein, occurrence of *NRAS* mutations activating both MAPK and PI3K-AKT pathways makes unnecessary the further activation of BRAF and PI3K (upstream effectors of the MAPK and PI3K-AKT pathways, respectively). Analogously, oncogenic *BRAF* mutations are able to more intensively activate ERK protein, main last effector downstream the MAPK pathway, when inactivation of the mechanisms controlling senescence and apoptosis concomitantly occurs.

In an attempt to simplify such complex processes underlying the different phases of development and progression of melanoma, the main pathogenetic molecular alterations may be grouped in the following way:

- oncogenic *BRAF* mutations, genomic rearrangements (mainly represented by allelic deletions) at the 9p21 chromosome, and increased expression levels of the AKT3 protein are the main alterations involved into the phase of stimulation of the proliferation for normal melanocytes (*initial preneoplastic phase*);
- impairments of the mechanisms controlling the cell senescence, apoptosis and cell survival (which particularly include alterations in the different components of *CDKN2A* pathways: functional deficit of $p16^{CDKN2A}$ gene, amplification of *CDK4-Cyclin D1/CCND1* loci, inattivation of *TP53* gene through a deregulation of the $p14^{CDKN2A}$-MDM2-p53 functional cascade), oncogenic mutations in *NRAS* gene, activating mutations and, to a lesser extent, gene amplifications of *cKIT* are the main alterations involved into the phase of acquisition of the malignant phenotype which underlay the development of melanoma (*intermediate neoplastic phase*);

- complete silencing of *p16*^{CDKN2A} gene, functional loss of PTEN, activation of the PI3K-AKT pathway, and amplification of the *MITF* gene are the main alterations involved into the phase of acquisition of a more aggressive and invasive phenotype which underlay the progression and dissemination of melanoma (*final metasticase phase*).

All these findings clearly indicate the existence of a complex molecular machinery that provides checks and balances in normal melanocytes, allowing a physiologically controlled cell proliferation. Progression from normal melanocytes to malignant metastatic cell in melanoma patients is the result of a combination of down- or up-regulations of the various effectors acting into the different molecular pathways. According to this, it has been proposed a linear model of pathogenesis of melanoma based on the sequential accumulation of most of the previously-described molecular alterations (Figure 2A) [7, 13, 93]. In a limited fraction of cases, it has been recently hypothesized a second non-linear model of melanomagenesis based on accumulation of the same genetic alterations in tissue stem cells, with generation of malignant cells directly forming RGP or VGP or metastatic melanoma lesions (Figure 2B) [94]. This latter hypothesis has been derived by the evidence of some inconsistencies of the linear model in subgroups of melanomas (i.e., incidence of *BRAF* mutations higher in VGP lesions than that found in RGP lesions [94]).

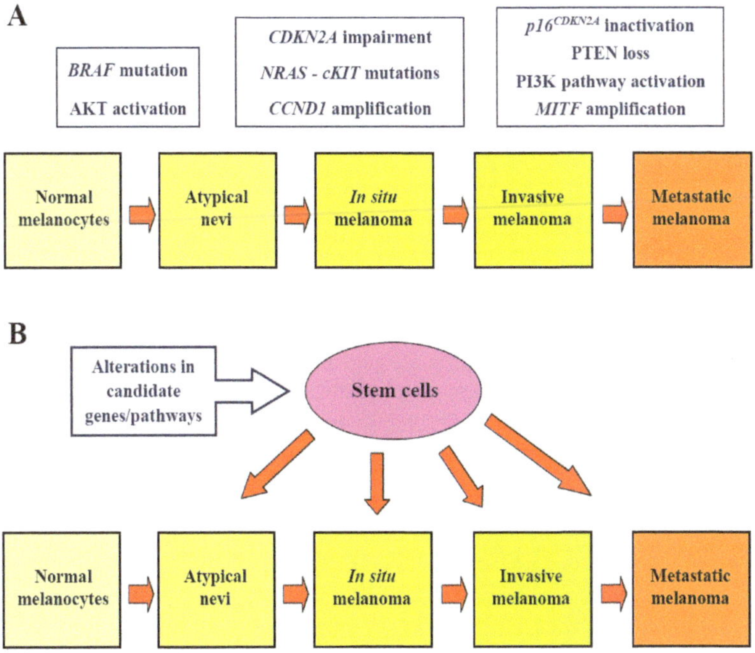

Figure 2. Models of development and progression for melanoma. A, sequential model. B, non-linear model.

Nevertheless, all these evidence represent a strong indication that the different molecular pathways associated with the melanomagenesis does correspond to different subsets of melanoma patients, with distinguished biological and clinical behavior of the disease. Identification of such different patients' subsets should be introduced in clinical trials, in order to better assess the classification of all predictive and prognostic factors associated with the disease as well as more accurately address patients to the most effective therapeutic intervention according to their biological and molecular status.

On the basis of the presence of the specific molecular features, a discrimination of the main subtypes of melanoma, along with the more appropriate therapeutic option for each subtype, could be schematically reported.

1. Subtype MAPK

Prevalence of *BRAF* mutations, with tendency to increased expression level of activated ERK (phospoERK$_{1-2}$) in melanoma tissues. This subtype benefits by the treatment with inhibitors of BRAF.

After failure of BAY 43-9006 (which is not specific for mutated BRAF, but suppresses activity of several different kinases [95]), a second generation BRAF inhibitor (Vemurafenib, also known as PLX4032 or RO5185426) was highly specific for ^{V600E}BRAF mutation and appeared very promising from the clinical point of view [96]. Very recently, results from a phase III study comparing the vemurafenib to dacarbazine have been indeed reported, indicating a relative reduction of 63% in the risk of death and of 74% in the risk of either death or disease progression, as compared with dacarbazine [97]. Preliminary data using an additional ^{V600E}BRAF inhibitor compound, Dabrafenib (previously known as GSK2118436), seemed to point out that this molecule is also active on ^{V600K}BRAF and ^{V600D}BRAF mutations [98]; actually, treatment with such a compound is under evaluation in a phase III study among BRAF mutation positive stage III-IV melanoma patients.

However, preliminary data seem to indicate that a large variety of induced alterations may drive resistance to BRAF inhibitors: upregulation of the receptor tyrosine kinase (RTK) effectors [99], mutation in *NRAS* gene and platelet-derived growth factor receptor β (PDGFRβ) [99], amplification of the *CCND1/Cyclin D1* gene or lack of phosphatase-and-tensin homologue (PTEN) function [100], mutations in downstream *MEK* gene [101], activation of MAPK pathway agonists such as COT kinase [102], or enhancement of the IGF-1R/PI3K signaling [103]. These findings highlight the need for combination therapy.

The MEK inhibitors (AS703026, E6201, GSK1120212, GDC0973, MEK162) as single agents have activity against melanoma, in patients either carrying BRAF mutations and unexposed to prior BRAF inhibitor therapy or presenting NRAS mutations [30]. A new combination of MEK and BRAF inhibitors as first line therapy for BRAF mutated melanoma patients naïve to prior anti-BRAF treatment is showing great promise [30].

The *BRAF* mutations may coexist with additional molecular alterations, with subsequent constitution of further biological and molecular subgroups of melanoma patients:

a. Impairment of the $p16^{CDKN2A}$-CDK4/CCND1-RB or $p14^{CDKN2A}$-MDM2-TP53 pathways, with reduced expression of the $p16^{CDKN2A}$ protein and tendency to amplification of the *CDK4/CCND1* gene loci or inactivation of the TP53 gene (with consequent functional loss of the p53 protein), respectively. This subtype benefits by the treatment with inhibitors of the cyclin-dependent kinases.

Melanoma patients carrying genetic alterations affecting $p16^{CDKN2A}$ could potentially be treated with inhibitors of CDK4/CDK6. There are currently no validated therapeutic options for melanoma with mutated $p14^{CDKN2A}$. Conversely, several CDK4 inhibitors (Alvocidib, AT-7519, P1446A-05, PD-0332991, Flavopiridol/alvocidib/HMR 1275, P276-00, R547, SNS-032/ BMS-387032, UCN-01, ZK 304709/MTGI) are currently under investigation for a variety of cancer types, including metastatic melanoma, and results are awaited. For p53, there are currently no drugs, approved or in trials, against such a target. Conversely, an anti-sense agent (Oblimersen) targeted at nuclear Bcl-2 has been evaluated in trials, failing to demonstrate a significant clinical benefit among patients with melanoma [104].

b. Amplification of *MITF* ± associated with reduction of the protein expression levels.

No drug targeting MITF has been developed; however, expression of MITF has been demonstrated to be reduced by compounds inhibiting the multiple histone deacetylase (HDAC) complex [105]. Ongoing trials based on HDAC-inhibitors [LBH589 (Panobinostat) or Valproic acid (Vorinostat)] will elucidate whether a clinical benefit could be obtained by down-regulating intracellular level of MITF protein.

c. Activation of NF-kB.

Proteasome inhibitors, such as Bortezomib (Velcade, previously known as PS-341), represent a new class of anticancer therapeutic agents which inhibit degradation of important cell cycle and/or regulatory proteins, including IkB [106-107]. Bortezomid has been demonstrated to contribute in maintaining integrity of the complexes sequestering NF-kB into the cytoplasm, thus reducing the NF-kB activity [106-107]. Phase 2 studies combinating Bortezomib with other chemotherapeutic agents, including paclitaxel, carboplatin, or temozolomide equally have been established [108-109]. A compound that more directly targets the NF-kB pathway is BMS-345541 (4(2'-aminoethyl) amino-1,8-dimethylimidazo(1,2-a)quinoxaline), identified as a selective inhibitor of the catalytic subunits of IKK that binds at an allosteric site of the enzyme [110].

Since mutational activation of BRAF in human melanomas has been demonstrated to contribute to constitutive induction of NF-kB activity through an increase of the IKK activity [111], inhibition of BRAF signaling using the above mentioned inhibitors may decrease the NF-kB transcriptional activity and sensitize melanoma cells to apoptosis.

2. Subtype NRAS

Prevalence of *NRAS* mutation, with markedly increased expression level of activated ERK ($phospoERK_{1-2}$) and eventual activation of AKT. This subtype benefits by the treatment with inhibitors of MEK or mTORC.

To date, two approaches have been considered in developing drugs against RAS. The first is based on the block of farnesylation. A small clinical trial using an inhibitor of the farnesyl transferase enzyme failed to be efficacious in a melanoma cohort; however, patients included into such a study were not selected on the basis of their *NRAS* mutation status [112-113]. In the light of recent successes of the target therapies based on anti-BRAF or anti-cKIT inhibitors, a more stringently selected cohort carrying alterations in *NRAS* gene would have increased responsiveness. On the other hand, a direct targeting of RAS has been demonstrated to be very difficult [114]; this is the reason why therapeutic strategies have focused on inhibiting downstream effectors into the pathways activated by RAS (i.e., MEK inhibitors for the MAPK pathway - see above - and mTORC inhibitors for the PI3K-AKT pathway - see below), which represent the second treatment approach against RAS.

3. Subtype cKIT

Prevalence of *cKIT* mutations ± gene amplification and/or increased protein expression levels. This subtype benefits by the treatment with inhibitors of cKIT (in particular, patients carrying gene mutations, with some sequence variants - such as K642E e L576P - which are highly responsive).

Activating cKIT mutations have been implicated in a variety of cancers, mainly represented by gastrointestinal stromal tumors (GIST) and chronic myelogenous leukemia (CML). This is the reason why several drugs targeting cKIT have been developed and tested in clinical trials, including Imatinib (approved for Philadelphia chromosome–positive CML and cKIT-positive GIST) and Sunitib (approved for advanced kidney cancer and Imatinib-resistant GIST) as well as Nilotinib and Dasatinib (approved for CML and Philadelphia chromosome-positive acute lymphoblastic leukemia).

The inhibitors of cKIT that may have a therapeutic benefit in melanoma, by inducing cell cycle arrest and apoptosis as well as significantly inhibiting cell migration and invasion of tumor cells, are:

Imatinib mesylate, formerly known as STI571, is designated chemically as 4-benzamide methanesulfonate. The efficacy of imatinib varies with the site of cKIT mutation; moreover, this drug can inhibit both the wild-type receptor activated by ligand and mutated receptor in the absence of ligand. However, imatinib is less effective at inhibiting the receptor with mutations in the enzymatic site (exon 17 mutations) [79];

Nilotinib (AMN107), which has been rationally designed based on the imatinib mesylate scaffold to have a more selective action. On this regard, Nilotinib inhibits both wild-type and cKIT mutants in exon 11 (V560del and V560G), exon 13 (K642E), double mutants involving exons 11, 13, and 17 as well as imatinib-resistant cKIT mutant (V560del/V654A) cells [115];

Dasatinib, which is a piperazinyl ethanol exhibiting increased potency but reduced selectivity compared with imatinib mesylate, has been demonstrated to inhibit both wild type and mutant cKIT in a dose-dependent manner, causing inhibition of cell migration and invasion through reduction of the phosphorylation of either Src kinase and FAK pathway [116-117].

4. Subtype mTORC

Prevalence of PTEN loss (± *PI3K* mutations, which are mostly infrequent) and phosphorylation of AKT, with absence of concurrent mutations in *BRAF* gene. This subtype mainly benefits by the treatment with inhibitors of mTOR.

In melanoma cells, three potential targets may be considered for therapeutic intervention against this pathway: AKT, PI3K and mTOR. Restoration of functional PTEN or interfering with AKT and PI3K activity would increase chemosensitivity to apoptotic agents and improve the efficacy of anti-tumor treatment. Several inhibitors of PI3K (BKM120, BEZ235, BGT226, GDC0941, PX-866, SF1126, and XL147) and AKT (GSK690693, MK2206, and VQD-002) have been developed; results of ongoing trials are thus awaited. To date, clinical trials using agents against the PI3K/AKT pathway have failed to demonstrate significant efficacy [118]. However, one therapeutic approach which seems to inhibit this pathway is based on the use of mTOR inhibitors [119]: rapamycin, Temsirolimus (CCI-779), Everolimus (RAD001), Sirolimus and AZD8055. While controversial data have been reported for rapamycin (suppressing disease progression in some patients with glioblastoma but ineffective in controlling the disease in others) [120], a limited advantage in response rates has been so far described for Temsirolimus [121]. It is to be underlined that none of the trials with mTOR inhibitors included patients specifically selected for alterations in the AKT/PI3K pathway. Several clinical trials are investigating specific combinations of mTOR inhibitors and chemotherapy drugs in the treatment of melanoma.

5. Subtype GNAQ/GNA11

Prevalence of *GNAQ/GNA11* mutations, with increased expression level of phosphoERK. This subtype benefits by the treatment with inhibitors of MEK.

The *GNAQ* and *GNA11* genes encodes specific GTP binding proteins that mediate signal transduction from the inner cell surface to the MAPK pathway through activation of the protein kinase C (PKC) enzyme [122]. Somatic mutations in *GNAQ* gene have been observed in about 90% of blue naevi, 50% of malignant blue naevi and 50% of primary uveal melanoma; conversely, the *GNA11* mutations have been found in less than 10% of blue nevi, about one third of primary uveal melanomas, and about 60% of metastatic uveal melanoma [122]. Since mutations in these two genes have non been detected among all the remaining types of melanoma (cutaneous, acral, mucosal), a clinical trial aimed at testing efficacy of a MEK inhibitor, Dabrafenib/GSK1120212, has been focused on patients with metastatic uveal melanoma carrying *GNAQ* and/or *GNA11* mutations [123].

4. Diagnostic panel of molecular alterations

The most prevalent molecular alterations within the heterogeneous patterns of biological features which characterize the distinct subtypes of melanoma are here summarized, according to the anatomical site of melanoma onset, the degree of exposure to the sun, and the histologic characteristics of the tumor lesions.

- Acral melanoma

Mutation ± amplification of *cKIT*; amplification of *CDK4* or *CCND1* (associated with increased expression levels of the related proteins); amplification of the 11q13, 22q11-13, and/or 5p15 genomic loci.

- Melanoma of the head and neck district and melanoma on skin with chronic sun-induced damage (CSD)

Amplification of *CDK4* and/or *CCND1*; increased expression levels of p53 protein; mutation ± amplification of *cKIT* (in about 5% of cases).

- Melanoma of the trunk and melanoma on skin without chronic sun-induced damage (non-CSD)

Mutation of *BRAF* or, alternatively, *NRAS* (with eventual coexistence of molecolar alterations which may ba associated with BRAF mutations; see above); tendency to reduced expression of the p53 protein; occurrence of specific polymorphisms in *MC1R* gene.

- Mucosal melanoma

Mutation ± amplification of *cKIT*; amplification of *CDK4* or *CCND1* (associated with increased expression levels of the related proteins); mutation of *BRAF* (in less than 10% of cases).

- Uveal melanoma

Mutation ± amplification of *cKIT*; mutation of *GNAQ* and/or *GNA11*.

Knowledge of the principal molecular alterations to be tested in patients with such distinct subtypes of melanoma will be of great clinical importance, because it is likely to result in separate targeted therapeutic approaches and prevention strategies. To date, it has been already developed a panel of molecular tests to be performed in patients with melanoma from different anatomical locations (Figure 3). This initial "*flow-chart*" will surely become more detailed and enriched on the basis of the progressive identification and validation of additional genetics and molecular alterations correlated with the disease.

Finally, recent meta-analyses tried to define the prognostic role of majority of molecular alterations previously described [124-125]:

- negative prognostic factors

loss of p53; over-expression of iNOS, AP-2, MMP-2 and metallothioneine; increased proliferation index (high expression levels of Ki-67);

- positive prognostic factors

reduced expression or loss of $p16^{CDKN2A}$; over-expression of Bcl-2 and ATF-2 (± associated with simultaneous increases expression of beta-catenin, fibronectin and p21 proteins).

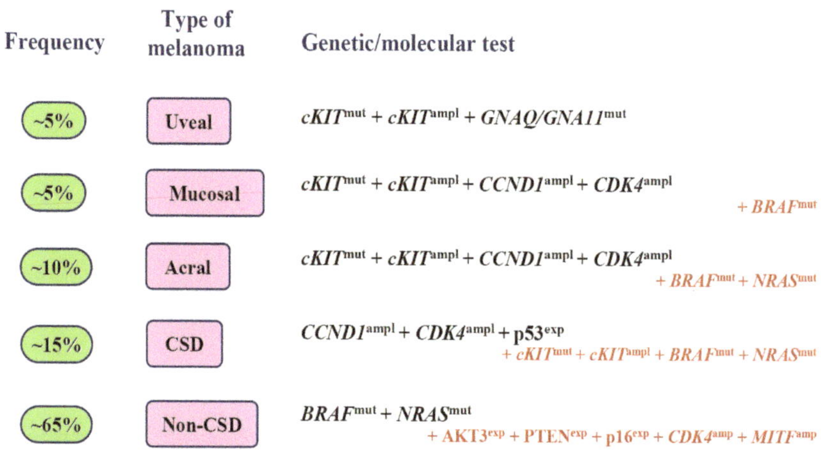

Figure 3. Principal genetic and molecular tests on tumor tissues for the different types of melanoma. Amp, gene amplification detected by *fluorescence in situ hybridization* (FISH) analysis. Exp, protein expression level detected by immunohistochemistry. Mut, gene sequence variation detected by mutation analysis. In red, tests for less prevalent alterations.

5. Conclusion

Taken together all the described molecular mechanisms involved in melanoma genesis and progression, data seem to emphasize the fact that in melanoma, but probably in all types of cancer, it is unlikely that targeting a single component in the signalling pathway will yield significant anti-tumour responses. For this purpose, molecular analyses could help clinicians to define the prognosis (prognostic value) as well as to make a prediction, identifying the subsets of patients who would be expected to be more or less likely to respond to specific therapeutic interventions (predictive value).

In other words, it is becoming evident that combination therapies targeting simultaneously several signaling pathways might be a winning therapeutic strategy to treat melanoma patients. Preclinical studies using combination of anti BRAF and AKT3 siRNA demonstrated a significantly higher reduction of tumor growth compared to single agent administration [126-127]. There is also evidence of synergism among MEK and PI3K inhibitors as well as promising results have been obtained by combinations of the mTOR inhibitors and sorafenib or MEK inhibitors [121, 128-129]. In contrast to single agent activity, these combinations of target drugs resulted in recovering of apoptosis by complete down-regulation of the anti-apoptotic proteins Bcl-2 and Mcl-1. Cooperation between BRAF and MEK inhibitors has also been demonstrated in preclinical studies with a consistent increase of apoptosis and abrogation of ERK activation compared to BRAF inhibitor alone [130]. Such cooperation was based on the observation that MEK activation was not abrogated in melanoma cells that develop resistance to BRAF inhibitors [131-134]. BRAF and MEK targeted synergic therapy is currently tested in a phase I clinical trial (NCT01072175) which combines the selective RAF inhibitor GSK2118436 with the MEK inhibitor GSK1120212 in patients with BRAF mutant tumors [135].

After decades without perspective, the history of medical treatment for the advanced melanoma is rapidly changing. Combined therapeutic approaches do represent the next challenge for treatment of patients with such a disease.

Acknowledgments

Authors are always grateful to patients for their cooperation into the various studies. Work was funded by Regione Autonoma della Sardegna and Ricerca Finalizzata Ministero della Salute.

Author details

Giuseppe Palmieri[1*], Maria Colombino[1], Maria Cristina Sini[1], Paolo Antonio Ascierto[2], Amelia Lissia[3] and Antonio Cossu[3]

*Address all correspondence to: gpalmieri@yahoo.com

1 Unit of Cancer Genetics, Institute of Biomolecular Chemistry (ICB), National Research Council (CNR), Traversa La Crucca, 3 - Baldinca Li Punti, Sassari, Italy

2 Unit of Medical Oncology and Innovative Therapy, Istituto Nazionale Tumori Fondazione "G. Pascale", Via Mariano Semmola, Napoli, Italy

3 University Hospital Health Unit - Azienda Ospedaliero Universitaria (AOU), Via Matteotti, Sassari, Italy

References

[1] Curado MP, Edwards B, Shin HR, Storm H, Ferlay J, Heanue M, Boyle P (eds). Cancer Incidence in Five Continents, Vol. IX, International Agency for Research on Cancer (IARC) Scientific Publications, No. 160, Lyon, IARC, 2007.

[2] Linos E, Swetter S, Cockburn MG, et al. Increasing burden of melanoma in the United States. J Invest Derm. 2009;129: 1666-74

[3] Rigel DS. Epidemiology of melanoma. Semin. Cutan. Med. Surg. 2010; 29: 204-209

[4] Welch HG, Woloshin S, Schwartz LM. Skin biopsy rates and incidence of melanoma: population based ecological study. BMJ 2005: 331: 481;

[5] de Vries E, Coebergh JW. Melanoma incidence has risen in Europe. BMJ. 2005: 331: 698

[6] Jhappan C, Noonan FP, Merlino G. Ultraviolet radiation and cutaneous malignant melanoma. Oncogene 2003: 22: 3099-3112

[7] Thompson JF, Scolyer RA, Kefford RF. Cutaneous melanoma. The Lancet 2005: 365: 687-701

[8] Cho E, Rosner BA, Feskanich D, Colditz GA. Risk factors and individual probabilities of melanoma for whites. J Clin Oncol. 2005: 23: 2669-2675

[9] Balch CM, Buzaid AC, Soong SJ, Atkins MB, Cascinelli N, Coit DG, Fleming ID, Gershenwald JE, Houghton A Jr, Kirkwood JM, McMasters KM, Mihm MF, Morton DL, Reintgen DS, Ross MI, Sober A, Thompson JA, Thompson JF. Final version of the American Joint Committee on Cancer Staging System for Cutaneous Melanoma. J Clin Oncol 2001; 19: 3635-48

[10] Bastian BC, Olshen AB, LeBoit PE, Pinkel D. Classifying melanocytic tumors based on DNA copy number changes. Am J Pathol 2003;163:1765-70

[11] Haluska FG, Tsao H, Wu H, Haluska FS, Lazar A, Goel V. Genetic alterations in signaling pathways in melanoma. Clin Cancer Res. 2006; 12: 2301-7

[12] Curtin JA, Fridlyand J, Kageshita T, Patel HN, Busam KJ, Kutzner H, Cho KH, Aiba S, Bröcker EB, LeBoit PE, Pinkel D, Bastian BC. Distinct sets of genetic alterations in melanoma. N Engl J Med. 2005; 353:2135-47

[13] Palmieri G, Capone ME, Ascierto ML, Gentilcore G, Stroncek DF, Casula M, Sini MC, Palla M, Mozzillo N, Ascierto PA. Main roads to melanoma. J Transl Med. 2009; 7: 86

[14] Miller AJ, Mihm MC. Melanoma. N Engl J Med 2006; 355, 51-65

[15] Giehl K. Oncogenic Ras in tumor progression and metastasis. Biol Chem. 2005;386:193–205

[16] Heidorn SJ, Milagre C, Whittaker S, et al. Kinase-dead BRAF and oncogenic RAS cooperate to drive tumor progression through CRAF. Cell. 2010 Jan 22;140:209-21

[17] Rajagopalan H, Bardelli A, Lengauer C, Kinzler KW, Vogelstein B, Velculescu VE. Tumorigenesis: RAF/RAS oncogenes and mismatch-repair status. Nature. 2002;418:934

[18] Quinlan MP, Settleman J. Isoform-specific ras functions in development and cancer. Future Oncol. 2009; 5:105-16

[19] Heidorn SJ, Milagre C, Whittaker S, et al. Kinase-dead BRAF and oncogenic RAS cooperate to drive tumor progression through CRAF. Cell. 2010; 140:209-21

[20] Davies H, Bignell GR, Cox C, Stephens P, Edkins S, Clegg S, Teague J, Woffendin H, Garnett MJ, Bottomley W, Davis N, Dicks E, Ewing R, Floyd Y, Gray K, Hall S, Hawes R, Hughes J, Kosmidou V, Menzies A, Mould C, Parker A, Stevens C, Watt S, Hooper S, Wilson R, Jayatilake H, Gusterson BA, Cooper C, Shipley J, Hargrave D, Pritchard-Jones K, Maitland N, Chenevix-Trench G, Riggins GJ, Bigner DD, Palmieri G, Cossu A, Flanagan A, Nicholson A, Ho JW, Leung SY, Yuen ST, Weber BL, Seigler HF, Darrow TL, Paterson H, Marais R, Marshall CJ, Wooster R, Stratton MR, Futreal PA. Mutations of the BRAF gene in human cancer. Nature. 2002; 417:949-54

[21] Smalley KSM. A pivotal role for ERK in the oncogenic behaviour of malignant melanoma? Int J Cancer 2003; 104:527-32

[22] McGary EC, Chelouche Lev D, Bar-Eli M. Cellular adhesion pathways and metastatic potential of human melanoma. Cancer Biol Ther 2002; 5: 459-465

[23] Kuphal S, Bauer R, Bosserhoff AK. Integrin signaling in malignant melanoma. Cancer Metastasis Reviews 24: 195–222, 2005

[24] Pollock PM, Harper UL, Hansen KS, Yudt LM, Stark M, Robbins CM, Moses TY, Hostetter G, Wagner U, Kakareka J, Salem G, Pohida T, Heenan P, Duray P, Kallioniemi O, Hayward NK, Trent JM, Meltzer PS. High frequency of BRAF mutations in nevi. Nat Genet. 2003, 33:19-20

[25] Michaloglou C, Vredeveld LC, Soengas MS, Denoyelle C, Kuilman T, van der Horst CM, Majoor DM, Shay JW, Mooi WJ, Peeper DS. BRAFE600-associated senescence-like cell cycle arrest of human naevi. Nature 2005; 436, 720–724

[26] Patton EE, Widlund HR, Kutok JL, Kopani KR, Amatruda JF, Murphey RD, Berghmans S, Mayhall EA, Traver D, Fletcher CD, Aster JC, Granter SR, Look AT, Lee C, Fisher DE, Zon LI. BRAF mutations are sufficient to promote nevi formation and cooperate with p53 in the genesis of melanoma. Curr Biol. 2005;15:249–54

[27] Wajapeyee N, Serra RW, Zhu X, et al. Oncogenic BRAF induces senescence and apoptosis through pathways mediated by the secreted protein IGFBP7. Cell. 2008;132:363–374

[28] Dhomen N, Reis-Filho JS, da Rocha Dias S, et al. Oncogenic Braf induces melanocyte senescence and melanoma in mice. Cancer Cell. 2009;15:294–303

[29] Smalley KS, Lioni M, Dalla Palma M, Xiao M, Desai B, Egyhazi S, Hansson J, Wu H, King AJ, Van Belle P, Elder DE, Flaherty KT, Herlyn M, Nathanson KL. Increased cyclin D1 expression can mediate BRAF inhibitor resistance in BRAF V600E-mutated melanomas. Mol Cancer Ther. 2008; 7: 2876-83

[30] Ascierto PA, Grimaldi AM, Curti B, Faries MB, Ferrone S, Flaherty K, Fox BA, Gajewski TF, Gershenwald JE, Gogas H, Grossmann K, Hauschild A, Hodi FS, Kefford R, Kirkwood JM, Leachmann S, Maio M, Marais R, Palmieri G, Morton DL, Ribas A, Stroncek DF, Stewart R, Wang E, Mozzillo N, Marincola FM. Future Perspectives in

melanoma research. Meeting report from the "Melanoma Research: a bridge from Naples to the World. Napoli, December 5th-6th 2011". J. Transl Med. 10: 83, 2012

[31] Pomerantz J, Schreiber-Agus N, Lie´ geois NJ. The Ink4a tumor suppressor gene product, 19Arf, interacts with MDM2 and neutralizes DM2's inhibition of p53. Cell 1998; 92: 713-23

[32] Zhang Y, Xiong Y, Yarbrough WG. ARF promotes MDM2 degradation and stabilizes p53: ARF-INK4a locus deletion impairs both the Rb and p53 tumor suppression pathways. Cell 1998: 92: 725–734

[33] Palmieri G, Capone ME, Ascierto ML, Gentilcore G, Stroncek DF, Casula M, Sini MC, Palla M, Mozzillo N, Ascierto PA. Main roads to melanoma. J Transl Med. 7: 86, 2009

[34] Soufir N, Avril MF, Chompret A, Demenais F, Bombled J, Spatz A, Stoppa-Lyonnet D, Bénard J, Bressac-de Paillerets B. Prevalence of p16 and CDK4 germline mutations in 48 melanoma-prone families in France. The French Familial Melanoma Study Group. Hum Mol Genet. 1998; 7: 209-16

[35] Sauter ER, Yeo UC, von Stemm A, Zhu W, Litwin S, Tichansky DS, Pistritto G, Nesbit M, Pinkel D, Herlyn M, Bastian BC. Cyclin D1 is a candidate oncogene in cutaneous melanoma. Cancer Res. 2002; 62:3200-6

[36] Box NF, Terzian T: The role of p53 in pigmentation, tanning and melanoma. Pigment Cell Melanoma Res 2008, 21:525-533

[37] Hocker TL, Singh MK, Tsao H. Melanoma genetics and therapeutic approaches in the 21st century: moving from the benchside to the bedside. J Invest Dermatol. 2008; 128:2575-95

[38] Bennett DC. How to make a melanoma: what do we know of the primary clonal events? Pigment Cell Melanoma Res. 2008; 21:27-38

[39] Sini MC, Manca A, Cossu A, Budroni M, Botti G, Ascierto PA, Cremona F, Muggiano A, D'Atri S, Casula M, Baldinu P, Palomba G, Lissia A, Tanda F, Palmieri G. Molecular alterations at chromosome 9p21 in melanocytic nevi and melanoma. Br. J. Dermatology 158: 243-250, 2008

[40] Meyle KD, Guldberg P. Genetic risk factors for melanoma. Hum Genet. 2009; 126: 499-510

[41] Fargnoli MC, Gandini S, Peris K, Maisonneuve P, Raimondi S. MC1R variants increase melanoma risk in famiglie with CDKN2A mutations: A meta-analysis. Eur J Cancer 2010; 46: 1413-20

[42] Scott MC, Wakamatsu K, Ito S, et al. Human melanocortin 1 receptor variants, receptor function and melanocyte response to UV radiation. J Cell Sci. 2002; 115: 2349-55

[43] Levy C, Khaled M, Fisher DE. MITF: master regulator of melanocyte development and melanoma oncogene. Trends Mol. Med. 2006;12, 406–414

[44] Hauser JE, Kadekaro AL, Kavanagh RJ, et al. Melanin content and MC1R function independently affect UVR-induced DNA damage in cultured human melanocytes. Pigment Cell Res. 2006; 19:303-14

[45] Landi MT, Bauer J, Pfeiffer RM, et al. MC1R germline variants confer risk for BRAF-mutant melanoma. Science 2006; 313:521-2

[46] Fargnoli MC, Pike K, Pfeiffer RM, et al. MC1R variants increase risk of melanomas harboring BRAF mutations. J Invest Dermatol. 2008; 128:2485-90

[47] Thomas NE, Kanetsky PA, Edmiston SN, et al. Relationship between germline MC1R variants and BRAF-mutant melanoma in a North Carolina population-based study. J Invest Dermatol. 2010; 130:1463-5

[48] Scherer D, Rachakonda PS, Angelini S, et al. Association between the germline MC1R variants and somatic BRAF/NRAS mutations in melanoma tumors. J Invest Dermatol. 2010; 130:2844-8

[49] Hacker E, Hayward NK, Dumenil T, et al. The association between MC1R genotype and BRAF mutation status in cutaneous melanoma: findings from an Australian population.J Invest Dermatol. 2010; 130:241-8

[50] Wu H, Goel V, Haluska FG. PTEN signaling pathways in melanoma. Oncogene. 2003; 22: 3113-22

[51] Vivanco I, Sawyers CL. The phosphatidylinositol 3-kinase AKT pathway in human cancer. Nat Rev Cancer. 2002;2:489-501

[52] Plas DR, Thompson CB. Akt-dependent transformation: there is more to growth than just surviving. Oncogene. 2005;24:7435–7442

[53] Aziz SA, Davies M, Pick E, Zito C, Jilaveanu L, Camp RL, Rimm DL, Kluger Y, Kluger HM. Phosphatidylinositol-3-kinase as a therapeutic target in melanoma. Clin Cancer Res. 2009; 15: 3029-36

[54] Mirmohammadsadegh A, Marini A, Nambiar S, et al. Epigenetic silencing of the PTEN gene in melanoma. Cancer Res. 2006; 66: 6546-52

[55] Goel VK, Lazar AJ, Warneke CL, Redston MS, Haluska FG. Examination of mutations in BRAF, NRAS, and PTEN in primary cutaneous melanoma. J Invest Dermatol. 2006; 126:154-60

[56] Tsao H, Goel V, Wu H, et al. Genetic interaction between NRAS and BRAF mutations and PTEN/MMAC1 inactivation in melanoma. J Invest Dermatol 2004; 122: 337–41

[57] Garraway LA, Widlund HR, Rubin MA, Getz G, Berger AJ, Ramaswamy S, Beroukhim R, Milner DA, Granter SR, Du J, Lee C, Wagner SN, Li C, Golub TR, Rimm DL, Meyerson ML, Fisher DE, Sellers WR. Integrative genomic analyses identify MITF as a lineage survival oncogene amplified in malignant melanoma. Nature. 2005; 436:117-22.

[58] Carreira S, Goodall J, Aksan I, et al. Mitf cooperates with Rb1 and activates p21Cip1 expression to regulate cell cycle progression. Nature 2005;433: 764-769

[59] Loercher AE, Tank EM, Delston RB, Harbour JW. MITF links differentiation with cell cycle arrest in melanocytes by transcriptional activation of INK4A. J Cell Biol 2005;168: 35-40

[60] Wellbrock C, Marais R: Elevated expression of MITF counteracts B-RAF stimulated melanocyte and melanoma cell proliferation. J Cell Biol 2005;170: 703-708

[61] McGill GG, Horstmann M, Widlund HR, et al. Bcl2 regulation by the melanocyte master regulator Mitf modulates lineage survival and melanoma cell viability. Cell 2002;109:707-718.

[62] Du J, Widlund HR, Horstmann MA, et al. Critical role of CDK2 for melanoma growth linked to its melanocyte-specific transcriptional regulation by MITF. Cancer Cell 2004;6: 565-576

[63] Wellbrock C, Rana S, Paterson H, et al. Oncogenic BRAF regulates melanoma proliferation through the lineage specific factor MITF. PLoS ONE 3:2734,2008

[64] Ekmekcioglu S, Tang CH, Grimm EA. NO news is not necessarily good news in cancer. Curr Cancer Drug Targets. 2005; 5:103-15

[65] Massi D, De Nisi MC, Franchi A, Mourmouras V, Baroni G, Panelos J, Santucci M, Miracco C. Inducible nitric oxide synthase expression in melanoma: implications in lymphangiogenesis. Mod Pathol. 2009; 22:21-30

[66] Grimm EA, Ellerhorst J, Tang CH, Ekmekcioglu S. Constitutive intracellular production of iNOS and NO in human melanoma: possible role in regulation of growth and resistance to apoptosis. Nitric Oxide. 2008; 19:133-7

[67] Sikora AG, Gelbard A, Davies MA, Sano D, Ekmekcioglu S, Kwon J, Hailemichael Y, Jayaraman P, Myers JN, Grimm EA, Overwijk WW. Targeted inhibition of inducible nitric oxide synthase inhibits growth of human melanoma in vivo and synergizes with chemotherapy. Clin Cancer Res. 2010; 16:1834-44

[68] Tschugguel W, Pustelnik T, Lass H, Mildner M, Weninger W, Schneeberger C, Jansen B, Tschachler E, Waldhör T, Huber JC, Pehamberger H: Inducible nitric oxide synthase (iNOS) expression may predict distant metastasis in human melanoma. Br J Cancer 1999, 79:1609-1612

[69] Ahmed B, Van den Oord JJ: Expression of the inducible isoform of nitric oxide synthase in pigment cell lesions of the skin. Br J Dermatol 2000, 142:432-40

[70] Ekmekcioglu S, Ellerhorst JA, Prieto VG, Johnson MM, Broemeling LD, Grimm EA. Tumor iNOS predicts poor survival for stage III melanoma patients. Int J Cancer. 2006; 119:861-6

[71] Dhawan P, Richmond A. A novel NF-kappa B-inducing kinase-MAPK signaling pathway up-regulates NF-kappa B activity in melanoma cells. J Biol Chem 2002; 277:7920-8

[72] Uffort DG, Grimm EA, Ellerhorst JA. NF-kappaB mediates mitogen-activated protein kinase pathway-dependent iNOS expression in human melanoma. J Invest Dermatol. 2009; 129:148-54

[73] Baldwin AS. Control of oncogenesis and cancer therapy resistance by the transcription factor NF-kB. J Clin Invest 2001;107:241–246

[74] Madonna G, Dansky Ullman C, Gentilcore G, Palmieri G, Ascierto PA. NF-kappaB as potential target in the treatment of melanoma. J. Transl Med. 2012; 10: 53

[75] Chaturvedi MM, Sung B, Yadav VR, Kannappan R, Aggarwal BB. NF-kB addiction and its role in cancer: 'one size does not fit all'. Oncogene. 2011; 30:1615-30.

[76] Kim HJ, Hawke N, Baldwin AS. NF-kappaB and IKK as therapeutic targets in cancer. Cell Death Differ. 2006; 13:738-47

[77] McNulty SE, del Rosario R, Cen D, et al. Comparative expression of NFkappaB proteins in melanocytes of normal skin vs. benign intradermal naevus and human metastatic melanoma biopsies. Pigment Cell Res. 2004; 17:173-80

[78] Clifford D, Mol, Kheng B. Lim. Structure of a c-Kit product complex reveals the basis for kinase transactivation. J. Biol Chem 2003; 278: 31461-64

[79] Smalley KS, Sondak VK, Weber JS. c-KIT signaling as the driving oncogenic event in sub-groups of melanomas. Histol Histopathol. 2009; 24:643-50.

[80] Alexeev V, Yoon K. Distinctive role of the cKit receptor tyrosine kinase signaling in mammalian melanocytes. J Invest Dermatol. 2006; 126: 1102-1110

[81] Shen SS, Zhang PS, Eton O, Prieto VG. Analysis of protein tyrosine kinase expression in melanocytic lesions by tissue array. J Cutan Pathol 2003; 30: 539-547

[82] Stefanou D, Batistatou A, Zioga A. Immunohistochemical expression of vascular endothelial growth factor (VEGF) and CKIT in cutaneous melanocytic lesions. Int J Surg Pathol 2004; 12: 133-138.

[83] Curtin JA, Busam K, Pinkel D, Bastian BC. Somatic activation of KIT in distinct subtypes of melanoma. J. Clin. Oncol. 2006; 24: 4340-43

[84] Beadling C, Jacobson-Dunlop E, Hodi FS, Le C, Warrick A, Patterson J, Town A, Harlow A, Cruz F 3rd, Azar S, Rubin BP, Muller S, West R, Heinrich MC, Corless CL. Kit gene mutations and copy numbering melanoma subtypes .Clin Cancer Res 2008; 14: 6821-6828

[85] Riviera RS, Nagatsuka H, Gunduz M, Cengiz B, Gunduz E, Siar CH, Tsujigiwa H, Tamamura R, Han K N, Nagai N. C-kit protein expression correlated with activating mutations in KIT gene in oral mucosal melanoma.Virchows Arch. 2008; 452: 27-32

[86] Postow MA, Harding J, Wolchok JD. Targeting immune checkpoints: releasing the restraints on anti-tumor immunity for patients with melanoma. Cancer J. 2012; 18:153-9

[87] Melero J, Hervas-Strubbs S, Glennie M et al. Immunostimulatory monoclonal antibodies for cancer therapy. Nat Rev Cancer 2007; 7:95-106

[88] Ascierto PA, Marincola FM, Ribas A. Anti-CTLA4 monoclonal antibodies: the past and the future in clinical application. J Transl Med. 2011 Nov 13;9:196

[89] Ozao-Choy J, Ma G, Kao J, Wang GX, Meseck M, Sung M, Schwartz M, Divino CM, Pan PY, Chen SH. The novel role of tyrosine kinase inhibitor in the reversal of immune suppression and modulation of tumor microenvironment for immune-based cancer therapies. Cancer Res. 2009 Mar 15;69(6):2514-22

[90] Lee KM, Chuang E, Griffin M, et al. Molecular basis of T cell inactivation by CTLA-4. Science. 1998; 282: 2263–2266

[91] Hodi FS, O'Day SJ, McDermott DF, Weber RW, Sosman JA, Haanen JB, Gonzalez R, Robert C, Schadendorf D, Hassel JC, Akerley W, van den Eertwegh AJ, Lutzky J, Lorigan P, Vaubel JM, Linette GP, Hogg D, Ottensmeier CH, Lebbé C, Peschel C, Quirt I, Clark JI, Wolchok JD, Weber JS, Tian J, Yellin MJ, Nichol GM, Hoos A, Urba WJ. Improved survival with ipilimumab in patients with metastatic melanoma. N Engl J Med. 2010; 363:711-23

[92] Robert C, Thomas L, Bondarenko I, O'Day S, M D JW, Garbe C, Lebbe C, Baurain JF, Testori A, Grob JJ, Davidson N, Richards J, Maio M, Hauschild A, Miller WH Jr, Gascon P, Lotem M, Harmankaya K, Ibrahim R, Francis S, Chen TT, Humphrey R, Hoos A, Wolchok JD. Ipilimumab plus dacarbazine for previously untreated metastatic melanoma. N Engl J Med. 2011; 364:2517-26

[93] Miller AJ, Mihm MC. Melanoma. N Engl J Med 2006; 355: 51-65

[94] Zabierowski SE, Herlyn M. Melanoma stem cells: the dark seed of melanoma. J Clin Oncol. 2008; 26: 2890-4

[95] Eisen T, Ahmad T, Flaherty KT, Gore M, Kaye S, Marais R, Gibbens I, Hackett S, James M, Schuchter LM, Nathanson KL, Xia C, Simantov R, Schwartz B, Poulin-Costello M, O'Dwyer PJ, Ratain MJ. Sorafenib in advanced melanoma: a phase II randomised discontinuation trial analysis. Br J Cancer 2006; 95: 581-86

[96] Flaherty KT, Puzanov I, Kim KB, Ribas A, McArthur GA, Sosman JA, O'Dwyer PJ, Lee RJ, Grippo JF, Nolop K, Chapman PB. Inhibition of mutated, activated BRAF in metastatic melanoma. N Engl J Med 2010; 363, 809-19

[97] Chapman PB, Hauschild A, Robert C, Haanen JB, Ascierto P, Larkin J, Dummer R, Garbe C, Testori A, Maio M, Hogg D, Lorigan P, Lebbe C, Jouary T, Schadendorf D, Ribas A, O'Day SJ, Sosman JA, Kirkwood JM, Eggermont AM, Dreno B, Nolop K, Li J, Nelson B, Hou J, Lee RJ, Flaherty KT, McArthur GA; BRIM-3 Study Group. Im-

proved survival with vemurafenib in melanoma with BRAF V600E mutation. N Engl J Med. 2011; 364:2507-16.

[98] Falchook GS, Long GV, Kurzrock R, Kim KB, Arkenau TH, Brown MP, Hamid O, Infante JR, Millward M, Pavlick AC, O'Day SJ, Blackman SC, Curtis CM, Lebowitz P, Ma B, Ouellet D, Kefford RF. Dabrafenib in patients with melanoma, untreated brain metastases, and other solid tumours: a phase 1 dose-escalation trial. Lancet. 2012; 379:1893-901

[99] Nazarian R, Shi H, Wang Q, Kong X, Koya RC, Lee H, Chen Z, Lee MK, Attar N, Sazegar H, Chodon T, Nelson SF, McArthur G, Sosman JA, Ribas A, Lo RS. Melanomas acquire resistance to B-RAF(V600E) inhibition by RTK or N-RAS upregulation. Nature 2010; 468: 973-77

[100] Smalley KS, Sondak VK. Melanoma--an unlikely poster child for personalized cancer therapy. N Engl J Med. 2010; 363:876-8

[101] Wagle N, Emery C, Berger MF, Davis MJ, Sawyer A, Pochanard P, Kehoe SM, Johannessen CM, Macconaill LE, Hahn WC, Meyerson M, Garraway LA. Dissecting therapeutic resistance to RAF inhibition in melanoma by tumor genomic profiling. J Clin Oncol. 2011; 29: 3085-96.

[102] Johannessen CM, Boehm JS, Kim SY, Thomas SR, Wardwell L, Johnson LA, Emery CM, Stransky N, Cogdill AP, Barretina J, Caponigro G, Hieronymus H, Murray RR, Salehi-Ashtiani K, Hill DE, Vidal M, Zhao JJ, Yang X, Alkan O, Kim S, Harris JL, Wilson CJ, Myer VE, Finan PM, Root DE, Roberts TM, Golub T, Flaherty KT, Dummer R, Weber BL, Sellers WR, Schlegel R, Wargo JA, Hahn WC, Garraway LA. COT drives resistance to RAF inhibition through MAP kinase pathway reactivation. Nature 2010; 468, 968-72

[103] Villanueva J, Vultur A, Lee JT, Somasundaram R, Fukunaga-Kalabis M, Cipolla AK, Wubbenhorst B, Xu X, Gimotty PA, Kee D, Santiago-Walker AE, Letrero R, D'Andrea K, Pushparajan A, Hayden JE, Brown KD, Laquerre S, McArthur GA, Sosman JA, Nathanson KL, Herlyn M. Acquired resistance to BRAF inhibitors mediated by a RAF kinase switch in melanoma can be overcome by cotargeting MEK and IGF-1R/PI3K. Cancer Cell 2010; 18, 683-95

[104] Bedikian AY, Millward M, Pehamberger H, Conry R, Gore M, Trefzer U, Pavlick AC, DeConti R, Hersh EM, Hersey P, Kirkwood JM, Haluska FG; Oblimersen Melanoma Study Group. Bcl-2 antisense (oblimersen sodium) plus dacarbazine in patients with advanced melanoma: the Oblimersen Melanoma Study Group. J Clin Oncol. 2006; 24:4738-45

[105] Yokoyama S, Feige E, Poling LL, Levy C, Widlund HR, Khaled M, Kung AL, Fisher DE. Pharmacologic suppression of MITF expression via HDAC inhibitors in the melanocyte lineage. Pigment Cell Melanoma Res. 2008; 21:457-63

[106] Adams J. The proteasome: a suitable antineoplastic target. Nat Rev Cancer 2004;4:349–60

[107] Amiri KI, Horton LW, LaFleur BJ, Sosman JA, Richmond A. Augmenting chemosensitivity of malignant melanoma tumors via proteasome inhibition: Implication for bortezomib (VELCADE, PS-341) as a therapeutic agent for malignant melanoma. Cancer Res 2004;64:4912–4918

[108] Su Y, Amiri KI, Horton LW, Yu Y, Ayers GD, Koehler E, Kelley MC, Puzanov I, Richmond A, Sosman JA. A phase I trial of bortezomib with temozolomide in patients with advanced melanoma: toxicities, antitumor effects, and modulation of therapeutic targets. Clin Cancer Res 2010;16:348-57

[109] Croghan GA, Suman VJ, Maples WJ, Albertini M, Linette G, Flaherty L, Eckardt J, Ma C, Markovic SN, Erlichman C. A Study of Paclitaxel, Carboplatin, and Bortezomib in the Treatment of Metastatic Malignant Melanoma. Cancer 2010;116:3463-8

[110] López-Guerra M, Roué G, Pérez-Galán P, Alonso R, Villamor N, Montserrat E, Campo E, Colomer D. p65 activity and ZAP-70 status predict the sensitivity of chronic lymphocytic leukemia cells to the selective IkappaB kinase inhibitor BMS-345541. Clin Cancer Res. 2009; 15:2767-76

[111] Liu J, Suresh Kumar KG, Yu D, Molton SA, McMahon M, Herlyn M, Thomas-Tikhonenko A, Fuchs SY. Oncogenic BRAF regulates β-Trcp expression and NF-kB activity in human melanoma cells. Oncogene 2007; 26:1954–1958

[112] Niessner H, Beck D, Sinnberg T, Lasithiotakis K, Maczey E, Gogel J, Venturelli S, Berger A, Mauthe M, Toulany M, Flaherty K, Schaller M, Schadendorf D, Proikas-Cezanne T, Schittek B, Garbe C, Kulms D, Meier F. The farnesyl transferase inhibitor lonafarnib inhibits mTOR signaling and enforces sorafenib-induced apoptosis in melanoma cells. J Invest Dermatol. 2011; 131:468-79

[113] Hong DS, Sebti SM, Newman RA, Blaskovich MA, Ye L, Gagel RF, Moulder S, Wheler JJ, Naing A, Tannir NM, Ng CS, Sherman SI, El Naggar AK, Khan R, Trent J, Wright JJ, Kurzrock R. Phase I trial of a combination of the multikinase inhibitor sorafenib and the farnesyltransferase inhibitor tipifarnib in advanced malignancies. Clin Cancer Res. 2009; 15:7061-8

[114] Konstantinopoulos PA, Karamouzis MV, Papavassiliou AG. Post-translational modifications and regulation of the RAS superfamily of GTPases as anticancer targets. Nat Rev Drug Discov. 2007; 6:541-55

[115] Tran A, Tawbi HA. A potential role for nilotinib in KIT-mutated melanoma. Expert Opin Investig Drugs. 2012; 21:861-9

[116] Serrels A, Macpherson IR, Evans TR, Lee FY, Clark EA, Sansom OJ, Ashton GH, Frame MC, Brunton VG. Identification of potential biomarkers for measuring inhibition of Src kinase activity in colon cancer cells following treatment with dasatinib. Mol Cancer Ther. 2006; 5: 3014–3022

[117] Gnoni A, Marech I, Silvestris N, Vacca A, Lorusso V. Dasatinib: an anti-tumour agent via Src inhibition. Curr Drug Targets. 2011; 12:563-78

[118] Courtney KD, Corcoran RB, Engelman JA. The PI3K pathway as drug target in human cancer.J Clin Oncol. 2010; 28:1075-83

[119] Abraham RT, Eng CH. Mammalian target of rapamycin as a therapeutic target in oncology.Expert Opin Ther Targets. 2008; 12:209-22

[120] Cloughesy TF, Yoshimoto K, Nghiemphu P, Brown K, Dang J, Zhu S, Hsueh T, Chen Y, Wang W, Youngkin D, Liau L, Martin N, Becker D, Bergsneider M, Lai A, Green R, Oglesby T, Koleto M, Trent J, Horvath S, Mischel PS, Mellinghoff IK, Sawyers CL. Antitumor activity of rapamycin in a Phase I trial for patients with recurrent PTEN-deficient glioblastoma. PLoS Med. 2008; 5:e8

[121] Margolin KA, Moon J, Flaherty LE, Lao CD, Akerley WL 3rd, Othus M, Sosman JA, Kirkwood JM, Sondak VK. Randomized phase II trial of sorafenib with temsirolimus or tipifarnib in untreated metastatic melanoma (S0438). Clin Cancer Res. 2012; 18:1129-37

[122] Van Raamsdonk CD, Griewank KG, Crosby MB, Garrido MC, Vemula S, Wiesner T, Obenauf AC, Wackernagel W, Green G, Bouvier N, Sozen MM, Baimukanova G, Roy R, Heguy A, Dolgalev I, Khanin R, Busam K, Speicher MR, O'Brien J, Bastian BC. Mutations in GNA11 in uveal melanoma. N Engl J Med. 2010; 363:2191-9

[123] Khalili JS, Yu X, Wang J, Hayes BC, Davies MA, Lizee G, Esmaeli B, Woodman SE. Combination Small Molecule MEK and PI3K Inhibition Enhances Uveal Melanoma Cell Death in a Mutant GNAQ- and GNA11-Dependent Manner. Clin Cancer Res. 2012 Jul 19

[124] Gould Rothberg BE, Bracken MB, Rimm DL. Tissue biomarkers for prognosis in cutaneous melanoma: a systematic review and meta-analysis. J Natl Cancer Inst. 2009; 101:452-74

[125] Gould Rothberg BE, Berger AJ, Molinaro AM, Subtil A, Krauthammer MO, Camp RL, Bradley WR, Ariyan S, Kluger HM, Rimm DL. Melanoma prognostic model using tissue microarrays and genetic algorithms. J Clin Oncol. 2009; 27:5772-80

[126] Cheung M, Sharma A, Madhunapantula SV, Robertson GP. Akt3 and mutant V600E B-Raf cooperate to promote early melanoma development. Cancer Res. 2008; 68, 3429–3439

[127] Tran MA, Gowda R, Sharma A, Park EJ, Adair J, Kester M, Smith NB, Robertson GP. Targeting V600EB-Raf and Akt3 using nanoliposomal small interfering RNA inhibits cutaneous melanocytic lesion development. Cancer Res. 2008; 68, 7638–7649

[128] Lasithiotakis KG, Sinnberg TW, Schittek B, Flaherty KT, Kulms D, Maczey E, Garbe C, Meier FE. Combined inhibition of MAPK and mTOR signaling inhibits growth, induces cell death, and abrogates invasive growth of melanoma cells. J Invest Dermatol. 2008;128:2013-23

[129] Davies MA, Fox PS, Papadopoulos NE, Bedikian AY, Hwu WJ, Lazar AJ, Prieto VG, Culotta KS, Madden TL, Xu Q, Huang S, Deng W, Ng CS, Gupta S, Liu W, Dancey

JE, Wright JJ, Bassett RL, Hwu P, Kim KB. Phase I study of the combination of sorafenib and temsirolimus in patients with metastatic melanoma. Clin Cancer Res. 2012;18:1120-8

[130] Paraiso KH, Fedorenko IV, Cantini LP, Munko AC, Hall M, Sondak VK, Messina JL, Flaherty KT, Smalley KS. Recovery of phospho-ERK activity allows melanoma cells to escape from BRAF inhibitor therapy. Br J Cancer. 2010; 102:1724-30

[131] Heidorn SJ, Milagre C, Whittaker S, Nourry A, Niculescu-Duvas I, Dhomen N, Hussain J, Reis-Filho JS, Springer CJ, Pritchard C, Marais R. Kinase-dead BRAF and oncogenic RAS cooperate to drive tumor progression through CRAF. Cell 2010;140:209-21

[132] Poulikakos PI, Zhang C, Bollag G, Shokat KM, Rosen N. RAF inhibitors transactivate RAF dimers and ERK signalling in cells with wild-type BRAF. Nature. 2010; 464:427-30

[133] Poulikakos PI, Persaud Y, Janakiraman M, Kong X, Ng C, Moriceau G, Shi H, Atefi M, Titz B, Gabay MT, Salton M, Dahlman KB, Tadi M, Wargo JA, Flaherty KT, Kelley MC, Misteli T, Chapman PB, Sosman JA, Graeber TG, Ribas A, Lo RS, Rosen N, Solit DB. RAF inhibitor resistance is mediated by dimerization of aberrantly spliced BRAF(V600E). Nature 2011; 480: 387-90

[134] Hatzivassiliou G, Song K, Yen I, Brandhuber BJ, Anderson DJ, Alvarado R, Ludlam MJ, Stokoe D, Gloor SL, Vigers G, Morales T, Aliagas I, Liu B, Sideris S, Hoeflich KP, Jaiswal BS, Seshagiri S, Koeppen H, Belvin M, Friedman LS, Malek S. RAF inhibitors prime wild-type RAF to activate the MAPK pathway and enhance growth. Nature 2010;464:431-5

[135] Arkenau H-T, Kefford R, Long GV. Targeting BRAF for patients with melanoma. Br J Cancer 2011; 104: 392-398

Chapter 3

Melanoma Genetics: From Susceptibility to Progression

Guilherme Francisco, Priscila Daniele Ramos Cirilo,
Fernanda Toledo Gonçalves,
Tharcísio Citrângulo Tortelli Junior and
Roger Chammas

Additional information is available at the end of the chapter

1. Introduction

Melanoma genetics has been for a long time a great challenge to cancer biologists, in part due to a complete lack of a single candidate gene to melanoma development. Different from breast and colorectal cancers, where BRCA-1/2 and *APC*/mismatch repair genes, respectively, characterize familial clusters of cancer susceptibility (reaching penetrance rates as high as 90% in some cases), in melanomas, the mutation rate of the most commonly altered genes associated with disease progression do not exceed 60% of the cases in familial clusters. Among the "classical melanoma genes" are those coded at the *CDKN2A locus* (coding for p14 and p16, both related to cell cycle arrest), BRAF (specially the V600E mutation), a downstream transducer of the RAS signaling pathway and critical for the cellular response to growth signals, and mutations in NRAS, somewhat related to initiation and progression of melanoma.

However, alterations in those genes, either by mutations or by epigenetic alterations do not account for all melanoma cases. Moreover, the mutations found in the classical melanoma genes are not typical UV signature mutations (such as C to T transitions). This observation poses an interesting problem in melanoma biology. Extensive epidemiological data indicates that intermittent exposure to UV radiation, mainly UVB is a major etiologic factor for melanoma development. On the other hand, genes commonly mutated in melanomas lack UV signature mutations. Thus, evidence so far for the presence of UVB-generated signature mutations in melanoma that could be defined as driver mutations has been less than compelling. Two critical questions need therefore to be answered; (1) If the classical melanoma genes do not account for the majority of cases, what other genes are involved in melanomagenesis? And, (2) what is the real relationship between the mutagenic potential of UV radiation and melanoma genetics?

In the following pages, we will discuss the new findings about the biology of this neoplasia, besides discussing the known genes involved in melanomagenesis. A systematic review of to date GWAS data, deep-sequencing data and functional genomics will serve as the background for this discussion. As examples, GWAS studies have identified genetic variations in genes related to pigmentation that confer susceptibility to melanomas. The importance of these studies resides in the identification of new variants that can represent low penetrance susceptibility genes. Other classes of genes that have emerged as critical genes to melanoma are DNA repair genes, especially NER genes (Nucleotide Excision Repair – a pathway that repair typical UV DNA damages). New studies have identified polymorphisms in those genes that confer higher risk to melanoma development. This susceptibility, in an interesting manner, seems to be influenced by the UV index of a certain region. On the other hand, microarray studies have suggested that DNA repair genes may be critical to metastasis sucess of melanomas, through stabilization of a "metastatic genome". Deep-sequencing studies of melanoma cells have also identified genes and patterns of mutational status that correlate with UV signatures, bringing new clues to melanoma genetics. Are these driver or passenger mutations? The importance of other genes and pathways is also highlighted. One good example of a gene involved with melanoma progression is the *Microphthalmia*-associated *transcription factor* (*MITF*). *MITF* has been found to be expressed in several melanomas and its function is related to a diversity of cell processes, contributing to melanoma progression. The importance of *TP53* gene and its pathways in melanocyte/melanoma biology is also discussed. The *TP53* gene has intrigued biologists for a long time, since its mutational frequency is very low in melanomas, differently from other skin cancers, which harbor a high frequency of p53 mutations, which in turn are UV-type mutations. Functional data indicate however that the p53 pathway is dysfunctional in melanomas. What are the bases for this malfunction in this critical pathway for genome stability?

Thus, in this chapter we discuss both the "old" and the "new" genetics of melanoma susceptibility and progression. A discussion that will allow for the readers a systematic overview of what is known about the classical melanoma genetics, at the same time that may provide the basis to explore the new concepts that are emerging in this field.

2. UV exposure, deep-sequencing and melanomas – Understanding the melanoma development in depth

Skin constitutes the first defense barrier in protection of internal environment and it is therefore subjected to several aggressions by pathogenic microorganisms or by chemical or physical damaging agents. Among these several agents, sunlight ultraviolet radiation (UV) is considered the most potent carcinogenic factor for skin cancers, although the precise relationship between dose, time and nature of sunlight exposure to skin cancer development remains controversial [1]. Ultraviolet radiation can be classified according to its wavelength in UVA

(320-400 nm), UVB (280-320 nm) and UVC (200-280 nm). Despite the fact that UVA is more abundant in sunlight (90 %), UVB is about 1000-fold more efficient to cause sunburns and DNA damage than UVA [2]. Skin exposure to UV light affects epidermal and dermal cell survival and proliferation, besides other cutaneous functions [3]. Acute effects of UV exposure are usually the most harmful, including DNA damage, apoptosis, erythema, immunosuppression, all factors contributing to aging and skin cancer [4].

One of the main effects of UV exposure on cancer development is direct damages to DNA. Photoreactions due to absorption of UV (mainly UVB) by DNA lead to the establishment of covalent linkages of adjacent pyrimidine bases (cytosine or thymine) thus forming cyclobutane pyrimidine dimers (CPD) and 6-4 photoproducts. CPDs are constituted by the ligation of C-4 and C-5 carbons in both pyrimidines, whereas 6-4 photoproducts are produced between C-6 and C-4 carbons of two adjacent pyrimidines, more frequently between TC and CC residues. CPDs are also considered more carcinogenic than 6-4 photoproducts, the frequency of CPD formation is three times higher and are less efficiently repaired [5]. If not repaired, both photoproducts lead to genetic mutations such as C→T and CC→TT transitions, besides single and double strand breaks on DNA [6]. Other genotoxic agents associated with excessive exposure to UV are reactive oxygen species (ROS), characterizing an indirect effect of radiation [7]. ROS can promote deanimation and adduct formation, leading to errors in base pairing and, thus, mutations and chromosomal reorganization, contributing to carcinogenic process.

Epidemiologic studies have indicated that a pattern of intense and intermittent exposure to sunlight is a major risk factor for developing melanoma [8]. History of skin sunburns have been frequently used as measure to intermittent exposure and can be a marker for high risk of melanoma development. One or more severe sunburns on younger ages increase the risk of melanoma [9-11]. Besides the clear risk attributed to sunlight and thus UV exposure in melanomagenesis, the lack of a typical signature of UV mutation in genes classically related to melanoma development and progression had intrigued researchers for years. First, *CDKN2A* and *CDK4* genes had inheritable mutations and thus not showed typical UV mutations. Even somatic alterations in *CDKN2A* show very low levels of UV mutations and the majority of *CDKN2A* alterations in melanomas are epigenetic silencing and homozygous deletions [12]. Regarding *NRAS*, another "old gene" involved with melanoma progression, the most commonly described mutation lies in codon 61 and does not correspond to typical UV mutations (CAA(Gln) to AAA(Lys) or CAA(Gln) to CGA(Arg)) and can be found in about 10% of somatic melanomas [13]. Regarding *BRAF* mutation, the most prevalent V600E (found in about 40% of melanomas – [14]), shows a transversion of thymine substituted by adenine. Finally, regarding the *PTEN* gene, increased allelic loss can be detected ranging to 40 to 60% of melanoma cases; less than 10% of melanoma samples show mutations in *PTEN*, the extensive majority consisting of frameshift mutations [15]. All those cited reports are the opposite to the high frequency of typical UV mutations in critical genes related to the other two skin cancers, namely basal cell carcinomas and squamous cell carcinomas, such as *TP53* [16].

In a seminal study, a comparison of four distinct sets of melanomas at the genomic level gave important clues about the role of UV in melanomagenesis [17]. The authors compared the number of copies of DNA and the mutational status of two critical genes to melanoma development, *BRAF* and *NRAS* in a panel consisting of 126 melanomas from four groups differing among them according the degree of exposure to ultraviolet light: 30 melanomas from skin with chronic sun-induced damage; 40 melanomas from skin without such damage; 36 melanomas from palms, soles, and subungual (acral) sites; and 20 mucosal melanomas. The results indicated that melanomas from sun-protected areas (acral and mucosal) had more frequent chromosomal aberrations including amplifications and losses compared to sun-exposed melanomas. Frequent amplification was identified in *CCND1* gene (cyclin D1 gene) and *CDK4* gene (more frequent in acral and mucosal melanomas). Moreover, deletions of the *CDKN2A* locus in were found in 50 percent of all melanomas, making it the most commonly lost genomic region, being also more frequent in acral and mucosal melanomas). Mutations in *BRAF* gene were significantly more common in the group of melanomas that were on skin without chronic sun-induced damage than in the other three groups. Therefore, there are distinct patterns of genetic alterations in the four groups of primary melanomas. The differences in both chromosomal aberrations and the frequency of mutations of specific genes suggest that these tumors develop through different mechanistic routes, and likely respond to different selective influences.

The unanswered question about the real impact of UV light on melanoma genetics began to be solved with the development of new technologies in DNA sequencing, the so called "deep-sequencing method". With this technology, the researchers could perform large-scale sequencing, covering the whole genome. In one of the first studies using deep-sequencing methods, the authors reported more than 1000 mutations using 210 diverse human cancers, including melanomas [18]. This study covered 274 megabases (Mb) and was restricted to 518 protein kinase genes. The results showed that melanomas (in that case, melanoma cell lines), had a high prevalence of mutations showing a mean number of 18.54 mutations per Mb of DNA. The main result from this first study was that of 144 mutations in melanomas, more than 90% was C to T mutations, the typical transition of UV-related mutations. Most somatic mutations found were classified as "passengers" mutations, i.e. those which do not contribute directly to carcinogenesis. "Driver" mutations, those mutations that contribute to carcinogenesis, were found in approximately 120 genes.

A second study, in this time a comprehensive catalogue of the whole genome of a melanoma cell line and a lymphoblastoid cell line from the same person, provided the first catalogue of somatic mutations from an individual cancer [19]. The numbers generated by the deep-sequencing are impressive. The study identified 33345 somatic mutations, where 32325 were single base mutations and 510 were double-base mutations. A total of 292 somatic base substitutions were in protein-coding sequences and of these, 187 were non-synonymous mutations leading to amino acid changes, including 172 missense mutations and 15 nonsense. Several individual substitutions highlighted novel candidate cancer genes such as mutations in *SPDEF* gene, which codes to an ETS transcription factor family, described as associated with some cancers types [20]. Moreover, mutations in *MMP28* gene (a member of matrix metalloproteinases) and in *UVRAG* (a putative tumor suppressor gene – [21]) were found. In addition, a 12-kilobase internal homozygous deletion was found in PTEN gene.

Of the total number of mutations found (33345), almost 25000 were C to T mutations, and of the 510 dinucleotide substitutions, 360 were CC to TT changes [19]. The mutational spectrum observed is consistent with UV-associated mutations, fact that denotes the influence of UV on melanoma development. C to T and CC to TT changes were significantly more frequent in CpG dinucleotides than the expected by chance. The mutational pattern also indicated a strong relation of UV mutations with the nucleotide excision DNA repair pathway (NER) due to the high frequency of mutations in non-transcribed strands when compared to mutational frequency in transcribed strands. The transcription-coupled repair (a sub-pathway of NER system), which operates in transcribed strands, is credited to be more efficiently in repair UV lesions when compared to NER system that operates in non-transcribed strands. Finally, besides the majority of C to T mutations, the second commonest mutation frequency was substitution of G to T. High production of ROS can lead to oxidized guanines and in turn causes G to T changes. As UV exposure can also lead to ROS production, is tempting to suggest that besides the direct DNA damage caused by UV, contributing to C to T changes, indirect effects such as ROS production also may contribute to melanoma carcinogenesis. Thus, this first entire catalogue of mutations in melanoma by whole genome sequencing supports the notion that UV exposure plays a critical role in melanoma development.

A third whole genome sequencing study also confirmed the elevated mutational rate in melanomas, that in mean was about 30 mutations per Mb, and the C to T mutations were the most frequent, once again reinforcing the role of UV irradiation in melanomas [22]. However, the great advantage of the study was using metastatic melanoma samples and also including melanomas from different body areas. Thus, the authors could present an interesting panel of mutational rate across the different melanoma subtypes. As example, acral melanomas showed mutational rates comparable to other solid tumor types (3 mutations per Mb), whereas melanomas from the trunk showed higher mutational rates. The sequencing of a melanoma from an individual with history of chronic sun exposure exhibited the higher mutational rate across the samples analyzed (111 somatic mutations per Mb). Moreover, that melanoma with the higher mutational rate showed 93% of C to T substitutions, while acral melanomas showed only 36% of such mutations. These data strongly support the contribution of sun exposure in melanoma etiology. From the most significantly genes, the authors identified frequent mutations in *PREX2* gene, mutated in 11 of the 25 melanomas samples. PREX2 is involved with PTEN pathway modulating its function [23]. Functional analysis by expressing the mutant forms of PREX2 in melanocytes injected in immunodeficient significantly accelerated *in vivo* tumorigenesis, suggesting that PREX2 mutations contribute to melanoma progression. Whole genome sequence of acral melanomas also identified low frequency of mutations (2.16 per Mb in the primary tumor and 1.95 per Mb in metastasis sample) [24].

Additional studies from exome sequencing have identified new genes related to melanoma development and also chemoresistance. From exome sequencing study performed in seven melanomas the authors found a total of 4933 somatic mutations, 3611 of which were located in protein-coding regions in 2586 genes [25]. Confirming previous results, C to T transitions were the most representative mutations (ranging from 73 to 87% of all mutations). In order to get a more comprehensive view of melanoma genome, the authors looked to genes involved with MAPK pathway, which includes NRAS and BRAF. Two of seven melanomas analyzed showed a somatic G to A transition at homologous site in the *MAP2K1* and *MAP2K2* genes, kinases that are downstream targets of BRAF. In an independent set of 127 melanomas, 8% confirmed the existence of damaging mutations in either gene. Following functional studies with either gene demonstrated a constitutive activation and resulted in ERK1/2 phosphorylation and the oncogenic activity of such mutations was also evaluated in transformation assays. Moreover, in four of the seven melanomas, mutations were found in *FAT4*, *DSC1* and *LRP1B* genes, which might be candidate genes, as suggested by the authors [25].

In an independent study [26], other melanoma exome sequencing also identified mutations in genes participating of MAPK pathway, more precisely *MAP3K5* and *MAP3K9*. Validation of such data indicated mutations in *MAP3K5* in 8 of 85 melanoma cell lines and mutation in 13 of 85 cell lines to *MAP3K9*. Functional analysis of such mutations indicated a significantly reduction in kinase activity of both proteins. Moreover, such mutations in both genes resulted in decreased levels of phosphorylated MEK-ERK and JNK, pathways involved with apoptosis, differentiation, survival and senescence. Interestingly, decreased expression of MAP3K5 and MAP3K9 by siRNA method led to chemoresistance to temozolomide [26]. A third exome sequencing study, using a large sample size (147 melanomas from sun-exposed areas), identified a recurrent UV-signature in *RAC1* gene in 9.2% of cases. Biochemical and functional analysis of mutated RAC1 showed that such alteration promotes melanocyte proliferation and migration [27].

All of these genome sequence studies identified a great number of mutations, however most mutations are passenger mutations. In order to differentiate passenger from driver mutations, Linda Chin coordinated an effort to sequence exons and introns of melanoma samples, comparing their frequency in order to identify positively selected genes, based on enrichment of mutations in exons [28]. The authors identified positive selection in melanoma genes including well-know genes such as *BRAF, NRAS, PTEN, TP53, p16* and also indentify new candidate genes, such as *PPP6C, RAC1* (previously described in [26]), *SNX31, TACC1* and *STK19*. Noteworthy, to *PPP6C* (a subunit of PP6C protein phosphatase), a candidate to tumor suppressor gene, showed 60% of mutations clustered within a 12 amino acid region flanking an arginine at codon 264. Regarding *RAC1*, the mutant forms also indicated gain-of-function. The study also indicated the role of UV in the advent of melanoma driver mutations. Of 262 driver mutations found in 21 genes identified by the study, 46% were caused by C to T mutations (37%) or G to T (9%), alterations characteristics of UVB/UVA-induced mutations. These numbers increased to 67% by excluding mutations in *BRAF* or *NRAS* genes.

Innovative strategies exploiting deep sequencing will contribute to the understanding of the diversity of pathways involved with melanoma. We anticipate that studies of melanomas arising in different ethnic groups, and mainly from individuals who migrated from low-UV index regions to high-UV index regions in the globe will help us understanding more about the genes involved in melanomagenesis.

3. Melanoma genetics: Susceptibility genes

When we talk about susceptibility genes to diseases, especially to cancer, we are talking about inheritable genetic alterations. Such alterations in critical genes related to tumor suppression contribute to modulate the susceptibility to certain tumors. Inheritable alterations can be classified as mutations or polymorphisms (also known as single nucleotide polymorphism – SNP). Both genetic alterations have different features such as: (i) related to population allelic frequency (mutations < 1% and polymorphisms > 1%); (ii) related to its impact to gene functionality, where mutations cause deleterious alterations to the function while polymorphisms may modify the function, however not in a deleterious manner; (iii) related to penetrance, where mutations exerts its deleterious function in a high penetrance to development of the disease. Conversely, polymorphisms exert its function in a low penetrance to disease and may be more susceptible to environmental influence; (iv) age of tumor onset, where high penetrance mutated genes contribute to disease development in younger ages while polymorphisms are related to older ages to cancer development. Temporally, high susceptibility genes to melanoma were well established through the years, however low susceptibility genes have been identified recently. Appreciation of high penetrance genes came from multiple studies of melanoma-predisposed families studies; in which linkage analysis, cytogenetic and candidate gene studies helped to identify those genes. However, the high-penetrance genes account for 5 to 10% melanoma cases, indicating that other genes, including low penetrance genes may modulate the susceptibility. The development of new technologies has contributed to identify new susceptible genes and understand their roles to melanoma. In this section we discuss the "old" and the "new" genetics for melanoma susceptibility.

3.1. High penetrance genes: "The old genetics" for melanoma

3.1.1. CDKN2A – The classical susceptibility gene

The best-established gene for melanoma susceptibility is the *CDKN2A* (cyclin-dependent kinase inhibitor 2A gene) locus, which is located in chromosome 9p21. Involvement of a 9p locus in melanomas was first indicated by cytogenetically detectable loss or translocation of this region. Subsequent loss of heterozigosity (LOH) studies and later studies indicated the existence of a tumor suppressor gene in this region. Germline mutations in this locus have been described among melanoma-predisposed families since 1995, and approximately 40% of familial melanomas cases harbor *CDKN2A* mutations [29]. The *CDKN2A* locus encodes for two different proteins, which are related to cell cycle control and tumor suppression. The two proteins are produced by alternative reading frame of four exons [30]. The proteins produced by *CDKN2A* locus, p16/Ink4a and p14/Arf, are involved with regulation of cell cycle from G1 to S phase, besides the ability of p14/Arf to induce apoptosis [30]. Regarding p16/Ink4a, its main function is to bind to CDK4 and to inhibit its kinase activity. By inhibiting CDK4 activity, p16/Ink4a avoids the phosphorylation of retinoblastoma (*Rb*) tumor suppressor gene, acting therefore as a negative regulator of E2F function. Thus, loss-of-function mutations or loss of p16/Ink4a expression, allow for CDK4 to phosphorylate Rb, thereby releasing E2F activity in the transition of G1 to S phase.

The role of p14/Arf in tumor suppression is related to regulation of p53 pathway. Its function is related to binding to HDM-2 protein and inhibition of its activity. The MDM-2 protein is a key regulator of p53 protein due to its ability to ubiquitinate p53, leading to p53 degradation. Thus, by p14/Arf function, MDM-2 is depleted and p53 is stabilized. Inactivation of p14/Arf functions is associated with MDM-2 accumulation, which in turn leads to p53 degradation and consequently loss of its tumor suppressor function. In summary, loss-of-function alterations in *CDKN2A* simultaneously impair two of the most critical pathways in tumor suppression, the Rb and p53 pathways. Most germline mutations in *CDKN2A* locus are missense mutations, usually found in exons 1α and exon 2, although mutations in 5′ UTR and intron regions are also found, affecting thus translation initiation and splicing events [31]. Overall, *CDKN2A* mutations have been found in 20 – 40% of families with 3 or more affected members and in 10% of families with 2 melanoma cases. However the frequency can vary according to different populations, fact that can be explained by different founder mutations in some of those populations. The low mutation detection rate has suggested that other susceptibility genes exist in melanomas. Moreover, the penetrance of mutations in *CDKN2A* shows geographical variations [32].

Some studies have suggested that the penetrance of the *CDKN2A* mutations may be modulated by other genetic risk modifiers. Certain MC1R variants (discussed below) increase melanoma risk in familial melanomas harboring mutations in *CDKN2A* [33]. As MC1R, a gene strongly related to skin color, plays a role as a modifier gene, it seems logical that other pigmentation genes might similarly act as genetic modifiers to *CDKN2A* penetrance. Environmental factors, such as relative exposure to UV radiation may contribute to the variability in penetrance of *CDKN2A* mutations according to geographical reasons, as suggested by previous studies [32].

3.1.2. CDK4 – The second line in melanoma susceptibility

Another well known gene associated with melanoma susceptibility is the *CDK4* gene. The gene is located in chromosome 12q13 and codes for cyclin-dependent kinase. Mutations in the *CDK4* gene were just described in 15 families with melanoma predisposition [34], where just two known mutations are described and located in codon, Arg24Cys e Arg24His. Curiously, these mutations can be also found in sporadic melanomas. Although less frequent than the inheritable mutations in *CDKN2A* locus, patients harboring mutations in *CDK4* usually show the same clinical characteristics as patients with mutations in *CDKN2A* such as mean age at diagnostics, mean number of melanomas and mean number of nevi [35]. These clinical similarities (phenocopies) shown by mutations in different genes may be explained by the same pathway that *CDK4* and p16 protein share together the Rb (retinoblastoma) tumor suppressor pathway. Both CDK4 mutant variants described above are unable to bind p16, and therefore CDK4 activity is not inhibited. The functional consequence is then phosphorylation of Rb, leading to Rb inactivity and thus allowing the cell to progress on cell cycle. Only in a few reports the whole *CDK4* gene was sequenced. Expansion of *CDK4* sequencing, including the whole gene, instead of only codon 2, might help to identify new mutations in non-9p-linked melanoma families.

3.1.3. *Evidence of new susceptibility locus and other critical genes that confer risk to melanoma*

Different from other familial cancer, such as breast and HNPCC colon cancers, a unique candidate gene seems not responsible to all familial cases of melanoma. As cited above, up to 40% of familial melanomas could be attributed to *CDKN2A* mutations. This fact opens the possibility to other susceptibility genes with high penetrance. A study performed in families with no *CDKN2A* and *CDK4* mutations identified a possible candidate locus in 1p22 chromosome [36]. Subsequent analysis of this locus in additional pedigrees supported this previous evidence. Moreover, LOH studies also indicated a putative tumor suppressor gene is this region, however, sequence analysis has not identified any mutations [37].

Other germline mutations in critical genes responsible for cancer susceptibility, which melanoma is not a clinically feature, also increase the risk for melanoma, where some melanoma cases have been reported. Individuals harboring germline mutations in *RB1* gene (Retinoblastoma); *TP53* and *CHEK2* genes (Li-Fraumeni and Li-Fraumeni Like syndrome respectively); *NF1* gene (Neurofibromatosis type 1); *Xeroderma Pigmentosum* genes (XP) and *BRCA2* were also associated with melanoma. Even melanomas cases were reported in such syndromes. The absolute low number of melanomas reported in these syndromes, especially in Li-Fraumeni syndrome, creates a debate regarding whether melanomas could be a rare manifestation of these cancer syndromes. A detailed discussion on the role of these genes and melanoma was published elsewhere [38].

3.2. Low penetrance genes: The "new genetics" of melanoma

The great development in low penetrance genes search for melanoma risk came with the development of genome-wide association studies (GWAS). With GWAS, several hundreds of thousands DNA variants can be detected and larger samples sizes can be used, thus increasing the power of analysis. A great advantage of using GWAS is the possibility to identify variants that are not located in protein coding regions. Coupled with the development of GWAS, the use of meta-analysis has also contributed to identify new low penetrance genes. Meta-analysis is a widely accepted method that summarizes the results from multiple published studies, then producing results with larger sample size and increasing statistical power. We discuss below the main findings regarding low-penetrance genes and melanoma of GWAS and meta-analysis studies in melanoma.

3.2.1. *MC1R gene – Coloring the knowledge of melanoma susceptibility*

The *MC1R* (melanocortin 1 receptor) is a critical gene related to human skin pigmentation. *MC1R* codes for a transmembrane protein receptor that binds to α-melanocyte stimulating hormone (α-MSH), upon binding the activation of adenylate cyclase is triggered and consequently intracellular cAMP levels increases, then leading to a switch in melanin production from pheomelanin pigments to eumelanin (a photoprotective pigment). The activation of MC1R is an integral part of the tanning response following UV irradiation.

The *MC1R* gene is highly polymorphic, a fact that denotes the huge variation in pigmentation phenotypes and skin colors in humans. This huge variation can create different haplotypes (many of them with amino acid substitutions) which have been show to modify the receptor functions altering the ratios of pheomelanin and eumelanin. The high levels of pheomelanin associated with some *MC1R* variants cause the red hair and fair skin phenotype. In European and Asian populations, there is considerable diversity of *MC1R* haplotypes, while in African populations the variation is less common, indicating an evolutional pressure to keep the high levels of eumelanin [39]. Germline variants that compromise the signaling of MC1R are present in about 80% of red hair and fair skin individuals; about 20% in individuals with brown or black hair and less than 4% in persons with a robust tanning response [40].

Epidemiological studies have indicated that red hair and fair skin are host characteristics predisposing to melanoma [11]. This phenotype is known to be more sensitive to harmful effects of UV exposure, mainly because the low capacity of tanning in red hair and fair skin individuals. As certain *MC1R* variants are strongly associated with skin color, and the type of skin color is associated with melanoma risk, it is not surprising therefore than some *MC1R* polymorphisms could influence susceptibility to melanoma development. Molecular epidemiology studies have reported melanoma patients as significantly harboring some *MC1R* variants more than control healthy subjects. Individuals that carry *MC1R* variants present a 2.2-to-3.9 fold risk to develop melanomas. Notably, there is an additive effect on having multiple variants, for example carriers of two *MC1R* variants have a 4.1-to-4.8 fold risk of developing melanoma [41-44].

In a recent meta-analysis, of 9 *MC1R* variants analyzed (V60L, D84E, V92M, R142H, R151C, I155T, R160W, R163Q, D294H), all variants were associated with melanoma risk. The odds ratio (OR) and the 95% confidence interval (95% CI), ranged from 1.18 (95% CI 1.04 – 1.35) to V60L to 2.40 (95% CI 1.64 - 3.51) to R142H [45]. Besides the risk values, the study showed a critical variation of a certain polymorphism among control and case populations. As example, to V60L variant, the frequency ranged from 5% in controls to 19.75 in cases, while to R160W, this variation was from 3.95% in controls to 11.64% in cases. The meta-analysis also validated the risk of melanoma associated with the so-called RHC and NRHC phenotypes [45]. The RHC phenotype (from red hair color) is defined by a nonfunctional melanocortin receptor, which leads to accumulation of pheomelanin, phenotype associated with fair skin, red hair, freckles and poor tanning ability [46]. Conversely, variants giving rise to receptors with a weak or without loss of function are called NRHC (from nonred hair color) convert pheomelanin into eumelanin less efficiently than control individuals. The RHC is composed by the variants R151C, R160W and D294H, a dominant effect of these variants is observed and the odds ratio to development of melanoma is 2.44 (95% CI 1.72 – 3.45) while to NRHC variants, the attributed odds ratio is 1.29 (95% CI 1.10 – 1.51) [45].

3.2.2. *MITF*

As it is well established, melanin is one of the major protective factors against ultraviolet radiation DNA damage that results in melanoma development. The formation of this pigment is triggered by melanocyte-stimulating hormone, a peptide hormone coded by the the proopiomelancortin gene (*POMC*). Melanocyte-stimulating hormone binding to *MC1R* also results in the induction of microphthalmia-associated transcription factor (MITF) [47;48]. This transcription factor is coded by *MITF* gene located in chromosome 3 (3p14.2-p14.1) and it regulates a suite of genes involved in cell cycle control and melanogenesis [49]. These functions allow MITF to mediate differentiation and survival of melanocytes while limiting their uncontrolled progression. It was observed by Cheli et al. (2010) [49] that loss of *MITF* in the germline abolishes melanocyte formation in mice, whereas its loss in established melanocyte gives rise to their expansion [49]. MITF achieves this partly via inducing senescence through expression of p16INK4a, p21, and anti-apoptosis genes such as B-cell lymphoma 2 (*BCL2*) and apex nuclease 1 (*APEX1*) [49]. Recently, two independent groups identified a rare functional non-synonymous SNP (E318K) in *MITF* gene that alters MITF transcriptional activity, and it is associated with a large population-wide melanoma risk estimated between odds ratio 2.19 (95% CI 1.41, 3.45) and 4.78 (95% CI 2.05, 11.75) ([50],[51]; respectively). *MITF* gene is also associated with increased nevus count and non-blue eye color, consistent with its enhanced transcriptional ability. Adjusting for these traits reduced (odds ratio 1.82, 95% CI 0.85, 3.92) but did not abolish E318K association with melanoma [50].

There is a positive feedback loop in melanocytes caused by UV radiation damage, which increases melanin production and blocks cell cycle progression via MITF until DNA damage is no longer detected [48]. Given its protective nature, melanoma researchers have spent significant effort testing skin coloration genes derived from animal studies or genetic association studies identified as targets of *MITF*, or highlighted by human pigmentation GWAS [52;53].

3.2.3. *Other pigmentation genes*

SLC45A2

Genetic epidemiological studies have recently identified a subset of other pigmentation genes that are associated with risk for melanoma and other cutaneous malignancies as well as photosensitivity for MITF-regulated solute carrier family 45 member 2 gene - *SLC45A2* [54;55]. This gene is located in chromosome 5p, comprised of seven exons spanning 40 kb, and encodes a 530 amino acid protein presumably located in the melanosome membrane [56-57]. The protein SLC45A2 probably directs the traffic of melanosomal proteins and other substances to the melanosomes [57]. The mutation 1122C>G in *SLC45A2*gene, which results in non-synonymous amino acid change (Phe374Leu) has been related with pigmentation variation and ethnic ancestry in different populations [58]. However, according to meta-analysis that summarize some association studies [54;55], this mutation confers protection from cutaneous melanoma in individuals with a fair phenotype in populations from South European regions (France, Italy and Spain) – OR =0.41 (95% CI: 0.33–0.50). This meta-analysis may explain the incidence of melanoma in cases with skin phototypes III–IV, dark eye and hair color, absence of ephelides, lentigines and with a low number of nevi [57].

ASIP

Another pigmentation gene extensively studied in melanoma is *ASIP*, located in chromosome 20q11.22, which encodes agouti signaling protein. Agouti signalling protein (ASIP) was first described to inhibit eumelanogenesis in human melanocytes [59]. The protein ASIP is a MC1R ligand of 132 amino acids that antagonises the function of the transmembrane receptor [60]. According with a recent review [34], in a large study of European population descendants, a significant association was found between two SNP haplotype (rs1015362 and rs4911414), at the *ASIP* locus and cutaneous melanoma, with a modest OR =1.45 [61]. In another study [62], the haplotype near *ASIP* with same SNPs was associated with fair skin color (OR, 2.28; 95% CI, 1.46-3.57) as well as the risks of melanoma (OR 1.68; 95% CI 1.18-2.39). Similar results were described [63] in a German population study with increased risk to melanoma development in carriers of the rs4911414 variant (OR 1.27; 95% CI 1.03–1.57). An Australian genome-wide association study [64] also indicated the presence of a melanoma susceptibility locus on chromosome 20q11.22, with an OR of 1.72 for *ASIP* SNPs, (rs910873 and rs1885120). As the *ASIP* gene encodes the antagonist melanocortin receptor, polymorphisms of this gene can alter the protein conformation or decreased level of ASIP mRNA in melanocytes. As a consequence of low ASIP protein levels, its inhibiting effect is diminished, while eumelanogenesis is increased. If there are some altered ratio of pheomelanin and eumelanin caused by huge variation in *MC1R* gene, the high level of pheomelanin synthesis will increase, resulting in phenotypes with increased risk of cutaneous melanoma (red hair and fair skin phenotype).

TYR

The gene *TYR*, located in 11q14-q21, coded tyrosinase, which is a copper-dependent enzyme that catalyzes the first two steps during melanogenesis. The protein is required for the synthesis of both types of melanin, eumelanin and pheomelanin. While a basal activity of the enzyme leads to pheomelanin synthesis, a switch to eumelanogensis occurs upon increased protein activity. It has been reported that TYR presents higher enzymatic activity in a neutral environment than in acidic conditions. This formed the basis for the assumption that a neutral environment is required for the formation of eumelanosomes instead of pheomelanosomes and that the pH value is a control mechanism for melanin synthesis [65]. In a recent review of the literature [34] polymorphisms in *TYR* gene has also been implicated in cutaneous malignant melanoma susceptibility, where variants in coding region (rs1126809) of the gene increased melanoma risk (OR 1.27; 95% CI 1.16: 1.40 and OR 1.22 ; 95% CI 1.14 : 1.31) ([66] [67]; respectively).

Genome-wide association studies (GWAS) have unveiled single nucleotide polymorphisms (SNPs) or genetic variants in other genes involved with pigmentation pathways that can contribute to melanoma susceptibility. Examples follow; two pore segment channel 2 (*TPCN2*), KIT ligand (*KITLG*), solute carrier family 24, member 5 (*SLC24A5*), interferon regulatory factor 4 (*IRF4*), oculocutaneous albinism II (*OCA2*), HECT and RLD domain containing E3 ubiquitin protein ligase 2 (*HERC2*) and tyrosinase-related protein 1 (*TYRP1*) pigmentation genes. These findings emphasize the contribution of pigmentation pathways to melanoma predisposition and tumorigenesis through gene-environment interactions. Since pigmentation genes in the melanin synthesis pathway also confer risk for cutaneous malignancy, a better understanding of the operative molecular mechanisms involved in this relationship has the potential to impact individual risk assessment for cutaneous malignant melanoma in the future [68].

3.2.4. DNA repair genes – Polymorphisms contributing to a mutator phenotype?

Epidemiological and experimental data suggest that UV radiation is the main carcinogenic agent responsible for melanoma development. While UV-B radiation (290–320 nm) induces critical damage to DNA in the form of cyclobutane pyrimidine dimers (CPD) and pyrimidine photoproducts, UV-A radiation (320–400 nm) induces single strand breaks and generates free radicals that cause oxidative damage [69]. While UV-induced DNA damage often activates distinct DNA repair pathways that maintain genome integrity, the main processes involve the Base Excision Repair (BER), which operates mainly to repair damage caused by oxidative stress and single strand breaks and Nucleotide Excision Repair (NER) that acts to neutralize photoproducts such as CPD and 6–4 dimers [2].

The differences in DNA repair capacity among individuals are genetically determined in function of mutations and polymorphisms in many genes implicated in these pathways and it has been examined in relation to cutaneous malignant melanoma. According with a recent review [34], some studies found significant association between variations in DNA repair genes and melanoma. The gene *XPD,* located in 19q13.3, codes a protein that is involved in transcription-coupled nucleotide excision repair and is an integral member of the basal transcription factor BTF2/TFIIH complex. The SNP 13181 A>C in exon 23 of the gene, with amino acid change in protein (Lys751Gln) was described as a risk factor for cutaneous melanoma susceptibility, with an OR of 1.12 (95% CI, 1.03-1.21) [70]. Other polymorphisms in members of XP family genes involved with NER pathway were also described. Another recent study found melanoma protection for the *XPG* (13q33) 1104 His/His genotype (OR 0.32; 95% CI 0.13-0.75), and increased risk for three polymorphisms in chromosome 3p25 at *XPC* gene (OR 3.64; 95% CI 1.77-7.48) (PAT+; IV-6A and 939Gln), which represent a haplotype for *XPC* [71].

In other repair pathways significant association has been described, for example variants in exon 7 of *XRCC3* (14q32.3). This gene encodes a member of the RecA/Rad51-related protein family that participates in homologous recombination to maintain chromosome stability and repair DNA damage. T241M *XRCC3* was associated with an increased risk for cutaneous melanoma [72]. Individuals who carry variant alleles had a decreased risk of cutaneous melanoma (OR 0.83, 95% CI, 0.79-0.98) [72]. Same results were found in a previous study [73]. An additional study reported a significant association between *MGMT* haplotypes and cutaneous melanoma risk, with a greater risk observed among 84Phe or 143Val carriers, who have a lower alkylation-damage repair capacity due to the variant alleles [74].

A summary of the main founds regarding low penetrance genes and melanoma risk can be found in Table 1.

Gene/ Polymorphism	rs	OR (95% CI)	References
MC1R - V60L	1805005	1.10 (1.04-1.35)	[45]
MC1R - D84E	1805006	1.67 (1.21-2.30)	[45]
MC1R - V92M	2228479	1.32 (1.04-1.68)	[45]
MC1R - R142H	11547464	2.40 (1.64-3.51)	[45]
MC1R - R151C	1805007	1.93 (1.54-2.41)	[45]
MC1R - I155T	1110400	1.39 (1.05-1.83)	[45]
MC1R - R160W	1805008	1.55 (1.21-1.97)	[45]
MC1R - R163Q	885479	1.21 (1.02-1.42)	[45]
MC1R - D294H	1805009	1.89 (1.39-2.56)	[45]
MITF - E318K	149617956	2.19 (1.41-3.45) 4.78 (2.05-11.75)	[50] [51]
SLC45A2 - F374L	16891982	0.41 (0.33-0.50)	[57]
ASIP - haplotype G;T	1015362/ 4911414	1.45 ($P = 1.2 \times 10^{-9}$) 1.68 (1.18-2.39) 1.27 (1.03-1.57)	[61] [62] [63]
ASIP - haplotype G;G	910873/ 1885120	1.72 (1.53, 2.01)	[64]
TYR - R402Q	1126809	1.27 (1.16-1.40) 1.22 (1.14-1.31)	[66] [67]
XPD - K751Q	1052559	1.12 (1.03-1.21)	[70]
XPG - D1104H	17655	0.32 (0.13-0.75)	[71]
XPC - IV11-6C/A		3.10 (1.65–5.83)	[71]
XPC - K939Q	2228001	2.89 (1.52–5.50)	[71]
XPC - PAT(-/+)		3.27 (1.75–6.12)	[71]
XPC haplotype PAT+; 6A,Gln allele		3.64 (1.77–7.48)	[71]
XRCC3 - T241M	861539	0.83 (0.79-0.98) 2.36 (1.44–3.86)	[72] [73]
MGMT haplotype L84F/ I143V	12917/ 2308321	1.75 (1.11-2.76)	[74]

Table 1. Summary of low-penetrance candidate melanoma susceptibility genes

4. Melanoma genetics: Progression genes

4.1. "Old genetics" of melanoma progression

The here called "old-genetics" of melanoma progression consist of known genes which its functions are well described and are also related to several other cancer types, mainly due to its function in controlling survival and proliferation pathways. An overview of such "old-genetics" of melanoma is shown in Figure 1.

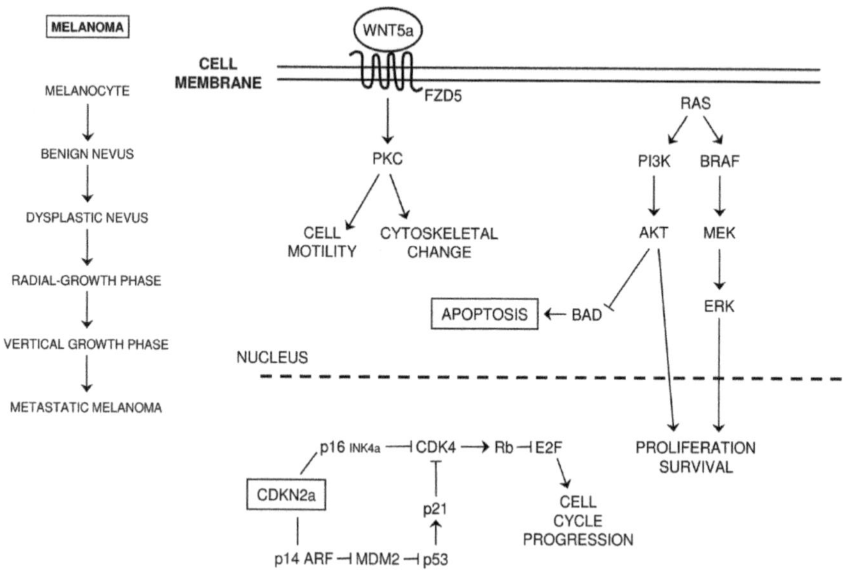

Figure 1. A schematic view of the main genes and pathways related to melanoma progression. The genes and pathways described are the here called "old genetics" of melanoma progression. Arrows indicate activation and blunt arrows indicate inhibition.

4.1.1. Mitogen-Activated Protein Kinases (MAPK) pathway – MAPing the first melanoma progression pathway

Several molecular pathways are activated/deactivated during tumor formation and some of them are responsible for the development of specific phases of tumor progression. Among them, is the Mitogen-activated protein kinases (MAPK) pathway. The pathway consists in a chain-like activation cascade of serine/threonine-specific protein kinases, where one protein must be phosphorylated to activate another. The proteins involved in this pathway are the RAS oncogene, discovered in the early 80s, with three known isoforms (H-Ras, K-RAS and N-RAS); RAF kinase, with also three isoforms (A-RAF, B-RAF and C-RAF or RAF-1); MEK kinase and ERK kinase, which have cytoplasmic targets or can phosphorylate transcription factors in the nucleus. The MAPK pathway is one of the most well-known pathways involved not only in melanoma formation, but probably in most types of tumors. The pathway is responsible to conduct an extracellular signal, like growth signal, from receptors in cell surface towards cell nucleus. After activation of RAS, the first protein of the cascade, a multitude of cellular responses, like protein synthesis, regulation of cell survival, differentiation and proliferation can be observed, showing the importance of this pathway for melanoma progression. Mutations in MAPK pathway are necessary for the development of early stages melanomas, as the transfection of constitutively activated MEK into immortalized melanocytes is sufficient to induce tumorigenesis in nude mice, activation of the angiogenic switch, and increased production of the pro-angiogenic factor, vascular endothelial growth factor (VEGF), and matrix metalloproteinases (MMPs) [75].

The most common mutations found in MAPK proteins in melanomas are in RAS protein, more specific in N-RAS and in RAF proteins, in B-RAF. The RAS proteins are members of a large superfamily of low molecular-weight GTP-binding proteins. The activation state of RAS proteins depends on whether they are bound to GTP (in which case, they are active and are able to engage downstream target enzyme) or GDP (in which case, they are inactive and fail to interact with these effectors). In normal cells, the activity of RAS proteins is controlled by the ratio of bound GTP to GDP [76]. N-RAS mutations can be found in over 15% of all melanoma cases and are most commonly the result of the substitution from leucine to glutamine at position 61 [77]. It is correlated to the vertical growth phase of melanoma progression. Although initially thought to occur mainly at the plasma membrane, there is increasing evidence that isoform-specific RAS signaling can take place at different cellular compartments and within different regions of the plasma membrane. Such compartmentalization and trafficking of endogenous RAS oncogenes is likely to play an important role in regulating downstream signaling processes involved in tumorigenesis [78]. For its activation and function as a signal transducer, N-RAS needs to be modified by a farnesylation near its C-terminal domain. Several farnesylation inhibitors were tested in the clinics and all results were disappointing [79]. In part, the failure of the clinical trials can be explained due to the fact that the farnesylation inhibitors may work in Rho (a subfamily of RAS superfamily) rather than RAS, or the fact that the inhibitors works on normal and mutated RAS.

Other important component of MAPK pathway that is mutated in melanomas is the RAF kinase B-RAF, the primer mediator of RAS protein. Some reports have shown that over 60% of all melanoma cases have mutation in B-RAF [80]. RAF mutations occur in the kinase domains and the most common mutation found in melanomas, approximately 80%, is the substitution of valine at position 600 with glutamic acid also called B-RAF^{V600E} mutation. This mutation creates a constitutively active status for B-RAF, independently of a previous activation by RAS oncogene and extracellular stimulus and it is more frequently found in skin of individuals with intermittent sun exposure than unexposed or chronically sun-damaged skin. Interestingly, B-RAF mutation frequency in benign melanocytic nevi seems to be equal or even higher than in that for melanomas. The frequency also varies, like melanomas, from 0% in Spitz nevi up to 90% in intradermal nevi. These differences, between B-RAF mutation in nevi and melanomas make the assessment of the impact of these mutations on prognosis difficult to determine [38]. B-RAF mutation in nevi might be a critical step in melanoma development, suggesting its importance in early stages of the disease.

Melanomas usually do not have B-Raf^{V600E} mutation at the same time they have mutations in any RAS isotype. However, some small proportions of cases carry mutation in both B-RAF and any RAS isoform, but in these cases, B-RAF mutation almost never is in V600E locus [81]. Recently, a link between B-RAF and the cell cycle controller E2F has been shown. B-RAF is able to phosphorylate the retinoblastoma (Rb) protein and release E2F transcription factor family to work [82]. E2F family is a classic cell cycle controller, but can also induce DNA repair, regulates autophagy and MMPs expression. The link between MAPK pathway and E2F transcription factor family may provide new strategies for melanoma treatment. New drugs using the B-Raf^{V600E} mutation as a target is currently being used in the clinics. Vemurafenib (PLX-4032) is a novel treatment for metastatic disease for melanomas with the V600E mutation. Vemurafenib treatment has demonstrated improved progression-free and prolonging overall survival in three months, compared with chemotherapy in a randomized trial, and represents a new standard of care in patients with advanced melanoma harboring a BRAF-V600 mutation [83]. However, Vemurafenib treatment induces several resistance pathways in B-Raf^{V600E} cells and is expected to failure after a few months, but it is the best treatment for melanoma disease so far. Among the resistance pathway induced by the drug are MEK activation by MAP3K8 [84], up regulation of N-RAS [85] and activation of fibroblast growth factor receptor 3 (FGFR3) [86].

4.1.2. PI3K pathway – Supporting MAPK pathway to melanoma progression

RAS can also activate other effectors pathways rather than RAF. RAS can interact directly with phosphatidylinositol 3-kinases (PI3Ks), activating other molecular pathways. One of the pathways activated by PI3Ks is the AKT/PKB pathway, which has a strong anti-apoptotic function by phosphorylating various targets and seems to be an important part of the survival signal that is generated by RAS activation.

MAPK activation is necessary for early stages melanomas, but is not sufficient for the development of advanced disease. Other molecular mechanisms are necessary for melanoma invade other tissues and survive in different microenvironments. AKT/PKB seems to be important for the development of radial growth melanomas, from cell lines which are characterized as radial growth melanomas. In this model, AKT overexpression induced VEGF expression and switched to a more glycolytic metabolism [87]. The AKT family consists of three members, AKT1–3 and 43–50% of melanomas have a selective constitutively active AKT3. AKT3 overexpression may occur as a result of copy number increases in the long arm of chromosome 1. Another mechanism for PI3K/AKT pathway activation in melanoma is through the acquisition of activating E17K mutations in AKT3. AKT has a critical role in cancer development through its ability to block apoptosis through the direct phosphorylation of BAD as well as through its effects in many other pathways, including the inhibition of forkhead signaling and the inhibition of glycogen synthase kinase-3. One of the most critical regulators of AKT is the phosphatase and tensin homolog (PTEN), which degrades the products of PI3K, preventing AKT activation. The mechanism by which the PI3K/AKT pathway is activated in melanoma may involve the loss of expression or functional inactivation of PTEN [88]. However, PI3K pathway mutations, though more heterogeneous, were present in 41% of the melanoma, with PTEN being the highest mutated gene of the PI3K pathway in melanomas (22%) [89].

PTEN is a tumor suppressor gene located in chromosome 10q23.3 and is a dual specificity phosphatase capable of dephosphorylating both tyrosine phosphate and serine/threonine phosphate residues in proteins. It also functions as a major lipid phosphatase, counteracting PI3K by dephosphorylating the second messengers phosphatidylinositol-3,4,5-triphosphate

(PIP3) and phosphatidylinositol-3,4-diphosphate (PIP2), which are required for the activation of AKT/PKB [17]. PTEN can work in other pathways than AKT/PKB. PTEN is involved in cell migration, spreading, and focal adhesion formation through direct dephosphorylation and inactivation of focal adhesion kinase (FAK). Also, PTEN inhibits Shc phosphorylation, preventing the association of Shc with Grb2/Sos and activation of the Ras/Raf/MEK1/MAPK pathway. PTEN suppresses the stabilization of hypoxia-mediated HIF-1α, which when stabilized through the PI3K/AKT pathway, upregulates VEGF expression suggesting a possible role for PTEN in angiogenesis [88]. An interesting study sequenced the PTEN gene from melanomas from patients harboring the *Xeroderma Pigmentosum* syndrome [90]. A total of 59 melanomas from 8 XP patients showed a mutation rate of 56% in *PTEN* gene. A detailed look for the mutational spectrum revealed that 91% of the melanomas with mutations had 1 to 4 UV type mutations (C to T changes) occurring at adjacent pyrimidines. Functional analyses also indicated impared PTEN function caused by the mutations. The study showed critical data to the understanding of melanoma progression in XP patients.

4.1.3. WNT5A – Progression to the edges, leading to melanoma metastasis

The metastatic disease does not have fixed histopathological subclasses. That is why there is a need to look for genetic profiles that could predict a behavior in advanced stages. WNT5A, a protein of Wnt family, was identified as the gene that best defined the new subclasses of tumors. The Wnt family of proteins has over 19 members, all of which are secreted, that are very closely structurally related. The activation of Wnt signaling can have very different results depending on which members of the family are involved. Wnt proteins work through three different pathways: the β-catenin pathway, the Wnt/Ca2+ pathway and the planar cell polarity pathway. The activation of WNT5A in melanomas uses the non-canonical pathway Wnt/Ca2+ together with Frizzled receptors, activating phospholipase C, which translocate to the membrane and hydrolyzes membrane phospholipids, initiating phosphatidylinositol signaling [91]. *In vitro* analysis of melanoma cell lines differing in WNT5A expression levels showed that WNT5A overexpression is correlated with increased motility and invasiveness of the cell [91]. WNT5A correlates with high aggressive metastatic disease and its activation is mediated through PKC pathways which are associated to cytoskeletal organization and invasion. WNT5A protein expression in human melanoma biopsies directly correlates with increasing tumor grade while inversely correlating with patient survival [92]. Members of the Wnt pathways have been identified in melanoma. WNT5A and others members like Rho pathway and frizzled 7 may play an important role in transition of melanoma from VGP to metastases. It is very likely that the temporal activation of Wnt pathways is very important for melanoma development and progression. It would not be surprising if β-catenin expression was an early event, and metastatic cells need to down regulate expression of this protein prior to invading, and escaping the immune system. WNT5A may provide a survival advantage to melanoma cells, despite the fact that in others tumor it may act as a tumor suppressor. Thus, its early expression may result in suppression of tumorigenesis, whereas if it is expressed at a later stage, it becomes a potent inducer of migration and motility. Wnt signaling and its effects on melanoma establishment and progression are complex, and surely temporal and context dependent [92].

4.2. "New genetics" of melanoma progression

Melanoma is a complex genetic disease. Recent studies have begun to characterize the mechanisms underlying melanoma plasticity, relating to intratumoral switching between varying malignant capacities, such as proliferation, invasion, or tumorigenesis. The rate at which somatic and germline genetic alterations have been cataloged in melanoma has accelerated greatly in recent years. The ability to modulate genes and proteins of interest, even when pharmacologic agents are not available, has provided preclinical evidence that many putative oncogenes represent potential therapeutic targets [93]. At the same time, the notorious resistance of melanoma to treatments with its strong potential to metastasize represents the major clinical obstacle in the treatment of these tumors. These observations allow the scientists to improve staging and subtype classification and lead them to design better therapeutic agents and approaches. New insights about genetics of melanoma, including high-throughput strategies such as gene expression microarrays, comparative genomic hybridization, mutation analysis by deep sequencing and microRNAs gene regulation have helped researchers to elucidate the crucial cell-signaling pathways or validate the already postulated pathways as modified in melanomas. The genes and pathways discussed below for the "new genetics" of melanoma progression are represented in Figure 2.

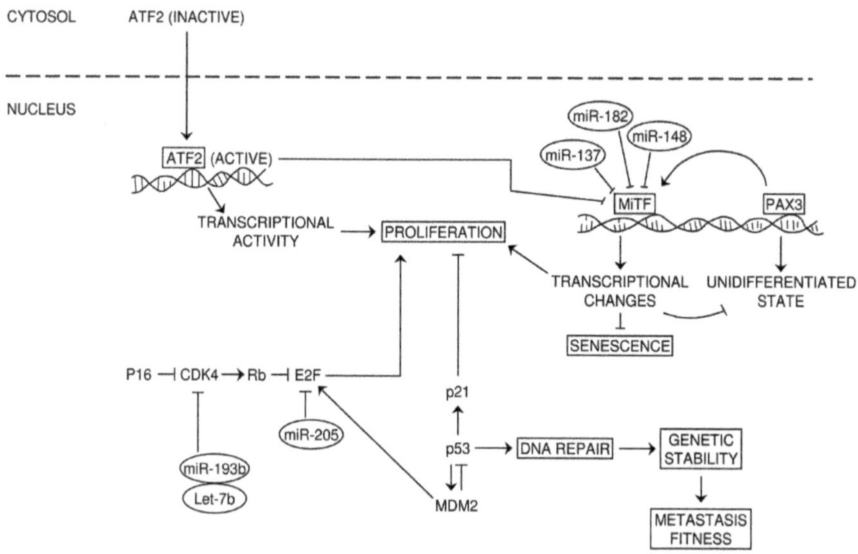

Figure 2. A schematic view of the main genes and pathways related to melanoma progression. The genes and pathways described are the here called "new genetics" of melanoma progression. Arrows indicate activation and blunt arrows indicate inhibition.

4.2.1. Activating Transcription Factor 2 (ATF2) – Helping melanoma progression activation

The ATF2 (Activating Transcription Factor-2 or cAMP response element [CRE]) it was first identified as an inducible enhancer of genes that can be transcribed in response to increased cAMP levels and mediates various transcriptional regulatory effects, for example, ATF2/Jun complex is implicated in multiple cellular processes [94,95]. The ATF2 transcriptional targets genes is divided into (a) regulation of transcription factors and proteins engaged in stress and DNA damage response (b) regulation of genes associated with growth and tumorigenesis (c) regulation of genes important for maintenance and physiological homeostasis [94]. In addition to its function as a transcription factor, ATF2 was found to play an important role in DNA damage response. After damage occurs, ATF2 is phosphorylated by ATM and its results in rapid localization of ATF2 to ionizing radiation (IR) induced foci (IRIF), which contain DNA repair proteins and chromatin-modifying enzymes. Furthermore, ATF2 phosphorylated is required for an intact intra-S-phase checkpoint response necessary to stop DNA replication [96]. In recent years, the study of ATF2 activity in melanoma cells has revealed a probably oncogenic function. In the early '90s, Ronai and Weinstein [97] elucidated the cellular response to UV irradiation. The authors characterized a UV-responsive element (URE;TGACAACA) and soon after, its binding proteins, AP1 and ATF family members [98]. Interesting, the URE was found within the promoter sequences of stress-responsive genes, including c-jun, DNA polymerase B, and cyclin A, as well as on regulatory regions of viruses that respond to UV irradiation [99]. Differences in transcriptional activities of URE-bound proteins were found after UV-irradiation of keratinocytes, melanocytes and melanoma, and also in repair deficient cells of patients with *Xeroderma pigmentosum*, or Cockayne syndrome [for review 9]. In 1998, the Ronai´s group investigated which of the CREB-associated proteins is directly involved in modifying specific characteristics of melanoma phenotypes. They demonstrate that ATF2 is the primary binding protein and regulator of URE-mediated transcription and it contributes specifically to radiation resistance of human melanoma cells.

An approach to selectively inhibit ATF2 activity in human melanoma was designed, based on peptides derived from ATF2 trans-activating domain which affect ATF2 transcriptional activity. In an attempt to sensitize melanoma cells to UV irradiation, Ronai *et al.* investigated the ability of cells to enter in apoptosis competing by endogenous ATF2 expression with ATF2-derived peptide(s) alone and/or combined with inhibition of p38 activity (one Mitogen-activated Protein Kinases that is responsive to stress stimuli) via its pharmacological inhibitor (SB203580) [100]. The expression of a 50-amino acid peptide derived from the NH2-terminal domain of ATF2 ($ATF2^{50-100}$) was sufficient to sensitize melanoma cells to radiation. Combination of this peptide with SB203580 induced programmed cell death in late stage melanoma cells via Fas signaling, whereas Fas ligand/receptor interactions play an important role in the progression of cancer. In 2002, experimental mouse models validated the expression of this peptide. The $ATF2^{50-100}$ not only sensitized melanoma cells to apoptosis but efficiently inhibited tumor growth and metastasis [101]. Analysis of mouse cell lines derived from melanomas formed in the HGF/SF (Hepatocyte Growth Factor/Scatter Factor) transgenic mouse, revealed that the proliferation rate in culture increased with increased ATF-2 activity [102], confirming the role of ATF2 in melanoma development. Along these lines, B16 mouse melanoma cells exhibit higher levels of phosphorylated ATF2 compared to immortalized non-malignant mouse melanocytes. Following treatment with retinoic acid, ATF2 phosphorylation was reduced, resulting in c-Jun dimerization with c-Fos and promoting a shift from proliferation towards differentiation [103]. Additional experiments showed that delivery of ATF2 inhibitory peptides elicited efficient inhibition of melanoma tumor growth [104].

Even with these encouraging results, one question remains unanswered: how ATF2 inhibition induces apoptosis in melanoma cells? It was demonstrated that $ATF2^{50-100}$ induced apoptosis by sequestering ATF2 to the cytoplasm, thereby inhibiting its transcriptional activities [105]. In addition, mutations within the c-Jun N-terminal kinases (JNK) binding region of $ATF2^{50-100}$ or expression of TAM67, a dominant negative of the Jun family of transcription factors, or JunD-RNA interference attenuate inhibition of melanoma tumorigenicity by $ATF2^{50-100}$. The JNKs are kinases responsive to stress stimuli, such as ultraviolet irradiation used in this study. These results were crucial to show that inhibition of ATF2 in concert with increased JNK/Jun activities is central for the sensitization of melanoma cells to apoptosis and inhibition of their tumorigenicity. Furthermore, $ATF2^{50-100}$ increases ATF2 localization within the cytoplasm. Indeed, one study evaluating the ATF2 as a prognostic marker among patients with melanomas validated this result. A study to determine the prognostic value of ATF2 evaluating the pattern and level of its expression in a tissue microarray was conducted [106]. Cytoplasmic ATF2 expression was associated with primary tumor rather than metastases and with better patient survival whereas nuclear ATF2 expression was associated with metastatic tumor and with poor survival. Nuclear ATF2 seems to be transcriptionally active while cytoplasmic ATF2 probably represents an inactive form. These findings support one preclinical finding in which transcriptionally active ATF2 is involved in tumor progression-proliferation in melanoma, suggesting that ATF2 might be a useful prognostic marker in early-stage melanoma. Although the use peptide $ATF2^{50-100}$ have shown good results to sensitize melanoma cells to treatments, Ronai group´s continued investigating peptides with smaller size but producing the same effect. In 2004, Bhoumik *et al.* [107] presented one peptide with only 10aa - $ATF2^{51-60}$. This peptide sensitizes melanoma cells to spontaneous apoptosis and inhibits the *in vivo* growth. Furthermore, the $ATF2^{51-60}$ expression coincides with activation of caspase 9, an important molecule activated during apoptosis. This study points to mechanisms underlying the activities of the ATF2 peptide while highlighting its possible use in drug design.

Based on these findings, ATF2 present oncogenic action, but could it act as one tumor suppressor molecule? Although genetic changes in ATF2 have not been identified in human tumors, many data sustain the notion that ATF2 is not only oncogenic, whereas its altered expression and sub cellular localization is associated with tumor stage and prognosis in melanomas, but it also acts as a tumor suppressor molecule, under specific conditions. This hypothesis arose from independent studies with skin and mammary tumors. Studies from a mouse mammary tumor model revealed that loss of ATF2 *per se*, does not promote mammary tumor formation, but heterozygous mouse *ATF2* mutants developed mammary tumors when crossed with p53 mutant mice, indicating that ATF2 may have a suppressor function only when combined with a p53 mutant background [108]. Likewise, loss of ATF2 transcriptional activities in keratinocytes promotes faster development of skin papillomas. Deletion of functional *ATF2* in keratinocytes was achieved using a K14-cre mouse which was crossed with mutant ATF2 mice. Exposure of K14-ATF2 mutant mice to DMBA (a carcinogen that causes Ras mutation) followed by application of TPA (a tumor promoter) resulted in faster formation of papillomas which were bigger, compared with mice bearing wild-type (WT) *ATF2* in their keratinocytes [109]. Importantly, mice in which *ATF2* was deleted only in keratinocytes did not develop papillomas, differently from WT mice when treated with the carcinogens DMBA or TPA alone. Therefore, ATF2 can limit tumor development by cooperating with existing oncogenes and inactivated tumor suppressor genes.

Present knowledge positions ATF2 as important transcription factor and DNA damage response protein, which is also implicated in the regulation of cellular growth control. Along the growing complexity of understanding ATF2 regulation and function are the observations that point to its ability to elicit oncogenes or tumor suppressor functions, depending on the tissue type. Based on these findings, it was proposed one model for ATF2 oncogenic *versus* tumor suppressor functions. Future studies will reveal the nature of these major differences, and further delineate the important role ATF2 plays in cellular growth control prior and following DNA damage, as in transformation and cancer development. In addition, the ATF2 function findings highlight the importance of transcriptional regulation, which enables the sensitization of melanoma to treatment and inhibits their growth and metastasis *in vivo*.

4.2.2. Microphthalmia-associated Transcription Factor (MITF) the conductor of melanoma players

Microphthalmia locus displays important roles for biology and pathology of pigmentation of the skin, as well as eye development and degeneration. Ever since, many other mutant alleles of the locus have been found in mice and other vertebrates [for review 110].The human *MITF* gene (3p14.2-p14.1) was cloned in 1994 [111] and so far, *MITF-A*, *MITF-B*, *MITF-H*, and *MITF-M* splice variants were described [112;113]. MITF contains a basic DNA binding domain and binds to DNA sequences primarily consisting of a 5′-CATGTG-3′ or 5′-CACGTG-3′ motif [114-116]. Ten isoforms of MITF have been described [117], but the m-MITF isoform is exclusively expressed in melanocytes. All MITF isoforms have a central transcriptional activation domain. MITF acts as a transcription factor which controls proliferation and apoptosis and plays a central role in the differentiation, growth, and survival of cells of the melanocytic lineage [118]. MITF is the main transcription activator for key genes involved in melanogenesis (*TYR*, *TYRP1*, *MLANA*, *SILV*), but its function can switch, in balance with *POU3F2*, to activate proliferation and inhibit invasion [119].

Recent observations of reversible phenotypic heterogeneity in melanoma have proposed a novel "phenotypic plasticity model" of cancer, whereas MITF seems to be one of the central players in melanoma phenotypic plasticity. The "dynamic epigenetic model" or rheostat model proposes that variations in the tumor microenvironment result in epigenetic lesions, leading to alterations observed in melanomas [for review 120]. In this model, high expression levels of MITF regulate genes involved with differentiation and cell cycle arrest. When MITF is expressed at average levels, melanoma cells proceed through cell cycle, while reduction of MITF to low levels switches off the cell proliferation program, inducing cell cycle arrest, and promotes invasion and metastasis. For example, prolonged MITF depletion leads melanomas to either quiescence or senescence [121]. So, MITF regulates distinct functions in melanocytic cells at different levels of expression. While MITF lower levels are commonly observed in melanoma cells rather than in melanocytes, high levels of MITF activate the expression of differentiation-associated genes implicated on melanosome function and promote a differentiation-associated cell cycle arrest via up regulation of the p16 (*CDKN2A*) and p21 (*CDKN1A*) cyclin-dependent kinase inhibitors ([122-124]. Chromatin immunoprecipitation of MITF from 501 melanoma cell line followed by high-throughput deep sequencing and RNA sequencing from MITF-depleted cells, showed *TYROSINASE, MET, LIG1, BRCA1, CCND1,* and *CCNB1* genes transcriptionally-regulated by *MITF*. Thus, MITF-depleted cells exhibit diminished capacity to passage through S-phase and repair DNA damage. These data highlight the multitasking role of MITF that, in addition to differentiation, survival, and its anti-proliferative roles, also includes a role in the S phase, controling mitosis and suppressing senescence. In an opposite way, increased MITF levels reduce melanoma cell proliferation even in the presence of oncogenic BRAF [124]. MITF can cooperate with $BRaf^{V600E}$ to transform immortalized melanocytes by expression of telomerase (TERT), dominant-negative p53 and activated Cdk4 [121]. These data indicates that, although MITF alone cannot transform normal human melanocytes, it can cooperate with $BRaf^{V600E}$ to contribute to the transformation process, functioning as a "lineage-specific oncogene", because it provides essential survival functions and contributes to proliferation. In this context, and bearing in mind that ERK is hyperactivated in melanoma and required for proliferation and survival, it is striking that MITF is targeted for degradation after its phosphorylation by ERK [125]. Indeed, constitutive activation of ERK by $BRaf^{V600E}$ in melanocytes results in constant down regulation of MITF [for review 126].

One interesting example from different levels of MITF action came from an elegant translational study [127]. The authors demonstrated that the transcription factor ATF2 negatively regulates *MITF* transcription in melanocytes and around 50% of melanoma cells. Increased MITF expression (upon inhibition of ATF2), effectively attenuated the ability of $BRaf^{V600E}$-melanocytes to exhibit a transformed phenotype. This effect was partially rescued when MITF expression was also blocked. The development of melanoma in mice carrying genetic changes seen in human tumors was inhibited upon inactivation of ATF2 in melanocytes. Melanocytes from mice lacking active ATF2 increased levels of MITF, confirming that ATF2 negatively regulates MITF and implicating this newly discovered regulatory link in melanomagenesis. Additionally, primary melanoma specimens that exhibit a high nuclear ATF2-to-MITF ratio were found to be associated with metastatic disease and poor prognosis, substantiating the significance of MITF control by ATF2. Taken together, these findings provide a genetic evidence for the role of ATF2 in melanoma development and indicate an ATF2 function as a regulator of MITF expression, which is central to understanding MITF control at the early phases of melanocyte transformation.

Another possible mechanism that could explain the different levels of expression of *MITF* observed in melanoma cells is DNA copy number alterations (CNAs). Copy number alterations involving "driver genes" can modulate substantially their expression

[128]. Melanoma genomes frequently contain somatic copy number alterations that can significantly perturb the expression level of affected genes. Recently, accurate strategies have been used to identify new genes and/or focus on molecular pathways already described as affected in melanomas (*BRAF, PTEN* and *MITF* alterations) [129]. By using integrative strategy of SNP (Single Nucleotide Polymorphism) array-based genetic, which has higher genomic resolution than CGH arrays, with gene expression signatures derived from NCI60 cell lines identified *MITF* as the target of novel melanoma amplification [121]. *MITF* amplification was more prevalent in metastatic disease and correlated with decreased overall patient survival. *BRAF* mutation and p16 inactivation was accompanied by *MITF* amplification in melanoma cell lines. Moreover, it was described that ectopic MITF expression in conjunction with the $BRAF^{V600E}$ mutant transformed primary human melanocytes, reinforcing the MITF as a melanoma oncogene. Although *MITF* amplification (10–100-fold) is observed around 10–16% of metastatic melanomas (in which *BRAF* is mutated), *MITF* levels are only increased about 1.5-fold compared with cells without amplification [121], again suggesting that MITF levels must be maintained within narrow limits. However, because only 10–16% of *BRAF*-mutated melanomas have *MITF* amplification, this raises the crucial question of how the remaining 84–90% counteracts MITF degradation mediated by hyperactivated ERK. One mechanism could involve β-catenin (molecule which regulates cell growth and adhesion between cells). β-catenin can induce MITF expression through a LEF-1/TCF binding site in the MITF promoter [130]. Although mutations in β-catenin are rare in melanoma [131], nuclear and/or cytoplasmic localization of β-catenin was found in 28% of metastatic melanoma [132]. Therefore, regardless the mechanism of activation, MITF was shown to be a key mediator of switching between the slow-growing invasive phenotype and the proliferative phenotype in melanoma cells.

Recent studies have shown the role of germline mutations associated with MITF function. Evidence for germline mutations in melanomas comes from studies with relatives of patients with melanoma with increased risk of melanoma development, indicating the presence of mutations in genes with high penetrance [for review 133]. A study conducted by Bertolotto et al. involving patients with melanoma and renal cell carcinoma (RCC) supports the hypothesis of genetic predisposition for both cancers [51]. MITF stimulates the transcription of HIF1A, the pathway of which is targeted by kidney cancer susceptibility genes, indicating that MITF might have a role in conferring a genetic predisposition to co-occurring melanoma and RCC. A germline missense substitution in *MITF* (Mi-E318K) was identified occurring at a significantly higher frequency in genetically enriched patients affected with melanoma, RCC or both cancers. Overall, patients bearing the Mi-E318K genotype had more than fivefold increased risk of developing melanoma, RCC or both cancers. The E318K variant was significantly associated with melanoma in a large case–control sample. The variant allele was significantly over-represented in cases with a family history of melanoma, multiple primary melanomas, or both. The variant allele was also associated with increased nevus count and no blue eye colour. In addition, Mi-E318K enhanced MITF protein binding to the HIF1A promoter and increased its transcriptional activity. Gene expression profiling from RCC cell line identified a Mi-E318K signature related to cell growth, proliferation and inflammation. Therefore, the mutant MITF present all features of a gain-of-function variant associated with tumorigenesis.

4.2.3. MITF as therapeutic strategy?

The understanding of the tumor stage, microenvironment, and mechanisms employed in phenotype switching have significant implications for clinical strategies in melanoma management. The description of *BRAF* and *KIT* mutations provided the first basis for a molecular classification of cutaneous melanoma and brought up insights about therapeutic approaches. Therapies based on BRAF moves on direction of regulatory approval and incorporation as standard therapy for patients with metastatic disease, as well as targeting mutated *KIT* has also been established for melanoma patients. *NRAS* mutations have been known to be present in a subset of melanomas and represent a complicated subgroup for targeted therapies. Matching patient subgroups defined by genetic aberrations in the phosphoinositide 3-kinase (PI3K) and p16/cyclin dependent kinase 4 (CDK4) pathways with appropriate targeted therapies has not yet been realized. So, an increasing understanding of lineage-specific transcriptional regulators, as MITF, and how they could play a role in melanoma pathophysiology provided other clues to therapies. Modulating MITF in a direct way with pharmacologic inhibitors would be challenging, particularly if the interaction of MITF with certain promoter regions on specific genes is desired. Reduction of MITF activity sensitizes melanoma cells to different chemotherapeutic agents [for review 121]. Targeting MITF combined with BRAF or cyclin-dependent kinase inhibitors is an exciting therapeutic strategy for melanoma patients.

One therapeutic strategy is target one or more of the post-translational processes that determine MITF activity, stability, or degradation. Another approach is targeting the melanocyte-specific mechanisms controlling MITF expression. Nonspecific histone deacetylases seem to function in such a manner [134]. Furthermore, MITF and its target genes have been used as diagnostic markers for melanoma [135]. As cited above, MITF-M isoform is involved in the *in vivo* growth control and contribute to the phenotype of human melanoma whereas MITF-M may qualify as a marker capable of identifying subgroups of melanoma patients with different tumor biology and prognosis [136]. Many MITF transcriptional targets are emerging, and it is likely that their identification may bring therapeutic strategies based on lineage-specific conditions. One candidate is cyclin dependent kinase 2 (CDK2). This molecule seems to contribute to deregulate cell cycle control via its transcriptional control by MITF, which is unique in the melanocyte lineage due to its genomic location adjacent to a *MITF*. Another molecule that seems to be regulated by MITF is BCL2 and it may contribute to resistance to apoptosis in melanomas [134].

4.2.4 DNA repair genes – Dual effect of DNA repair genes in melanoma progression

Exposure to UV radiation from sunlight induces DNA damage, which can lead to melanocyte carcinogenesis when not efficiently corrected. UV radiation may induce direct alterations through formation of pyrimidine dimmers, indirect alterations through formation of reactive oxygen species that may oxidize DNA bases and also induce DNA breaks. In a scenario where such alterations may facilitate the carcinogenic process, DNA repair systems are critical to suppress malignant transformation. There are different DNA repair systems inside the cells, which may repair a variety of DNA lesions, since mismatch base pairing formation during replication process, oxidized DNA bases, bulky addictions, intra and interstrand damages and single and double strand breaks. The main DNA repair systems are: Base excision repair (BER), Nucleotide Excision Repair (NER), Mismatch Repair (MMR), Homologous Repair (HR) and Non-Homologous End-Joinning Repair (NHEJ) [137].

The critical role of DNA repair systems in cancer suppression is observed in a diversity of cancer predisposition syndromes which the main cause is due to mutations in DNA repair genes. Mutations in genes of nucleotide excision repair (NER), which preferentially corrects UV damages, caused the so-called *Xeroderma Pigmentosum* syndrome. The affected individuals have a one thousand fold greater chances of developing skin cancer under the age of 20 years [138], including melanomas, compared to DNA repair proficient individuals.

As discussed above, genetic variants that may alter the functionality of DNA repair genes, mainly genes from NER repair systems, may also modulate the susceptibility for melanoma. DNA repair systems were pointed as a functional network that could contribute to melanocyte carcinogenesis process by complete inactivating (such as in XP patients) or by differential functionality due to genetic variants associated with environmental factors such as UV exposure. However, this intuitive thought regarding the role of DNA repair systems restrict to the initials steps of melanoma development has changed in the last years. A study published in 2008 [139] has suggested a new role of DNA repair systems in melanoma progression and metastasis. Aiming at the better understanding of primary melanoma to metastasis progression, the authors used a collection of frozen primary melanomas to study their gene expression by microarray. Those patients that had primary melanomas included in the study had a follow up for four years. After that, 26 of 60 patients showed metastasis while the other 34 patients did not. Gene expression of primary melanomas that originated metastasis (called M+ by the authors) was compared with the gene expression of primary melanomas that did not originate metastasis (M-). The results indicated a high and robust significant expression of genes involved with DNA replication ($p = 4.02 \times 10^{-14}$) and DNA repair genes ($p = 1.4 \times 10^{-16}$) in those M+ primary melanomas. Besides the high expression of such class of genes, a strong correlation with Breslow index was also observed. To certain genes, its high expression was positively correlated to tumor thickness. To genes with low expression in M+ primary melanomas compared to M- melanomas, a negative correlation with tumor thickness was observed.

The study indentified a total of 48 genes with higher expression in M+, which are related to DNA repair genes and genes related to maintenance of genetic stability in replication process [139]. Among those genes, genes from the BER repair systems (a repair system strongly related to repair oxidized bases and single strand breaks) such as *OGG1* and *EXO1* were high expressed. A possible biological interpretation is that the high expression of these genes could facilitate tumor growth and invasiveness, since base oxidation is the most frequent spontaneous and deleterious lesions observed in actively replicating cells. Overexpression of genes of

MMR repair systems was also observed. Since the inactivation of the MMR system leads to DNA damage hypersensitivity, it is likely that over-expression of the MMR system could improve the cellular resistance to DNA lesions. However, the main results indicate an over-expression of genes related to rescue of stalled DNA replication forks, DNA double strand breaks and interstrand crosslink repair. These processes, acting on the S-phase checkpoint and post-replicative repair mechanisms, are essential for cell proliferation and survival by correcting eventual damages and replicative stress, such as cancer cells may exhibit higher rate of DNA synthesis. Thus, by maintaining an elevate activity of such DNA repair systems and checkpoints in S-phase during replicative stress, metastatic cancer cells can grow and survive, and further be resistant to chemotherapy.

As example, a gene overexpressed in M+ melanomas was *TOP2A*, an enzyme that plays a role in replication and chromosome segregation by solving torsional stress [140]. Moreover, cells over-expressing *TOP2A* were more resistant to chemotherapeutic drugs such as alkylating agents [141]. Finally, over-expression of genes related to FANC-BRCA pathways (genes acting in double strand breaks repair and rescue of blocked replication forks) in melanomas M+ suggest the critical role that these process exerts on keeping the genetic stability in cancer cells with metastatic fitness. These findings demonstrate an important duality of DNA repair genes in tumor progression. First, the development of malignant cells from normal cells has been credited to a reduction or lack of DNA repair genes, thereby allowing the accumulation of mutations and subsequent transformation of the cells. This concept is well documented, since the relationship of individuals with genetic predisposition to certain tumors, where such predisposition may be is attributed to genes related to DNA repair or pathways that do support to DNA repair pathways [142]. However, at some point in the progression of melanoma, genetic stability appears to be a crucial factor to ensure that the tumor cells maintain the genetic repertoire that guarantees the ability of invasion and metastasis. Thus, melanoma cells with higher expression of DNA repair genes, would have greater capacity for metastasis due to maintenance of genetic capability. The genetic stability suggested [139] is not limited to the repair genes. Genes linked to telomere stability, as well as genes that ensure proper chromosome separations were also highly expressed in melanomas M+. Another important implication based on the results is that high expression of repair gene may be responsible for the characteristic low response of metastatic melanoma to chemotherapy, since many of the chemotherapeutic agents used to treat melanoma act causing DNA damage. It was also observed a higher expression of genes correlated to resistance to chemotherapeutic agents such as cisplatin and dacarbazine (e.g., *BRCA1, XRCC5, XRCC6*). In addition, other genes related to the maintenance of DNA replication machinery were also highly expressed, leading to translesion replication, thereby preventing the apoptosis signal being secondary to the arrest of DNA/RNA polymerase.

Following studies, confirmed the high expression of FANC DNA repair genes in melanoma samples when compared to normal skin and non-melanoma skin cancers [143]. Moreover, there is a positive correlation regarding FANC genes and melanoma thickness by Breslow index. Conversely, NER genes were significantly decreased in melanomas, albeit its expression was not correlated with melanoma thickness. Immunohistochemistry of independent melanoma and non-melanoma skin cancers, confirmed the results previous discovered in gene expression regarding FANC genes and melanomas. Interestingly, down regulation of NER genes may have contributed to initial steps of melanomagenesis, however, the high expression of gene products of DNA repair pathways, mainly those regarding to solve double strand breaks, may be related to melanoma progression.

In another study, expression of DNA repair genes was associated with prognosis, disease relapse, tumor thickness and response to chemotherapy in melanomas [144]. In that study, high expression of genes *RAD51, RAD52 and TOP2A* was significantly associated to poor relapse-free survival. Expression of *RAD51* was 1.22 times greater in tumors from patients who relapsed versus those who did not; the fold changes between tumors from relapsers and non-relapsers for *RAD52* and *TOP2A* were 1.16 and 1.12 respectively. *RAD54B, RAD52, TOP2A* and *RAD51* were also overexpressed in tumours from patients who died versus surviving patients. As reported by the studies cited above [139;143], expression of DNA repair genes was also correlated with tumor thickness and to mitotic rate. Finally, when the chemotherapy response was analyzed, *RAD51* and *TOP2A* had significantly higher expression in tumors from non-responders compared to responders [144]. Finally, the results described point to new methods for melanoma treatment, where in addition to chemotherapy and radiotherapy for melanoma cells, the development of new drugs capable to modify the activity of proteins related to DNA repair, may increase the efficiency of treatment.

4.2.5. PAX3 – Back to stemness?

The *PAX* family genes (from Paired Box) consist of transcriptional factors highly conserved and also essential to development of different tissues during embryogenesis as well as essential to maintenance of stem cells in the adult organism. Indeed, *PAX* genes are related to regulation of several processes such as proliferation, migration, avoiding apoptosis and sustaining stemness phenotype in undifferentiated cells. There are nine PAX proteins, of which PAX3 is a particularly interesting protein for its function in regulating the development of melanocytes and other cell types.

Together with SOX10, PAX3 regulate transcription of MITF [145] and c-RET [146] in melanocytes. PAX3 is a key transcription factor during the development of the neural crest and its derivatives in the embryo. The neural crest cells detach from the dorsal neural epithelium and give origin to a diverse set of cells, including melanocytes. PAX3 starts its expression in neural crest precursors that are further committed with melanocytic cells lineage, such as melanoblasts [147]. PAX3 exerts its activity by expressing MITF and repressing Dct (Dopachrome-tautomerase), thus leading to an undifferentiated cell state [148]. When MITF levels reach a threshold, a complex consisting of MITF and β-catenin binds to Dct promoter, abolishing PAX3 inhibition, which leads to Dct expression and melanocyte differentiation. It is thought that upon terminal differentiation, the expression of PAX3 is reduced as suggested by initial studies that reported no expression of PAX3 in normal skin melanocytes [148;149] PAX3 expression has been described in nevi, in most primary melanoma tumors, melanoma cell lines [150-152]. The first study described the expression of PAX3 in 8/8 melanoma cell lines [150]. The study also showed that PAX3 was commonly expressed in primary melanoma samples (21/58) but significantly less frequently in benign pigmented lesions (9/75). However, the following studies found PAX3 expression in melanoblasts localized in hair follicles and also in mature melanocytes in hair follicles, in 100% of the nevi examined, 94% of primary melanomas and in 90% of metastatic melanomas examined [151;152].

A most complete study performed in melanocytic lesions [152], analyzed PAX3 expression in normal skin, nevi, primary melanoma and melanoma metastases by immunohistochemistry. PAX3 was expressed in all samples and in normal cells. PAX3 expression showed a pattern of distribution characteristic of melanocytes (at epidermal-dermal boundary and along the hair follicle). Moreover, PAX3-positive cells were fewer and had a weaker staining in normal skin, as compared to nevi and melanomas. Co-expression of PAX3 with MITF was also observed in all samples, however, in normal skin some cells expressed only MITF, highlighting the differences in melanocyte phenotype. PAX3-positive cells were also co-stained with markers of less or more melanocyte differentiation, such as HES1 and Melan-A respectively. The samples indicated PAX3-positive cells co-stained with either markers, showing then a variable differentiation status of epidermal and follicular melanocytes, however a higher proportion of PAX3 and Melan-A positive cells. Finally, to further describe the phenotype of PAX3-positive melanocytes and melanoma cells, antiapoptotic factor BCL2L1 and melanoma progression marker MCAM were also analyzed in those cells. Regarding BCL2L1, a high similar proportion of PAX3-positive cells were also BCL2L1 positive cells, in all samples, with exception of melanoma metastases. These results suggest a role for PAX3 in regulation of survival of melanocytes and melanomas. Regarding MCAM, all melanocytic lesions showed its expression. Co-staining of MCAM and PAX3 increased in proportion from nevi to primary melanoma to melanomas metastases. As suggested above, PAX3 also plays a role in regulating genes involved in protecting cancer cells from apoptosis, as indicated by studies where the down-regulation of PAX3 increased the levels of apoptosis [153;154]. One of the mechanisms by which PAX3 may be involved with resistance to apoptosis resides in the fact that PAX3 interacts with the enhancer element of Bcl-XL gene, triggering its activation [155]. Another mechanism described for the anti-apoptotic role of PAX3 is via the regulation of tumor supressor PTEN [156]. In melanoma cells, the down regulation of PAX3 showed a dose-dependent reduction of proliferation and induction of apoptosis when cells were treated with cisplatin [157]. Indeed, PAX3 down-regulation lead to increase in p53 protein and also caspase3 (a critical protein involved with apoptosis).

Functional studies have clarified the PAX3 function on melanocytes/melanomas [158]. PAX3, acting synergistically with SOX10, play a role in the regulation of MET expression. MET is a transmembrane receptor tyrosine kinase activated by Hepatocyte Growth Factor (HGF) and plays a role in normal development and in cell migration, growth, survival, differentiation, angiogenesis [159]. The HGF-MET pathway is involved in melanocyte biology acting on survival and maintenance of specific genes. MET is commonly over-expressed in melanoma and is associated with a more aggressive phenotype in terms of invasion and metastasis [160;161]. A strong correlation of expression of MET with PAX3 and SOX10 in primary melanomas was observed [158]. Thus, the expression of PAX3 may facilitate melanoma progression and metastasis through the expression of MET, a classical proto-oncogene involved in invasion, metastasis, resistance of apoptosis, and tumor cell expansion.

PAX3 activities as a transcription factor were also analyzed by comparing melanocytic and melanoma cell lines [162]. Initially, PAX3 binding to promoter regions of specific genes was analyzed and a enrichment of binding in melanoma cells was observed in genes such as HES1, SOX9 and NES (genes related to maintenance of stemness phenotype), CCNA2 and TPD52 (genes related to proliferation), BCL2L1, PTEN and TGFB1 (genes related to survival) and MCAM, CSPG4 and CXCR4 (genes related to migration). Conversely, in melanocytic cell lines, enrichment of PAX3 binding was just observed in HES1, SOX9, MCAM, TGFB1 and CSPG4, however quantitative analysis indicated lower PAX3 binding activity in melanocyte promoters, as compared to melanomas. Finally, a correlation of PAX3 promoter binding levels in melanocyte/melanoma cell line with gene expression of those genes indicated up-regulation of SOX9, NES, CCNA2, TPD52, TGFB1, MCAM, CSPG4 and CXCR4 in melanoma. Regarding BCL2L1 and PTEN, lower levels were observed in melanoma. In general, the study described a correlation between PAX3 binding to the target gene and its expression level, identified possible PAX3-regulated genes and also suggested the differential activity of PAX3 in transcriptional activity in melanocytes and melanoma cells. The interpretation of the results indicates critical features of the PAX3 function. Those genes up-regulated are genes related to cancer progression (SOX9 and NES), genes involved with cell motility, spread and metastatic potential (MCAM, CSPG4 and CXCR4) and with proliferation (TPD52). Moreover, down regulation of PTEN also contributes to melanoma progression due to tumor suppression activity of PTEN. Decreased of CDK2, BCL2 and MelanA (a melanocyte differentiation marker) gene expression and inhibition of cell growth was observed with PAX3 knock-down in melanoma cell lines, although the results were strongly cell line dependent [157]. Moreover, an induced cell cycle arrest in S and G2/M phases and increase in apoptosis was also observed in PAX3 knock-down melanoma cells, and in one cell line. Silencing of PAX3 induced terminal differentiation.

In general, there is convincing evidence that PAX3 is expressed in melanomas and in melanocytic lesions, such as nevi. Indeed, PAX3 expression in melanomas may play a role in progression regulating processes such as survival, proliferation, metastases and participating in the maintenance of stemness. However, PAX3 seems expressed in a subset of differentiated melanocytes. Further clarification of PAX3 function in these cells is necessary. Environmental stimuli may be related to PAX3 expression in melanocytic lesions, as reported by up-regulation of PAX3 under UV-induced loss of TFG-β signaling from keratinocytes [163]. Thus, PAX3 may be a good target gene to understanding the melanomagenesis process and more studies regarding its function are required.

4.2.6 TP53 gene and melanoma – What is its function?

The *TP53* gene is thought to be the "guardian of the genome" due to its pleiotropic function in protecting cells from genotoxic events, acting on cell cycle control, DNA repair and also triggering apoptosis. In general, *TP53* is frequently mutated in a diversity of cancer types and its inactivation confers advantage to tumor initiation and progression. Regarding the sources of mutagenic agents to TP53, sun exposure is a potent mechanism of induction of *TP53* mutations as suggested by the frequent occurrence of such mutations in skin cancers such as basal cell carcinomas (BCC) and squamous cell carcinomas (SCC). In such skin cancers, UV-related mutations (C to T and CC to TT transitions) are frequently described in *TP53* and in other genes, confirming then the role of UV exposure in skin cancers. As melanocytes from exposed skin areas have UV-exposure as the major environmental factor to its tumorigenesis, one could expect a high frequency of UV-related mutations in *TP53* in melanomas, as those found in the melanoma genome [19] and *PTEN* gene [90].

However, the proportion of primary melanomas harboring *TP53* mutations is frequently low, around 7% of melanoma samples, although ranging from 0 to 24% between individual studies [38]. Data from meta-analysis of 645 melanoma specimens showed that only 13.2% were *TP53* mutants, and more than half were UV signature changes [164]. Curiously, *TP53* mutations have been described in some nevi and in melanomas from XP patients [165]. In fact, on one hand *TP53* inactivating mutations play a role in cancer progression, however, on the other hand, TP53 mutations in melanomas are frequently low. With this duality in mind, interesting question arises: What is the function of *TP53* in melanoma initiation and progression? Moreover, is there a positive pressure to keep wild-type *TP53* in melanomas? Recent functional studies start to address these questions. Indeed, inactivation of p53 pathway may be relevant for melanocyte transformation [166]. Study from melanocytes indicated that murine cells engineered to have high levels of p53 developed less pigmented lesions, primary melanomas and metastases [167]. Besides this feature, melanomas from elevated p53 levels had lower size and growth rate, indicating a role for p53 as a suppressor of tumor development. Regarding human melanocytes and melanoma cells, pharmacological activation of p53 by a specific inhibitor of HDM-2, led cells to cell cycle arrest in low doses and to apoptosis in high doses. In addition, chemical activation of p53 in primary human melanocytes and melanoma cells demonstrated that these cells were far more sensitive to cell cycle arrest than to apoptosis. Moreover, *CDKN1A* (also known as p21) was identified as the predominant network operating in such tumor suppressor activity in melanocytes and melanomas [167]. In summary, such study indicated an anti-proliferative role of p53, both *in vivo* and *in vitro*, as the preferential mode for tumor suppression in melanocytes, indicating then the "need" for p53 supression to allow melanomagenesis. However, as mutations are infrequent in *TP53* from melanomas, a possible way to inactivate p53 pathway is by regulating its activity. One possible mechanism for the inactivation of the p53 pathway in melanoma may be attributed to mutations in the *CDKN2A* locus. As discussed above, *CDKN2A* is frequently mutated, lost or even epigenetically silenced in melanomas. Besides p16 protein, the locus also codes for p14ARF protein, which is regulates HDM-2 protein, the classical negative regulator of p53. Thus, one manner to contribute to melanoma progression through inactivation of p53-dependent pathways is by inactivation of p14 protein, or even by amplification of *HDM-2* gene. Under both circumstances, abundance of p53 protein decreases. However, p14 mutations are frequently associated with familial melanomas, which does not explain the somatic cases, *HDM-2* amplification in melanomas occurs in a very low frequency (ranging 3 to 5% - [168]) and high-level expression of wild-type p53 can be found in melanoma tissues and cell lines [169].

Some reports have indicated that high expression of p53 can be found in both melanoma samples and melanoma cell lines. In addition, others reports have also indicated that this high expression does not correlate with p53 functionality. Melanoma cell lines harboring wild-type p53 showed transcriptional inactivity [169], a feature of melanoma cell lines that corroborates with data showing different gene expression of p53 targets in melanomas compared with nevi, strongly suggesting a dysfunctional p53 [166]. Moreover, melanoma cell lines with wild-type p53 shows an absent p53 DNA-binding activity [170]. All these reports indicate that downstream mechanisms could be operating to down-regulate p53 pathway in melanomas. One of the challenges of melanoma genetics in the coming years is to identify and characterize those downstream mechanisms, which certainly will improve our knowledge about p53 dysfunction in melanoma biology as well as identifying possible windows for melanoma treatment. There are at this moment critical candidates genes to act as negative regulator of p53 activity. Proteins such as iASPP (Inhibitor of apoptosis-stimulating protein of p53) [171], delta Np73 [172], YB-1 [173] and Parc protein [174] has been described as p53 inhibitors. Alternatively, posttranslational modifications may also be responsible to p53 transcriptional silencing, such as phosphorylation, acetylation, methylation, sumoylation and neddlyation. Some findings have suggested that accumulation and increase in wild type p53 expression during melanoma progression may be indicative of dysfunctional p53 activity, reflecting posttranslational p53 modifications. Cytoplasmatic functions of transcriptionally inactive p53 have also emerged as a good hypothesis to a new p53 activity in either limit or promote tumor growth [175].

Additional reports have also confirmed the p53 transcriptional inability in melanomas [176]. The results from such study showed that p53 downstream genes involved in apoptosis have low expression in melanoma metastases and melanoma cell lines. Conversely, genes involved with cell cycle were over-expressed in melanoma cell lines. Curiously, little difference between melanomas with wild-type p53 and mutant p53 could be observed regarding expression of p53 target genes, which confirm the notion that possible negative regulators are involved in the suppression of the p53 pathway. Even with down-regulation of p53 by using short-harpin method, there was limited effect on p53 target genes in p53 wild-type melanomas, however to melanocytes, p53 inhibition leads to alteration of several p53-dependent transcripts. An interesting feature observed was related to the proliferative capacity in melanocytes and melanomas, down regulation of p53 in melanocytes resulted in a gene expression similar to melanomas and increased proliferation rates while in melanomas, down regulation of p53 contributed to decreased proliferation, corroborating the results described by an independent study [177] (discussed below).

Although melanomas may have an inability to exert p53 full transcriptional capability, the p53 accumulation observed in such melanomas may still have basal activity. A central question is to understand the role of this basal p53 transcriptional activity in progression of melanomas. Recent functional studies start to address this interesting question. Melanoma cells are described as largely adapted to certain stress such as endoplasmic reticulum (ER) stress [178], a situation where melanomas acquire resistance to ER stress-induced apoptosis as well as resistance to chemotherapy [179]. This adaptative response may be attributed to expression of Mcl-1 protein, which acts antagonizing the pro-apoptotic proteins PUMA and NOXA. Under ER stress, melanoma cells accumulate p53, which in turn (even in basal activity) induces the transcription of the microRNA miR149* [180]. The p53-dependent expression of miR149* decrease the activity of GSK3α, resulting in Mcl-1 increase and consequent resistance to apoptosis. Moreover, decrease of miR149* elevated the rate of cell death in these melanoma cells and inhibited melanoma growth in a xenograft model. Finally, elevated expression of miR149 was found in melanoma samples, associated with decrease of GSK3α and increase of Mcl-1.

Other elegant functional study indicated critical features of p53 role in melanocytes and melanoma cells [177]. First, the study indicated that p53 may be dispensable for melanoma cells due to lack of increase in DNA damage and enhanced proliferative potential in p53 depleted cells. Conversely, depletion of p53 in melanocytes increased mitotic defects. This last result is consistent with animal models in which genetic depletion of p53 cooperates with cell transformation [167]. Indeed, in melanoma cells p53 is kept in a basal state of functionality. This basal activity showed to be critical to melanoma growth, as: (i) basal p53 activity leads to HDM-2 expression, which in turn keeps the basal levels of p53; (ii) this basal level of p53 avoids the activation of a p53-dependent pro-senescence program; (iii) in a basal state, p53 does not induce expression of p21, which in turn does not inhibits E2F1. The following E2F1 activation contributes to melanoma cell proliferation; (iv) expression of HMD-2 leads to activation of E2F1 in a p53-independet manner, contributing to melanoma cell proliferation. Instead, the "so-called" HDM-2 addiction in melanoma cells seems not to be related to melanocytes due to maintenance of viability and absence of senescence when p53 is activated by MDM-2 depletion. In summary, this study [177] elucidates new functions of the p53-HDM-2 axis in melanomas. Besides, the p53-HDM-2 axis in melanomas is now suggested as a promising target for melanoma treatment, since the use of specific HDM-2 antagonist rescues the p53 activity, leading to melanoma growth suppression and melanoma cell death [181].

The identification of negative p53 regulators that keep p53 pathway dysfunctional seems critical for a better understanding of the involvement of p53-dependent pathways in melanomagenesis and progression. Further functional studies will elucidate the intriguing questions regarding the real function of p53 to melanoma biology: Why has TP53 low frequency of mutations? How is p53 basal state maintained? What are p53 functions in melanomas?

4.2.7. MicroRNAs and melanoma – Another level of gene expression in melanomas

MicroRNAs (miRNAs) are small non-coding RNAs (21–23 nucleotides) encoded in the genome of plants, invertebrates, and vertebrates. These small molecules bind imperfectly to the 3′ untranslated (3′UTR) regions of target messenger RNAs (mRNAs) thus, miRNAs are central regulators of gene expression and can act both in a positive and a negative way to control protein levels in the cell. More than a thousand miRNAs exist in the human genome and each one can potentially regulate hundreds of mRNAs. Target prediction algorithms can be helpful in identifying potential mRNA targets of the miRNA of interest and further they should be validated by functional studies [182]. MicroRNAs play an important role in many cellular processes, such as differentiation, proliferation, apoptosis, and stress response. Additionally, they are key regulators in many diseases, including cancer [183]. These molecules regulate pathways in cancer by targeting various oncogenes and tumor suppressors and there is an increasing body of evidence suggesting that genomic instability regions harbor miRNA genes [184]. The first study to associate genomic instability regions, miRNAs and cancer was published in 2002 [185]. The authors found frequent deletions at 13q14 involving miR-15 and miR-16 genes in B-cell from chronic lymphocytic leukaemia. Since then, hundreds miRNAs have been reported acting as oncogenes or tumour suppressor genes in a wide variety of cancers [for review 183]. The first miRNAs described as involved in cancer formation was miR-let-7 [186] and further the family of miRs let 7a and let 7b were reported to play a role in melanomas [for review 187]. For example, miR-let 7-b acts as a negative regulator of melanoma cell proliferation via regulation of cyclin D1, whereas miR-let-7a was demonstrated to regulate the expression of integrin-β3 and the Ras [188]. So, modulation of miRNA expression is increasingly thought to be an important mechanism by which tumour suppressor proteins and oncoproteins exert some of their effects. Studies assessing the role of miRNAs in melanomas are still very recent and many efforts have been made to identify the 'melano-miRs'. Despite the increasing number of studies (NCBI searching in September 2012 retrieved 162 results) a small number of miRNAs were identified to regulate genes involved specifically in melanomagenesis and some of them will be discussed here.

The linking between expression of miR-137 and *MITF* expression, a crucial gene involved in melanomas and already presented above have been described [189]. However, *MITF* seems to be also regulated by miR-182, miR-148, and miR-340, respectively [190;191]. Additionally, melanoma tumors preferentially express *MITF* mRNA isoforms with shorter 3′UTR, "to avoid" miRNA post-transcriptional regulation. Although the translation of the transcripts can be regulated by miRNAs the transcriptional regulation of miRNAs is still poorly known [192]. Some studies have searched for miRNA promoters that are specific to melanoma progression [193]. In an opposite way, the authors identified miRNAs that are specifically regulated by *MITF* transcription factor/oncoprotein and identified miR-146a, miR-221/222 and miR-363 as MITF-regulated. This high-throughput identification of miRNA promoters and enhancer regulatory elements sheds light on evolution of miRNA transcription and permits rapid identification of transcriptional networks of miRNAs, inclusive in melanomas. Moreover, expression of *MITF* has been recently shown to be involved in the regulation of DICER, the central regulator of miRNA maturation and key enzyme involved in the formation of the RNA-induced silencing complex. MITF binds and activates a conserved regulatory element upstream of DICER's transcriptional start site upon melanocyte differentiation [194]. Moreover, when DICER was knocked out, melanocytes failed to survive [194].

Besides miRNAs "*MITF* regulators" or miRNAs "regulated by MITF", other molecules with known target genes in melanoma are also regulated by miRNAs. Recently an interesting review focusing on miRNAs that act in major pathways of formation of melanomas: RAS-RAF-MEK-ERK, $p16^{INK4A}$-CDK4-RB, PIK3-AKT and the MITF pathway was published [195]. As cited, mutation $BRaf^{V600E}$ occurs in 50–70% of sporadic melanomas which active constitutively the MEK/ERK signaling pathway, promoting tumor progression and metastasis through enhanced cell proliferation, survival, motility and invasion. Two studies have investigated the correlation between B-Raf mutational status and miRNA expression in melanomas and only one study linking three miRNAs to BRaf^{V600E} [196]. Recently, [197] a network of 420 miRNAs deregulated in B-Raf/MKK/ERK pathway in melanoma cells whereas majority of which modulate the expression of key cancer regulatory genes and functions was identified. In addition to MEK/ERK pathway, new insights about miRNAs and p16^{INK4A}-CDK4-RB pathway have been described. The mains senescence pathway associated with miRNAs are p53/p21 and p16/Rb pathways [for review 198]. Several miRNAs have been shown to be involved in the regulation of pathways involved in cellular senescence exerting negative effects on cell cycle progression, such as E2F family of transcription factors acting in cell cycle [198-200]. Recent studies reported that E2F1 to E2F3 are targets of several miRNAs, such as miR-34a [201]. In addition, miR-205 in human melanoma cells induces senescence by targeting E2F1 [202] and miR-203 also induces senescence by targeting E2F3 in melanoma cells [203]. Therefore, miRNA/E2F interaction is an important mechanism that leads melanomas cells to senescence.

Other studies have identified a cluster of miRNAs that are either involved in melanomagenesis or predictors of survival. A study has identified the miR-506–514 cluster as a transforming oncogene that regulates melanoma progression and melanocyte transformation [204]. Moreover, the authors showed that ectopic expression of this cluster in melanocytes was sufficient to transform them, activating cell growth, cell proliferation and migration/invasion along with inhibiting apoptosis. Although this study did not identify any direct gene targets of the miRNAs, further investigation is necessary because this cluster may reveal pathways that contribute to both the initiation and the maintenance of melanoma. As presented above, studies showed the increased expression of the miR-221/222 cluster associated with melanoma progression [for review 205]. A cascade involving *PLZF* transcription factor as a repressor of miR-221 and miR-222 by direct binding to their putative regulatory region was described [206]. These miRNAs regulate directly *KIT* and *CDKN1B*, respectively resulting in cell cycle inhibition and differentiation. Thus, over-expression of these miRNAs cluster increases proliferation and tumourigenesis and activates invasion/migration in melanomas.

Approaches investigating miRNAs expression are also based on gene silencing by CpG methylation. Since miRNAs precursor genes are usually within regions of coding genes (intron sequences, for example), dysfunction of these protein-coding genes by epigenetic mechanisms may also be expected to cause aberrant regulation of the miRNA target genes [207]. For example, miRNA-34a is highly methylated in melanoma cell lines and primary tumors and additionally, it was described that *MET* transcript is miRNA-34a target [for review 188]. Besides miR-34a, the miR-34b, belonging to the same family, seems to have an important effect on melanomas. A group of epigenetically regulated miRNA genes in melanoma cells, and confirmed the upstream hypermethylated CpG island sequences of several miRNAs genes in cell lines derived from different stages of melanoma, but not in melanocytes and keratinocytes was identifies [208]. Among them, miR-34b expression reduced cell invasion and motility rates of melanoma cell lines. After deep sequencing, the authors identified network modules that are potentially regulated by miR-34b, and which suggest a mechanism for the role of miR-34b in regulating normal cell motility and cytokinesis. Additionally, this same group identified the epigenetic regulation of miR-375 in human melanomas. Melanoma cells were treated with one demethylating agent (5-aza-2'-deoxycytidine) and it was identified the miR-375 highly methylated. Ectopic expression of miR-375 inhibited melanoma cell proliferation, invasion, and cell motility, and induced cell shape changes, suggesting that miR-375 may have an important function in the development and progression of human melanomas [209].

All of these studies investigated the biological functions of miRNAs and their contribution to melanomagenesis. Other studies have attempted to identify miRNAs signatures for diagnostic and prognostic, melanoma progression by comparing the expression profiles in different stages of transformation, and others focused on specific pathways. Some of these studies will be presented here. In 2007, assays were performed using the well established NCI-60 cancer cell line panel and normal tissue [210]. The study was able to discriminate between the malignancies, including melanomas cell lines whereas miR-146, miR-204 and miR-211 miRNAs shown to be highly expressed in melanomas. Large cohorts of miRNAs associated with malignant transformation as well as with the progression and with metastatic colonization in melanocytes and subsets of melanoma cell lines also was identified [211]. Subsequently, down regulation of miRNA-200c in melanocytes, melanoma cell lines, and patient samples could be reported, whereas miRNA-205 and miRNA-23b were markedly reduced among patient samples [212]. In contrast, miR-146a and miR-155 were upregulated in all analyzed patients but none of the cell lines. Using deep sequencing approach of a diverse set of melanoma and pigment cell libraries it was identified 539 known mature sequences along with the prediction of 279 novel miRNAs candidates [213]. Some of these novel candidate miRNAs may be specific to the melanocytic lineage and as such could be used as biomarkers in the early detection of distant metastases by measuring the circulating levels in blood. The expression of 611 miRNAs in 59 metastatic specimens was profiled and the authors were able to identify a "miRNA classifier" consisting of miR-150, miR-342-3p, miR-455-3p, miR-145, miR-155 and miR-497 that were considered predictors of post-recurrence survival [214]. Similarly the analyses of the miRNA expression profiling from melanoma lymph node metastases reported a unique signature consisting of down regulation of miR-191, combined with up regulation of miR-193a, miR-193b, miR-365, miR-338 and let-7. Together, this miRNAs also serves as predictors of short-term survival in melanoma patients [215]. These findings indicate that miRNAs are differentially expressed in melanoma subtypes and that their dysfunction can be impacted by inherited gene variants, supporting the hypothesis that miRNA dysfunction reflects biological differences in melanoma. Recently, the use of microarray analysis of formalin-fixed and paraffin-embedded samples from different stages of melanomagenesis identified differentially expressed microRNAs [216]. The miR-203 and miR-205 were differentially expressed between primary and metastatic melanomas and functional *in vitro* assays validated this found. So, these results indicated that differentially expressed miRNAs that could be useful as diagnostic or prognostic markers for melanoma.

As such, miRNAs represent a new class of molecules that might prove to be powerful cancer biomarkers useful in future staging systems and used as stratification criteria in clinical trials as well as treatment of patients with disseminated disease. It was demonstrated that miR-214 is over-expressed in metastatic melanoma cell lines as well as tumor specimens. MiR-214 regulates the expression of two transcription factors, AP-2c and AP-2a [217]. These molecules have been previously shown to play major roles in melanoma metastasis via regulation of genes involved in invasion and angiogenesis. Histological examination of skin biopsies remains the standard method for melanoma diagnosis and prognosis. Significant morphological overlap between benign and malignant lesions complicates diagnosis, and tumour thickness is not always an accurate predictor of prognosis. For purpose of clinical management, the microRNA profiling of clinical melanoma subtypes samples considering the somatic and inherited mutations associated with melanomas, including the presence of one variant in a miRNA binding site in the 3'UTR of the *KRAS* oncogene has been evaluated [218]. The authors showed that miR-142-3p, miR-486, miR-214, miR-218, miR-362, miR-650 and miR-31 were significantly correlated with acral as compared to non-acral melanomas. In addition, the *KRAS*-variant was enriched in non-acral melanoma and that miR-137 under expression was significantly associated with melanomas with the *KRAS*-variant. Recently, it was develop one *in situ* measurement methodology to evaluate the miR-205 in a cohort of human melanomas [219]. Based on previous findings, the authors hypothesized that decreased miR-205 would be associated with more aggressive tumors. So, multiplexing miR-205 qISH (quantitative *in situ* hybridization) with immunofluorescent assessment of S100/GP100 (melanocytic markers), the authors evaluated quantitatively the miR-205 expression. Outcome was assessed on the Yale Melanoma Discovery Cohort consisting of 105 primary melanoma specimens and then, validated the results on an independent set of 206 primary melanomas. Measurement of melanoma cell miR-205 levels shows a significantly shorter melanoma-specific survival in patients with their low expression and it was significantly independent of stage, age, gender, and Breslow depth. Low levels of miR-205 expression in melanoma cell quantified by ISH show worse outcome, supporting the role of miR-205 as a tumor suppressor miRNA. This promising result indicates that the quantification of miR-205 *in situ* suggests its potential use for future prognostic or predictive models. Studies investigating the various roles of miRNAs in melanocytes and melanoma are gaining momentum and should continue to provide fertile ground for both clinical and basic research.

5. Conclusions

In this chapter we proposed to discuss the melanoma genetics, starting from the genes that may confer susceptibility to the genes that may be involved with progression. Moreover, we addressed the already known genes (here called as "old genetics") as well as new genes that have been discovered as involved in melanoma (here called as "new genetics). It is noteworthy that the new technologies such as GWAS and deep-sequencing have improved our knowledge about melanoma genetics. Nowadays we have critical information about the disease, such as the clear involvement of UV in carcinogenic process and the many pathways that contribute significantly to it. As could be observed, conversely to other cancer types where single genes has great impact on susceptibility and progression, such as BRCA in breast and ovarian, mismatch repair pathways and colorectal cancer or *TP53* to Li-Fraumeni syndrome, a single gene cannot be pointed as "the melanoma gene". Huge amplitude of genetic pathways may be related to melanoma progression and this same amplitude may be responsible for melanoma metastasis and chemoresistance, making this neoplasia of complex management. However, in a biologist point of view such huge amplitude makes this neoplasia fascinating to understand, challenging researchers to approach the problem in creative ways.

It is tempting to assume that the more we know about melanoma biology, including melanoma genetics, much more efficacious melanoma prevention and treatment will be. Heterogeneity within the very same tumor will certainly hamper treatment. We will need to take it in account in the days of personalized medicine. To this, improvement of technologies, coordinated studies of gene-environment interactions, allied to functional studies and critical clinical trials, will be necessary for the adequate translation of this body of information into patient benefit.

Acknowledgements

The authors thank Cristina Grandal for helping with figures editing.

Author details

Guilherme Francisco[1,2], Priscila Daniele Ramos Cirilo[1,2], Fernanda Toledo Gonçalves[3], Tharcísio Citrângulo Tortelli Junior[1,2] and Roger Chammas[1,2]

*Address all correspondence to: guilherme@lim24.fm.usp.br

*Address all correspondence to: rchammas@usp.br

1 Department of Radiology and Oncology, School of Medicine, University of São Paulo, Brazil

2 Center of Translational Research in Oncology, São Paulo State Cancer Institute (ICESP), São Paulo, Brazil

3 Department of Ethical and Legal Medicine, School of Medicine, University of São Paulo, Brazil

References

[1] Jhappan C, Noonan FP, Merlino G. Ultraviolet radiation and cutaneous malignant melanoma. Oncogene 2003; 22:3099-112.

[2] Costa RM, Chiganças V, Galhardo R da S, Carvalho H, Menck CF. The eukaryotic nucleotide excision repair pathway. Biochimie 2003;85(11):1083-99.

[3] Kadekaro AL, Kavanagh RJ, Wakamatsu K, Ito S, Pipitone MA, Abdel-Malek ZA. Cutaneous photobiology. The melanocyte vs. the sun: who will win the final round? Pigment Cell Res 2003; 16:434-47.

[4] Brash DE, Ziegler A, Jonason AS, Simon JA, Kunala S, Leffell DJ. Sunlight and sunburn in human skin cancer: p53, apoptosis, and tumor promotion. J Investig Dermatol Symp Proc 1996; 1:136-42.

[5] You YH, Lee DH, Yoon JH, Nakajima S, Yasui A, Pfeifer GP. Cyclobutane pyrimidine dimers are responsible for the vast majority of mutations induced by UVB irradiation in mammalian cells. J Biol Chem 2001; 276:44688-94.

[6] Cleaver JE, Crowley E. UV damage, DNA repair and skin carcinogenesis. Front Biosci 2002; 7:1024-43.

[7] Sander CS, Chang H, Hamm F, Elsner P, Thiele JJ. Role of oxidative stress and the antioxidant network in cutaneous carcinogenesis. Int J Dermatol 2004; 43:326-35.

[8] Nelemans PJ, Groenendal H, Kiemeney LA, Rampen FH, Ruiter DJ, Verbeek AL. Effect of intermittent exposure to sunlight on melanoma risk among indoor workers and sun-sensitive individuals. Environ Health Perspect 1993; 101:252-5.

[9] Weinstock MA, Colditz GA, Willett WC, Stampfer MJ, Bronstein BR, Mihm MC Jr, Speizer FE. Nonfamilial cutaneous melanoma incidence in women associated with sun exposure before 20 years of age. Pediatrics 1989; 84:199-204.

[10] Elwood JM. Melanoma and sun exposure: contrasts between intermittent and chronic exposure. World J Surg 1992; 16:157-65.

[11] Luiz OC, Gianini RJ, Gonçalves FT, Francisco G, Festa-Neto C, Sanches JA, et al. Ethnicity and cutaneous melanoma in the city of Sao Paulo, Brazil: a case-control study. PLoS One 2012;7(4):e36348.

[12] Law MH, Macgregor S, Hayward NK. Melanoma genetics: recent findings take us beyond well-traveled pathways. J Invest Dermatol 2012;132(7):1763-74.

[13] Eskandarpour M, Hashemi J, Kanter L, Ringborg U, Platz A, Hansson J. Frequency of UV-inducible NRAS mutations in melanomas of patients with germline CDKN2A mutations. J Natl Cancer Inst 2003;95(11):790-8.

[14] Mann GJ, Pupo GM, Campain AE, Carter CD, Schramm SJ, Pianova S, et al. BRAF Mutation, NRAS Mutation, and the Absence of an Immune-Related Expressed Gene Profile Predict Poor Outcome in Patients with Stage III Melanoma. J Invest Dermatol 2012 Aug 30. doi: 10.1038/jid.2012.283.

[15] Birck A, Ahrenkiel V, Zeuthen J, Hou-Jensen K, Guldberg P. Mutation and allelic loss of the PTEN/MMAC1 gene in primary and metastatic melanoma biopsies. J Invest Dermatol 2000;114(2):277-80.

[16] Giglia-Mari G, Sarasin A. TP53 mutations in human skin cancers. Hum Mutat 2003;21(3):217-28.

[17] Curtin JA, Fridlyand J, Kageshita T, Patel HN, Busam KJ, Kutzner H, et al. Distinct sets of genetic alterations in melanoma. N Engl J Med 2005;353(20):2135-47.

[18] Greenman C, Stephens P, Smith R, Dalgliesh GL, Hunter C, Bignell G, et al. Patterns of somatic mutation in human cancer genomes. Nature 2007;446(7132):153-8.

[19] Pleasance ED, Cheetham RK, Stephens PJ, McBride DJ, Humphray SJ, Greenman CD, et al. A comprehensive catalogue of somatic mutations from a human cancer genome. Nature 2010;463(7278):191-6.

[20] Sood AK, Saxena R, Groth J, Desouki MM, Cheewakriangkrai C, Rodabaugh KJ, et al. Expression characteristics of prostate-derived Ets factor support a role in breast and prostate cancer progression. Hum Pathol 2007;38(11):1628-38.

[21] Liang C, Feng P, Ku B, Dotan I, Canaani D, Oh BH, Jung JU. Autophagic and tumour suppressor activity of a novel Beclin1-binding protein UVRAG. Nat Cell Biol 2006;8(7): 688-99.

[22] Berger MF, Hodis E, Heffernan TP, Deribe YL, Lawrence MS, Protopopov A, et al. Melanoma genome sequencing reveals frequent PREX2 mutations. Nature 2012;485(7399):502-6.

[23] Fine B, Hodakoski C, Koujak S, Su T, Saal LH, Maurer M, et al. Activation of the PI3K pathway in cancer through inhibition of PTEN by exchange factor P-REX2a. Science 2009;325(5945):1261-5.

[24] Turajlic S, Furney SJ, Lambros MB, Mitsopoulos C, Kozarewa I, Geyer FC, et al. Whole genome sequencing of matched primary and metastatic acral melanomas. Genome Res 2012;22(2):196-207.

[25] Nikolaev SI, Rimoldi D, Iseli C, Valsesia A, Robyr D, Gehrig C, et al. Exome sequencing identifies recurrent somatic MAP2K1 and MAP2K2 mutations in melanoma. Nat Genet 2011;44(2):133-9.

[26] Stark MS, Woods SL, Gartside MG, Bonazzi VF, Dutton-Regester K, Aoude LG, et al. Frequent somatic mutations in MAP3K5 and MAP3K9 in metastatic melanoma identified by exome sequencing. Nat Genet 2011;44(2):165-9.

[27] Krauthammer M, Kong Y, Ha BH, Evans P, Bacchiocchi A, McCusker JP, et al. Exome sequencing identifies recurrent somatic RAC1 mutations in melanoma. Nat Genet 2012;44(9):1006-14. doi: 10.1038/ng.2359.

[28] Hodis E, Watson IR, Kryukov GV, Arold ST, Imielinski M, Theurillat JP, et al. A landscape of driver mutations in melanoma. Cell 2012;150(2):251-63.

[29] Hansson J. Familial cutaneous melanoma. Adv Exp Med Biol 2010;685:134-45.

[30] Hayward NK. Genetics of melanoma predisposition. Oncogene 2003;22(20):3053-62.

[31] Maubec E, Chaudru V, Mohamdi H, Blondel C, Margaritte-Jeannin P, Forget S, et al. Familial melanoma: Clinical factors associated with germline CDKN2A mutations according to the number of patients affected by melanoma in a family. J Am Acad Dermatol 2012.

[32] Bishop DT, Demenais F, Goldstein AM, Bergman W, Bishop JN, Bressac-de Paillerets B, et al. Geographical variation in the penetrance of CDKN2A mutations for melanoma. J Natl Cancer Inst 2002;94(12):894-903.

[33] Box NF, Duffy DL, Chen W, Stark M, Martin NG, et al. MC1R genotype modifies risk of melanoma in families segregating CDKN2A mutations. Am J Hum Genet 2001;69(4): 765-73.

[34] Ward KA, Lazovich D, Hordinsky MK. Germline melanoma susceptibility and prognostic genes: A review of the literature. J Am Acad Dermatol 2012.

[35] Goldstein AM, Struewing JP, Chidambaram A, Fraser MC, Tucker MA. Genotype-phenotype relationships in U.S. melanoma-prone families with CDKN2A and CDK4 mutations. J Natl Cancer Inst 2000;92(12):1006-10.

[36] Gillanders E, Juo SH, Holland EA, Jones M, Nancarrow D, Freas-Lutz D, et al. Localization of a novel melanoma susceptibility locus to 1p22. Am J Hum Genet 2003;73(2): 301-13.

[37] Walker GJ, Indsto JO, Sood R, Faruque MU, Hu P, Pollock PM, et al. Deletion mapping suggests that the 1p22 melanoma susceptibility gene is a tumor suppressor localized to a 9-Mb interval. Genes Chromosomes Cancer 2004;41(1):56-64.

[38] de Snoo FA, Hayward NK. Cutaneous melanoma susceptibility and progression genes. Cancer Lett 2005;230(2):153-86.

[39] Harding RM, Healy E, Ray AJ, Ellis NS, Flanagan N, Todd C, et al. Evidence for variable selective pressures at MC1R. Am J Hum Genet 2000;66(4):1351-61.

[40] Valverde P, Healy E, Jackson I, Rees JL, Thody AJ. Variants of the melanocyte-stimulating hormone receptor gene are associated with red hair and fair skin in humans. Nat Genet 1995;11(3):328-30.

[41] Valverde P, Healy E, Sikkink S, Haldane F, Thody AJ, Carothers A, et al. The Asp84Glu variant of the melanocortin 1 receptor (MC1R) is associated with melanoma. Hum Mol Genet 1996;5(10):1663-6.

[42] Ichii-Jones F, Lear JT, Heagerty AH, Smith AG, Hutchinson PE, Osborne J, et al. Susceptibility to melanoma: influence of skin type and polymorphism in the melanocyte stimulating hormone receptor gene. J Invest Dermatol 1998;111(2):218-21.

[43] Palmer JS, Duffy DL, Box NF, Aitken JF, O'Gorman LE, Green AC, et al. Melanocortin-1 receptor polymorphisms and risk of melanoma: is the association explained solely by pigmentation phenotype? Am J Hum Genet 2000;66(1):176-86.

[44] Kennedy C, ter Huurne J, Berkhout M, Gruis N, Bastiaens M, Bergman W, et al. Melanocortin 1 receptor (MC1R) gene variants are associated with an increased risk for cutaneous melanoma which is largely independent of skin type and hair color. J Invest Dermatol 2001;117(2):294-300.

[45] Williams PF, Olsen CM, Hayward NK, Whiteman DC. Melanocortin 1 receptor and risk of cutaneous melanoma: a meta-analysis and estimates of population burden. Int J Cancer 2011;129(7):1730-40.

[46] Smith R, Healy E, Siddiqui S, Flanagan N, Steijlen PM, Rosdahl I, et al. Melanocortin 1 receptor variants in an Irish population. J Invest Dermatol 1998;111(1):119-22.

[47] Buscà R, Ballotti R. Cyclic AMP a key messenger in the regulation of skin pigmentation. Pigment Cell Res. 2000;13(2):60-9.

[48] Law MH, Macgregor S, Hayward NK. Melanoma genetics: recent findings take us beyond well-traveled pathways. J Invest Dermatol. 2012;132(7):1763-74.

[49] Cheli Y, Ohanna M, Ballotti R, Bertolotto C. Fifteen-year quest for microphthalmia-associated transcription factor target genes. Pigment Cell Melanoma Res 2010;23(1): 27-40.

[50] Yokoyama S, Woods SL, Boyle GM, Aoude LG, MacGregor S, Zismann V, et al. A novel recurrent mutation in MITF predisposes to familial and sporadic melanoma. Nature 2011;480(7375):99-103.

[51] Bertolotto C, Lesueur F, Giuliano S, Strub T, de Lichy M, Bille K, et al. A SUMOylation-defective MITF Germline Mutation Predisposes to Melanoma and Renal Carcinoma. Nature 2011;480(7375):94-98.

[52] Sulem P, Gudbjartsson DF, Stacey SN, Helgason A, Rafnar T, et al. Two newly identified genetic determinants of pigmentation in Europeans. Nat Genet 2008;40(7):835-7.

[53] Meng S, Zhang M, Liang L, Han J. Current opportunities and challenges: genome-wide association studies on pigmentation and skin cancer. Pigment Cell Melanoma Res 2012;25(5):612-7.

[54] Fernandez LP, Milne RL, Pita G, Avilés JA, Lázaro P, Benítez J, et al. SLC45A2: a novel malignant melanoma-associated gene. Hum Mutat 2008;29(9):1161-7.

[55] Guedj M, Bourillon A, Combadières C, Rodero M, Dieudé P, Descamps V, et al. Variants of the MATP/SLC45A2 gene are protective for melanoma in the French population. Hum Mutat 2008;29(9):1154-60.

[56] Newton JM, Cohen-Barak O, Hagiwara N, Gardner JM, Davisson MT, King RA, et al. Mutations in the human orthologue of the mouse underwhite gene (uw) underlie a new form of oculocutaneous albinism, OCA4. Am J Hum Genet 2001;69(5):981-8.

[57] Ibarrola-Villava M, Hu HH, Guedj M, Fernandez LP, Descamps V, Basset-Seguin N, et al. MC1R, SLC45A2 and TYR genetic variants involved in melanoma susceptibility in Southern European populations: Results from a Meta-analysis. Eur J Cancer 2012;48(14):2183-91.

[58] Graf J, Hodgson R, van Daal A. Single nucleotide polymorphisms in the MATP gene are associated with normal human pigmentation variation. Hum Mutat 2005;25(3): 278-84.

[59] Suzuki I, Tada A, Ollmann MM, Barsh GS, Im S, Lamoreux ML, et al. Agouti signaling protein inhibits melanogenesis and the response of human melanocytes to alpha-melanotropin. J Invest Dermatol 1997;108(6):838-42.

[60] Scherer D, Rachakonda PS, Angelini S, Mehnert F, Sucker A, Egberts F, et al. Association between the germline MC1R variants and somatic BRAF/NRAS mutations in melanoma tumors. J Invest Dermatol. 2010 Dec;130(12):2844-8.

[61] Gudbjartsson DF, Sulem P, Stacey SN, Goldstein AM, Rafnar T, Sigurgeirsson B, et al., ASIP and TYR pigmentation variants associate with cutaneous melanoma and basal cell carcinoma. Nat Genet 2008;40(7):886-91.

[62] Nan H, Kraft P, Hunter DJ, Han J. Genetic variants in pigmentation genes, pigmentary phenotypes, and risk of skin cancer in Caucasians. Int J Cancer 2009;125(4):909-17.

[63] Maccioni L, Rachakonda PS, Scherer D, Bermejo JL, Planelles D, Requena C, et al. Variants at chromosome 20 (ASIP locus) and melanoma risk. Int J Cancer 2012. doi: 10.1002/ijc.27648.

[64] Brown KM, Macgregor S, Montgomery GW, Craig DW, Zhao ZZ, Iyadurai K, et al. Common sequence variants on 20q11.22 confer melanoma susceptibility. Nat Genet 2008;40(7):838-40.

[65] Ancans J, Tobin DJ, Hoogduijn MJ, Smit NP, Wakamatsu K, Thody AJ. Melanosomal pH controls rate of melanogenesis, eumelanin/phaeomelanin ratio and melanosome maturation in melanocytes and melanoma cells. Exp Cell Res 2001;268(1):26-35.

[66] Bishop DT, Demenais F, Iles MM, Harland M, Taylor JC, Corda E, et al. Genome-wide association study identifies three loci associated with melanoma risk. Nat Genet 2009;41(8):920-5.

[67] Chatzinasiou F, Lill CM, Kypreou K, Stefanaki I, Nicolaou V, Spyrou G, et al. Comprehensive field synopsis and systematic meta-analyses of genetic association studies in cutaneous melanoma. J Natl Cancer Inst 2011;103(16):1227-35.

[68] Pho LN, Leachman SA. Genetics of pigmentation and melanoma predisposition. G Ital Dermatol Venereol 2010;145(1):37-45.

[69] Schuch AP, Menck CF. The genotoxic effects of DNA lesions induced by artificial UV-radiation and sunlight. J Photochem Photobiol B 2010;99(3):111-6.

[70] Mocellin S, Verdi D, Nitti D. DNA repair gene polymorphisms and risk of cutaneous melanoma: a systematic review and meta-analysis. Carcinogenesis 2009;30(10):1735-43.

[71] Gonçalves FT, Francisco G, de Souza SP, Luiz OC, Festa-Neto C, Sanches JA, et al., European ancestry and polymorphisms in DNA repair genes modify the risk of melanoma: a case-control study in a high UV index region in Brazil. J Dermatol Sci 2011;64(1):59-66.

[72] Figl A, Scherer D, Nagore E, Bermejo JL, Botella-Estrada R, Gast A, et al. Single-nucleotide polymorphisms in DNA-repair genes and cutaneous melanoma. Mutat Res 2010;702(1):8-16.

[73] Winsey SL, Haldar NA, Marsh HP, Bunce M, Marshall SE, Harris AL, et al. A variant within the DNA repair gene XRCC3 is associated with the development of melanoma skin cancer. Cancer Res 2000;60(20):5612-6.

[74] Gu F, Qureshi AA, Kraft P, Guo Q, Hunter DJ, Han J. Polymorphisms in genes involved in DNA repair, cell growth, oxidative stress and inflammatory response, and melanoma risk. Br J Dermatol 2009;161(1):209-12.

[75] Govindarajan B, Bai X, Cohen C, Zhong H, Kilroy S, Louis G, et al. Malignant transformation of melanocytes to melanoma by constitutive activation of mitogen-activated protein kinase kinase (MAPKK) signaling. J Biol Chem 2003;278(11):9790-9795.

[76] Downward J. Targeting RAS signalling pathways in cancer therapy. Nat Rev Cancer 2003;3(1):11-22.

[77] Brose MS, Volpe P, Feldman M, Kumar M, Rishi I, Gerrero R, et al. BRAF and RAS mutations in human lung cancer and melanoma. Cancer Res 2002;62(23):6997-7000.

[78] Dhillon AS, Hagan S, Rath O, Kolch W. MAP kinase signalling pathways in cancer. Oncogene 2007;26(22):3279-90.

[79] Beeram M, Patnaik A, Rowinsky EK. Regulation of c-Raf-1: therapeutic implications. Clin Adv Hematol Oncol 2003;1:476–481.

[80] Davies H, Bignell GR, Cox C, Stephens P, Edkins S, Clegg S, et al., Mutations of the BRAF gene in human cancer. Nature 2002;417:949–954.

[81] R. Kumar, S. Angelini, K. Hemminki, Activating BRAF and N-Ras mutations in sporadic primary melanomas: an inverse association with allelic loss on chromosome 9, Oncogene 22 2003 9217–9224.

[82] Singh S, Davis R, Alamanda V, Pireddu R, Pernazza D, Sebti S, et al. Rb-Raf-1 interaction disruptor RRD-251 induces apoptosis in metastatic melanoma cells and synergizes with dacarbazine. Mol Cancer Ther 2010;9(12):3330-41.

[83] Fisher R, Larkin J. Vemurafenib: a new treatment for BRAF-V600 mutated advanced melanoma. Cancer Manag Res 2012;4:243-52.

[84] Johannessen CM, Boehm JS. COT drives resistance to RAF inhibition through MAP kinase pathway reactivation. Nature 2010;468(7326):968-72.

[85] Nazarian R, Shi H. Melanomas acquire resistance to B-RAF(V600E) inhibition by RTK or N-RAS upregulation. Nature 2010;468(7326):973-7.

[86] Yadav V, Zhang X. Reactivation of Mitogen-activated Protein Kinase (MAPK) Pathway by FGF Receptor 3 (FGFR3)/Ras Mediates Resistance to Vemurafenib in Human B-RAF V600E Mutant Melanoma. J Biol Chem 2012;287(33):28087-98.

[87] Govindarajan B, Sligh JE, Vincent BJ, Li M, Canter JA, Nickoloff BJ, et al. Overexpression of Akt converts radial growth melanoma to vertical growth melanoma. J Clin Invest 2007;117(3):719-29.

[88] Bogenrieder T, Herlyn M. The molecular pathology of cutaneous melanoma. Cancer Biomark 2010;9(1-6):267-86.

[89] Shull AY, Latham-Schwark A, Ramasamy P, Leskoske K, Oroian D, Birtwistle MR, et al., Novel Somatic Mutations to PI3K Pathway Genes in Metastatic Melanoma. PLoS One 2012;7(8):e43369.

[90] Wang Y, Digiovanna JJ, Stern JB, Hornyak TJ, Raffeld M, Khan SG, et al. Evidence of ultraviolet type mutations in xeroderma pigmentosum melanomas. Proc Natl Acad Sci U S A 2009;106(15):6279-84.

[91] Weeraratna AT. A Wnt-er wonderland--the complexity of Wnt signaling in melanoma. Cancer Metastasis Rev 2005;24(2):237-50.

[92] Bittner M, Meltzer P. Molecular classification of cutaneous malignant melanoma by gene expression profiling. Nature 2000;406(6795):536-40.

[93] Flaherty KT, Fisher DE. New Strategies in Metastatic Melanoma: Oncogene-Defined Taxonomy Leads to Therapeutic Advances. Clinical Cancer Research 2011;17(15): 4922-4928.

[94] Bhoumik A, Lopez-Bergami P, Ronai Z. ATF2 on the Double—Activating Transcription Factor and DNA Damage Response Protein. Pigment Cell Research 2007;20(6):498-506.

[95] Hai T, Curran T. Cross-Family Dimerization of Transcription Factors Fos/Jun and ATF/ CREB Alters DNA Binding Specificity. Proceedings of the National Academy of Sciences of the United States of America 1991;88(9):3720-3724.

[96] Bhoumik A, Ronai Z. ATF2: A Transcription Factor that Elicits Oncogenic or Tumor Suppressor Activities. Cell Cycle 2008;7(15):2341-2345.

[97] Ronai ZA, Weinstein IB. Identification of Ultraviolet-Inducible Proteins that Bind to a TGACAACA Sequence in the Polyoma Virus Regulatory Region. Cancer Research 1990;50(17):5374-5381.

[98] Rutberg SE, Goldstein IM, Yang YM, Stackpole CE ,Ronai Z. Expression and Transcriptional Activity of AP-1, CRE, and URE Binding Proteins in B16 Mouse Melanoma Subclones. Molecular Carcinogenesis 1994;10(2) 82-87.

[99] Ronai Z, Yang Y, Fuchs SY, Adler V, Sardana M, Herlyn M. ATF2 Confers Radiation Resistance To Human Melanoma Cells. Oncogene 1998;16(4) 523-531.

[100] Bhoumik A, Ivanov V, Ronai Z. Activating Transcription Factor 2-derived Peptides Alter Resistance of Human Tumor Cell Lines to Ultraviolet Irradiation and Chemical Treatment. Clinical Cancer Research 2001;7(2):331-342.

[101] Bhoumik A, Huang TG, Ivanov V, Gangi L, Qiao RF, Woo SL, et al. An ATF2-Derived Peptide Sensitizes Melanomas to Apoptosis and Inhibits their Growth and Metastasis. The Journal of Clinical Investigation 2002;110(5): 643-650.

[102] Recio JA, Merlino G. Hepatocyte Growth Factor/Scatter Factor Activates Proliferation in Melanoma Cells through p38 MAPK, ATF-2 and Cyclin D1. Oncogene 2002;21(7): 1000-1008.

[103] Huang Y, Minigh J, Miles S, Niles RM. Retinoic Acid Decreases ATF-2 Phosphorylation and Sensitizes Melanoma Cells to Taxol-Mediated Growth Inhibition. Journal of Molecular Signaling 2008;3(3):1-11.

[104] Bhoumik A, Gangi L, Ronai Z. Inhibition of Melanoma Growth and Metastasis by ATF2-Derived Peptides. Cancer Research 2004;64(22):8222–8230.

[105] Bhoumik A, Jones N, Ronai Z. Transcriptional Switch by Activating Transcription Factor 2-Derived Peptide Sensitizes Melanoma Cells to Apoptosis and Inhibits their Tumorigenicity. Proceedings of the National Academy of Sciences of the United States of America 2004 23;101(12):4222-4227.

[106] Berger AJ, Kluger HM, Li N, Kielhorn E, Halaban R, Ronai Z, Rimm DL. Subcellular Localization of Activating Transcription Factor 2 in Melanoma Specimens Predicts Patient Survival. Cancer Research 2003;63(23): 8103-8107.

[107] Bhoumik A, Gangi L, Ronai Z. Inhibition of Melanoma Growth and Metastasis by ATF2-Derived Peptides. Cancer Research 2004;64(22):8222-8230.

[108] Maekawa T, Shinagawa T, Sano Y, Sakuma T, Nomura S, Nagasaki K, et al. Reduced Levels of ATF-2 Predispose Mice to Mammary Tumors. Molecular and Cellular Biology 2007;27(5):1730-1744.

[109] Bhoumik A, Fichtman B, Derossi C, Breitwieser W, Kluger HM, Davis S, et al. Suppressor role of activating transcription factor 2 (ATF2) in skin cancer. Proceedings of the National Academy of Sciences of the United States of America 2008;105(5): 1674-1679.

[110] Steingrimsson E, Copeland NG, Jenkins NA. Melanocytes and the Microphthalmia Transcription Factor Network. Annual Review of Genetics 2004;38:365–411.

[111] Tachibana M, Perez-Jurado LA, Nakayama A, Hodgkinson CA, Li X, Schneider M, Miki T, et al. Cloning of MITF, The Human Homolog of the Mouse Microphthalmia Gene and Assignment to Chromosome 3p14.1-p12.3. Human Molecular Genetics 1994;3(4): 553-557.

[112] Fuse N, Yasumoto K, Takeda K, Amae S, Yoshizawa M, Udono T, Takahashi K, et al. Molecular Cloning of cDNA Encoding a Novel Microphthalmia-Associated Transcription Factor Isoform with a Distinct Amino-Terminus. Journal of Biochemistry 1999;126(6):1043-1051.

[113] Udono T, Yasumoto K, Takeda K, Amae S, Watanabe K, Saito H, et al. Structural Organization of the Human Microphthalmia-Associated Transcription Factor Gene

Containing Four Alternative Promoters. Biochimica et Biophysica Acta 2000;1491(1-3): 205-219.

[114] Lowings P, Yavuzer U, Goding CR. Positive and Negative Elements Regulate a Melanocyte-Specific Promoter. Molecular and Cellular Biology 1992;12(8):3653–3662.

[115] Yasumoto KI, Mahalingam H, Suzuki H, Yoshizawa M, Yokoyama K, Shibahara S. Transcriptional Activation of the Melanocyte-Specific Genes by the Human Homolog of the Mouse Microphthalmia Protein. Journal of Biochemistry 1995;118(5):874–881.

[116] Cheli Y, Ohanna M, Ballotti R, Bertolotto C. Fifteen-Year Quest for Microphthalmia-Associated Transcription Factor Target Genes. Pigment Cell and Melanoma Research 2010;23(1):27–40.

[117] Boeckmann B, Blatter MC, Famiglietti L, Hinz U, Lane L, Roechert B, Bairoch A. Protein Variety And Functional Diversity: Swiss-Prot Annotation in its Biological Context. Comptes Rendus Biologies 2005;328(10-11):882–899.

[118] Goding CR. Mitf from Neural Crest to Melanoma: Signal Transduction and Transcription in the Melanocyte Lineage. Genes and Development 2000;14(14):1712–1728.

[119] Hoek KS, Goding CR. Cancer Stem Cells versus Phenotype-Switching in Melanoma. Pigment Cell and Melanoma Research 2010;23(6):746–759.

[120] Bell RE, Levy C. The three M's: Melanoma, Microphthalmia-Associated Transcription Factor and microRNA. Pigment Cell and Melanoma Research 2011;24(6):1088-1106.

[121] Garraway LA, Widlund HR, Rubin MA, Getz G, Berger AJ, Ramaswamy S Beroukhim R, et al. Integrative Genomic Analyses Identify MITF as a Lineage Survival Oncogene Amplified in Malignant Melanoma. Nature 2005;436(7047):117–122.

[122] Carreira S, Goodall J, Denat L, Rodriguez M, Nuciforo P, Hoek KS Testori A, Larue L, Goding CR. Mitf Regulation of Dia1 Controls Melanoma Proliferation and Invasiveness. Genes and Development 2006;20(24):3426–3439.

[123] Goding CR. A Picture of Mitf in Melanoma Immortality. Oncogene 2011;30(20): 2304-2306.

[124] Wellbrock C, Marais R. Elevated Expression Of MITF Counteracts B-RAF-Stimulated Melanocyte And Melanoma Cell Proliferation. The Journal of Cell Biology 2005;170(5): 703–708.

[125] Wu M, Hemesath TJ, Takemoto CM, Horstmann MA, Wells AG, Price ER, Fisher DZ, Fisher DE. c-Kit Triggers Dual Phosphorylations, Which Couple Activation and Degradation of the Essential Melanocyte Factor Mi. Genes and Development 2000;14(3):301–312.

[126] Gray-Schopfer V, Wellbrock C, Marais R. Melanoma Biology and New Targeted Therapy. Nature 2007;22 445(7130):851-857.

[127] Shah M, Bhoumik A, Goel V, Dewing A, Breitwieser W, Kluger H, et al. A role for ATF2 in regulating MITF and melanoma development. PLoS Genetics 2010;6(12):e1001258.

[128] Akavia UD, Litvin O, Kim J, Sanchez-Garcia F, Kotliar D, Causton HC, Pochanard P, Mozes E, Garraway LA, Pe'er D. An integrated approach to uncover drivers of cancer. Cell 2010;143(6):1005-1017.

[129] Valsesia A, Rimoldi D, Martinet D, Ibberson M, Benaglio P, Quadroni M, et al. Network-guided analysis of genes with altered somatic copy number and gene expression reveals pathways commonly perturbed in metastatic melanoma. PLoS One 2011;6(4):e18369.

[130] Takeda K, Yasumoto K, Takada R, Takada S, Watanabe K, Udono T, et al. Induction of Melanocyte-Specific Microphthalmia-Associated Transcription Factor by Wnt-3a. The Journal of Biological Chemistry 2000;275(19):14013–14016.

[131] Omholt K, Platz A, Ringborg U, Hansson, J. Cytoplasmic and Nuclear Accumulation of b-Catenin is Rarely Caused by CTNNB1 Exon 3 Mutations in Cutaneous Malignant Melanoma. International Journal of Cancer 2001;92(6):839–842.

[132] Rimm DL, Caca K., Hu, G., Harrison, F. B. & Fearon, E. R. Frequent Nuclear/Cytoplasmic Localization of b-Catenin without Exon 3 Mutations in Malignant Melanoma. The American Journal of Pathology 1999;154(2):325–329.

[133] Bishop JN, Harland M, Randerson-Moor J, Bishop DT. Management of Familial Melanoma. The Lancet Oncology 2007;8(1):46-54.

[134] Flaherty KT, Fisher DE. New Strategies in Metastatic Melanoma: Oncogene-defined Taxonomy Leads to Therapeutic Advances. Clinical Cancer Research 2011;17(15): 4922-4928.

[135] Levy C, Khaled M, Fisher DE. MITF: Master Regulator Of Melanocyte Development And Melanoma Oncogene. Trends in Molecular Medicine 2006;12(9):406-414.

[136] Selzer E, Wacheck V, Lucas T, Heere-Ress E, Wu M, Weilbaecher KN, Schlegel W, Valent P, Wrba F, Pehamberger H, Fisher D, Jansen B. The Melanocyte-Specific Isoform of the Microphthalmia Transcription Factor Affects the Phenotype of Human Melanoma. Cancer Research 2002;62(7):2098-2103.

[137] Sancar A, Lindsey-Boltz LA, Unsal-Kaçmaz K, Linn S. Molecular mechanisms of mammalian DNA repair and the DNA damage checkpoints. Annu Rev Biochem 2004;73:39-85.

[138] DiGiovanna JJ, Kraemer KH. Shining a light on xeroderma pigmentosum. J Invest Dermatol 2012;132(3 Pt 2):785-96.

[139] Kauffmann A, Rosselli F, Lazar V, Winnepenninckx V, Mansuet-Lupo A, Dessen P, et al. High expression of DNA repair pathways is associated with metastasis in melanoma patients. Oncogene 2008;27(5):565-73.

[140] Wang L, Eastmond DA. Catalytic inhibitors of topoisomerase II are DNA-damaging agents: induction of chromosomal damage by merbarone and ICRF-187. Environ Mol Mutagen 2002;39(4):348-56.

[141] Eder JP Jr, Chan VT, Ng SW, Rizvi NA, Zacharoulis S, Teicher BA, et al. DNA topoisomerase II alpha expression is associated with alkylating agent resistance. Cancer Res 1995 Dec 15;55(24):6109-16.

[142] Sarasin A. An overview of the mechanisms of mutagenesis and carcinogenesis. Mutat Res 2003;544(2-3):99-106.

[143] Kao WH, Riker AI, Kushwaha DS, Ng K, Enkemann SA, Jove R, et al., Upregulation of Fanconi anemia DNA repair genes in melanoma compared with non-melanoma skin cancer. J Invest Dermatol 2011;131(10):2139-42.

[144] Jewell R, Conway C, Mitra A, Randerson-Moor J, Lobo S, Nsengimana J, et al. Patterns of expression of DNA repair genes and relapse from melanoma. Clin Cancer Res 2010;16(21):5211-21.

[145] Bondurand N, Pingault V, Goerich DE, Lemort N, Sock E, Le Caignec C, et al., Interaction among SOX10, PAX3 and MITF, three genes altered in Waardenburg syndrome. Hum Mol Genet 2000;9(13):1907-17.

[146] Lang D, Epstein JA. Sox10 and Pax3 physically interact to mediate activation of a conserved c-RET enhancer. Hum Mol Genet 2003;12(8):937-45.

[147] Medic S, Ziman M. PAX3 across the spectrum: from melanoblast to melanoma. Crit Rev Biochem Mol Biol 2009;44(2-3):85-97.

[148] Lang D, Lu MM, Huang L, Engleka KA, Zhang M, et al. Pax3 functions at a nodal point in melanocyte stem cell differentiation. Nature 2005;433(7028):884-7.

[149] Scholl FA, Kamarashev J, Murmann OV, Geertsen R, Dummer R, Schäfer BW. PAX3 is expressed in human melanomas and contributes to tumor cell survival. Cancer Res 2001;61(3):823-6.

[150] Plummer RS, Shea CR, Nelson M, Powell SK, Freeman DM, Dan CP, Lang D. PAX3 expression in primary melanomas and nevi. Mod Pathol 2008;21(5):525-30.

[151] He S, Yoon HS, Suh BJ, Eccles MR. PAX3 Is extensively expressed in benign and malignant tissues of the melanocytic lineage in humans. J Invest Dermatol 2010;130(5): 1465-8.

[152] Medic S, Ziman M. PAX3 expression in normal skin melanocytes and melanocytic lesions (naevi and melanomas). PLoS One 2010;5(4):e9977.

[153] Bernasconi M, Remppis A, Fredericks WJ, Rauscher FJ 3rd, Schäfer BW. Induction of apoptosis in rhabdomyosarcoma cells through down-regulation of PAX proteins. Proc Natl Acad Sci U S A 1996;93(23):13164-9.

[154] Borycki AG, Li J, Jin F, Emerson CP, Epstein JA. Pax3 functions in cell survival and in pax7 regulation. Development 1999;126(8):1665-74.

[155] Margue CM, Bernasconi M, Barr FG, Schäfer BW. Transcriptional modulation of the anti-apoptotic protein BCL-XL by the paired box transcription factors PAX3 and PAX3/FKHR. Oncogene 2000;19(25):2921-9.

[156] Kubic JD, Mascarenhas JB, Iizuka T, Wolfgeher D, Lang D. GSK-3 Promotes Cell Survival, Growth, and PAX3 Levels in Human Melanoma Cells. Mol Cancer Res 2012;10(8):1065-76.

[157] He SJ, Stevens G, Braithwaite AW, Eccles MR. Transfection of melanoma cells with antisense PAX3 oligonucleotides additively complements cisplatin-induced cytotoxicity. Mol Cancer Ther 2005;4(6):996-1003.

[158] Mascarenhas JB, Littlejohn EL, Wolsky RJ, Young KP, Nelson M, Salgia R, Lang D. PAX3 and SOX10 activate MET receptor expression in melanoma. Pigment Cell Melanoma Res 2010;23(2):225-37.

[159] Gentile A, D'Alessandro L, Lazzari L, Martinoglio B, Bertotti A, Mira A, et al. Met-driven invasive growth involves transcriptional regulation of Arhgap12. Oncogene 2008;27(42):5590-8.

[160] Cruz J, Reis-Filho JS, Silva P, Lopes JM. Expression of c-met tyrosine kinase receptor is biologically and prognostically relevant for primary cutaneous malignant melanomas. Oncology 2003;65(1):72-82.

[161] Puri N, Ahmed S, Janamanchi V, Tretiakova M, Zumba O, Krausz T, et al. c-Met is a potentially new therapeutic target for treatment of human melanoma. Clin Cancer Res 2007;13(7):2246-53.

[162] Medic S, Rizos H, Ziman M. Differential PAX3 functions in normal skin melanocytes and melanoma cells. Biochem Biophys Res Commun 2011;411(4):832-7.

[163] Yang G, Li Y, Nishimura EK, Xin H, Zhou A, Guo Y, et al. Inhibition of PAX3 by TGF-beta modulates melanocyte viability. Mol Cell 2008;32(4):554-63.

[164] Hocker T, Tsao H. Ultraviolet radiation and melanoma: a systematic review and analysis of reported sequence variants. Hum Mutat 2007;28(6):578-88.

[165] Ragnarsson-Olding BK, Karsberg S, Platz A, Ringborg UK. Mutations in the TP53 gene in human malignant melanomas derived from sun-exposed skin and unexposed mucosal membranes. Melanoma Res 2002;12(5):453-63.

[166] Yu H, McDaid R, Lee J, Possik P, Li L, Kumar SM, et al. The role of BRAF mutation and p53 inactivation during transformation of a subpopulation of primary human melanocytes. Am J Pathol 2009;174(6):2367-77.

[167] Terzian T, Torchia EC, Dai D, Robinson SE, Murao K, Stiegmann RA, et al. p53 prevents progression of nevi to melanoma predominantly through cell cycle regulation. Pigment Cell Melanoma Res 2010;23(6):781-94.

[168] Muthusamy V, Hobbs C, Nogueira C, Cordon-Cardo C, McKee PH, Chin L, Bosenberg MW, et al. Amplification of CDK4 and MDM2 in malignant melanoma. Genes Chromosomes Cancer 2006;45(5):447-54.

[169] Houben R, Hesbacher S, Schmid CP, Kauczok CS, Flohr U, Haferkamp S, et al. High-level expression of wild-type p53 in melanoma cells is frequently associated with inactivity in p53 reporter gene assays. PLoS One 2011;6(7):e22096.

[170] Haapajärvi T, Pitkänen K, Laiho M. Human melanoma cell line UV responses show independency of p53 function. Cell Growth Differ 1999;10(3):163-71.

[171] Bergamaschi D, Samuels Y, Sullivan A, Zvelebil M, Breyssens H, Bisso A, et al. iASPP preferentially binds p53 proline-rich region and modulates apoptotic function of codon 72-polymorphic p53. Nat Genet 2006;38(10):1133-41.

[172] Grob TJ, Novak U, Maisse C, Barcaroli D, Lüthi AU, Pirnia F, et al. Human delta Np73 regulates a dominant negative feedback loop for TAp73 and p53. Cell Death Differ 2001;8(12):1213-23.

[173] Homer C, Knight DA, Hananeia L, Sheard P, Risk J, Lasham A, et al. Y-box factor YB1 controls p53 apoptotic function. Oncogene 2005;24(56):8314-25.

[174] Nikolaev AY, Li M, Puskas N, Qin J, Gu W. Parc: a cytoplasmic anchor for p53. Cell 2003;112(1):29-40.

[175] Kastan MB, Berkovich E. p53: a two-faced cancer gene. Nat Cell Biol 2007;9(5):489-91.

[176] Avery-Kiejda KA, Bowden NA, Croft AJ, Scurr LL, Kairupan CF, Ashton KA, et al. P53 in human melanoma fails to regulate target genes associated with apoptosis and the cell cycle and may contribute to proliferation. BMC Cancer 2011;11:203.

[177] Verhaegen M, Checinska A, Riblett MB, Wang S, Soengas MS. E2F1-dependent oncogenic addiction of melanoma cells to MDM2. Oncogene 2012;31(7):828-41.

[178] Hersey P, Zhang XD. Adaptation to ER stress as a driver of malignancy and resistance to therapy in human melanoma. Pigment Cell Melanoma Res 2008;21(3):358-67.

[179] Griffith TS, Chin WA, Jackson GC, Lynch DH, Kubin MZ. Intracellular regulation of TRAIL-induced apoptosis in human melanoma cells. J Immunol 1998;161(6):2833-40.

[180] Jin L, Hu WL, Jiang CC, Wang JX, Han CC, Chu P, et al. MicroRNA-149*, a p53-responsive microRNA, functions as an oncogenic regulator in human melanoma. Proc Natl Acad Sci U S A 2011;108(38):15840-5.

[181] Ji Z, Njauw CN, Taylor M, Neel V, Flaherty KT, Tsao H. p53 rescue through HDM2 antagonism suppresses melanoma growth and potentiates MEK inhibition. J Invest Dermatol 2012;132(2):356-64.

[182] Glud M, Gniadecki R. MicroRNAs in the Pathogenesis of Malignant Melanoma. Journal of the European Academy of Dermatology and Venereology 2012, doi: 10.1111/j. 1468-3083.2012.04579.x.

[183] Kong YW, Ferland-McCollough D, Jackson TJ, Bushell M. MicroRNAs in Cancer Management. The Lancet Oncology 2012;13(6):249-258.

[184] Zhang L, Huang J, Yang N, Greshock J, Megraw MS, Giannakakis A, et al.. MicroRNAs Exhibit High Frequency Genomic Alterations in Human Cancer. Proceedings of the National Academy of Sciences of the United States of America 2006;103(24):9136-9141.

[185] Calin GA, Dumitru CD, Shimizu M, Bichi R, Zupo S, Noch E, et al. Frequent Deletions and Down-Regulation of Micro-RNA Genes miR-15 and miR-16 at 13q14 in Chronic Lymphocytic Leukemia. Proceedings of the National Academy of Sciences of the United States of America 2002;99(24):15524–15529.

[186] Johnson SM, Grosshans H, Shingara J, Byrom M, Jarvis R, Cheng A, et al. RAS is Regulated by the let-7 microRNA Family. Cell 2005;120(5):635–647.

[187] Mueller DW, Bosserhoff AK. Role of miRNAs in the Progression of Malignant Melanoma. British Journal of Cancer 2009;101(4):551–556.

[188] Bar-Eli M. Searching for the 'melano-miRs': miR-214 Drives Melanoma Metastasis. The EMBO Journal 2011;30(10):1880-1881.

[189] Bemis LT, Chen R, Amato CM, Classen EH, Robinson SE, Coffey DG, et al. MicrorRNA-137 Targets Microphtalmia-Associated Transcription Factor in Melanoma Cell Lines. Cancer Research 2008;68(5):1362–1368.

[190] Segura MF, Hanniford D, Menedez S, Reavie L, Zou X, Alvarez-Diaz S, et al. Aberrant miR-182 Expression Promote Melanoma Metastasis by Repressing FOX03 and Microphtalmia-Associated Transcription Factor. Proceedings of the National Academy of Sciences of the United States of America 2009;106(6):1814–1819.

[191] Haflidadóttir BS, Bergsteinsdóttir K, Praetorius C, Steingrímsson E. miR-148 regulates Mitf in Melanoma Cells. PLoS One 2010;5(7):e11574.

[192] Goswami S, Tarapore RS, Teslaa JJ, Grinblat Y, Setaluri V, Spiegelman VS. MicroRNA-340-mediated Degradation of Microphthalmia-Associated Transcription Factor mRNA is Inhibited by the Coding Region Determinant-Binding Protein. The Journal of Biological Chemistry 2010;285(27):20532-20540.

[193] Ozsolak F, Poling LL, Wang Z, Liu H, Liu XS, Roeder RG, et al. Chromatin structure analyses identify miRNA promoters. Genes and Development 2008;22(22):3172–3183.

[194] Levy C, Khaled M, Robinson KC, Veguilla RA, Chen PH, Yokoyama S, et al. Lineage-Specific Transcriptional Regulation of DICER by MITF in Melanocytes. Cell 2010;141(6): 994–1005.

[195] Glud M, Gniadecki R. MicroRNAs in the pathogenesis of malignant melanoma. J Eur Acad Dermatol Venereol. 2012 May 23. doi: 10.1111/j.1468-3083.2012.04579.x

[196] Chan E, Patel R, Nallur S, Ratner E, Bacchiocchi A, Hoyt K, et al. MicroRNA Signatures Differentiate Melanoma Subtypes. Cell Cycle 2011;10(11):1845–1852.

[197] Couts KL, Anderson EM, Gross MM, Sullivan K, Ahn NG. Oncogenic B-Raf Signaling in Melanoma Cells Controls a Network of microRNAs with Combinatorial Functions. Oncogene 2012, doi: 10.1038/onc.2012.209.

[198] Liu FJ, Wen T, Liu L. MicroRNAs as a Novel Cellular Senescence Regulator. Ageing Research Review 2012;11(1):41–50.

[199] Gorospe M, Abdelmohsen K. MicroRegulators Come of Age in Aenescence. Trends in Genetics 2011;27(6):233–241.

[200] Bueno MJ, Malumbres M. MicroRNAs and the Cell Cycle. Biochimica et Biophysica Acta 2011;1812(2):592–601.

[201] Tazawa H, Tsuchiya N, Izumiya M, Nakagama H. Tumor-suppressive miR-34a induces senescence-like growth arrest through modulation of the E2F pathway in human colon cancer cells. Proceedings of the National Academy of Sciences of the United States of America 2007;104(39):15472-15427.

[202] Dar AA, Majid S, de Semir D, Nosrati M, Bezrookove V, Kashani-Sabet M. miRNA-205 Suppresses Melanoma Cell Proliferation and Induces Senescence Via Regulation of E2F1 Protein. The Journal of Biological Chemistry 2011;286(19):16606-16614.

[203] Noguchi S, Mori T, Otsuka Y, Yamada N, Yasui Y, Iwasaki J, et al. Anti-oncogenic microRNA-203 induces senescence by targeting E2F3 protein in human melanoma cells. The Journal of Biological Chemistry 2012;287(15):11769-11777.

[204] Streicher KL, Zhu W, Lehmann KP, Georgantas RW, Morehouse CA, Brohawn P, et al. A novel oncogenic role for the miRNA-506-514 cluster in initiating melanocyte transformation and promoting melanoma growth. Oncogene 2012;31(12):1558-1570.

[205] Bonazzi VF, Stark MS, Hayward NK. MicroRNA Regulation of Melanoma Progression. Melanoma Research 2012;22(2):101-113.

[206] Felicetti F, Errico MC, Bottero L, Segnalini P, Stoppacciaro A, Biffoni M, et al. The Promyelocytic Leukemia Zinc Finger-microrna-221/-222 Pathway Controls Melanoma Progression Through Multiple Oncogenic Mechanisms. Cancer Research 2008;68(8): 2745-2754.

[207] Lujambio A, Ropero S, Ballestar E, Fraga MF, Cerrato C, Setién F, et al. Genetic Unmasking of an Epigenetically Silenced microRNA in Human Cancer Cells. Cancer Research 2007;67(4):1424–1429.

[208] Mazar J, Khaitan D, DeBlasio D, Zhong C, Govindarajan SS, Kopanathi S, et al.. Epigenetic Regulation of microRNA Genes and the Role of miR-34b in Cell Invasion and Motility in Human Melanoma. PLoS One 2011;6(9):e24922.

[209] Mazar J, DeBlasio D, Govindarajan SS, Zhang S, Perera RJ. Epigenetic Regulation of microRNA-375 and its Role in Melanoma Development in Humans. FEBS Letters 2011;585(15):2467-2476.

[210] Gaur A, Jewell DA, Liang Y, Ridzon D, Moore JH, Chen C, et al. Characterization of microRNA Expression Levels and Their Biological Correlates in Human Cancer Cell Lines. Cancer Research 2007;67(6):2456-2468.

[211] Mueller DW, Rehli M, Bosserhoff AK. miRNA Expression Profiling in Melanocytes and Melanoma Cell Lines Reveals miRNAs Associated with Formation and Progression of Malignant Melanoma. The Journal of Investigative Dermatology 2009;129(7) 1740–1751.

[212] Philippidou D, Schmitt M, Moser D, Margue C, Nazarov PV, Muller A, et al. Signatures of microRNAs and selected microRNA target genes in human melanoma. Cancer Research 2010;70(10):4163–4173.

[213] Stark MS, Tyagi S, Nancarrow DJ, Boyle GM, Cook AL, Whiteman DC, et al. Characterization of the Melanoma miRNAome by Deep Sequencing. PLoS One 2010;12(5):e9685.

[214] Segura MF, Belitskaya-Lévy I, Rose AE, Zakrzewski J, Gaziel A, Hanniford D, et al. Melanoma MicroRNA Signature Predicts Post-Recurrence Survival. Clinical Cancer Research 2010;16(5):1577-1586.

[215] Caramuta S, Egyházi S, Rodolfo M, Witten D, Hansson J, Larsson C, Lui WO. MicroRNA expression profiles associated with mutational status and survival in malignant melanoma. The Journal of Investigative Dermatology 2010;130(8):2062-2070.

[216] Xu Y, Brenn T, Brown ER, Doherty V, Melton DW. Differential expression of microRNAs during melanoma progression: miR-200c, miR-205 and miR-211 are downregulated in melanoma and act as tumour suppressors. Britsh Journal of Cancer 2012;106(3) 553-561.

[217] Penna E, Orso F, Cimino D, Tenaglia E, Lembo A, Quaglino E, et al. microRNA-214 Contributes to Melanoma Tumour Progression Through Suppression of TFAP2C. The EMBO Journal 2011;30(10):1990-2007.

[218] Chan E, Patel R, Nallur S, Ratner E, Bacchiocchi A, Hoyt K, et al. MicroRNA Signatures Differentiate Melanoma Subtypes. Cell Cycle 2011;10(11):1845-1852.

[219] Hanna JA, Hahn L, Agarwal S, Rimm DL. In Situ Measurement of miR-205 in Malignant Melanoma Tissue Supports its Role as a Tumor Suppressor microRNA. Laboratory Investigation 2012, doi: 10.1038/labinvest.2012.119.

Chapter 4

Low-Penetrance Variants and Susceptibility to Sporadic Malignant Melanoma

G. Ribas, M. Ibarrola-Villava, M.C. Peña-Chilet,
L.P. Fernandez and C. Martinez-Cadenas

Additional information is available at the end of the chapter

1. Introduction

Although malignant melanoma (MM) is mainly a sporadic disease, about 3 to 15% of the cases may show familial aggregation [1, 2]. The diagnosis of melanoma in different members of the same families does indeed suggest there is a genetically-based hereditary predisposition in a significant percentage of the cases. However, this predisposition has proven to be genetically heterogeneous. Only two high-penetrance genes had been described so far: *CDKN2A* and *CDK4* [1]. Yet mutations in these genes are found in only 30–40% of melanoma kindreds, indicating the existence of additional genes involved in melanoma predisposition [1]. Also, common low-penetrance alleles of the human pigmentation *MC1R* gene have been implicated in melanoma predisposition as well [3-13]. More recently, several other pigmentation genes, such as *ASIP, TYR, TYRP1, SLC45A2* and *OCA2* have also emerged as being potentially important in both normal human pigmentation variation and in melanoma susceptibility [14-17].

Other putative low-penetrance genes involved in melanoma predisposition are DNA repair genes belonging to the base excision repair (BER) and the nucleotide excision repair (NER) mechanisms. BER and NER pathways eliminate a wide variety of DNA damage, including ultraviolet (UV) photoproducts. Therefore, the ability of each individual to repair DNA damage following different causes might explain at least in part the variability in melanoma susceptibility. Although several studies have investigated the association between polymorphisms in NER genes and risk of melanoma, most of the study sizes were relatively small, and the results were not consistent [18-24]. On the other hand, genetic polymorphisms have been identified in several BER genes and studies suggest that some of these polymorphisms may be associated with cancer risk [25-29].

Further candidate low-penetrance genes allegedly linked to melanoma predisposition are members of the glutathione S-transferase (*GST*) gene family. GSTs are multifunctional enzymes involved in the detoxification of a wide range of reactive oxygen species (ROS) which, together with inflammatory response to UV exposure, contribute to skin carcinogenesis by oxidative stress mechanisms [30-32]. Since UV radiation can also indirectly induce oxidative stress via ROS, several *GST* genes have been considered as possible low-penetrance melanoma predisposition genes. Among the *GST* genes, *GSTM1*, *GSTT1* and *GSTP1* commonly harbor functional polymorphisms in the general population [33]. The frequencies of variants in the *GSTM1* and *GSTT1* genes have been studied in relation to susceptibility to melanoma; however, conflicting results have been reported [34-39].

In recent years, several genome-wide association studies (GWAS) have identified novel genomic *loci* associated with pigmentation and skin cancer [40-44]. GWAS are the ideal strategy to identify common, low-penetrance susceptibility *loci* without prior hypothesis bias due to gene role knowledge. Some of the associations detected were already known, such as *MC1R* with pigmentation and skin cancer, *ASIP*, *TYR*, *OCA2*, etc. However, several novel chromosomal regions and genes have been revealed using large cohorts of samples, such as *IRF4*, *PARP1*, *CASP8*, *CCND1* and others.

What follows is a summary of the results obtained in our laboratory after the screening of genes belonging to three different genetic pathways: pigmentation, DNA repair and oxidative stress. For the past few years, our group has been studying melanoma candidate genes in Spain, a southern European population, displaying a considerably darker skin than most of the other well-studied Caucasian populations, including Australian, North American and Northern Europe populations.

2. Research methods

2.1. Study subjects and data collection

A case-control collection of 946 non-related MM cases from several Spanish Hospitals and 353 volunteer cancer-free controls were recruited from 1 September 2004 to January 2011. All participants were Caucasians of Spanish origin. A standardized questionnaire was used to collect information on pigmentation characteristics (eye, hair and skin color, number of nevi, presence of solar lentigines, sun exposure habits and presence of childhood sunburns), Fitzpatrick's classification of skin type (extracted from the medical record of cases only), tumor localization, Breslow index (depth index), and personal or family history of cancer. All study subjects gave informed consent and the study was approved by the Ethics Committee of Gregorio Marañón General University hospital and Clínico University Hospital.

Genomic DNA from cases and controls was isolated from peripheral blood lymphocytes and diluted to a final solution of 50ng/ml. MagNA Pure LC Instrument DNA extracción was used according to the manufacturer's protocol (Roche Applied Science, Mannheim, Germany); the DNAzol procedure (Invitrogen, Eugene, OR, USA) or traditional saline method was used. DNA concentration was quantified in samples prior to genotyping by using Quant-iT PicoGreen dsDNA Reagent (Invitrogen, Eugene, OR, USA).

2.2. SNP genotyping

2.2.1. MC1R sequencing

MC1R variants were detected by automated gene sequencing. The *MC1R* coding region was amplified by PCR using two overlapping pairs of primers previously described [9]. PCR products were 671 and 610 bp in length, respectively, and they overlapped by 104 bp. PCR amplification was performed according to Matichard and cols [9]. Sequence analysis was performed on the ABI Prism system (Life Technology, Foster city, CA) using the BigDye Terminator Cycle Sequencing kit and the ABI 3700 automated DNA sequencer according to the manufacturer's instructions. The sequence results were analyzed using Polyphred, Phred Phrap and Consed software [45-47] or SeqScape in order to detect all possible changes. All detected changes were confirmed manually.

2.2.2. Gene and SNP selection

The rest of the genes in the study were analyzed by genotyping selected SNPs. Public databases were used to collect information about single nucleotide polymorphisms (SNPs): NCBI (http://www.ncbi.nlm.nih.gov), Ensembl (http://www.ensembl.org/index.html) and HapMap (http://www.hapmap.org). SNPs selected were located in exons, in putative promoter regions or had been reported to be associated with cancer in previous studies. All SNPs had a minor allele frequency (MAF) greater than or equal to 5%. As a quality control measure we included two sample duplicates and a non-template sample per 96-well plate. For some high-throughput platforms three DNA duplicates (two intra-assays and one inter-assay) were added. For all the studies performed genotypes were scored by two different personnel in the laboratory and no discrepancies were observed.

2.2.3. Taqman and kaspar assays

The PCR primers and probes were designed by Life Technology (Foster City, CA) using their Custom Taqman SNP genotyping assays or KASPAR SNP Genotyping System KBiosciences (Hoddesdon, Herts UK). The primer and allele-specific probe sequences for Taqman as well as those used for Kaspar assays are detailed elsewhere [6, 7, 14, 16, 17, 27].

PCR conditions used were according to the manufacturer's protocol (Life technology, Foster City, CA). After PCR, the genotype of each sample was automatically determined by measuring allele-specific final fluorescence in the ABI Prism 7900HT Detection System, using the SDS 2.1 software for allele discrimination (Life technology, Foster City, CA).

2.2.4. Sequenom

Genotyping assays were designed according to the Sequenom MassARRAY Assay Design software (version 3.0.0; Sequenom Inc., San Diego, CA, USA). Assay primers are detailed elsewhere [15, 27]. One duplicate sample, one father–mother–child trio and two negative controls were included across the plates to assess the accuracy of genotyping. SNPs were genotyped using iPLEX^{TM} chemistry on a MALDI-TOF Mass Spectrometer (Sequenom Inc, San Diego, CA, USA). PCR reactions were carried out according to their own instructions (Sequenom Inc.).

2.2.5. *Illumina*

A total of 384 SNPs were genotyped using the GoldenGate Genotyping Assay system according to the manufacturer's protocol (Illumina, San Diego, CA, USA) [16]. Genotyping was carried out using 350 ng of DNA per reaction. In addition, cases and control samples were always included in the same run. Genotypes were called using the proprietary software supplied by Illumina (BeadStudio, version 3.1.3.).

2.2.6. *Taqman quantitative real-time PCR*

The *GSTM1* and *GSTT1* copy number polymorphisms were determined using the TaqMan Quantitative real-time PCR. Assay designs were Hs02575461_cn (*GSTM1)* and Hs000100004_cn (*GSTT1)* and were used according to Life Technology instructions. After PCR, the genotype of each sample was automatically determined by measuring allele-specific final fluorescence in the ABI Prism 7900HT Detection System, using the SDS 2.3 software for allele discrimination (Life Technology, Foster City, Ca, USA). Analysis of PCR products was done using the COPY CALLER Software v1.0 (Life Technology, Foster City, USA) that allowed the classification of unambiguous homozygous (zero copies), heterozygous (one copy) and homozygous (two copies) *GSTM1* or *GSTT1* carrier individuals.

2.3. Statistical analysis

Associations between *MC1R* variants and melanoma risk were initially assessed individually using Fisher's exact test. Associations with melanoma were assessed using logistic regression. Estimating odds ratios (ORs), their associated 95% confidence intervals (CIs) and P-values were obtained using SPSS v19. Multivariate logistic regression was also applied, including age, sex, hair color, skin color, solar lentigines and childhood sunburn as covariates. Associations between the number of variants carried and various individual and tumor characteristics were assessed via logistic regression.

To study the effect of combined protective and risk genotypes, we reduced the sample set to 528 samples successfully genotyped for all the associated SNPs. We used a 2x2 contingency table and a t-student test between *SLC45A2* (rs35414) and both *SILV* (rs2069398) and *NOS1* (rs2682826), as well as with all three genes together. In addition, we studied the results between the risk alleles, *TYR* (rs17793678), *ADAMTS20* (rs1510521), *GSTP1* (rs1695) and *OCA2/HERC2* (rs12913832). Finally, we analyzed possible interactions between *MC1R* (0, 1 or 2 variants) and all previous risk and protective alleles

3. Results

3.1. MC1R

Of the 946 individuals studied, 559 (59.15%) carried at least one *MC1R* variant, including 388 (65.43%) of 593 cases and 171 (48.4%) of the 353 controls. A total of 36 *MC1R* variants were identified.

Among these, 25 variants were non-synonymous changes, 20 of which had been described previously [5] and 5 were identified for the first time: S41F, M128T, P268R, A285V and N281S. Six variants of the receptor have been traditionally associated with red hair color (RHC): D84E, R142H, R151C, R160W, I155T and D294H.

Similarly, another three variants have not been associated with RHC phenotype and have been designated as NRHC (V60L, V92M and R163Q). These amino acid changes have been studied in different populations because their frequency is greater than 1%.

The other variants detected in the *MC1R* gene have frequencies lower than 1% in control samples and included C35Y, F45L, a trinucleotide deletion that results in a new amino acid in position 54 (c.161delTGG, V54E), S83P, G89R, V92L, T95M, a nonsense change (Y152X), two nucleotide insertions (c.537insC, p.ins179C; and c.537insT, p.ins179T), R213W, R272M, K278E, and T308M, plus all novel ones described before. These rare variants have been designated as "ns_rare SNPs" in Figure 1. The synonymous variants included the most common change, T314T (A>G), and the rare changes I63I, Q233Q, I264I, F300F as well as I180I and S316S, the last two described for the first time. These synonymous variants are called "s_rare" with or without T314T in Figure 1. The estimated frequency of common *MC1R* variants and some combinations such as all synonymous changes with and without the common T314T and all non-synonymous rare variants, as well as the corresponding estimated OR for MM and associated P-values are shown in Figure 1.

Among the 36 changes detected, five were individually associated with melanoma risk: V60L, R151C, I155T, R160W and D294H ($P < 0.05$). The highest OR was estimated for I155T (OR 3.65, 95% CI: 1.40–9.52; P=0.006). The estimated OR associated with carrying one non-synonymous variant was 1.58 (95% CI: 1.19–2.097; P =0.0013); however, the OR for carrying two non-synonymous variants was 4.38 (95% CI: 2.72–7.05; P =1.33×10^{-9}). The MM associated OR among those Spanish patients carrying one RHC variant was 2.36 (95% CI: 1.71–3.26; P =1.86×10^{-7}). However if we consider individuals homozygous or compound heterozygous for two RHC variants, the OR increased to 12.76 (95% CI: 3.06–53.29; P =1.9×10^{-5}).

We considered blue /green eye color, blond /red hair color, solar lentigines and childhood sunburns as confounders in a multivariate model. *MC1R* variant analysis retained statistically significant results when adjusted for all potential confounders (OR: 1.77, 95% CI: 1.37–2.27; P =9.57×10^{-6}). Hair color, solar lentigines and childhood sunburns were independently associated with MM (OR: 2.11, 95% CI: 1.22–3.66, P=0.008; OR: 2.28 95% CI: 1.61–3.23, P=3.54×10^{-6}; OR: 4.77, 95% CI: 3.37–6.77, P =9.57×10^{-6}, respectively).

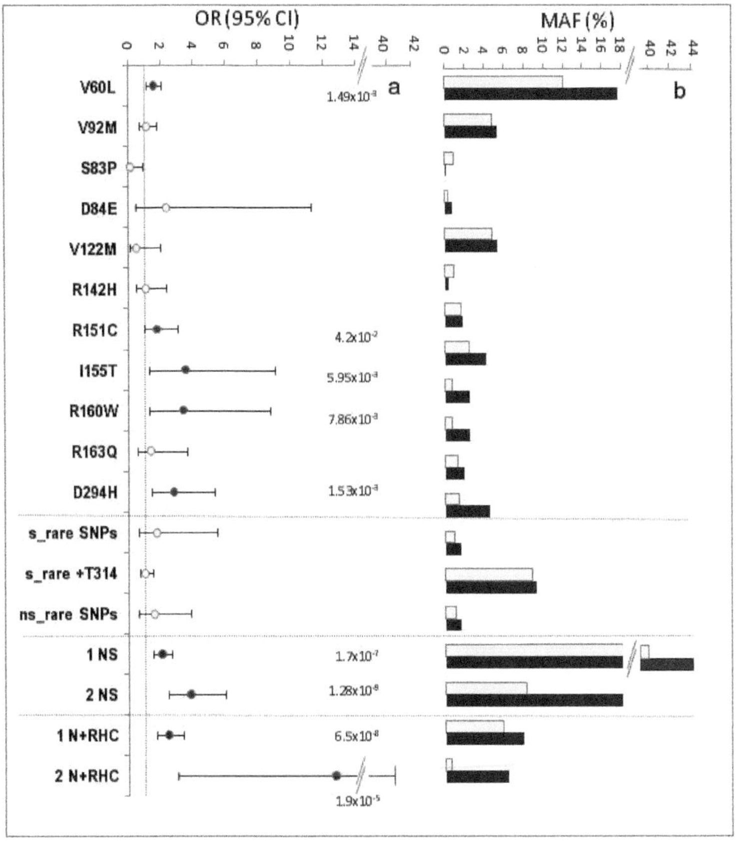

Figure 1. a) Summary of all *MC1R* variants associated with MM. Odds Ratios (OR), 95% confidence interval (95% CI) and P-values. b) Minor Allele Frequencies (MAF) of *MC1R* genetic variants. ns: non-synonymous variants :V60L, V92M, S83P, D84E,V122M, R142H, R151C, I155T R160W, R163Q and D294H; s_rare SNPs: synonymous variants with MAFs in controls lower than 1%: I63I, I180I, Q233Q, I264I, F300F and S316S; s_rare +T314T: same variants as before plus the addition of T314T; ns_rare SNPs: non-synonymous variants with less than 1% frequency in controls: C35Y;S41F, F45L, 54delTGG, G89R, V92L,T95M, M128T, Y152X, 179insTor C, R213W, P268R, T272M, K278E, N281S, A285V and T308M. Grey squares represent control data whereas black bars represent MM cases. Dark circles denote statistically significant values.

3.2. Other genes from pathways associated to melanoma

Several studies have been performed in order to evaluate other pigmentation-related genes and their relationship to MM susceptibility. The first results generated by Fernandez and cols. [4] analyzed the oculocutaneous albinism (OCA) genes: *TYR* (MIM#606933), *OCA2* (MIM#611409), *TYRP1* (MIM#115501) and *SLC45A2* (MIM#606202); the melanocyte protein *SILV* (MIM#155550) and *MC1R* inverse agonist *ASP* (MIM#600201).

Allele frequencies for each SNP and the P-value for their comparisons between case and control subjects are detailed in Figure 2. After discarding two of the selected SNPs, one in the *OCA2* gene due to its monomorphic nature in our sample collection, and one in the *SLC45A2* gene due to its departure from HWE, we observed evidence of differences in allele frequency for one SNP in the *SLC45A2* gene, corresponding to F374L (NCBI dbSNP rs16891982). The estimated OR per minor allele copy was 0.41 (95% CI, 0.24–0.70; P=0.001) with the minor allele being more frequent in controls than cases (16% vs. 7%; adjusted P=0.001).

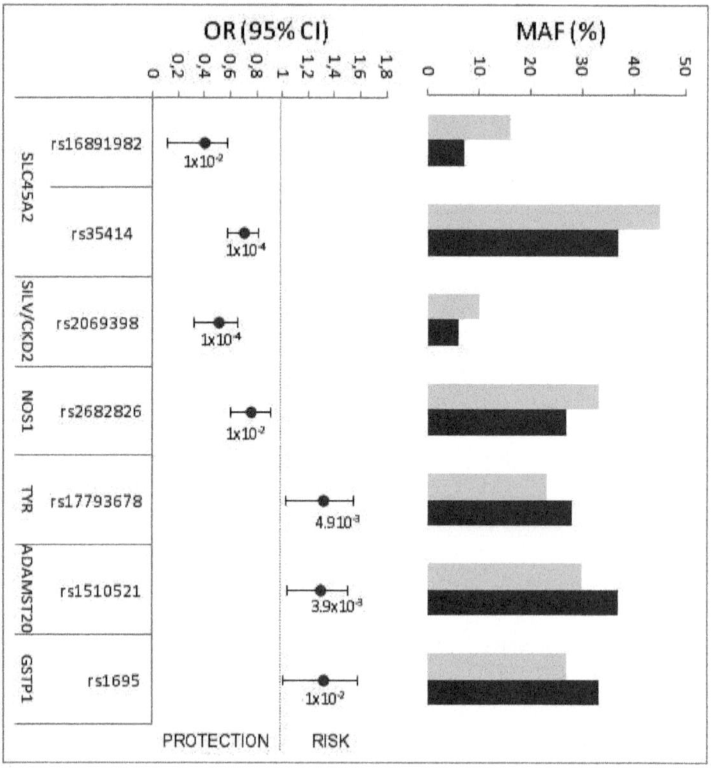

Figure 2. Odds ratios (OR), 95% confidence interval (95% CI), P-values and Minor Allele Frequency (MAF) for the best seven genetic variants in genes belonging to pigmentation, DNA repair and oxidative stress pathways. Grey bars represent control data while black bars represent MM cases. Dark circles denote statistically significant values. Exact P-values are indicated in number.

In a second study we genotyped 384 SNPs from 65 genes belonging mainly to the pigmentation pathway [16]. Ten SNPs located on six individual chromosomes (one in each of *ADAMTS20*, *TYR* and *SILV/CDK2*; two in each of *KIT* and *MYO7A*; and three in *SLC45A2*) constituted the top ten MM phase I associated SNPs in our sample after establishing a restrictive P-value threshold of 0.01. A phase II validation study was conducted to analyze the most significant SNP of each of the 6 candidate genes. One SNP, rs35414 in the *SLC45A2* gene, had an unadjusted P=0.002 in this phase II and overall OR of 0.75 (95% CI 0.67–0.84, P=0.0001) (Figure 2). None of the other five SNPs tested in phase II reached statistical significance at this stage. However, three of them, located in *TYR*, *SILV/CDK2* and *ADAMTS20* had an overall P<0.05 when phase I and II were considered together.

After analysis of genes in the pigmentation pathway, we conducted two studies where 16 genes belonging to both base excision repair (BER) and nucleotide excision repair (NER) pathways, as well as 14 genes involved in oxidative stress, including *GSTT1* and *GSTM1*, were screened for copy number variation [17, 27]. Two statistically significant results suggested a putative role of oxidative stress processes in the genetic predisposition to melanoma.

First of all, a novel variant in the *NOS1* oxidative stress gene (rs2682826) was detected (P=0.01). A second association pointed to *GSTP1* polymorphism rs1695, encoding the amino acid change I105V, and individually associated with MM (OR: 1.32, 95%CI: 1.06–1.63, P=0.01) found associated with melanoma for the first time. The best seven SNPs associated with MM in our population are shown in Figure 2. We could not detect any association between *GSTM1* or *GSTT1* deletions and MM risk.

3.3. Phenotypic characteristics

If we take into account *MC1R* and the associated phenotypic characteristics we detect the estimated ORs for melanoma associated with various phenotypic characteristics based on univariate analyses. MM risk was associated with the presence of blond or RHC (OR: 4.86, 95% CI: 2.35–10.03, P=2x10^{-5}), solar lentigines (OR: 1.71, 95% CI: 1.04–2.81, P =0.032) and childhood sunburn (OR: 10.41, 95%CI: 5.81–18.65, P=3x10^{-13}). No association with melanoma risk was observed for eye color, skin color or number of nevi.

The number of *MC1R* variants was statistically significantly associated with blond or RHC (OR: 1.80, 95% CI: 1.26–2.58, P=0.001), fair skin (OR: 1.42, 95% CI: 1.06–1.89, P=0.018) and with the presence of childhood sunburn (OR: 1.71, 95% CI: 1.28–2.27, P= 2x10^{-4}). The corresponding ORs for the number of functional *MC1R* variants were 2.32 (95% CI: 1.42–3.78, P=0.001) for blond or RHC, 1.58 (95% CI: 1.09–2.3, P= 0.014) for fair skin and 2.35 (95% CI: 1.6–3.45, P=5 x10^{-5}) for the presence of childhood sunburn.

We assessed whether *SLC45A2* polymorphisms were associated with various phenotypic characteristics. The F374L variant allele was associated with dark eye color, dark hair color, darker skin and absence of both solar lentigines and childhood sunburns. Finally, we tested for associations between *SLC45A2* SNPs and phototype, tumor location, and tumor depth among cases only (Table 5). The minor (G) allele of the F374L variant was found to be associated with phototypes III/IV (per allele OR, 3.25; 95% CI, 1.05–10.03; P=0.04). Additionally, *SLC45A2* SNPs rs35414 and rs35415 were also associated with dark skin color (P=0.028 and P=0.0485) and only rs35414 with dark hair color (P=0.0183).

Evidence of association with phenotypic characteristics for two *KIT* SNPs, rs759083 and rs13135792, were also present. Both SNPs appeared to be associated with both light hair color (P=0.0021 and P=0.0072) and childhood sunburns (P=0.0112 and P=0.0167).

Two different SNPs in *MYO7A* were associated with dark hair color (rs948970, P=0.04), and childhood sunburn (rs3758708, P=0.0474). One SNP in the *TYR* gene (rs17793678) was associated with light eye color (P=0.0239). Likewise, the *ADAMTS20* gene was associated with light eye color (P=0.0339), blond or red hair color (P=0.0353) and with number of nevi (rs1510521; P=0.0338). Finally, *SILV/CDK2* SNP rs2069398 was associated with absence of childhood sunburns (P=0.0353).

3.4. Gene-gene interactions

We explored the combined effects of the individually associated SNPs located in the six relevant genes studied: *SLC45A2, SILV, NOS1* (protective associated genes) and *TYR, ADAMTS20* and *GSTP1* (risk associated genes). Although in our series it does not show individual association with MM, we added rs12913832 from the *OCA2/HERC2* gene due to its strong association with eye color [6, 48] and the fact that it has been demonstrated to have epistatic effects with the *MC1R* gene [49].

3.4.1. Interaction between protective alleles

Two SNPs, rs16891982 and rs35414, located in the *SLC45A2* gene were associated with MM. Both of them could have been used to perform the interaction analyses; however, rs35414 was chosen due to its higher MAF. SNPs rs2069398, located in the *SILV/CDK2* gene region, and rs2682826 in *NOS1* were also included in the analyses. Interaction results are shown in Figure 3.

We observed some degree of epistatic protective interaction between rs35414 (*SLC45A2* gene) and rs2069398 (*SILV/CDK2* gene region) when considering rare allele carriers at both *loci*. A significant decrease in MM associated OR was observed when two (heterozygotes for both *SLC45A2* and *SILV*) or three (heterozygous for *SLC45A2* and minor homozygotes for *SILV*) rare alleles were present at both *loci* (OR: 0.54, 95% CI: 0.39–0.75, P=0.0003). Similarly, when three (minor homozygotes for *SLC45A2* and heterozygous for *SILV*) or four (minor homozygous for both *SLC45A2* and *SILV*) rare alleles were carried, a greater decrease in MM risk was observed (OR: 0.31, 95% CI: 0.18–0.55, P=0.0001). Results including joint genotypes for rs35414 and rs2069398 SNPs, individual status (heterozygous or minor homozygous), ORs with their corresponding 95% CIs and P-values are shown in Figure 3a.

In addition, we observed some degree of epistatic protective interaction between rs35414 (*SLC45A2*) and rs2682826 (*NOS1*) when considering heterozygote alleles at both *loci* (OR 0.23, 95% CI 0.16–0.55, P=0.0001). However, a trend toward protective effect was detected when both homozygous rare alleles were compared (OR: 0.50, 95% CI 0.18–1.20; P=0.1). This lack of statistically significant results is most probably due to the reduced number of samples in this category (21 MM cases vs. 17 controls). Results are shown in Figure 3b.

The interaction analyses between *NOS1* rs2682826 SNP and *SILV* rs20693989 SNP revealed a trend toward significance when both rare alleles are considered (OR: 0.19, 95% CI: 0.03–1.07, P=0.055). Results are shown in Figure 3c.

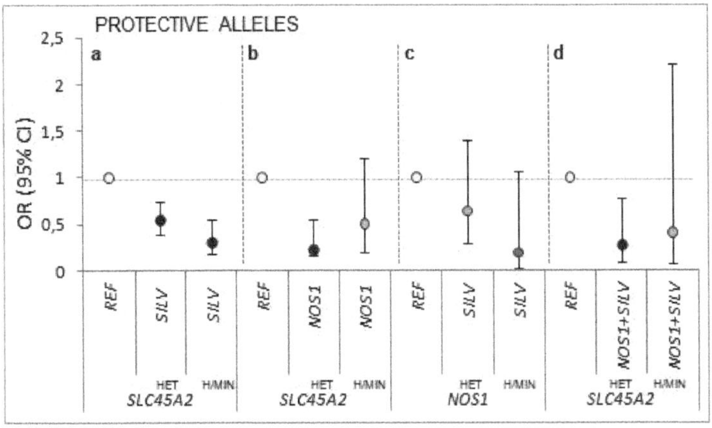

Figure 3. Interaction between protective allele variants and their effect on MM susceptibility. a) *SLC45A2* and *SILV*, b) *SLC45A2* and *NOS1*, c) *NOS1* and *SILV* and d) *SLC45A2*, *NOS1* and *SILV* all together. OR: odds ratios per minor allele; 95% CI: 95% confidence intervals; REF: reference value; HET: heterozygotes; and HMIN: minor homozygotes. For the genes labeled in vertical, we joined heterozygotes and minor homozygotes. Dark circles denote statistically significant results.

Finally, when the effect of the interaction between the three *loci* protectively associated with MM, rs35414 (*SLC45A2*), rs2682826 (*NOS1*) and rs2069398 (*SILV*) were analyzed, statistically significant results were observed. Individuals heterozygous for the three genes were more common in controls than in MM cases (OR: 0.09, 95% CI: 0.022–0.316, P=0.0001), showing a cumulative protective effect. The comparison with rare homozygous alleles in all three *loci* was statistically not relevant due to the small number of samples found (Figure 3d).

3.4.2. Interaction between risk alleles

In order to show the distinct combinations of MM risk alleles we performed two different analyses. The first comparison studied the effect in MM susceptibility by taking together four genotypes: rs17793678 (*TYR*), rs1510521 (*ADAMTS20]*; rs1695 (*GSTP1*), and rs12913832 (*OCA2/HERC2*). Results are shown in Figure 4a-d.

Some degree of epistatic risk interaction was seen between rs17793678 (*TYR*) and rs1510521 (*ADAMTS20*) when considering either heterozygous or rare alleles at both *loci*. We observed an increased risk effect when two or three rare alleles were present at both *loci* (rs17793678 heterozygotes and rs1510521 heterozygous, and minor homozygous carriers; OR: 1.41, 95% CI: 1.12–1.78, P=0.004). When three or four rare alleles (rs17793678 minor homozygotes and rs1510521 heterozygotes, and minor homozygous carriers) were analyzed together, we obtained an OR of 1.54 (95% CI 0.96–2.48) with a trend toward significance (P=0.088). Results are shown in Figure 4a.

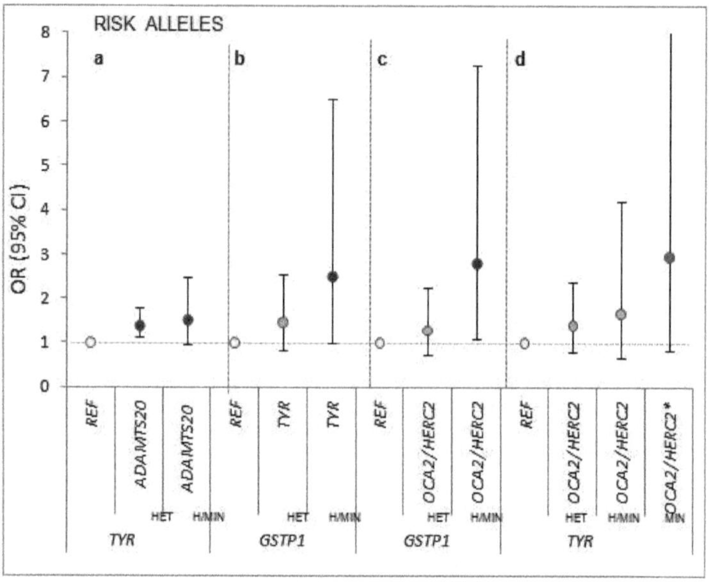

Figure 4. Interactions between risk allele variants and their effect on MM susceptibility. a) *TYR* and *ADAMTS20*, b) *GSTP1* and *TYR*, c) *GSTP1* and *OCA2/HERC2* and d) *TYR* and *OCA2/HERC2*. OR: odds ratios per minor allele; 95% CI: 95% confidence intervals; REF: reference value; HET: heterozygotes; H MIN: minor allele homozygotes; and MIN: only minor homozygotes for *TYR* and *GSTP1* respectively. For genes labeled in vertical we joined heterozygous and minor homozygous status. Dark circles denote statistically significant results.

A similar effect was observed when we compared rs1695 (*GSTP1*) with both rs1510521 (*ADAMTS20*) and rs12913832 (*OCA2/HERC2*) polymorphisms. We detected some degree of epistatic risk interaction when considering homozygous rare alleles at both *loci*. Results for rs1695 and rs1510521 showed an OR of 2.53 (95% CI 1.005–6.49, P=0.04, data shown in Figure 4b), while the interaction between rs1695 and rs12913832 had an OR of 2.81 (95% CI 1.11–7.27, P=0.018, see Figure 4c).

An additional comparison with rs17793678 (*TYR*) and rs12913832 (*HERC2/OCA2)* showed increasing epistasis as the number of risk alleles augmented, showing a trend toward significance only when homozygous minor alleles were considered at both *loci*, OR=2.95 (95% CI 0.84–11.326] (p=0.077). See Figure 4d. All other complex comparisons did not add further information.

For the second type of analyses we included the *MC1R locus* together with the previous four polymorphisms. As *MC1R* had already been associated with MM, it seemed biologically plausible that genetic interactions would be detected between risk variants within *MC1R* and other associated genes. Indeed, increased risks appeared when heterozygotes or rare alleles at *MC1R* were combined with heterozygotes plus rare homozygous at *GSTP1* (OR: 5.3, 95% CI: 2.80–417.42; P =1x10^{-4}, see Figure 5a), at *TYR* (OR: 6.42; 95% CI 2.32–18.64; P=0.0001, see Figure 5b), and at *OCA2/HERC2* (OR: 7.163; 95% CI 2.659–20.05; P=0.0001, see Figure 5c).

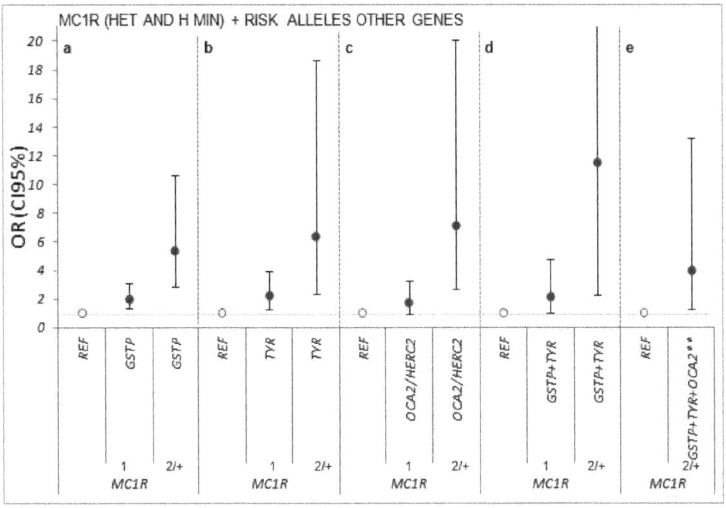

Figure 5. Interactions between risk allele variants on *MC1R* together with other risk associated genes alone or in multiple combinations, and their effect on MM susceptibility. a) *MC1R* and *GSTP1*, b) *MC1R* and *TYR*, c) *MC1R* and *OCA2/HERC2* and d) *MC1R*, *TYR* and *OCA2/HERC2*, e) *MC1R*, *GSTP1*, *TYR* and *OCA2/HERC2*. OR: odds ratios per minor allele; 95% CI: 95% confidence intervals; REF: reference value; HET: heterozygotes; H MIN: minor allele homozygotes. For the genes labeled in vertical we joined heterozygotes and minor homozygotes. Dark circles denote statistically significant results.

The last group of comparisons was done taking into consideration three and four genes at the same time. Firstly, we showed that combining *MC1R* genotypes with both *TYR* and *GSTP1* resulted in the highest MM associated risk (OR: 11.56, 95% CI 2.25–79.54, P=0.0001; data shown in Figure 5d). Secondly, we performed a final analysis taking into account only rare homozygotes of the four risk alleles and compared them, for MM association, with wild type genotype individuals. We obtained an OR of 4.008 (95% CI 1.25–13.2) with a P-value of 0.016 (see Figure 5e). There is not enough power to consider any other comparison with statistical significance.

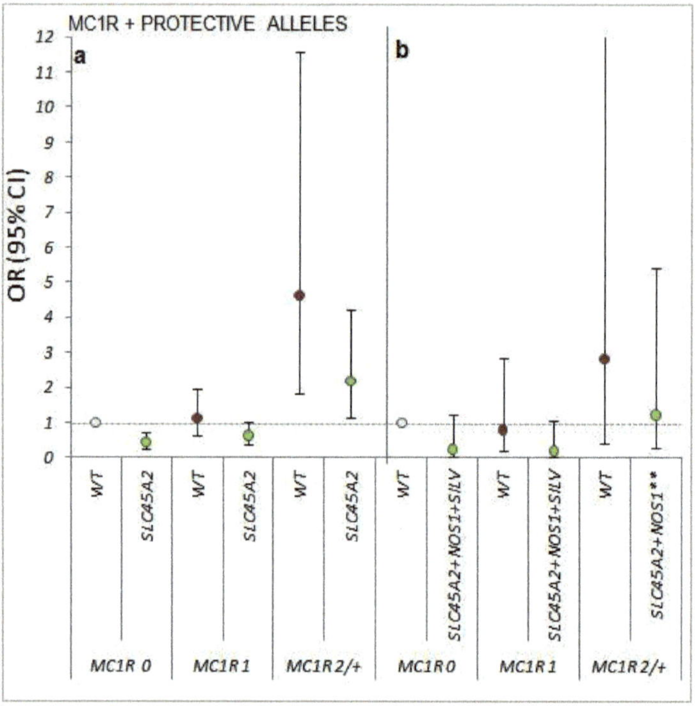

Figure 6. Interactions between risk variants on *MC1R* compared with protective alleles in a) *SLC45A2*, b) *SLC45A2*, *NOS1* and *SILV*, and their effect on MM susceptibility. OR: odds ratios per minor allele; 95% CI: 95% confidence intervals; WT: wild type alleles; *MC1R* 0: normal sequence in the *MC1R* gene; *MC1R* 1: carriers of 1 non-synonymous variant in *MC1R*; *MC1R* 2/+: carriers of two or more non-synonymous variants in the *MC1R* gene. For the genes labeled in vertical we have joined heterozygotes and minor homozygotes. Red circles represent carriers of risk alleles in *MC1R* whereas green circles correspond to carriers of risk alleles in *MC1R* and protective alleles either in *SLC45A2* alone or in combination.

3.4.3. Complex interactions

The role of *SLC45A2* and the other protective genes (*NOS1* and *SILV*) in melanoma predisposition was further analyzed in relation to *MC1R*, the main low-penetrance gene associated to melanoma. Since all these genes have been studied by our group, we analyzed the interaction effects between both *MC1R* and *SLC45A2 loci* (see Figure 6a) and between *MC1R* and all the protective alleles (see Figure 6b).

A great reduction of risk was detected when the rare protective alleles at *SLC45A2* were carried in individuals with two *MC1R* variants (OR: 2.20, 95% CI 1.14–4.23, P=0.02), in comparison to individuals carrying only two *MC1R* variants (OR: 4.64; 95% CI 1.85–11.58, P=0.001). Individuals having only one *MC1R* mutation plus the rare protective *SLC45A2* allele also showed a reduction in MM risk, although this decline does not seem to reach significant values (data shown in Figure 6a). These results confirmed the protective role of the rs35414 variant in *SLC45A2* regarding MM risk. Similar effects are observed when we included in the calculations the protective SNPs located in *NOS1* and *SILV*, however less statistically significant results were obtained due to the small number of samples in each class.

4. Discussion

Since *MC1R* genetic variability is strongly associated with the RHC phenotype [12], a large number of studies have investigated the involvement of this gene in MM susceptibility. *MC1R* is highly polymorphic, with more than 100 variants described in Caucasian populations [13]. Despite of its high variability, the synonymous changes are greatly reduced, with only three described in the literature: T314T (A>G), F300F (C>T) and C273C (C>T) [50, 51]. Results obtained from our laboratory confirmed the association between five *MC1R* polymorphic variants and MM risk in the Spanish population. We found 36 *MC1R* variants, this number being quite similar to the number found in other Mediterranean population studies (16 in France, 26–29 in Italy and 18 in Greece) [9, 11]. The most frequent Spanish variant is V60L with a frequency of 12.03%. This value is close to that reported in other populations (15.7% among Northern Italians, 12.4% among fair-skinned Australians and 15.0% among Northern Europeans) [52]. The RHC phenotype-associated variants (R151C, R160W and D294H) were present at frequencies of 0,71, 0.71 and 1.42%, respectively, in our population, compared to 9.9, 8.7 and 3.6%, respectively, reported in Northern European populations [52]. There were very few red-haired individuals among the control sample, and only 36 (6%) of MM cases had red hair. This finding is consistent with other results from Mediterranean populations and is at odds with red hair frequencies found in Northern European populations [12]. Red-haired subjects with no *MC1R* variants are not uncommon and have been seen in a Northern European population as well [53].

RHC variants have been consistently associated with MM in Northern European populations [3, 10, 12] and also in the Northern French population [9]. In Spain, we detected statistically significant individual associations for R151C, R160W and D294H. These three variants have been detected in the Northern French and Central Italian populations [9, 54]. We did not observe any MM risk associated with the rare RHC variant D84E (OR: 1.63, 95% CI: 0.02–128, P= 0.99), as detected in Northern Europeans [32, 55, 56], probably due to its low prevalence in Spain (0.28% in controls). The I155T variant has not been associated with MM in other populations to date, but this may also be due to its low frequency. However, our results clearly suggest that this rare variant increases risk of MM, at least in the Spanish population (OR: 3.51, 95% CI: 1.35–9.12, P= 0.006). While the associations of RHC with MM were expected, the case of V60L (an NRHC variant) was more intriguing, since its involvement in MM pathology has been generally unclear in Caucasian populations. However, V60L could play a role in MM susceptibility only in darker skinned populations since it has been found associated with MM in other Mediterranean populations such as France and Greece [9, 11]. The fact that NRHC variants could be important in MM risk is also supported by our finding that risk increased with the number of non-synonymous changes carried, regardless of whether they were RHC or NRHC. The presence of two non-synonymous changes implies that both copies of the MC1R protein are compromised. In addition, the presence of two NRHC increases by more than five times the risk of only one non-synonymous variant ($P=1.9x10^{-5}$). All these results taken together strongly support the role of the *MC1R* gene as highly linked to the susceptibility of developing MM in Mediterranean countries such as Spain [3, 5, 10, 52].

In recent years, *SLC45A2* has joined the group of genes (including *MC1R, OCA2,* and *ASP*) identified as being related to pigmentation, and it is now considered integral to pigmentation variation. Mutations in the *SLC45A2* or *MATP* gene (MIM #606202), which encodes the membrane-associated transporter, have recently been associated with the *OCA4* albinism subtype [57]. The non-synonymous variant F374L (rs16891982) has been reported to have a strong association with dark hair, skin and eye color in Europeans [58]. These phenotypic correlations were replicated in our analysis on the Spanish population and we also established for the first time its role in MM susceptibility [14]. We also found that other polymorphisms on *SLC45A2* other than rs16891982 were also associated with dark phenotypic characteristics [16], confirming the role of *SLC45A2* in pigmentation. A parallel work by Guedj and cols. [59] also detected association of this variant with melanoma in a French population, supporting our previous results. It has been proposed that the F374 allele causes a reduction of protein function that alters the intracellular trafficking of melanosomal proteins, creating an environment for decreased melanin production [58]. More than 90% of European genes carry the F374 allele, which is rare or absent in Africans. The remaining 10% of people of European descent with the Leucine ancestral allele (the most common in Africans) appear to have significantly more pigmented skin. There is a clear evidence of selective sweep of the chromosomal segment around the *SLC45A2* gene in the European population, which is consistent with our data [60]. The derived L374 allele shows unusually large allele frequency differences between Europeans and other populations, and has reduced haplotype diversity. These patterns are consistent with the action of recent natural selection on these genes in Europeans.

The *NOS1* gene is located on chromosome 12q24.2 and consists of 29 exons, encompassing more than 160kb of genomic DNA [61] and it is the main NO synthesizing enzyme in the central nervous system [62, 63]. The rs2682826 SNP is located in the 3′ UTR of exon 29 of the *NOS1* gene and was selected as the tag SNP of one of the most frequent haplotypes. However, rs2682826 seems to be the most likely functional SNP due to its location close to several miRNAs binding sites in 3′UTR region. Possibly, differences in protein translation might be elicited depending on the allele present in the mRNA of this gene. No other regulatory element close to this region seems to modulate this gene. We propose this SNP as a novel variant related to melanoma (P=0.01).

Despite not being able to detect association between MM and the absence of either *GSTM1* or *GSTT1* copies, minor homozygotes for rs1695 in the *GSTP1* gene appeared to be strongly associated with MM. The latter SNP encodes an amino acid change, I105V, that was described for the first time associated with MM (P =0.01) in our population. This finding is consistent with the hypothesis that patients with the *GSTP1* V105 variant enzyme have a reduced ability to detoxify compounds, which results in lower clearance and reduced efficacy. The *GSTP1* V105 variant is associated with a lower thermal stability and altered catalytic activity to a variety of substrates compared with those for *GSTP1* I105 [34].

It seemed biologically plausible that genetic interactions would be detected between several of the SNPs identified in our studies, and for that reason we grouped protective alleles located in the genes *SLC45A2, SILV/CDK2* and *NOS1*. On one hand, a great reduction of risk was detected when rare alleles at these *loci* were combined. The strongest protective combination was between *SLC45A2* and *SILV/CDK2*, followed by the combination of heterozygote samples at *SLC45A2* and *NOS1*. Other protective effects were seen, although they did not reach statistical significance due to the low number of samples in the analyzed categories.

In order to determine possible genetic interactions between *MC1R* and the rest of the genes studied, we compared individuals carrying risk variants in *TYR, ADAMTS20* or *OCA2/HERC2* with the *MC1R locus*. Indeed, increasing risk effects were observed in all comparisons when as more risk alleles accumulated in the same individuals. However, when *MC1R* was taken into consideration, the epistatic effect was far stronger, increasing from an OR of 4.38 when combined with *GSTP1* up to an OR of 11.56 when *MC1R, TYR* and *GSTP1* heterozygotes and homozygotes are considered together, and achieving risk effect values similar to having two *MC1R* RHC alleles. It is worth mentioning here that some genetic interactions, for instance between *MC1R* and *OCA2,* have already been described among pigmentation genes [49, 64].

Finally, we tried to see whether protective alleles were going to be able to reduce the risk induced by the accumulation of risk alleles. Some comparisons were not possible due to the absence of individuals in some of the categories. Therefore, we present only the results between *MC1R* risk alleles and the more robust protective gene, *SLC45A2,* alone or in combination with *NOS1* and *SILV.* We could indeed observe a great reduction in risk in individuals carrying two risk alleles in *MC1R* when simultaneously carrying protective alleles in the other genes. These results are important because the overall risk for an individual does not rely in only one gene but in the interaction of all his/hers genetic background and this should be considered in the future.

In summary, we found that five *MC1R* variants (V60L, R151C, I155T, R160W and D294H) are individually associated with MM risk in the Spanish population. Carrying two non-synonymous *MC1R* variants was associated with even higher risk, more than doubling the risk of carrying a single variant and having a five time higher risk than when carrying an NRHC variant. We described for the first time an association with the F374L variant, located on the *SLC45A2* gene, which appears to be a novel protective low-penetrance melanoma susceptibility gene. We therefore propose an integral study when trying to assert the MM risk of an individual, because the combination of rare alleles at several *loci* modulates the final risk/protective value that predisposes him/her to MM.

Acknowledgements

All these works were supported by several grants from the Ministerio de Educación y Ciencia (MEC) (SAF2007-65542-C02-01), Fundación Mutua Madrileña (FMMA 2009), and Ministerio Salud Carlos III (CP08/00069 and FI10_0405). LPF was funded by the Ministerio de Ciencia y Tecnología (MCT) and a grant from the Fondo de Investigación Sanitaria (FIS) FI05/00918; MI-V and MP-Ch were funded by the Spanish Ministerio de Educación y Ciencia under a grant FPI (BES-2008-009234) and by Generalitat Valenciana ValI+D under a grant (ACIF[2011/207) respectively. GR is funded by Ministerio de Salud Carlos III (MS08/00069). We thank the staff at the Spanish National Genotyping Centre in Santiago de Compostela and Madrid for their expert technical support with Sequenom and Illumina. Quantitative real-time PCR and Taqman was performed at the Unidad Central de Investigacion Medica (UCIM) of the Faculty of Medicine at the University of Valencia. Sequencing was done at the Sequencing Unit at CNIO and the Diagnostic and Genotyping Unit at UCIM, Faculty of Medicine at the University of Valencia.

Author details

G. Ribas[1], M. Ibarrola-Villava[1], M.C. Peña-Chilet[1], L.P. Fernandez[2] and C. Martinez-Cadenas[3]

1 Health Research Institute-INCLIVA, Av. Blasco Ibañez, Valencia, Spain

2 IIB Instituto de Investigaciones Biomédicas "Alberto Sols", Madrid, Spain

3 Department of Medicine, University of Castellon Jaume I, Castellon, Spain

References

[1] Bataille, V. Genetic epidemiology of melanoma. Eur J Cancer, 39: 1341-7, 2003

[2] Ferlay, J., Autier, P., Boniol, M., Heanue, M., Colombet, M., and Boyle, P. Estimates of the cancer incidence and mortality in Europe in 2006. Ann Oncol, 18: 581-92, 2007.

[3] Bastiaens, M. T., ter Huurne, J. A., Kielich, C., Gruis, N. A., Westendorp, R. G., Vermeer, B. J., and Bavinck, J. N. Melanocortin-1 receptor gene variants determine the risk of nonmelanoma skin cancer independently of fair skin and red hair. Am J Hum Genet, 68: 884-94, 2001

[4] Fernandez, L., Milne, R., Bravo, J., Lopez, J., Aviles, J., Longo, M., Benitez, J., Lazaro, P., and Ribas, G. MC1R: three novel variants identified in a malignant melanoma association study in the Spanish population. Carcinogenesis, 28: 1659-64, 2007

[5] Han, J., Kraft, P., Colditz, G. A., Wong, J., and Hunter, D. J. Melanocortin 1 receptor variants and skin cancer risk. Int J Cancer, 119: 1976-84, 2006.

[6] barrola-Villava, M., Fernandez, L. P., Pita, G., Bravo, J., Floristan, U., Sendagorta, E., Feito, M., Aviles, J. A., Martin-Gonzalez, M., Lazaro, P., Benitez, J., and Ribas, G. Genetic analysis of three important genes in pigmentation and melanoma susceptibility: CDKN2A, MC1R and HERC2/OCA2. Exp Dermatol, 19: 836-44, 2010

[7] Ibarrola-Villava, M., Hu, H. H., Guedj, M., Fernandez, L. P., Descamps, V., Basset-Seguin, N., Bagot, M., Benssussan, A., Saiag, P., Fargnoli, M. C., Peris, K., Aviles, J. A., Lluch, A., Ribas, G., and Soufir, N. MC1R, SLC45A2 and TYR genetic variants involved in melanoma susceptibility in Southern European populations: Results from a Meta-analysis. Eur J Cancer, 2012

[8] Kanetsky, P. A., Ge, F., Najarian, D., Swoyer, J., Panossian, S., Schuchter, L., Holmes, R., Guerry, D., and Rebbeck, T. R. Assessment of polymorphic variants in the melanocortin-1 receptor gene with cutaneous pigmentation using an evolutionary approach. Cancer Epidemiol Biomarkers Prev, 13: 808-19, 2004

[9] Matichard, E., Verpillat, P., Meziani, R., Gerard, B., Descamps, V., Legroux, E., Burnouf, M., Bertrand, G., Bouscarat, F., Archimbaud, A., Picard, C., Ollivaud, L., Basset-Seguin, N., Kerob, D., Lanternier, G., Lebbe, C., Crickx, B., Grandchamp, B., and Soufir, N. Melanocortin 1 receptor (MC1R) gene variants may increase the risk of melanoma in France independently of clinical risk factors and UV exposure. J Med Genet, 41: e13, 2004.

[10] Smith, R., Healy, E., Siddiqui, S., Flanagan, N., Steijlen, P. M., Rosdahl, I., Jacques, J. P., Rogers, S., Turner, R., Jackson, I. J., Birch-Machin, M. A., and Rees, J. L. Melanocortin 1 receptor variants in an Irish population. J Invest Dermatol, 111: 119-22, 1998.

[11] Stratigos, A. J., Dimisianos, G., Nikolaou, V., Poulou, M., Sypsa, V., Stefanaki, I., Papadopoulos, O., Polydorou, D., Plaka, M., Christofidou, E., Gogas, H., Tsoutsos, D., Kastana, O., Antoniou, C., Hatzakis, A., Kanavakis, E., and Katsambas, A. D. Melanocortin receptor-1 gene polymorphisms and the risk of cutaneous melanoma in a low-risk southern European population. J Invest Dermatol, 126: 1842-9, 2006

[12] Valverde, P., Healy, E., Jackson, I., Rees, J. L., and Thody, A. J. Variants of the melanocyte-stimulating hormone receptor gene are associated with red hair and fair skin in humans. Nat Genet, 11: 328-30, 1995.

[13] Wong, T. H., and Rees, J. L. The relation between melanocortin 1 receptor (MC1R) variation and the generation of phenotypic diversity in the cutaneous response to ultraviolet radiation. Peptides, 26: 1965-71, 2005

[14] Fernandez, L. P., Milne, R. L., Pita, G., Aviles, J. A., Lazaro, P., Benitez, J., and Ribas, G. SLC45A2: a novel malignant melanoma-associated gene. Hum Mutat, 29: 1161-7, 2008.

[15] Fernandez, L. P., Milne, R. L., Pita, G., Floristan, U., Sendagorta, E., Feito, M., Aviles, J. A., Martin-Gonzalez, M., Lazaro, P., Benitez, J., and Ribas, G. Pigmentation-related genes and their implication in malignant melanoma susceptibility. Exp Dermatol, 18: 634-42, 2009

[16] Ibarrola-Villava, M., Fernandez, L. P., Alonso, S., Boyano, M. D., Pena-Chilet, M., Pita, G., Aviles, J. A., Mayor, M., Gomez-Fernandez, C., Casado, B., Martin-Gonzalez, M., Izagirre, N., De la Rua, C., Asumendi, A., Perez-Yarza, G., Arroyo-Berdugo, Y., Boldo, E., Lozoya, R., Torrijos-Aguilar, A., Pitarch, A., Pitarch, G., Sanchez-Motilla, J. M., Valcuende-Cavero, F., Tomas-Cabedo, G., Perez-Pastor, G., Diaz-Perez, J. L., Gardeazabal, J., Martinez de Lizarduy, I., Sanchez-Diez, A., Valdes, C., Pizarro, A., Casado, M., Carretero, G., Botella-Estrada, R., Nagore, E., Lazaro, P., Lluch, A., Benitez, J., Martinez-Cadenas, C., and Ribas, G. A customized pigmentation SNP array identifies a novel SNP associated with melanoma predisposition in the SLC45A2 gene. PLoS One, 6: e19271, 2011.

[17] Ibarrola-Villava, M., Martin-Gonzalez, M., Lazaro, P., Pizarro, A., Lluch, A., and Ribas, G. Role of glutathione S-transferases in melanoma susceptibility: association with GSTP1 rs1695 polymorphism. Br J Dermatol, 166: 1176-83, 2012

[18] Baccarelli, A., Calista, D., Minghetti, P., Marinelli, B., Albetti, B., Tseng, T., Hedayati, M., Grossman, L., Landi, G., Struewing, J. P., and Landi, M. T. XPD gene polymorphism and host characteristics in the association with cutaneous malignant melanoma risk. Br J Cancer, 90: 497-502, 2004.

[19] Blankenburg, S., Konig, I. R., Moessner, R., Laspe, P., Thoms, K. M., Krueger, U., Khan, S. G., Westphal, G., Berking, C., Volkenandt, M., Reich, K., Neumann, C., Ziegler, A., Kraemer, K. H., and Emmert, S. Assessment of 3 xeroderma pigmentosum group C gene polymorphisms and risk of cutaneous melanoma: a case-control study. Carcinogenesis, 26: 1085-90, 2005

[20] Han, J., Colditz, G. A., Liu, J. S., and Hunter, D. J. Genetic variation in XPD, sun exposure, and risk of skin cancer. Cancer Epidemiol Biomarkers Prev, 14: 1539-44, 2005.

[21] Liu, D., O'Day, S. J., Yang, D., Boasberg, P., Milford, R., Kristedja, T., Groshen, S., and Weber, J. Impact of gene polymorphisms on clinical outcome for stage IV melanoma patients treated with biochemotherapy: an exploratory study. Clin Cancer Res, 11: 1237-46, 2005.

[22] Millikan, R. C., Hummer, A., Begg, C., Player, J., de Cotret, A. R., Winkel, S., Mohrenweiser, H., Thomas, N., Armstrong, B., Kricker, A., Marrett, L. D., Gruber, S. B., Culver, H. A., Zanetti, R., Gallagher, R. P., Dwyer, T., Rebbeck, T. R., Busam, K., From, L., Mujumdar, U., and Berwick, M. Polymorphisms in nucleotide excision repair genes and risk of multiple primary melanoma: the Genes Environment and Melanoma Study. Carcinogenesis, 27: 610-8, 2006.

[23] Tomescu, D., Kavanagh, G., Ha, T., Campbell, H., and Melton, D. W. Nucleotide excision repair gene XPD polymorphisms and genetic predisposition to melanoma. Carcinogenesis, 22: 403-8, 2001

[24] Wei, Q., Lee, J. E., Gershenwald, J. E., Ross, M. I., Mansfield, P. F., Strom, S. S., Wang, L. E., Guo, Z., Qiao, Y., Amos, C. I., Spitz, M. R., and Duvic, M. Repair of UV light-induced DNA damage and risk of cutaneous malignant melanoma. J Natl Cancer Inst, 95: 308-15, 2003

[25] Hu, Z., Ma, H., Chen, F., Wei, Q., and Shen, H. XRCC1 polymorphisms and cancer risk: a meta-analysis of 38 case-control studies. Cancer Epidemiol Biomarkers Prev, 14: 1810-8, 2005.

[26] Hung, R. J., Hall, J., Brennan, P., and Boffetta, P. Genetic polymorphisms in the base excision repair pathway and cancer risk: a HuGE review. Am J Epidemiol, 162: 925-42, 2005.

[27] Ibarrola-Villava, M., Pena-Chilet, M., Fernandez, L. P., Aviles, J. A., Mayor, M., Martin-Gonzalez, M., Gomez-Fernandez, C., Casado, B., Lazaro, P., Lluch, A., Benitez, J., Lozoya, R., Boldo, E., Pizarro, A., Martinez-Cadenas, C., and Ribas, G. Genetic polymorphisms in DNA repair and oxidative stress pathways associated with malignant melanoma susceptibility. Eur J Cancer, 47: 2618-25, 2011.

[28] Lockett, K. L., Hall, M. C., Xu, J., Zheng, S. L., Berwick, M., Chuang, S. C., Clark, P. E., Cramer, S. D., Lohman, K., and Hu, J. J. The ADPRT V762A genetic variant contributes to prostate cancer susceptibility and deficient enzyme function. Cancer Res, 64: 6344-8, 2004.

[29] Wilson, D. M., 3rd, and Bohr, V. A. The mechanics of base excision repair, and its relationship to aging and disease. DNA Repair (Amst), 6: 544-59, 2007.

[30] Baars, A. J., and Breimer, D. D. The glutathione S-transferases: their role in detoxification and toxification of xenobiotics. Ann Biol Clin (Paris), 38: 49-56, 1980.

[31] Lusini, L., Tripodi, S. A., Rossi, R., Giannerini, F., Giustarini, D., del Vecchio, M. T., Barbanti, G., Cintorino, M., Tosi, P., and Di Simplicio, P. Altered glutathione anti-oxidant metabolism during tumor progression in human renal-cell carcinoma. Int J Cancer, 91: 55-9, 2001

[32] Mossner, R., Anders, N., Konig, I. R., Kruger, U., Schmidt, D., Berking, C., Ziegler, A., Brockmoller, J., Kaiser, R., Volkenandt, M., Westphal, G. A., and Reich, K. Variations of the melanocortin-1 receptor and the glutathione-S transferase T1 and M1 genes in cutaneous malignant melanoma. Arch Dermatol Res, 298: 371-9, 2007

[33] Nebert, D. W., and Vasiliou, V. Analysis of the glutathione S-transferase (GST) gene family. Hum Genomics, 1: 460-4, 2004

[34] Bu, H., Rosdahl, I., Holmdahl-Kallen, K., Sun, X. F., and Zhang, H. Significance of glutathione S-transferases M1, T1 and P1 polymorphisms in Swedish melanoma patients. Oncol Rep, 17: 859-64, 2007.

[35] Dolzan, V., Rudolf, Z., and Breskvar, K. Genetic susceptibility to environmental carcinogenesis in Slovenian melanoma patients. Acta Dermatovenerol Alp Panonica Adriat, 15: 69-78, 2006.

[36] Heagerty, A. H., Fitzgerald, D., Smith, A., Bowers, B., Jones, P., Fryer, A. A., Zhao, L., Alldersea, J., and Strange, R. C. Glutathione S-transferase GSTM1 phenotypes and protection against cutaneous tumors. Lancet, 343: 266-8, 1994

[37] Kanetsky, P. A., Holmes, R., Walker, A., Najarian, D., Swoyer, J., Guerry, D., Halpern, A., and Rebbeck, T. R. Interaction of glutathione S-transferase M1 and T1 genotypes and malignant melanoma. Cancer Epidemiol Biomarkers Prev, 10: 509-13, 2001

[38] Lafuente, A., Molina, R., Palou, J., Castel, T., Moral, A., and Trias, M. Phenotype of glutathione S-transferase Mu (GSTM1] and susceptibility to malignant melanoma. MMM group. Multidisciplinary Malignant Melanoma Group. Br J Cancer, 72: 324-6, 1995.

[39] Shanley, S. M., Chenevix-Trench, G., Palmer, J., and Hayward, N. Glutathione S-transferase GSTM1 null genotype is not overrepresented in Australian patients with nevoid basal cell carcinoma syndrome or sporadic melanoma. Carcinogenesis, 16: 2003-4, 1995

[40] Amos, C. I., Wang, L. E., Lee, J. E., Gershenwald, J. E., Chen, W. V., Fang, S., Kosoy, R., Zhang, M., Qureshi, A. A., Vattathil, S., Schacherer, C. W., Gardner, J. M., Wang, Y., Bishop, D. T., Barrett, J. H., MacGregor, S., Hayward, N. K., Martin, N. G., Duffy, D. L., Mann, G. J., Cust, A., Hopper, J., Brown, K. M., Grimm, E. A., Xu, Y., Han, Y., Jing, K., McHugh, C., Laurie, C. C., Doheny, K. F., Pugh, E. W., Seldin, M. F., Han, J., and Wei, Q. Genome-wide association study identifies novel loci predisposing to cutaneous melanoma. Hum Mol Genet, 20: 5012-23, 2011.

[41] Barrett, J. H., Iles, M. M., Harland, M., Taylor, J. C., Aitken, J. F., Andresen, P. A., Akslen, L. A., Armstrong, B. K., Avril, M. F., Azizi, E., Bakker, B., Bergman, W., Bianchi-Scarra, G., Bressac-de Paillerets, B., Calista, D., Cannon-Albright, L. A., Corda, E., Cust, A. E., Debniak, T., Duffy, D., Dunning, A. M., Easton, D. F., Friedman, E., Galan, P., Ghiorzo, P., Giles, G. G., Hansson, J., Hocevar, M., Hoiom, V., Hopper, J. L., Ingvar, C., Janssen, B., Jenkins, M. A., Jonsson, G., Kefford, R. F., Landi, G., Landi, M. T., Lang, J., Lubinski, J., Mackie, R., Malvehy, J., Martin, N. G., Molven, A., Montgomery, G. W., van Nieuwpoort, F. A., Novakovic, S., Olsson, H., Pastorino, L., Puig, S., Puig-Butille, J. A., Randerson-Moor, J., Snowden, H., Tuominen, R., Van Belle, P., van der Stoep, N., Whiteman, D. C., Zelenika, D., Han, J., Fang, S., Lee, J. E., Wei, Q., Lathrop, G. M., Gillanders, E. M., Brown, K. M., Goldstein, A. M., Kanetsky, P. A., Mann, G. J., Macgregor, S., Elder, D. E., Amos, C. I., Hayward, N. K., Gruis, N. A., Demenais, F., Bishop, J. A., and Bishop, D. T. Genome-wide association study identifies three new melanoma susceptibility loci. Nat Genet, 43: 1108-13, 2011.

[42] Bishop, D. T., Demenais, F., Iles, M. M., Harland, M., Taylor, J. C., Corda, E., Randerson-Moor, J., Aitken, J. F., Avril, M. F., Azizi, E., Bakker, B., Bianchi-Scarra, G., Bres-

sac-de Paillerets, B., Calista, D., Cannon-Albright, L. A., Chin, A. W. T., Debniak, T., Galore-Haskel, G., Ghiorzo, P., Gut, I., Hansson, J., Hocevar, M., Hoiom, V., Hopper, J. L., Ingvar, C., Kanetsky, P. A., Kefford, R. F., Landi, M. T., Lang, J., Lubinski, J., Mackie, R., Malvehy, J., Mann, G. J., Martin, N. G., Montgomery, G. W., van Nieuwpoort, F. A., Novakovic, S., Olsson, H., Puig, S., Weiss, M., van Workum, W., Zelenika, D., Brown, K. M., Goldstein, A. M., Gillanders, E. M., Boland, A., Galan, P., Elder, D. E., Gruis, N. A., Hayward, N. K., Lathrop, G. M., Barrett, J. H., and Bishop, J. A. Genome-wide association study identifies three loci associated with melanoma risk. Nat Genet, 41: 920-5, 2009.

[43] Han, J., Kraft, P., Nan, H., Guo, Q., Chen, C., Qureshi, A., Hankinson, S. E., Hu, F. B., Duffy, D. L., Zhao, Z. Z., Martin, N. G., Montgomery, G. W., Hayward, N. K., Thomas, G., Hoover, R. N., Chanock, S., and Hunter, D. J. A genome-wide association study identifies novel alleles associated with hair color and skin pigmentation. PLoS Genet, 4: e1000074, 2008

[44] Macgregor, S., Montgomery, G. W., Liu, J. Z., Zhao, Z. Z., Henders, A. K., Stark, M., Schmid, H., Holland, E. A., Duffy, D. L., Zhang, M., Painter, J. N., Nyholt, D. R., Maskiell, J. A., Jetann, J., Ferguson, M., Cust, A. E., Jenkins, M. A., Whiteman, D. C., Olsson, H., Puig, S., Bianchi-Scarra, G., Hansson, J., Demenais, F., Landi, M. T., Debniak, T., Mackie, R., Azizi, E., Bressac-de Paillerets, B., Goldstein, A. M., Kanetsky, P. A., Gruis, N. A., Elder, D. E., Newton-Bishop, J. A., Bishop, D. T., Iles, M. M., Helsing, P., Amos, C. I., Wei, Q., Wang, L. E., Lee, J. E., Qureshi, A. A., Kefford, R. F., Giles, G. G., Armstrong, B. K., Aitken, J. F., Han, J., Hopper, J. L., Trent, J. M., Brown, K. M., Martin, N. G., Mann, G. J., and Hayward, N. K. Genome-wide association study identifies a new melanoma susceptibility locus at 1q21.3. Nat Genet, 43: 1114-8, 2011.

[45] Ewing, B., and Green, P. Base-calling of automated sequencer traces using phred. II. Error probabilities. Genome Res, 8: 186-94, 1998.

[46] Gordon, D., Abajian, C., and Green, P. Consed: a graphical tool for sequence finishing. Genome Res, 8: 195-202, 1998.

[47] Nickerson, D. A., Tobe, V. O., and Taylor, S. L. PolyPhred: automating the detection and genotyping of single nucleotide substitutions using fluorescence-based resequencing. Nucleic Acids Res, 25: 2745-51, 1997.

[48] Jannot, A. S., Meziani, R., Bertrand, G., Gerard, B., Descamps, V., Archimbaud, A., Picard, C., Ollivaud, L., Basset-Seguin, N., Kerob, D., Lanternier, G., Lebbe, C., Saiag, P., Crickx, B., Clerget-Darpoux, F., Grandchamp, B., Soufir, N., and Melan, C. Allele variations in the OCA2 gene (pink-eyed-dilution locus) are associated with genetic susceptibility to melanoma. Eur J Hum Genet, 13: 913-20, 2005.

[49] Duffy, D. L., Box, N. F., Chen, W., Palmer, J. S., Montgomery, G. W., James, M. R., Hayward, N. K., Martin, N. G., and Sturm, R. A. Interactive effects of MC1R and OCA2 on melanoma risk phenotypes. Hum Mol Genet, 13: 447-61, 2004.

[50] Harding, R. M., Healy, E., Ray, A. J., Ellis, N. S., Flanagan, N., Todd, C., Dixon, C., Sajantila, A., Jackson, I. J., Birch-Machin, M. A., and Rees, J. L. Evidence for variable selective pressures at MC1R. Am J Hum Genet, 66: 1351-61, 2000.

[51] Rana, B. K., Hewett-Emmett, D., Jin, L., Chang, B. H., Sambuughin, N., Lin, M., Watkins, S., Bamshad, M., Jorde, L. B., Ramsay, M., Jenkins, T., and Li, W. H. High polymorphism at the human melanocortin 1 receptor locus. Genetics, 151: 1547-57, 1999.

[52] Sturm, R. A., Teasdale, R. D., and Box, N. F. Human pigmentation genes: identification, structure and consequences of polymorphic variation. Gene, 277: 49-62, 2001.

[53] Sturm, R. A., Box, N. F., and Ramsay, M. Human pigmentation genetics: the difference is only skin deep. Bioessays, 20: 712-21, 1998.

[54] Fargnoli, M. C., Chimenti, S., Keller, G., Hofler, H., and Peris, K. Identification of four novel melanocortin 1 receptor (MC1R) gene variants in a Mediterranean population. Hum Mutat, 21: 655, 2003.

[55] Palmer, J. S., Duffy, D. L., Box, N. F., Aitken, J. F., O'Gorman, L. E., Green, A. C., Hayward, N. K., Martin, N. G., and Sturm, R. A. Melanocortin-1 receptor polymorphisms and risk of melanoma: is the association explained solely by pigmentation phenotype? Am J Hum Genet, 66: 176-86, 2000.

[56] Valverde, P., Healy, E., Sikkink, S., Haldane, F., Thody, A. J., Carothers, A., Jackson, I. J., and Rees, J. L. The Asp84Glu variant of the melanocortin 1 receptor (MC1R) is associated with melanoma. Hum Mol Genet, 5: 1663-6, 1996

[57] Sturm, R. A., and Frudakis, T. N. Eye color: portals into pigmentation genes and ancestry. Trends Genet, 20: 327-32, 2004.

[58] Graf, J., Hodgson, R., and van Daal, A. Single nucleotide polymorphisms in the MATP gene are associated with normal human pigmentation variation. Hum Mutat, 25: 278-84, 2005.

[59] Guedj, M., Bourillon, A., Combadieres, C., Rodero, M., Dieude, P., Descamps, V., Dupin, N., Wolkenstein, P., Aegerter, P., Lebbe, C., Basset-Seguin, N., Prum, B., Saiag, P., Grandchamp, B., and Soufir, N. Variants of the MATP/SLC45A2 gene are protective for melanoma in the French population. Hum Mutat, 29: 1154-60, 2008.

[60] Jackson, I. J. Identifying the genes causing human diversity. Eur J Hum Genet, 14: 979-80, 2006.

[61] Hall, A. V., Antoniou, H., Wang, Y., Cheung, A. H., Arbus, A. M., Olson, S. L., Lu, W. C., Kau, C. L., and Marsden, P. A. Structural organization of the human neuronal nitric oxide synthase gene (NOS1]. J Biol Chem, 269: 33082-90, 1994.

[62] Baranano, D. E., Ferris, C. D., and Snyder, S. H. Atypical neural messengers. Trends Neurosci, 24: 99-106, 2001

[63] Snyder, S. H., and Ferris, C. D. Novel neurotransmitters and their neuropsychiatric relevance. Am J Psychiatry, 157: 1738-51, 2000.

[64] Duffy, D. L., Zhao, Z. Z., Sturm, R. A., Hayward, N. K., Martin, N. G., and Montgomery, G. W. Multiple pigmentation gene polymorphisms account for a substantial proportion of risk of cutaneous malignant melanoma. J Invest Dermatol, 130: 520-8, 2010.

Chapter 5

Recombinant DNA Technology in Emerging Modalities for Melanoma Immunotherapy

Vitali Alexeev, Alyson Pidich,
Daria Marley Kemp and Olga Igoucheva

Additional information is available at the end of the chapter

1. Introduction

The history of immunotherapy of cancer dates back to 1890s when New York surgeon William Coley used Streptococcus and Serratia bacterial extracts to treat cancer. Up to the mid-1930s 'Coley's mixed toxins,'' were used to treat various tumors. Better understanding of the human immune system led to the identification of a number of tumor-associated antigens (TAAs) in the 1980s [1] and development of various immunotherapeutic approaches. Of particular relevance to melanoma immunotherapy was the identification of various antigens expressed specifically in melanocytes and, respectively, in the majority of melanomas. These melanoma-associated antigens include tyrosinase (Tyr), a key enzyme in melanin biosynthesis, tyrosinase-related proteins 1 and 2 (TRP1, TRP2), gp100 (aka pmel17), Melan-a, and MART1. These and several other melanoma-associated antigens formed the basis for the immunologic targeting of the tumor. Up to date, multiple peptide, dendritic cell, adjuvant, lymphocyte, antibody, DNA and virus-based strategies were tested in pre-clinical and clinical studies with varying degrees of success. In recent years, identification of the specific antigenic MHC class I epitopes, advancements in genetic engineering, gene delivery, and cell-based therapeutic approaches allowed development of the novel melanoma-targeting immuno-therapeutics.

2. Genetic engineering of antigen-specific T cells

2.1. Recombinant T cell receptors

Identification of the tumor-reactive T cells among a population of the tumor-infiltrating lymphocytes led to the development of the T cell-based therapies, particularly to the strategy known as adoptive T cells transfer. This strategy is based on the isolation of the tumor-infiltrating lymphocytes following analysis of their ability to target tumor cells and clonal expansion of tumor-reactive T cells via stimulation of cell proliferation with anti-CD3 and antiCD28 antibodies in the presence of IL-2. Upon obtaining a large quantity (> 10^8 cells), these cells are infused back to a tumor-bearing patient along with the lymphodepleting chemotherapy to temporary knock down circulating immunocytes and repetitive administration of the IL-2 (Fig. 1).

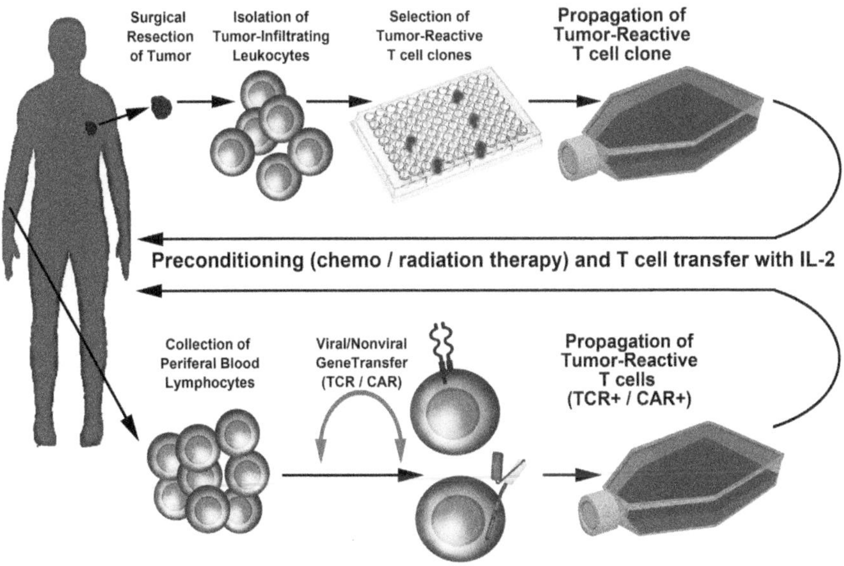

Figure 1. Clinical application of the T cell-mediated tumor immunotherapy. Diagram on the top depicts application of the Tumor-Infiltrating Lymphocytes (TILs). Diagram on the bottom illustrates application of the genetically engineered (TCR and CAR-modified) T cells.

Presently, 87 clinical trials using TIL are completed or on-going. These clinical trials are aimed at treatment of multiple cancers including: Malignant Melanoma, Nasopharyngeal Carcinoma, Hepatocellular Carcinoma, Breast Carcinoma, Leukemia, Lymphoma, Multiple Myeloma, Plasma Cell Neoplasm, Kidney Cancer, Metastatic Colorectal Cancer, Metastatic Gastric Cancer, Metastatic Pancreatic Cancer, Metastatic Hepatocellular Carcinoma, Cervical Cancer, Oropharyngeal Cancer, Vaginal Cancer, Anal Cancer, Penile Cancer, Non-Small Cell Lung Cancer, Brain and Central Nervous System Tumors. Several completed clinical trials on malignant melanoma clearly demonstrated that infusing TILs along with IL-2 and pre-conditioning with reduced-intensity circulating lymphocyte-depleting chemotherapy mediates tumor-targeting immune response in up to 50% of patients [2]. The highest response rate up to 70 % with up to 30% complete remission lasting for up to 3 years was reported when radiation sensitization was used in conjunction with the transfer of the tumor-reactive TILs.

Despite the success of the pioneering studies at the Surgery Branch of the US National Cancer Institute and the consequent clinical trials, this approach, although holding much promise in treating melanoma, is facing several challenges that limit broad application of the TIL-based immunotherapy. As TILs are isolated from resected tumors, the first and foremost requirement is the eligibility for surgery, which should be conducted, preferably, in the facility equipped for the isolation of TILs, identification and expansion of the tumor-reactive T cells. *Ex vivo* stimulation and propagation of TILs to large quantities required for the effective immunotherapy is time-consuming, labor-retaining, and expensive. Although recent clinical studies showed that infusion of the minimally cultured TILs without pre-selection for tumor reactivity provide a rather high response rate [3], the search for a better melanoma-targeting strategy is on-going.

Nevertheless, isolation of the individual melanoma-reactive T cell clones allowed the development of another immunotherapeutic approach – generation of the T cells expressing recombinant antigen specific T cell receptors (TCRs). TCRs are members of the immunoglobulin family proteins. Each TCR consists of 2 different membrane-anchored chains that are joined by the disulfide bridges to form heterodimer. About 95% of the T cells are characterized by the expression of the α and β chains, whereas the remaining 5% express γ and δ chains. Respectively, T cells expressing these receptors are often referred to as α/β and γ/δ T cells. Each chain is comprised of the variable and constant regions. The variable domain of both α- and β-chains have three hypervariable regions also known as complementarity determining regions (CDR), however, the β-chain has an additional area of hypervariability that is not involved in antigen binding. TCR α and γ chains are generated within T cells by VJ recombination, whereas β and δ chains by the V(D)J recombination. Currently, the majority of the TILs selected for the ability to target tumors are α/β T cells expressing respective TCR chains that determine T cell specificity to an antigenic peptides presented by the major histocompatability complex (MHC) proteins. Therefore, it was proposed that sequences encoding tumor antigen recognizing TCR chains can be obtained from tumor-reactive T cells and then used for the gene transfer into patient-derived lymphocytes, thereby creating large quantities of tumor-reactive T cells. The first TCRs specific to melanocytic antigens MART-1 and gp-100 were cloned in 1990s. Pioneering clinical studies using human peripheral blood lymphocytes transduced with these TCRs demonstrated melanoma regression in lymphodepleted patients [4] (Fig. 1). Although these and other initial clinical studies demonstrated a feasibility of the recombinant T cells-based approach, they also revealed multiple challenges. For example, the ability of recombinant TCR chains to interact and pair with the endogenous chains could lead to the generation of 4 different TCRs in a single cell (Fig. 2). Chain misparing decreases the expression of the function, tumor-reactive TCRs and therefore reduces T cell-mediated tumor targeting. To overcome misparing, several strategies were proposed. Recent pre-clinical and clinical studies demonstrated that replacement of the human TCR constant region with murine counterpart reduced misparing and allowed enhanced expression of the functional TCRs and improved T cell functional activity [5]. It was also reported that targeted mutagenesis and generation of the additional cystein residues in recombinant α and β chains permitted stronger pairing of these chains, higher expression of functional TCRs and improved T cell function [6, 7]. Recent studies also showed that targeting of the endogenous chains by siRNA allows higher expression of the functional recombinant TCR. Of particular interest is the proposed approach to encode siRNA along with the TCR chains to concurrently express recombinant and inhibit translation of the endogenous chains [8]. Protein engineering was also employed to improve pairing of the recombinant chains. Thus, substitution of specific amino acids within constant regions of the antigen-specific TCRs supported paring and enhanced functional activity of these receptors [9]. It remains to be determined which of these recombinant DNA-based methods will provide better targeting of melanoma (Fig. 2). Nevertheless, recent studies using chimeric murine-human hybrid highly avid tyrosinase-specific TCR demonstrated a favorable clinical outcome [10].

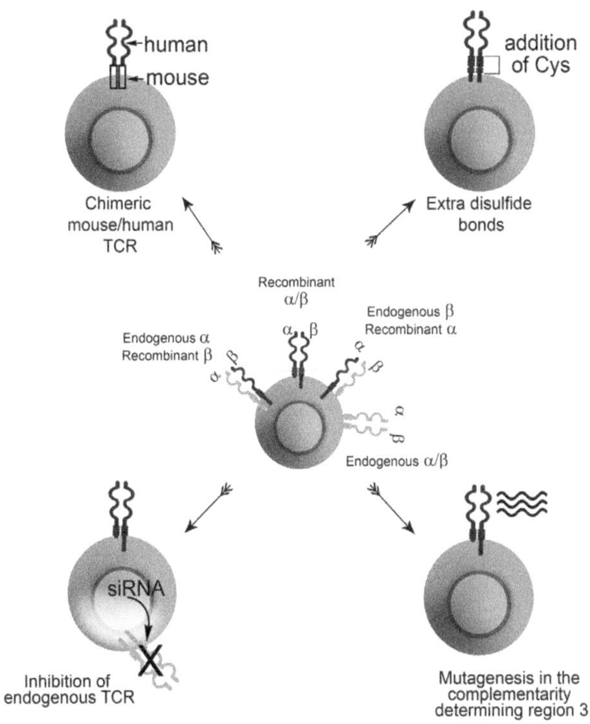

Figure 2. Strategies aimed at the improvement of the recombinant TCR pairing. Expression of the recombinant TCR may lead to the generation of 4 different TCRs within a cell (center). Different strategies designed to improve tumor-specific recombinant TCR pairing and activity include: generation of hybrid molecules containing the constant region from murine TCR, addition of disulfide bonds, alteration of the amino acid sequence within the TCR chains, and siRNA-mediated inhibition of the endogenous TCR gene expression (see text for details).

It is apparent that both α and β chains of the antigen-specific TCR should be expressed in each individual T cell. To date, internal ribosomal entry site (IRES) elements [11], double promoters [12], or co-infection with several viral vectors [13] were used to express several heterologous proteins in cells. However, these methods have their imperfections. For instance, in IRES-mediated co-expression, the upstream protein is usually more strongly transcribed than the downstream protein. Expression of the proteins from two different or biscistronic promoters or the use of multiples viruses also do not provide equal concurrent expression of multiple transgenes. A more promising approach involves the use of the self-processing viral peptide bridges such as 2A or 2A-like peptides described in Picornaviridae [14]. In picornavirus, these sequences share a highly conservative 18 amino acids motif mediating cleavage between C-terminal glycine and N-terminal proline of the 2B peptide. At present 2a and 2A-like sequences are commonly refer to as *cis*-acting hydrolase elements that allows ribosome skipping and cellular expression of multiple, discrete proteins in essentially equimolar quantities derived from a single ORF. To ensure concurrent expression of both α and β chains of the transgenic TCR an A2 sequence is most commonly used for quantitative co-expression of these heterologous proteins.

Transfer of the recombinant TCR genes into the T cells is another somewhat limiting factor for the broad application of the genetically engineered T cells for melanoma immuno-targeting. Currently, for human applications, a gene transfer platform that can mediate stable transfer of the TCR genes is retroviral system [15]. Lentiviral vectors and transposons were also tested [16, 17]. Use of retroviruses provided several advantages including a rather high infectivity and rapid integration of the transgene into host genome. With multiple vector backbones, virus packaging cell lines, and well-established GMP protocols, a retroviral system offers relative simplicity of viral vector construction and production of viruses. Since retroviruses can infect only dividing cells, stimulation of the T cell proliferation must be done prior to the gene transfer. Also, these viruses have limited capacity for the packaging. For instance, high virus titers cannot be obtained with larger retroviral vectors. Although an average size of a viral vector encoding typical α/β TCR is around 7 kb, this limits possible alternative approaches such as inclusion of various regulatory elements or another transgenes that may enhance T cell activation. Use of the viral system also presents certain safety concerns relevant to the random integration of the transgenes into the host genome that may result in the activation of oncogenes or inactivation of tumor suppressors. This may lead to the various adverse invents including development of a lymphoproliferative disease resembling leukemia due, in part, to the integration of the retroviral gene transfer vehicle near an oncogene [18, 19]. Thus far, the development of lymphoma-like symptoms has not been reported in patients treated with recombinant T cells. It is also essential to note that production of the TCR-encoding cGMP virus substantially increases the cost of the treatment with recombinant T cells. On the contrary to the retrovirus-based gene transfer, lentiviruses can infect non-dividing cells and therefore can be used for the gene transfer into quiescent T cells. Although "safe" lentiviral systems are developed to minimize the chance of producing replication-competent virus (eg. ViaraSafe from Cell Biolabs), transduction of patient-derived T cells for the adoptive transfer will always present some degree of risk.

Besides viral approaches, non-viral gene transfer may also be used for the expression of the TCRs in T cells. Recently, a Sleeping Beauty Transposon System was tested for the transduction of the T cells [17]. Sleeping Beauty Transposon System consists of two components - the transposon, composed of inverted terminal repeat sequences (IRs) with desired genetic material in between, and a SB transposase enzyme. Most recently, a number of IRs and hyperactive transposases with increasing enzymatic activities were developed to mediate transposition of transposon-encoding proteins into the genomic DNA [20]. Although transposition of SB transposons appears to be unregulated, it has certain advantages over viral based approaches. For instance, expression of transgenes, TCRs in particular, could be regulated by specific promoters that provide either T cell specific expression (eg. CD3 promoter; [21, 22]), or high level of expression (eg. elongation factor 1 promoter; [23,24]. Promoters may also be selected for further specific applications (discussed below). On the contrary to the viral gene transfer, non-viral systems also permit significantly simpler production of the cGMP-grade material (plasmid DNA) and lesser safety testing. Up to date, the Sleeping Beauty transposon-mediated approach was shown to mediate a long-term stable integration of the T-cell receptor genes targeting melanoma-derived antigen, MART-1, in laboratory settings (Fig. 3b). This system provided 50% efficiency of the TCR integration into the genome of the T cells and sustained functional reactivity of lymphocytes to the antigen-positive melanoma [25].

Other non-viral strategies could be useful in genetic engineering of the T cells. For example, integrase-mediated insertion of the genetic material may provide stable, site-directed integration of the transgenes (TCRs) into T cell genome. This strategy involves integrase from the *Streptomyces* phage ΦC31 that catalyzes unidirectional recombination between attP motifs in phage and attB sites in bacterial genomes. Usually attP and attB sites are cleaved and joined to each other, generating two hybrid sequences (attL and attR) that flank the integrated phage genome. However, ΦC31 integrase can also recognize several endogenous sequences in eukaryotic chromosomes as attP sites and integrate attB-bearing transgenes into them (Fig. 3c). Such pseudo attP sites were found in every mammalian genome with more than 100 ΦC31 integration sites identified in human cells. Thus far, only three preferred sites located in human Xq22.1, 8p22, 19q13.31 loci are commonly used by this enzyme [26, 27]. Therefore, ΦC31-integrase-based system is somewhat similar to the SB transposone system (Fig. 3b, c). Yet, it provides better specificity of the transgene integration. We recently tested whether ΦC31 can efficiently integrate transgenes into the T cells. Our initial data using GFP-encoding reporter plasmid with short (34bp) attB site demonstrated that nucleofection reaction provides rather efficient transduction of the transgene and ΦC31 integrase-encoding plasmids into T cells (Fig. 4a) and stable, integrase-dependent insertion of the reporter into both CD4+ and CD8+ T cells (Fig. 4b). Transduction of the T cells with tyrosinase-specific TCR (described in 10) ligated into the attB-harboring mammalian expression vector also resulted in the sustained expression of this melanoma-specific TCR and the ability of the T cells to target antigen-positive melanoma cells *in vitro* (Fig. 4c)

Collectively, viral and non-viral strategies for the genetic engineering of the T cells expressing melanoma-specific TCRs are suitable for the *ex vivo* production of large quantities (more than 10^8 cells) of the tumor-specific T cells that can be used for the adoptive T cell transfer. However, clinical utility of the non-viral approaches remains to be elucidated. In spite of T cell trans-

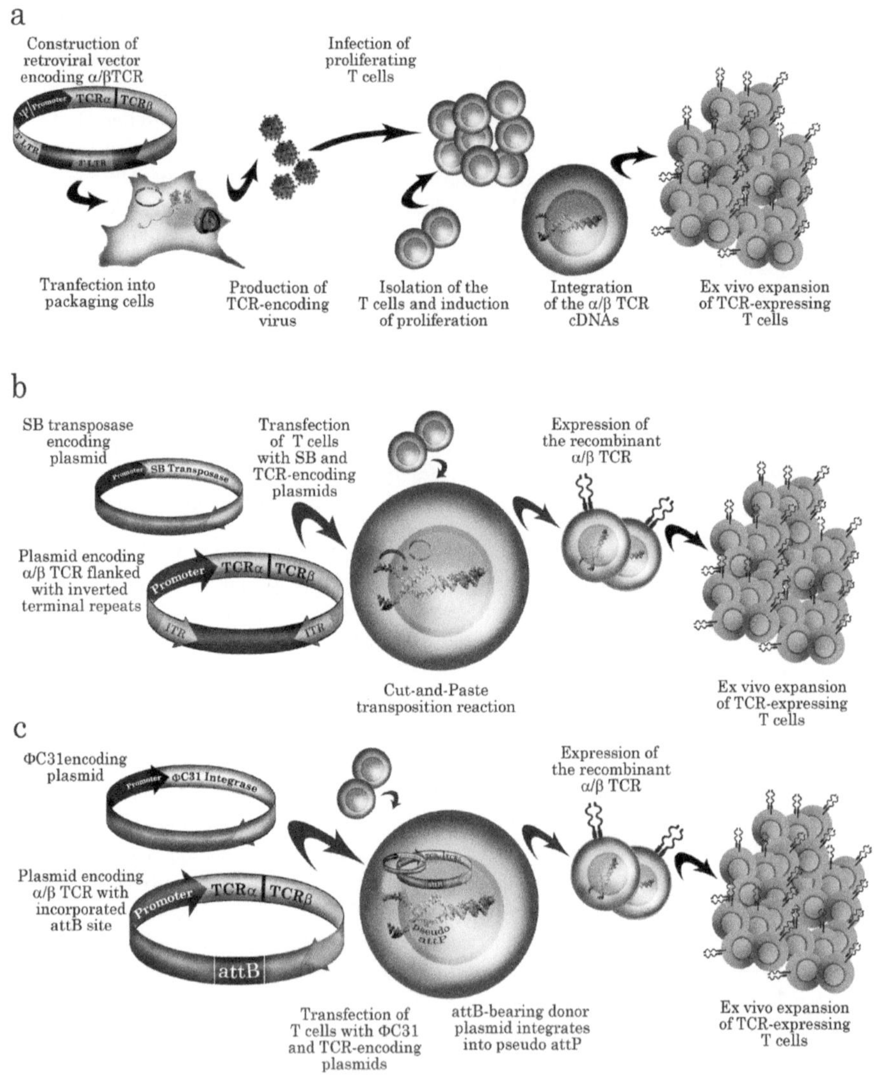

Figure 3. Schematic diagram depicting genetic engineering of the tumor-targeting T cells expressing recombinant TCR. Diagrams depict generation of the recombinant T cells via (a) retrovirus-mediated gene transfer, (b) Sleeping Beauty transposon-mediated gene transposition, and (c) ΦC31 integrase-mediated gene insertion (see text for details).

duction strategy, it is clear that the ability to generate melanoma-specific recombinant T cell receptors allowed significant advancement in the development of the clinically-applicable TCR-based approach for melanoma immunotherapy. Its primary advantages are in the use of

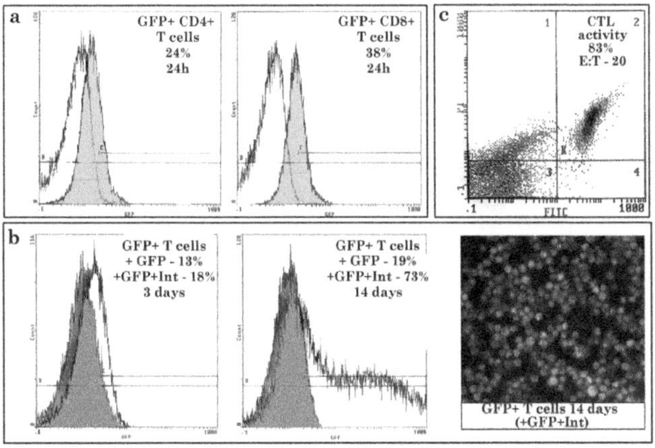

Figure 4. ΦC31 integrase-mediated genetic modification of the T cells. (a) Example showing typical nucleofection reaction of the reporter gene (GFP) into freshly isolated T cells 24 hours post Nucleofection (representative FACS profiles). (b) Analysis of the GFP expression after Nucleofection of the T cells in the presence of absence of the ΦC31 integrase-encoding plasmid (representative profiles and the direct fluorescent microscopy) 3 and 14 days after Nucleofection. (c) FACS-based analysis of the CTL activity of the recombinant T cells generated to express tyrosinase-specific TCR against human melanoma in vitro (representative profile). Times and percentages are indicated in the panels; Shaded Profiles – GFP-positive cells (see text for details).

a natural and a rather well-understood mechanism of the T cell function and the ability to select/generate multiple melanoma-reactive TCRs that can be used alone or in combination. Currently, several melanoma-targeting TCRs specific to tyrosinase, MART-1, and gp100 were cloned. One can envision generation of TCR-encoding cDNA banks that could be utilized for the generation of different melanoma-reacting T cells from the pool of patient-derived T cells to target several TAAs. However, this strategy has several disadvantages including restriction of specific TCRs to one HLA type, dependence from the expression and presentation of an antigen, limited intracellular signaling from the recombinant α/β TCRs, misparing of TCR chains, and the inability to target non-protein tumor antigens.

At present time, about 20 clinical studies involving melanoma-specific T cells expressing recombinant TCR were conducted in US alone (some of them reviewed in [28]). The result of some of the completed trials opened new perspectives for the improvement of the TCR-based strategies. For instance, adoptive transfer of the T cells genetically engineered to express highly avid MART-1-specific TCR has achieved objective clinical responses in a 13% of treated patients [29]. Analysis of CTL-resistant tumor cell revealed that these resistant clones exhibited hyperactivation of the NF-κB survival pathway and overexpression of the antiapoptotic Bcl-2, Bcl-x, Bcl-$_{xL}$, and Mcl-1 genes [30]. These studies suggest that sensitivity of melanoma to the recombinant T cells could be increased by the pharmacological inhibition of the NF-κB pathway and/or Bcl-2 family members. Multiple investigative studies are on-going to further improve recombinant TCR-based approach.

2.2. Chimeric antigen receptors

Independently, an alternative approach involving recombinant DNA technology was developed to generate tumor-targeting T cells. It utilizes fusion of the variable chain of the tumor-antigen-specific antibody, TCR constant region, and intracellular signaling domains. Initially, these structures were called T-bodies [31]. They are comprise of the single-chain antibody (sFv), TCR transmembrane domain and the intracellular signaling domain of the TCR-ζ. One of the first tumor associated antigens targeted by T cells expressing T-bodies was erbB2 (HER2/neu) receptor that is over-expressed in multiple cancers [32]. Later, a more general term – chimeric antigen receptors or CARs emerged. As compared to the TCRs, CARs allow overcoming dependency on HLA type, antigen presentation, and restricted intracellular signaling of the recombinant α/β TCRs. Initial studies with T-bodies (and recombinant TCRs) demonstrated a rather short lifespan of the engineered T cells and the inability of the recombinant receptors to fully support persistence of the T cell. To address this issue, several studies were conducted to identify the most potent CAR structures by testing several signaling molecules involved in T cell activation (Fig. 5). It was demonstrated that fusion of TCR-ζ with the intracellular domain of CD28 can augment cytokine production by CAR-expressing T cells upon encountering antigen and enhance antitumor efficacy [33]. Inclusion of CD134 (OX-40) into CAR structure also led to the elevated tumoricidal activity of the recombinant T cells [34]. Comparative analysis of the different CARs comprised of TCR-ζ signal transduction domain, CD28 and/or CD137 (4-1BB) intracellular domains demonstrated that addition of the CD137 supports T cell function to a greater extent as compared to other constructs [35]. Collectively, addition of these signaling domains to the CAR structure allowed overcoming (to certain extent) inefficient effector function and anergic status of the T cells.

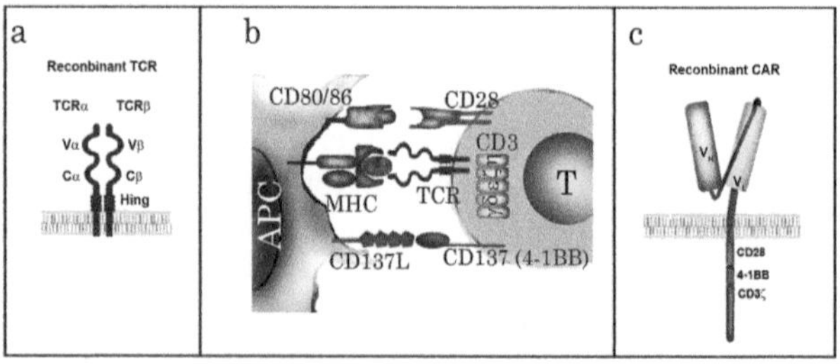

Figure 5. Recombinant TCR and CAR structures. (a) Diagram depicting recombinant TCR structure. (b) Diagram illustrating molecular interactions involved in TCR-mediated pro-proliferation and pro-survival intracellular signaling including engagement of the CD28, CD3, and CD137 (4-1BB). (c) Diagram depicting recombinant CAR structure with CD3ξ, CD137 (4-1BB), and CD28 signaling domains (see text for details).

As recognition of target cells by CAR depends on the antibody, CARs can recognize not only polypeptides but also non-protein molecules such as tumor-associated glycolipids and carbohydrates. However, antibody-mediated binding require surface expression of an antigen and strict selection of TAAs to avoid autoimmune side effects. Also, use of the mouse monoclonal antibody sequences in CAR design may lead to the unwanted immune recognition of the CAR-expressing T cells and limit long-term clinical use [36, 37]. Nevertheless, existence of a large number of the tumor antigen-specific antibodies and robust anti-tumor response by CAR-expressing T cells suggest great clinical utility of these recombinant molecules. Currently, in US alone there are 18 clinical trials aimed at treatment of various malignancies with CAR-engineered leukocytes, with 16 trials in the recruitment phase. Eight of them are aimed at targeting different B cell malignancies with anti-CD19-CAR. Three trials are intended to test HER2-specific CAR-modified T cells for the treatment of sarcoma, glioblastoma, and advanced Her2-positive lung malignancy.

With regard to melanoma, several CAR designs were tested for the ability to target this malignancy. Thus, recent studies demonstrated that treatment of melanoma xenografts in nude mice using engineered T cells expressing tandem CAR (CD28/TCRζ) specific to ganglioside GD3 with IL2 supplementation led to complete remissions of the established tumors in 50 % of treated animals [38]. As GD3 is often over-expressed in melanoma, this approach could be potent in eliminating melanoma in human patients.

Another attractive target for the CAR-mediated T cell therapy for melanoma is a high molecular weight melanoma-associated antigen (HMW-MAA) encoded by CSPG4 gene. This is a cell-surface proteoglycan expressed on more than 90% of the tumors. Recent studies on targeting of this antigen using CAR that is comprised of the anti- HMW-MAA antibody chain and intracellular signaling domains of the CD28, CD137, and CD3ζ demonstrated that T cell genetically modified to express this CAR were cytolytic to the HMW-MAA–positive melanoma cells, produced cytokine and proliferate *in vitro* [39]. The potential clinical utility of the CAR-mediated HMW-MAA targeting was emphasized by another recent animal study [40]. Analysis of a few human melanoma biopsies revealed the presence of less than 2% of specific tumor cells co-expressing CD20 and HMW-MAA. Implantation of tumors containing these CD20+ HMW-MAA+ cells into immuno-deficient mice resulted in a rapid growth of tumors. Targeting of these pre-established lesions with T cells expressing either CD20 or HMW-MAA-directed CAR showed elimination of lesions in nearly 90% of treated animals. CD20-specific engineered T cells were unable to eradicated melanoma lesions artificially expressing CD20 suggesting that native expression of the antigen is required for effective targeting. These studies provided additional evidence that direction of the T cells toward HMW-MAA via genetic engineering can permit effective elimination of tumor lesions.

As progression of most tumors including melanoma depends on the microenvironment, T-cell mediated targeting of the microenvironmental components could also be a viable strategy for melanoma immunotherapy. Particularly, tumor survival was shown to be dependent on the *de novo* formation of the intratumoral blood vessels characterised by high levels of the vascular endothelial growth factor receptor 2 (VEGFR2/KDR). Also, a number of studies associated high levels of VEGFR2 expression with various tumor stroma cells including subsets of macrophages, immature monocytes, immature dendritic cells and immuno-suppressive CD4+CD25+ regulatory T cells (Treg) [41-46]. Therefore, it was suggested that targeting of VEGFR2 – positive cells in tumor stroma may provide clinical benefits and tumor regression. In support of this notion, recent studies demonstrated that the direction of the T cells toward VEGFR-2 via CAR provide an effective means to eliminate pre-established experimental melanoma.

Thus, using an animal model, it was shown that after systemic transplantation, anti–VEGFR-2 CAR and IL-12–co-transduced T cells infiltrated the tumors, expanded and persisted within tumor mass leading to tumor regression [47]. The anti-tumor effect was dependent on targeting of IL-12–responsive host cells via activation of anti–VEGFR-2 CAR-T cells and release of IL-12. Based on this data, one clinical trial aimed at the assessment of safety and effectiveness of cell therapy was initiated to treat recurrent and relapsed cancer by using anti-VEGFR2 CAR-modified T cells.

Presently, there is an accumulating body of evidence suggesting clinical utility of the T cell genetically engineered to express melanoma antigen-specific CARs. It is likely that in the near future CAR-mediated targeting of different melanoma antigens will evolve into general practice of cancer immunotherapy.

3. DNA vaccination

Another immunotherapeutic approach directly relevant to recombinant DNA is genetic or DNA vaccination. The original idea of DNA vaccination emanated from the observations that intramuscular injection of DNA encoding influenza A virus protein resulted in the robust activation of the immune responses that protected the host from viral challenge [48]. Generally, DNA-mediated activation of immune response involves multiple processes. First, plasmid DNA should be delivered intracellularly and expressed in the host cells. Next, in most of cases the antigen has to be secreted from the cells and picked up by the dendritic cells (DC), processed and presented in the context of the MHC class II to the CD4+ T helper (Th) cells. Alternatively, if the antigen is expressed directly in the DCs, it could be processed intracellularly and presented via MHC class I molecules, leading to the activation of the CD8+ T cells and induction of the cytotoxic immune responses. Initial studies on DNA vaccination were carried out using an intramuscular route of vaccine administration (Fig. 6). This allowed high levels of antigen expression and secretion from the elongated muscle cells into perimysium, the resident site of the intramuscular DCs. Later, DNA vaccination through the skin was suggested to be superior over the intramuscular route. Skin has evolved as a barrier to prevent the entry of pathogens, with efficient immune surveillance complex including Langerhans cells, dendritic cells, lymphocytes, and other leukocytes. Skin is also rich in lymphatic vasculature network that provides an efficient route for DC and T cell trafficking. Depending on the physical methods of into-skin DNA delivery, DNA-based vaccines can be targeted to specific locations in the skin [49].

The DNA vaccination approach has several advantages over other types of vaccinations: (i) multiple expression vectors coding for different antigen and co-stimulatory molecules can be concurrently delivered into the skin (or the muscle); (ii) the use of cell-type-specific promoters can provide specificity of protein expression; (iii) protein expression from designed plasmids can be controlled by inducible promoters, the use of ubiquitous chromatin opening elements (UCOE), or chemically (e.g. sodium butyrate). Also of note is the relative simplicity and inexpensiveness of the cGMP grade DNA vaccine production and pre-clinical testing. These

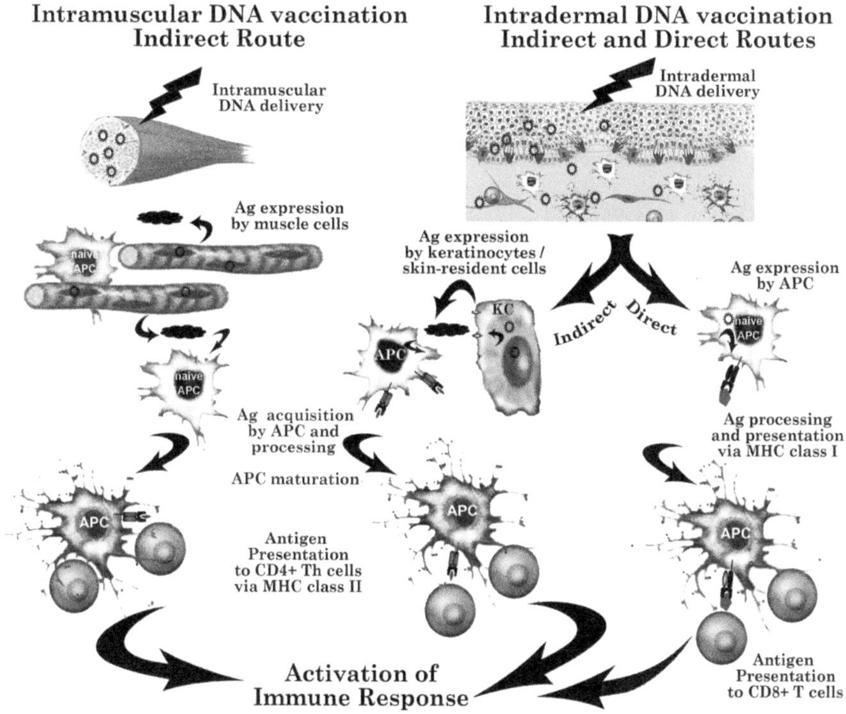

Figure 6. Intramuscular and Intradermal DNA vaccination. Intramuscular and intradermal sites are used for DNA vaccination. The former allows high level of antigen (Ag) expression in muscle cells and MHC class II Ag processing and presentation whereas the latter permits expression of the Ag in the Antigen-Presenting Cells (APC) and direct presentation of the antigenic peptides to the CD8+ cytotoxic T cells (see text for details).

attractive characteristics of DNA vaccines have prompted extensive research within the past 10 years.

Multiple studies on pre-clinical animal models of melanoma and other cancers have been conducted. Studies on the canine model of aggressive and metastatic melanoma (stages II-IV) demonstrated that xenogeneic vaccination of dogs with DNA vaccine coding for human tyrosinase led to an excellent clinical response in the majority of vaccinated dogs. A long-term survival of dogs with advanced stage IV disease with bulky lung metastases (on average 400 days) was observed [50]. Vaccinated dogs with stage II/III disease also had long-term survivals (on average 500 days) with no evidence of melanoma on necropsy. Overall, median survival time for all treated dogs was 389 days. Another canine model study [51] showed that xenogeneic DNA vaccination induces melanoma-specific antibody response, which coincides with observed clinical responses. As a result, in 2010 Merial, an animal health company has gained full-licensure from the U.S. Department of Agriculture (USDA) for ONCEPT™ Canine

Melanoma DNA Vaccine. Up to date, ONCEPT is the first and only USDA-approved therapeutic vaccine for the treatment of cancer in either animals or humans. (The first DNA vaccine was licensed by the USDA in 2005 for prevention of West Nile virus infection in horses).

However, presently only a few human clinical trials on DNA vaccination were conducted. One of such study, aimed at the evaluation of the immune response in patients with hormone-refractory prostate cancer showed that DNA vaccination with a prostate-specific antigen (PSA) encoding plasmid given with GM-CSF and IL-2 is safe in doses of up to 900 μg, and that the vaccination can induce cellular and humoral immune responses [52].

Similar to the reference above canine studies, DNA vaccines were shown to be effective in mouse melanoma models when mice were vaccinated with heterologous DNA encoding human melanoma-associated antigen gp-100 [53]. This vaccination regimen was augmented by the GM-CSF and was most effective in the prophylactic setting. It was also effective in suppressing pre-established melanoma. However, vaccinations with autologous mouse melanoma antigens were less successful. Nevertheless, the relative simplicity of modifying recombinant DNA allowed testing of various genetic alterations aimed at breaking the immunologic tolerance and enhancing immune responses to DNA vaccines. For example, concurrent vaccination with DNA encoding several melanoma-specific epitopes can be used. This approach was tested in several studies with different degree of success. As a result, vaccination of mice with $gp100_{25-33}$ and $TRP\text{-}2_{181-188}$ encoding minigene was effective in preventing melanoma development [54]. As many of the melanoma MHC class I epitopes were characterized for melanoma including those derived from tyrosinase, TRP1, TRP2, gp-100, MART-1, and MC-1R (some of them shared between mouse and human MHC molecules [55], one can envision generation of an ultimate genetic immunogen capable of targeting several melanoma-associated antigens.

Recombinant DNA technology has also allowed introduction of immuno-augmentation sequences into the DNA vaccine composition. Identified universal pan HLA DR helper binding epitope (PADRE; KXVAAWYLKA) was shown to enhance immunogenicity of both peptide and DNA vaccines [56, 57]. Other studies demonstrated augmentation of melanoma-specific immune responses via direct fusion of the DNA vaccine with the VP22 protein of the herpes simplex virus-1 [58].

Besides introducing immuno-enhancing alteration to the DNA vaccine, other strategies could be employed to enhance DNA vaccination efficacy including addition of the immuno-enhancing molecules to vaccine composition, alteration of the microenvironment at vaccine administration site, and use of the prime-boost immunization regimens. Recent studies demonstrated that antibody-mediated inhibition of the cytotoxic T lymphocyte antigen 4 (CTLA-4) enhances melanoma-specific immune response. This strategy was recently tested in treatment of stage III-IV melanoma and the drug (Ipilimumam) was approved by the FDA as first anti-melanoma immunotherapeutic [59, 60]. CTLA-4 presents its immuno-inhibitory function during activation of the T cells by the antigen-presenting cells. It also inhibits TCR-mediated intracellular signaling in activated T cells and down-modulating T cell mediated immunity. Therefore, it is possible that inhibition of CTLA-4 in conjunction with DNA vaccination may provide significant enhancement of the vaccine-mediated immune response induction. Although providing CTLA-4 inhibiting antibodies like Ipilimumab along with DNA vaccination is not feasible, other options could be explored. For example, recently characterized genetically engineered lipocalin (LCN2) exhibits a strong cross-species antagonistic activity to CTLA-4 [61]. It is likely that this molecule could be included into DNA vaccine composition to enhance DC-mediated activation of the T cells. Other immuno-modulatory strategies may include addition of CD40 ligand, which was shown to stimulate expression of maturation markers CD80, CD86 and IL-12 in APC [62, 63] and its ability to activate $CD8^+$ T cells and increase cell-mediated immunity [64, 65]. Addition of different cytokines and growth factors including GM-CSF, IL-2, IL12 for stimulation/support of the T cells was also tested in several studies (as exemplified in preceding paragraphs) and could be further explored. Alteration of microenvironment via application chemokines to recruit specific sets of the leukocytes to the vaccine administration site may also provide a favorable milieu for the launch of the effective DNA-vaccine induced immune response [66, 67]. These and many other strategies can be proposed; however, the clinical utility of the DNA vaccination combination with other approaches remains to be determined. Nevertheless, presently in the US alone, 10 clinical studies utilizing xenogenic (mouse) or human DNA vaccines coding for melanoma associated antigens have been completed. In these trials, tyrosinase, gp75, gp100, and TRP2 were used as antigens. Although most of these studies are already completed, currently no study results are posted nor are follow-up reports available on patient survival and characterization of immune response. Nevertheless, DNA vaccination remains to be a promising modality that could provide cost-effective and generic immunotherapy for patients with melanoma and other cancers.

4. Other strategies involving recombinant DNA technology

At the present time, almost every immuno-therapeutic approach utilizes recombinant DNA in one way or another. Understanding of the immuno-regulatory functions of DCs and the molecular mechanisms involved in the capture, processing and presentation of antigens by DCs allowed the development of the DC-based vaccines. Initially, in the mid 1990's, several pre-clinical and clinical studies were conducted using autologous DCs pulsed with melanoma-associated antigens. These studies demonstrated that antigen-loaded DC can trigger active melanoma specific immune responses [68, 69]. However, it became apparent that enforced expression of the antigens in DC rather than loading of these cells with peptides allows for presentation of the tumor-derived antigens via MHC class I complex and priming of the CD8+ T cells to elicit cytotoxic immune response. Moreover, to provide DC specific expression of the antigens, long and short CD11c promoters were characterized and used in several studies [70, 71]. These promoters allow effective and cell type specific expression of the antigens in DCs, as well as more efficient priming and activation of the T cells *in vitro* and *in vivo*. Considering a necessity of the direct interaction of the DC with T lymphocytes, application of T cell recruiting chemokines was also explored recently. These pioneering studies demonstrate that forced expression of the secondary lymphoid chemokine, CCL21, in antigen loaded DCs enhances their ability to recruit and activate T cells [72, 73]. One clinical phase I clinical trial using CCL21 transduced DCs pulsed with MART-1 and gp100 was completed in 2012. Altogether, a total of 64 clinical trials aimed at targeting of melanoma using dendritic cells are listed. Thirty nine of them are completed with no reports yet available. The majority of these trials in some way utilize recombinant DNA technology.

5. Conclusion

During last decade, various melanoma-specific immunotherapeutics that utilize recombinant DNA have been developed and tested in pre-clinical and clinical studies with varying degrees of clinical success. Many of these approaches, including recombinant TCRs and CARs, have already demonstrated promising clinical results, thus providing us with the hope that in the near future melanoma immunotherapy will become curable for melanoma patients.

Acknowledgements

Presented here data regarding clinical trials was obtained through registry and results database of publicly and privately supported clinical studies (clinicaltrials.gov). Experimental data presented on Fig. 4 was obtained in Dr. Alexeev's laboratory. Plasmid DNA encoding tyrosinase-specific TCR was kindly provided by Dr. S.A. Rosenberg (NCI, NIH). ΦC31 integrase-encoding plasmid was obtained from Dr. M.P. Calos (Stanford University, CA).

Author details

Vitali Alexeev[1*], Alyson Pidich[2], Daria Marley Kemp[1] and Olga Igoucheva[1]

*Address all correspondence to: vitali.alexeev@jefferson.edu

1 Department of Dermatology and Cutaneous Biology, Jefferson Medical College, Thomas Jefferson University, Philadelphia, Pennsylvania, USA

2 Temple University School of Medicine, Philadelphia, Pennsylvania, USA

References

[1] Knuth, A., Wolfel, T., Klehmann, E., Boon, T. and Meyer zum Buschenfelde, K.H. (1989) Cytolytic T-cell clones against an autologous human melanoma: specificity study and definition of three antigens by immunoselection. *Proceedings of the National Academy of Sciences of the United States of America*, 86, 2804-2808.

[2] Dudley, M.E., Yang, J.C., Sherry, R., Hughes, M.S., Royal, R., Kammula, U., Robbins, P.F., Huang, J., Citrin, D.E., Leitman, S.F. *et al.* (2008) Adoptive cell therapy for patients with metastatic melanoma: evaluation of intensive myeloablative chemoradiation preparative regimens. *J Clin Oncol*, 26, 5233-5239.

[3] Dudley, M.E., Gross, C.A., Langhan, M.M., Garcia, M.R., Sherry, R.M., Yang, J.C., Phan, G.Q., Kammula, U.S., Hughes, M.S., Citrin, D.E. *et al.* CD8+ enriched "young" tumor infiltrating lymphocytes can mediate regression of metastatic melanoma. *Clinical cancer research : an official journal of the American Association for Cancer Research*, 16, 6122-6131.

[4] Goff, S.L., Johnson, L.A., Black, M.A., Xu, H., Zheng, Z., Cohen, C.J., Morgan, R.A., Rosenberg, S.A. and Feldman, S.A. Enhanced receptor expression and in vitro effector function of a murine-human hybrid MART-1-reactive T cell receptor following a rapid expansion. *Cancer immunology, immunotherapy : CII*, 59, 1551-1560.

[5] Cohen, C.J., Zhao, Y., Zheng, Z., Rosenberg, S.A. and Morgan, R.A. (2006) Enhanced antitumor activity of murine-human hybrid T-cell receptor (TCR) in human lymphocytes is associated with improved pairing and TCR/CD3 stability. *Cancer research*, 66, 8878-8886.

[6] Cohen, C.J., Li, Y.F., El-Gamil, M., Robbins, P.F., Rosenberg, S.A. and Morgan, R.A. (2007) Enhanced antitumor activity of T cells engineered to express T-cell receptors with a second disulfide bond. *Cancer research*, 67, 3898-3903.

[7] Kuball, J., Dossett, M.L., Wolfl, M., Ho, W.Y., Voss, R.H., Fowler, C. and Greenberg, P.D. (2007) Facilitating matched pairing and expression of TCR chains introduced into human T cells. *Blood*, 109, 2331-2338.

[8] Okamoto, S., Mineno, J., Ikeda, H., Fujiwara, H., Yasukawa, M., Shiku, H. and Kato, I. (2009) Improved expression and reactivity of transduced tumor-specific TCRs in human lymphocytes by specific silencing of endogenous TCR. *Cancer research*, 69, 9003-9011.

[9] Govers, C., Sebestyen, Z., Coccoris, M., Willemsen, R.A. and Debets, R. T cell receptor gene therapy: strategies for optimizing transgenic TCR pairing. *Trends Mol Med*, 16, 77-87.

[10] Frankel, T.L., Burns, W.R., Peng, P.D., Yu, Z., Chinnasamy, D., Wargo, J.A., Zheng, Z., Restifo, N.P., Rosenberg, S.A. and Morgan, R.A. Both CD4 and CD8 T cells mediate equally effective in vivo tumor treatment when engineered with a highly avid TCR targeting tyrosinase. *J Immunol*, 184, 5988-5998.

[11] Douin, V., Bornes, S., Creancier, L., Rochaix, P., Favre, G., Prats, A.C. and Couderc, B. (2004) Use and comparison of different internal ribosomal entry sites (IRES) in tricistronic retroviral vectors. *BMC biotechnology*, 4, 16.

[12] Baron, U., Freundlieb, S., Gossen, M. and Bujard, H. (1995) Co-regulation of two gene activities by tetracycline via a bidirectional promoter. *Nucleic acids research*, 23, 3605-3606.

[13] Mastakov, M.Y., Baer, K., Kotin, R.M. and During, M.J. (2002) Recombinant adeno-associated virus serotypes 2- and 5-mediated gene transfer in the mammalian brain: quantitative analysis of heparin co-infusion. *Molecular therapy : the journal of the American Society of Gene Therapy*, 5, 371-380.

[14] Ryan, M.D., King, A.M. and Thomas, G.P. (1991) Cleavage of foot-and-mouth disease virus polyprotein is mediated by residues located within a 19 amino acid sequence. *J Gen Virol*, 72 (Pt 11), 2727-2732.

[15] Baum, C., Schambach, A., Bohne, J. and Galla, M. (2006) Retrovirus vectors: toward the plentivirus? *Molecular therapy : the journal of the American Society of Gene Therapy*, 13, 1050-1063.

[16] Frecha, C., Levy, C., Cosset, F.L. and Verhoeyen, E. (2010) Advances in the field of lentivector-based transduction of T and B lymphocytes for gene therapy. *Molecular therapy : the journal of the American Society of Gene Therapy*, 18, 1748-1757.

[17] Hackett, P.B., Largaespada, D.A. and Cooper, L.J. (2010) A transposon and transposase system for human application. *Molecular therapy : the journal of the American Society of Gene Therapy*, 18, 674-683.

[18] Hacein-Bey-Abina, S., von Kalle, C., Schmidt, M., Le Deist, F., Wulffraat, N., McIntyre, E., Radford, I., Villeval, J.L., Fraser, C.C., Cavazzana-Calvo, M. *et al.* (2003) A serious adverse event after successful gene therapy for X-linked severe combined immunodeficiency. *The New England journal of medicine*, 348, 255-256.

[19] Nam, C.H. and Rabbitts, T.H. (2006) The role of LMO2 in development and in T cell leukemia after chromosomal translocation or retroviral insertion. *Molecular therapy : the journal of the American Society of Gene Therapy*, 13, 15-25.

[20] Mates, L. (2011) Rodent transgenesis mediated by a novel hyperactive Sleeping Beauty transposon system. *Methods Mol Biol*, 738, 87-99.

[21] Chatterjee, M., Hedrich, C.M., Rauen, T., Ioannidis, C., Terhorst, C. and Tsokos, G.C. (2012) CD3-T Cell Receptor Co-stimulation through SLAMF3 and SLAMF6 Receptors Enhances RORgammat Recruitment to the IL17A Promoter in Human T Lymphocytes. *The Journal of biological chemistry*, 287, 38168-38177.

[22] Clevers, H., Lonberg, N., Dunlap, S., Lacy, E. and Terhorst, C. (1989) An enhancer located in a CpG-island 3' to the TCR/CD3-epsilon gene confers T lymphocyte-specificity to its promoter. *The EMBO journal*, 8, 2527-2535.

[23] Hahm, S.H., Yi, Y., Lee, D.K., Noh, M.J., Yun, L., Hwang, S. and Lee, K.H. (2004) Construction of retroviral vectors with enhanced efficiency of transgene expression. *Journal of virological methods*, 121, 127-136.

[24] Morita, S., Kojima, T. and Kitamura, T. (2000) Plat-E: an efficient and stable system for transient packaging of retroviruses. *Gene therapy*, 7, 1063-1066.

[25] Peng, P.D., Cohen, C.J., Yang, S., Hsu, C., Jones, S., Zhao, Y., Zheng, Z., Rosenberg, S.A. and Morgan, R.A. (2009) Efficient nonviral Sleeping Beauty transposon-based TCR gene transfer to peripheral blood lymphocytes confers antigen-specific antitumor reactivity. *Gene therapy*, 16, 1042-1049.

[26] Sclimenti, C.R., Thyagarajan, B. and Calos, M.P. (2001) Directed evolution of a recombinase for improved genomic integration at a native human sequence. *Nucleic acids research*, 29, 5044-5051.

[27] Groth, A.C., Olivares, E.C., Thyagarajan, B. and Calos, M.P. (2000) A phage integrase directs efficient site-specific integration in human cells. *Proceedings of the National Academy of Sciences of the United States of America*, 97, 5995-6000.

[28] Park, T.S., Rosenberg, S.A. and Morgan, R.A. (2011) Treating cancer with genetically engineered T cells. *Trends in biotechnology*, 29, 550-557.

[29] Morgan, R.A., Dudley, M.E., Wunderlich, J.R., Hughes, M.S., Yang, J.C., Sherry, R.M., Royal, R.E., Topalian, S.L., Kammula, U.S., Restifo, N.P. *et al.* (2006) Cancer regression in patients after transfer of genetically engineered lymphocytes. *Science*, 314, 126-129.

[30] Jazirehi, A.R., Baritaki, S., Koya, R.C., Bonavida, B. and Economou, J.S. (2011) Molecular mechanism of MART-1+/A*0201+ human melanoma resistance to specific CTL-killing despite functional tumor-CTL interaction. *Cancer research*, 71, 1406-1417.

[31] Eshhar, Z. (1997) Tumor-specific T-bodies: towards clinical application. *Cancer immunology, immunotherapy : CII*, 45, 131-136.

[32] Moritz, D., Wels, W., Mattern, J. and Groner, B. (1994) Cytotoxic T lymphocytes with a grafted recognition specificity for ERBB2-expressing tumor cells. *Proceedings of the National Academy of Sciences of the United States of America*, 91, 4318-4322.

[33] Koehler, H., Kofler, D., Hombach, A. and Abken, H. (2007) CD28 costimulation overcomes transforming growth factor-beta-mediated repression of proliferation of redirected human CD4+ and CD8+ T cells in an antitumor cell attack. *Cancer research*, 67, 2265-2273.

[34] Finney, H.M., Akbar, A.N. and Lawson, A.D. (2004) Activation of resting human primary T cells with chimeric receptors: costimulation from CD28, inducible costimulator, CD134, and CD137 in series with signals from the TCR zeta chain. *J Immunol*, 172, 104-113.

[35] Milone, M.C., Fish, J.D., Carpenito, C., Carroll, R.G., Binder, G.K., Teachey, D., Samanta, M., Lakhal, M., Gloss, B., Danet-Desnoyers, G. *et al.* (2009) Chimeric receptors containing CD137 signal transduction domains mediate enhanced survival of T cells

and increased antileukemic efficacy in vivo. *Molecular therapy : the journal of the American Society of Gene Therapy*, 17, 1453-1464.

[36] Kershaw, M.H., Westwood, J.A., Parker, L.L., Wang, G., Eshhar, Z., Mavroukakis, S.A., White, D.E., Wunderlich, J.R., Canevari, S., Rogers-Freezer, L. *et al.* (2006) A phase I study on adoptive immunotherapy using gene-modified T cells for ovarian cancer. *Clinical cancer research : an official journal of the American Association for Cancer Research*, 12, 6106-6115.

[37] Lamers, C.H., Willemsen, R., van Elzakker, P., van Steenbergen-Langeveld, S., Broertjes, M., Oosterwijk-Wakka, J., Oosterwijk, E., Sleijfer, S., Debets, R. and Gratama, J.W. (2011) Immune responses to transgene and retroviral vector in patients treated with ex vivo-engineered T cells. *Blood*, 117, 72-82.

[38] Lo, A.S., Ma, Q., Liu, D.L. and Junghans, R.P. (2010) Anti-GD3 chimeric sFv-CD28/T-cell receptor zeta designer T cells for treatment of metastatic melanoma and other neuroectodermal tumors. *Clinical cancer research : an official journal of the American Association for Cancer Research*, 16, 2769-2780.

[39] Burns, W.R., Zhao, Y., Frankel, T.L., Hinrichs, C.S., Zheng, Z., Xu, H., Feldman, S.A., Ferrone, S., Rosenberg, S.A. and Morgan, R.A. (2010) A high molecular weight melanoma-associated antigen-specific chimeric antigen receptor redirects lymphocytes to target human melanomas. *Cancer research*, 70, 3027-3033.

[40] Schmidt, P., Kopecky, C., Hombach, A., Zigrino, P., Mauch, C. and Abken, H. (2011) Eradication of melanomas by targeted elimination of a minor subset of tumor cells. *Proceedings of the National Academy of Sciences of the United States of America*, 108, 2474-2479.

[41] Duignan, I.J., Corcoran, E., Pennello, A., Plym, M.J., Amatulli, M., Claros, N., Iacolina, M., Youssoufian, H., Witte, L., Samakoglu, S. *et al.* Pleiotropic stromal effects of vascular endothelial growth factor receptor 2 antibody therapy in renal cell carcinoma models. *Neoplasia (New York, N.Y*, 13, 49-59.

[42] Larrivee, B., Pollet, I. and Karsan, A. (2005) Activation of vascular endothelial growth factor receptor-2 in bone marrow leads to accumulation of myeloid cells: role of granulocyte-macrophage colony-stimulating factor. *J Immunol*, 175, 3015-3024.

[43] Murdoch, C., Muthana, M., Coffelt, S.B. and Lewis, C.E. (2008) The role of myeloid cells in the promotion of tumour angiogenesis. *Nature reviews*, 8, 618-631.

[44] Suzuki, H., Onishi, H., Wada, J., Yamasaki, A., Tanaka, H., Nakano, K., Morisaki, T. and Katano, M. VEGFR2 is selectively expressed by FOXP3high CD4+ Treg. *European journal of immunology*, 40, 197-203.

[45] Udagawa, T., Puder, M., Wood, M., Schaefer, B.C. and D'Amato, R.J. (2006) Analysis of tumor-associated stromal cells using SCID GFP transgenic mice: contribution of local and bone marrow-derived host cells. *Faseb J*, 20, 95-102.

[46] Zhang, N., Fang, Z., Contag, P.R., Purchio, A.F. and West, D.B. (2004) Tracking angiogenesis induced by skin wounding and contact hypersensitivity using a Vegfr2-luciferase transgenic mouse. *Blood*, 103, 617-626.

[47] Chinnasamy, D., Yu, Z., Kerkar, S.P., Zhang, L., Morgan, R.A., Restifo, N.P. and Rosenberg, S.A. Local delivery of interleukin-12 using T cells targeting VEGF receptor-2 eradicates multiple vascularized tumors in mice. *Clinical cancer research : an official journal of the American Association for Cancer Research*, 18, 1672-1683.

[48] Ulmer, J.B., Donnelly, J.J., Parker, S.E., Rhodes, G.H., Felgner, P.L., Dwarki, V.J., Gromkowski, S.H., Deck, R.R., DeWitt, C.M., Friedman, A. *et al.* (1993) Heterologous protection against influenza by injection of DNA encoding a viral protein. *Science*, 259, 1745-1749.

[49] Alexeev, V. and Uitto, J. (2005) *DNA pharmaceuticals for skin diseases*. Wiley-VCH, Weinheim.

[50] Bergman, P.J., McKnight, J., Novosad, A., Charney, S., Farrelly, J., Craft, D., Wulderk, M., Jeffers, Y., Sadelain, M., Hohenhaus, A.E. *et al.* (2003) Long-term survival of dogs with advanced malignant melanoma after DNA vaccination with xenogeneic human tyrosinase: a phase I trial. *Clinical cancer research : an official journal of the American Association for Cancer Research*, 9, 1284-1290.

[51] Liao, J.C., Gregor, P., Wolchok, J.D., Orlandi, F., Craft, D., Leung, C., Houghton, A.N. and Bergman, P.J. (2006) Vaccination with human tyrosinase DNA induces antibody responses in dogs with advanced melanoma. *Cancer Immun*, 6, 8.

[52] Pavlenko, M., Roos, A.K., Lundqvist, A., Palmborg, A., Miller, A.M., Ozenci, V., Bergman, B., Egevad, L., Hellstrom, M., Kiessling, R. *et al.* (2004) A phase I trial of DNA vaccination with a plasmid expressing prostate-specific antigen in patients with hormone-refractory prostate cancer. *British journal of cancer*, 91, 688-694.

[53] Rakhmilevich, A.L., Imboden, M., Hao, Z., Macklin, M.D., Roberts, T., Wright, K.M., Albertini, M.R., Yang, N.S. and Sondel, P.M. (2001) Effective particle-mediated vaccination against mouse melanoma by coadministration of plasmid DNA encoding Gp100 and granulocyte-macrophage colony-stimulating factor. *Clin Cancer Res*, 7, 952-961.

[54] Xiang, R., Lode, H.N., Chao, T.H., Ruehlmann, J.M., Dolman, C.S., Rodriguez, F., Whitton, J.L., Overwijk, W.W., Restifo, N.P. and Reisfeld, R.A. (2000) An autologous oral DNA vaccine protects against murine melanoma. *Proceedings of the National Academy of Sciences of the United States of America*, 97, 5492-5497.

[55] Parkhurst, M.R., Fitzgerald, E.B., Southwood, S., Sette, A., Rosenberg, S.A. and Kawakami, Y. (1998) Identification of a shared HLA-A*0201-restricted T-cell epitope from the melanoma antigen tyrosinase-related protein 2 (TRP2). *Cancer research*, 58, 4895-4901.

[56] Bettahi, I., Dasgupta, G., Renaudet, O., Chentoufi, A.A., Zhang, X., Carpenter, D., Yoon, S., Dumy, P. and BenMohamed, L. (2009) Antitumor activity of a self-adjuvanting glyco-lipopeptide vaccine bearing B cell, CD4+ and CD8+ T cell epitopes. *Cancer immunology, immunotherapy : CII*, 58, 187-200.

[57] del Guercio, M.F., Alexander, J., Kubo, R.T., Arrhenius, T., Maewal, A., Appella, E., Hoffman, S.L., Jones, T., Valmori, D., Sakaguchi, K. *et al.* (1997) Potent immunogenic short linear peptide constructs composed of B cell epitopes and Pan DR T helper epitopes (PADRE) for antibody responses in vivo. *Vaccine*, 15, 441-448.

[58] Engelhorn, M.E., Guevara-Patino, J.A., Merghoub, T., Liu, C., Ferrone, C.R., Rizzuto, G.A., Cymerman, D.H., Posnett, D.N., Houghton, A.N. and Wolchok, J.D. (2008) Mechanisms of immunization against cancer using chimeric antigens. *Molecular therapy : the journal of the American Society of Gene Therapy*, 16, 773-781.

[59] Hodi, F.S., O'Day, S.J., McDermott, D.F., Weber, R.W., Sosman, J.A., Haanen, J.B., Gonzalez, R., Robert, C., Schadendorf, D., Hassel, J.C. *et al.* Improved survival with ipilimumab in patients with metastatic melanoma. *The New England journal of medicine*, 363, 711-723.

[60] Schartz, N.E., Farges, C., Madelaine, I., Bruzzoni, H., Calvo, F., Hoos, A. and Lebbe, C. Complete regression of a previously untreated melanoma brain metastasis with ipilimumab. *Melanoma research*, 20, 247-250.

[61] Schonfeld, D., Matschiner, G., Chatwell, L., Trentmann, S., Gille, H., Hulsmeyer, M., Brown, N., Kaye, P.M., Schlehuber, S., Hohlbaum, A.M. *et al.* (2009) An engineered lipocalin specific for CTLA-4 reveals a combining site with structural and conformational features similar to antibodies. *Proceedings of the National Academy of Sciences of the United States of America*, 106, 8198-8203.

[62] Feder-Mengus, C., Schultz-Thater, E., Oertli, D., Marti, W.R., Heberer, M., Spagnoli, G.C. and Zajac, P. (2005) Nonreplicating recombinant vaccinia virus expressing CD40 ligand enhances APC capacity to stimulate specific CD4+ and CD8+ T cell responses. *Human gene therapy*, 16, 348-360.

[63] Sato, T., Terai, M., Yasuda, R., Watanabe, R., Berd, D., Mastrangelo, M.J. and Hasumi, K. (2004) Combination of monocyte-derived dendritic cells and activated T cells which express CD40 ligand: a new approach to cancer immunotherapy. *Cancer immunology, immunotherapy : CII*, 53, 53-61.

[64] Peter, I., Nawrath, M., Kamarashev, J., Odermatt, B., Mezzacasa, A. and Hemmi, S. (2002) Immunotherapy for murine K1735 melanoma: combinatorial use of recombinant adenovirus expressing CD40L and other immunomodulators. *Cancer gene therapy*, 9, 597-605.

[65] Rousseau, R.F., Biagi, E., Dutour, A., Yvon, E.S., Brown, M.P., Lin, T., Mei, Z., Grilley, B., Popek, E., Heslop, H.E. *et al.* (2006) Immunotherapy of high-risk acute leukemia

with a recipient (autologous) vaccine expressing transgenic human CD40L and IL-2 after chemotherapy and allogeneic stem cell transplantation. *Blood*, 107, 1332-1341.

[66] Guo, J.H., Fan, M.W., Sun, J.H. and Jia, R. (2009) Fusion of antigen to chemokine CCL20 or CXCL13 strategy to enhance DNA vaccine potency. *International immunopharmacology*, 9, 925-930.

[67] Novak, L., Igoucheva, O., Cho, S. and Alexeev, V. (2007) Characterization of the CCL21-mediated melanoma-specific immune responses and in situ melanoma eradication. *Molecular cancer therapeutics*, 6, 1755-1764.

[68] Nestle, F.O., Alijagic, S., Gilliet, M., Sun, Y., Grabbe, S., Dummer, R., Burg, G. and Schadendorf, D. (1998) Vaccination of melanoma patients with peptide- or tumor lysate-pulsed dendritic cells. *Nature medicine*, 4, 328-332.

[69] 69.Thurner, B., Haendle, I., Roder, C., Dieckmann, D., Keikavoussi, P., Jonuleit, H., Bender, A., Maczek, C., Schreiner, D., von den Driesch, P. *et al.* (1999) Vaccination with mage-3A1 peptide-pulsed mature, monocyte-derived dendritic cells expands specific cytotoxic T cells and induces regression of some metastases in advanced stage IV melanoma. *The Journal of experimental medicine*, 190, 1669-1678.

[70] Brocker, T., Riedinger, M. and Karjalainen, K. (1997) Targeted expression of major histocompatibility complex (MHC) class II molecules demonstrates that dendritic cells can induce negative but not positive selection of thymocytes in vivo. *The Journal of experimental medicine*, 185, 541-550.

[71] Ni, J., Nolte, B., Arnold, A., Fournier, P. and Schirrmacher, V. (2009) Targeting antitumor DNA vaccines to dendritic cells via a short CD11c promoter sequence. *Vaccine*, 27, 5480-5487.

[72] Mule, J.J. (2009) Dendritic cell-based vaccines for pancreatic cancer and melanoma. *Annals of the New York Academy of Sciences*, 1174, 33-40.

[73] Terando, A., Roessler, B. and Mule, J.J. (2004) Chemokine gene modification of human dendritic cell-based tumor vaccines using a recombinant adenoviral vector. *Cancer gene therapy*, 11, 165-173.

Chapter 6

Diagnosis, Histopathologic and Genetic Classification of Uveal Melanoma

J.G.M. van Beek, A.E. Koopmans, R.M. Verdijk,
N.C. Naus, A. de Klein and E. Kilic

Additional information is available at the end of the chapter

1. Introduction

Uveal melanoma (UM) is the most common cause of primary eye cancer in the western world. During embryogenesis neural crest cells migrate to the neural tract where they develop into melanocytes. Melanomas of the uvea are derived from these melanocytes. UM may arise in the iris (5%), ciliary body (23%) or choroid (72%). Choroidal melanomas are the most common and usually display a discoid, dome-shaped or mushroom shaped growth pattern. Approximately 80% of the primary intraocular tumours are diagnosed as UM in patients above the age of 20 years, with a mean age of 60 years (Singh & Topham, 2003). Despite a shift towards more conservative eye treatments, survival has not improved during 1973 to 2008 (Singh et al, 2011). Growth of the primary tumour is related with histopathological features, as well as the genetic changes within these tumours. In this chapter we will not discuss iris melanoma, as this shows a different clinical and genetic behaviour, compared to ciliary body and choroidal melanoma. The clinical features, histopathological profile and genetic alterations of UM, as well as therapeutic options for primary tumours and metastases will be discussed.

2. Epidemiology

The incidence of UM ranges from 4.3 to 10.9 per million (Singh et al, 2009). For the past fifty years, the incidence has remained stable, unlike trends indicating a higher incidence of cutaneous melanoma. The incidence in Europe and United States is comparable to that in Australia and New Zealand. In Europe, a lower incidence is reported in Spain and the south of

Italy, about 2 per million, whereas registries in France, the Netherlands, Switzerland and Germany has intermediate values around 4 to 5 per million. The United Kingdom registered over 6 per million, and the highest incidence is up to > 8 per million in Norway and Denmark (Virgili et al, 2007).

3. Predisposing factors

Men and women with UM are more or less affected equally (Damato & Coupland, 2012; Singh et al, 2011). Iris melanoma is more common in women than in men (Damato & Coupland, 2012). Several phenotypes, like blue or grey eyes and fair skin have been suggested to predispose for UM (Schmidt-Pokrzywniak et al, 2009). This might explain why Caucasians are approximately 150 times more frequently affected than Africans (Margo et al, 1998; Singh et al, 2005a). In Asians UM is less common (Biswas et al, 2002).

From all the parts of the uvea the iris is most exposed to ultraviolet light, because of filtering effects of the lens and retinal pigment epithelium (RPE), the choroid receives less light (Singh et al, 2004). Although several epidemiologic and case control studies have been performed to investigate the influence of sunlight exposure on UM, the results are not conclusive (Guenel et al, 2001; Holly et al, 1990; Pane & Hirst, 2000; Shah et al, 2005; Vajdic et al, 2002). UM may occur as a part of familial syndromes, like xeroderma pigmentosa, Li-Fraumeni syndrome and familial breast and ovarian cancer. Of all UM 0.6% is considered to be familial (Singh et al, 1996). In a retrospective study 0.0017% of the primary UM patients were in the setting of familial atypical mole and melanoma syndrome (FAMM). These patients were relatively young with a mean age of 40 years (Singh et al, 1995). Furthermore, an association of neurofibromatosis type 1 and UM has been suggested, since both are of neural crest origin, however this association remains unclear (Honavar et al, 2000). Ocular and oculodermal melanocytosis (Nevus of Ota), dysplastic nevi and cutaneous melanoma are correlated with an increased risk of UM development (Carreno et al, 2012; Gonder et al, 1982; Hammer et al, 1995; Richtig et al, 2004; Singh et al, 1998; Toth-Molnar et al, 2000; van Hees et al, 1994). Additionally, in UM patients ocular and oculodermal melanocytosis are about 35 to 70 times more common (Carreno et al, 2012; Singh et al, 1998).

4. Clinical presentation

Depending on de location and size of the tumour, patients can present with visual complaints. Most UMs are detected during a routine ophthalmic examination. Approximately 30% of the patients have no symptoms at time of diagnosis, and if there are any complaints these consist mostly of blurred vision, floaters, photopsias and visual field loss (Damato, 2010) (figure 1). Usually patients do not present with severe ocular pain, however, this can occur secondary to inflammation or neovascular glaucoma.

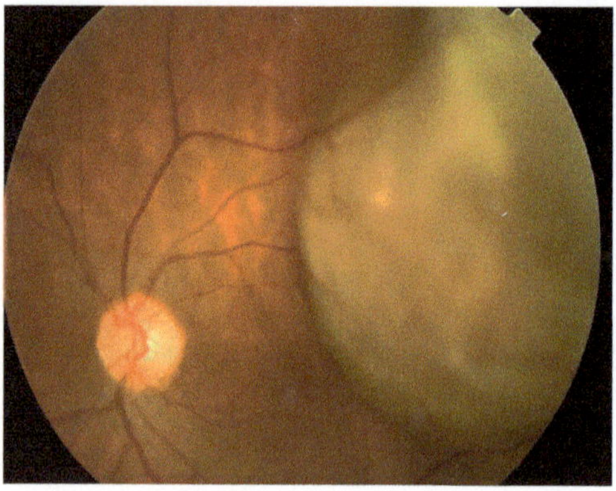

Figure 1. A large amelanotic uveal melanoma leads to a visual field defect.

5. Diagnosis

Diagnosis of UM is based on a combination of clinical examination with slit lamp biomicroscopy, indirect ophthalmoscopy (figure 1, 2a, 3a) and ultrasonography (US) (figure 2b, 3b). Iris melanomas are readily detectable by slit lamp biomicroscopy, whereas ciliary body tumours are hidden behind the iris and can be visualized by US. Choroidal tumours, depending on their location, are diagnosed by dilated indirect ophthalmoscopy and US. In suspect cases of intravenous fluorescein angiography can be helpful in differentiating melanomas from other diagnoses. Also optical coherence tomography (OCT) and autofluorescence can provide additional information (Lavinsky et al, 2007; Shields et al, 2008). In selected cases, when in doubt, an intraocular biopsy is taken of the tumour.

Indirect ophthalmoscopy through a dilated pupil provides a correct diagnosis in more than 95% of the cases (Char et al, 1980). Accuracy of the right diagnosis is established to be over 99% by experienced clinicians with US, ophthalmoscopy, and fluorescein angiography and confirmed by histopathology (Collaborative Ocular Melanoma Study Group, 1990). The ability to differentiate melanoma from other lesions has improved over the last decades. When comparing studies of 1964 and 1973, in 19% of the enucleated patients with the clinical diagnosis melanoma no histopathological evidence of a melanoma was found (Ferry, 1964; Shields, 1973). The accuracy in diagnosing medium to small sized tumours is quite challenging. Nine percent of presumed melanomas are found to have another diagnosis by fine needle aspiration biopsy (Char & Miller, 1995). Most important is to minimise the delay in referring patients with melanoma to a specialised centre. It is reported that in 29% of the patients a melanoma is missed during the first visit by an ophthalmologist, and that 31.5% of the patients referred to an oncology centre with the diagnosis of melanoma actually had a mimicking lesion (Eskelin & Kivelä, 2002; Khan & Damato, 2007).

5.1. Characteristics

Melanoma are generally pigmented, but one fourth are relatively non-pigmented or amelanotic (figure 1). Melanoma can develop into two different directions: towards the vitreous and outwards, through the underlying sclera. Having broken through Bruch's membrane, into the vitreous, UMs achieve a characteristic shape, even pathognomonic, like a 'collar button' or 'mushroom'. Small melanomas can appear flat or dome shaped.

5.2. Clinical prognostic factor

Well-known clinical prognostic factors are age and location of the tumour. Older patients tend to have a worse prognosis (Shields et al, 2012). One study found that UMs were located predominantly posterior and temporal or had a preference for macular zone, while others found a more equal distribution of melanoma (Krohn et al, 2008; Li et al, 2000; Shields et al, 2009b). Patients with larger tumours, tumours that ruptured through Bruch membrane and in patients who have developed metastasis, the tumours were significantly more often located anterior to the equator (Krohn et al, 2008).

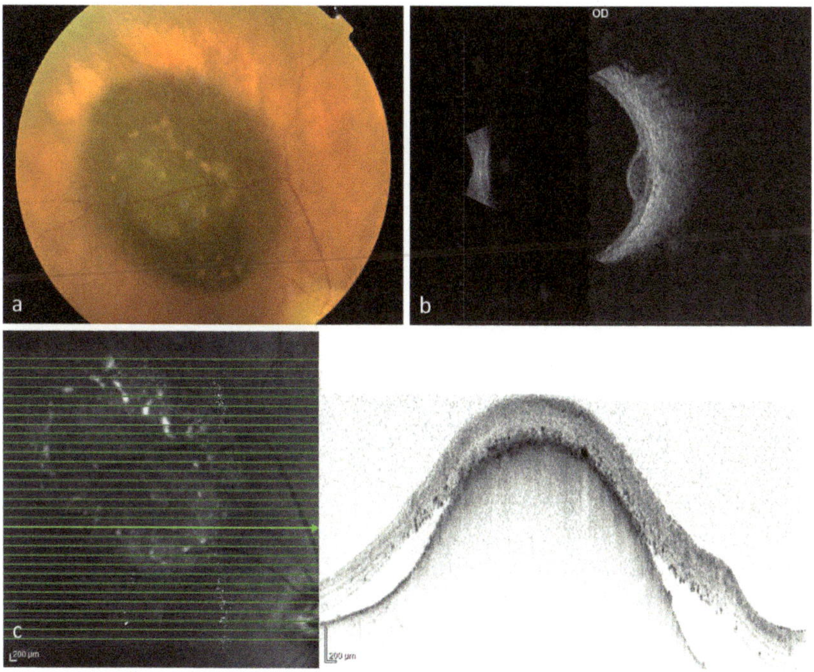

Figure 2. a: A dark pigmented uveal melanoma with orange pigment; 2b: On B-scan ultrasonography acoustic hollowing and choroidal excavation is present, 2c: Subretinal fluid and retinal pigment epithelial alterations are visible on optical coherence tomography scan at the top of the tumour.

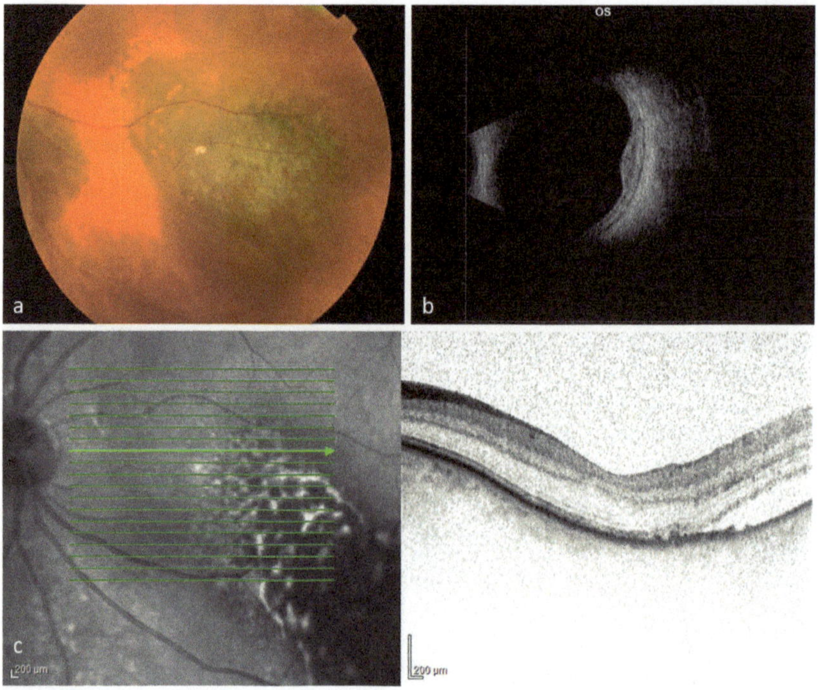

Figure 3. a: Pigmented uveal melanoma with orange pigment (lipofuscin); 3b: A homogeneous grey scale in the tumour and choroidal excavation on B-scan ultrasonography; 3c: Optical coherence tomography of the same tumour with subretinal fluid.

The most important clinical prognostic factor is tumour size, and is often used for selection of the treatment. There are several treatment options, which will be discussed later in this chapter. UM are subdivided into different categories depending on the apical size and diameter, however, many centres use their own definition. Most widely used definition is suggested by the COMS study. Small melanomas are 1.0 - 2.5 mm in apical height and > 5.0 mm in largest basal dimension (Collaborative Ocular Melanoma Study Group, 1997). Medium tumours are defined as tumours 2.5 to 10 mm in apical height and ≤ 16 mm in largest basal diameter. Large tumours are ≥ 2 mm in apical height and > 16 mm in maximal basal diameter, or a melanoma > 10 mm in apical height, regardless of the basal diameter (Collaborative Ocular Melanoma Study Group, 2003). One large study described that each increase in millimeter of tumour thickness increased the risk for metastasis by 5% (Shields et al, 2009b). The mortality rate for small (< 2 - 3 mm height), medium (3 - 8 mm height) and large (> 8 mm height) melanoma was 16%, 32% and 53% in 5 years, respectively, and has not changed in recent years (Diener-West et al, 1992). This supports the model of tumour doubling time of melanoma and its' related metastasis. The model suggests that micrometastasis already exist several years before diagnosis of the primary tumour (Eskelin et al, 2000). This emphasizes the importance of identifying small melanoma and reducing the risk of metastases.

5.3. Clinical predictive factors of small melanoma

In general, choroidal nevi have a less than 5 mm basal diameter and are minimal in height (< 2 mm), although several definitions of nevi have been proposed. Due to different examination methods and definitions, the prevalence of nevi is between 0.2% and 30% (Gass, 1977; Wilder, 1946). Overall in a Caucasian population the incidence is 6.5% (Sumich et al, 1998). Whenever, growth of a nevus is measured on US in a short time a transformation into a small melanoma is suspected. On the other hand benign nevi can also grow slowly. Mashayekhi *et al* observed in 31% of nevi a slight growth, without evidence of development into a melanoma over a mean follow up of 15 years (Mashayekhi et al, 2011). As described by Singh and co-workers, assuming that all melanoma result from nevi, 1 out of 8845 choroidal nevi can undergo malignant transformation into melanoma in the Caucasian population in the USA (Singh et al, 2005b). In Australia this is estimated 1 out of 4300 nevi (Sumich et al, 1998).

It is important to differentiate melanoma form other choroidal pathologies, such as choroidal nevi, by identifying indicators of potential malignancy which may differentiate nevi from small UM. Shields *et al* constructed a mnemonic "TFSOM", i.e. "to find small ocular melanoma" to assist in identifying small choroidal melanoma at risk for growth (Shields et al, 1995). The letters of the mnemonic indicate: Thickness > 2 mm, subretinal Fluid, Symptoms, Orange pigment and Margin to the optic disc. Tumours with no, one or more than two factors have 4%, 36% or > 45% chance of growth, respectively (Shields et al, 2000). A tumour with a thickness of more than 2 mm is considered suspect of being a melanoma rather than a nevus. Subretinal fluid is the strongest indicator of malignancy. Exudative retinal detachment, overlying or adjacent to the tumour, is associated with tumour growth (Augsburger et al, 1989). Presence of symptoms, as mentioned earlier or a change in symptoms is a risk factor for malignancy. Orange pigment is formed on melanomas of the posterior pole, although this can also be seen on the surface of presumed benign nevi and haemangioma. Orange pigment is an accumulation of lipofuscin within the RPE. In amelanotic tumours it appears brown-black of colour. Besides orange pigment as a risk factor, a tumour margin within 3 mm of the optic disc is also suspect for malignant potential (figure 4a).

Later "Using Helpful Hints Daily" was added to "TFSOM" mnemonic (Shields et al, 2009a). These features indicate a low acoustic profile or Ultrasound Hollowness, absence of a Halo around the tumour and absence of Drusen over the tumour. US hollowness is shown in 25% of nevi that transformed into melanoma, compared to the 4% with growth without US hollowness (Shields et al, 2009a). A halo around a tumour is a pigmented lesion with a surrounding depigmentation, as can also be noticed in dysplastic nevi. Drusen suggest a chronic lesion and usually indicate that the tumour is benign, however this is not conclusive.

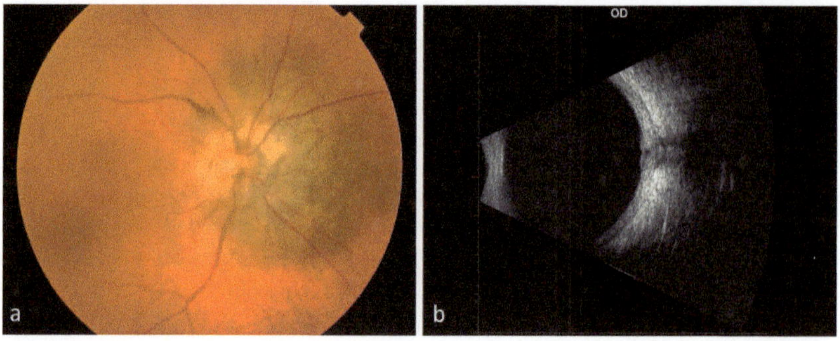

Figure 4. a: Peripapillary nevus, barely elevated, with margin located < 3 mm to the optic disc in the right eye of a 72 year-old man; 4b: High reflectivity on B-scan ultrasonography.

5.4. Ancillary testing

5.4.1. Ultrasonography

US is a non-invasive tool and helps to establish the diagnosis of UM, despite media opacities or whether the tumour is located far peripherally. UM shows characteristic low to medium internal reflectivity on A-scan. B-scan US is primarily used to plan therapy based on the first measurement, and to periodically measure tumour prominence (height) and basal diameter for follow-up. The B-scan can identify possible extraocular extension as an empty area behind the sclera. On B-scan US the internal structure of the tumour is typically seen as a relative homogeneous grey scale, although this pattern is not specifically diagnostic (figure 3b). At the base of the tumour an acoustically silent zone (called acoustic hollowing) is seen, as well as choroidal excavation and shadowing in the orbit (figure 2b). Eighty-eight percent of the UM show US hollowness or low acoustic reflectivity (Boldt et al, 2008). Choroidal excavation is not observed in all melanomas and varies from 42% to 70% (Coleman et al, 1974; Sobottka et al, 1998; Verbeek, 1985). US provides accurate measurements with an interobserver variability of 0.5 mm (Char et al, 1990).

5.4.2. Fluorescein angiography

The diagnostic value of fluorescein angiography in UM is limited. Fluorescein angiography does not show pathognomonic patterns and is especially helpful in differentiating lesions, which simulate melanoma. The pigmentation, size and effect on the RPE of the tumour influence the fluorescein angiogram. It is of little help in some medium to large melanomas that have an intrinsic tumour circulation. This 'double circulation' (simultaneous visualization of retinal and choroidal circulation) consists of late staining of the lesion and multiple pin-point leaks at the level of the RPE, which is evident in the early phase of the angiogram. Blockage of background fluorescence and late staining, when fluorescein leaks from the vessels can be seen on an angiogram as well (Atmaca et al, 1999). Characteristic signs are hypofluorescence in the early phase followed by diffuse hyperfluorescence and hyperfluorescent spots (due to changes in RPE). In the late phase the dye accumulates in the tumour tissue and hyperfluorescents (figure 5b). Hypofluorescent spots correspond with deposits of orange pigment on the surface of the tumour.

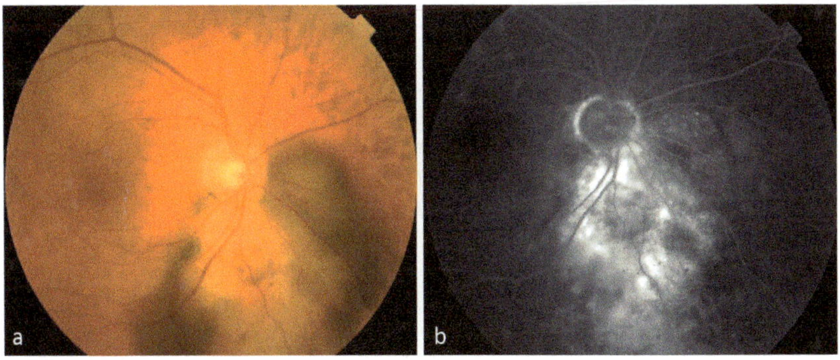

Figure 5. a: A partly pigmented and non-pigmented uveal melanoma; 5b: Fluorescein angiogram with blockage of the background and fluorescein leaking from the vessels.

5.4.3. Indocyanine green angiography

Indocyanine green angiography is designed to visualize the choroidal vessels and provides more information than fluorescein angiography. Whether an evident pattern can be seen on an angiogram depends on the pigmentation, thickness, disruption through Bruch's membrane and vascularisation of the tumour (Atmaca et al, 1999). More fluorescence is seen in less pigmented and larger tumours. The choroidal vasculature can be better visualised with indocyanine green than fluorescein. On indocyanine green late staining is observed, because of the leaking of indocyanine green in the extracellular space of the tumour (Frenkel et al, 2008; Guyer et al, 1993; Stanga et al, 2003).

5.4.4. Optical coherence tomography and fundus autofluorescence

OCT and fundus autofluorescence imaging have limited use in detecting changes in the choroid, however, both techniques are non-invasive and of help in identifying subtle changes in the RPE, retina and vitreoretinal interface. By means of an OCT subretinal fluid can be visualized and quantified, small tumours can be measured, whereas with fundus autofluorescence orange pigment can be shown. Spectral domain OCT can be useful in the detection of subretinal deposits, vitreous seeding and transretinal tumour extension (Heindl et al, 2009).

Although OCT itself is not useful in diagnosing uveal melanoma, it aids in differentiating other pigmented lesions from melanomas (Schaudig et al, 1998). For example, melanocytoma tend to have a high reflective signal anteriorly, corresponding with the nerve fibre layer, and an optical shadowing posteriorly (Muscat et al, 2001). In most choroidal nevi no characteristic or subtle patterns of autofluorescence were observed (Lavinsky et al, 2007; Shields et al, 2008). Choroidal melanoma and related retinal and RPE changes, show different autofluorescence patterns, and secondary changes, such as subclinical retinal detachments associated with presence of small amounts of subretinal fluid can discriminate small choroidal melanoma and nevi at risk for growth (Muscat et al, 2004). Like some nevi UM show brighter hyperautofluorescence in overlying orange pigment, RPE detachment and subsequently decreased brightness in subretinal fluid and drusen (Shields et al, 2008) (figures 2c and 3c).

5.4.5. Magnetic resonance imaging and computed tomography

Magnetic resonance imaging (MRI) and computed tomography (CT) can be of additional value in the differential diagnosis of UM. On CT an UM appears as a hyperdense lesion with moderate contrast enhancement. Tumours thinner than 2 mm are not detectable on CT. Besides that, CT is less accurate than US in differentiating melanoma and is more expensive (Mafee et al, 1986; Peyster et al, 1985). For extrascleral extension CT is inferior to US (Scott et al, 1998). On the other hand, MRI seems more sensitive and more specific than US for detection of extraocular extension of UM (Hosten et al, 1997). A choroidal melanoma appears hyperintense on a T1 and hypointense on a T2 weighted scan. As this can also be the appearance of a melanocytoma, MRI is not specific for uveal melanoma. Due to the higher expenses of CT and MRI and the superiority of US, both techniques are not routinely used for diagnostic evaluation.

5.5. Differential diagnosis

About 54 different conditions are able to simulate UM. The most frequent diagnosis is choroidal nevus, accounting for 49% of the approximately 1739 presumed melanoma patients referred to a large tertiary Oncology Department in the USA (Shields et al, 2005b). The differentiation between small melanomas and choroidal nevi remains a clinical challenge. Clinical features that are more prevalent in *choroidal nevi* than in melanomas are drusen and RPE changes, whereas retinal detachment, choroidal neovascularisation or haemorrhagic retinal detachment can occur in both. On B-scan US, nevi have a high internal reflectivity (figure 4b). Also orange pigment and subretinal fluid, which are features of potential malignancy as mentioned previously, can be present in nevi. Ten percent of the nevi have orange pigment and 18% have subretinal fluid.

Congenital hypertrophy of the retinal pigment epithelium (CHRPE) has sharper edges than melanoma and usually sharply bordered nonpigmented areas (lacunae), or a depigmentated or pigmented halo within. The lesions might be slightly elevated and are black or grey of colour. CHRPE is a benign lesion and is typically located in the peripheral fundus. On the other hand, adenocarcinomas arising from a CHRPE have been reported (Shields et al, 2009e).

Optic disc melanocytoma is a heavily pigmented benign lesion with a fibrillated or feathery margin. Although it can occur anywhere in the uveal tract, the tumour is most often located unilateral and on or nearby the optic disc. Optic disc melanocytoma is a variant of melanocytic nevus. Most patients (75%) have no visual complaints, whereas patients with visual loss were related to neuroretinitis from tumour necrosis and secondary subretinal fluid of the fovea (Shields et al, 2006; Shields et al, 2004). In addition, visual field defects have been described (Meyer et al, 1999; Shields et al, 2006). Ocular melanocytosis is associated with melanocytoma in 8% of cases, and melanocytoma enlargement is noticed in 57% within 8 years (Lee et al, 2010) and 32% within 10 years (Shields et al, 2004). Although malignant transformation is extremely rare, it has been reported (Meyer et al, 1999; Shields et al, 2004).

Hyperplasia of the RPE is a common ocular finding, which is idiopathic or develops in response to trauma, inflammation, haemorrhage and retinal detachment. It is characterised as a black irregular usually small retinal lesion consisting of proliferated RPE cells. Intraretinal pigmented spicules can be seen, and when it manifests as a subretinal localized mass, a melanoma can be suspected.

Choroidal haemangioma is a benign tumour consisting of blood vessels with a typical red to orange colour. Some areas of increased pigmentation can be observed, which makes it difficult to differentiate from melanoma. On angiography typical early hyperfluorescence is shown and on US a characteristic high internal reflectivity is present.

Choroidal metastases are the most common intraocular malignancies. The prevalence of uveal metastases from all forms of carcinoma is between 2% and 9%, with a mean of 7% for breast cancer and 5% for lung cancer (Kanthan et al, 2007). The origin of choroidal metastases is predominantly breast cancer in woman and lung cancer in man. Less frequently patients are diagnosed with other primary tumours, such as gastrointestinal tract, kidney, skin and prostate carcinoma (Shields et al, 1997). Choroidal metastases typically develop after the diagnosis of breast cancer and in some cases systemic metastases have already been detected. In 66% to 97% of lung cancer patients, choroidal metastases are detected after the primary tumour has been diagnosed (Kanthan et al, 2007). In conclusion, uveal metastases can also be observed before the diagnosis of breast or lung cancer (Demirci et al, 2003; Singh et al, 2012). The median interval between diagnosis of the primary tumour and uveal metastasis is 1 - 4.5 years (Amer et al, 2004; Ratanatharathorn et al, 1991; Rosset et al, 1998; Rottinger et al, 1976; Tsina et al, 2005). Choroidal metastases are creamy yellow, flat or elevated and often multilobulated lesions that can occur bilateral. More than half of the patients may develop subretinal fluid (Demirci et al, 2003). The lesion can show clumps of brown pigmentation, known as leopard spots and RPE alterations. Metastases grow in a different fashion than primary UMs, they infiltrate and replace the normal choroidal architecture more diffusely. On US metastases from breast carcinoma show a higher internal reflectivity than UM (Sobottka et al, 1998).

Choroidal osteoma is a rare ossifying benign lesion of the choroid that appears as a yellowish to orange well-defined, juxtapapillary or macular choroidal tumour. These lesions mostly occur in young women with a mean age of 26 years; usually it occurs unilateral, although in 20-30% of cases it appears to be bilateral. Over time an osteoma may enlarge and decalcify partially or totally (Ross & Kemp, 2009; Shields et al, 2005a). There is a 31% chance of developing choroidal neovascularisation after 10 years (Shields et al, 2005a). On B-scan US a highly reflective lesion that shadows the orbit can be seen.

Peripheral exudative hemorrhagic chorioretinopathy (PEHC) lesions, unilateral and often bilateral, have peripheral (> 3 mm outside the fovea) subretinal or sub-RPE haemorrhage that arises from choroidal neovascularisation. In the periphery signs of macular degeneration, such as lipid exudation, subretinal fluid and fibrosis can be observed (Mantel et al, 2009; Shields et al, 2009c). Also in the macula drusen, RPE alterations or choroidal neovascularisation can be present, which is then consistent with macular degeneration (Shields et al, 2009c). On B-scan internal lesion characteristics show a solid or hollow acoustic quality and no choroidal excavation (Mantel et al, 2009; Shields et al, 2009d). The majority of the peripheral lesions resolve spontaneously over time, leaving a scar.

Hemorrhagic detachment of the retina and RPE may also simulate melanoma.

Choroidal haemorrhage may be distinguished from UM by partially or totally resorption of the haemorrhage over a few weeks, and on US an after-movement can be noticed by kinetic evaluation. Key features are elevated eye pressure, forward movement of diaphragm combined with severe pain (Yang et al, 2003).

Posterior nodular scleritis is rare, but often underdiagnosed. It is twice as common in women as in men, and in 35% of the patients it occurs in both eyes. The most common symptoms are periocular pain, pain with eye movement and decreased vision. The differentiation between scleritis and melanoma can be made by US. On B-scan echogenic scleral nodules, fluid in Tenon's capsule, swelling of the optic disc and serous retinal detachment are found (McCluskey et al, 1999).

Intraocular leiomyoma is a rare benign amelanotic tumour of the uvea and mimics an UM. It presents as a dome-shaped lesion, showing light translucency and often contains dilated episcleral vessels, with a predilection in young females (Shields et al, 1994). Sometimes the diagnosis cannot be made by non-invasive examination and intraocular biopsy is necessary (Richter et al, 2003).

Adenoma of the RPE is infrequently diagnosed before enucleation. RPE adenoma is dome-shaped and has in contrast to melanoma a higher internal reflectivity on A-scan US (Nakamura et al, 2012). Compared to UM, RPE adenoma has more frequently retinal feeder vessels, retinal or subretinal exudates and exudative retinal detachment (Wei et al, 2010).

6. Classification and histopathologic features

UMs develop from melanocytes of the uvea that are derived from neural crest cells. Initially Callender and colleagues described several melanoma cell types, (Callender, 1931) currently three histopathological uveal melanoma categories are being recognised: spindle, epithelioid and mixed cell type (Campbell et al, 1998). Haematoxylin and eosin (H&E) staining is used to differentiate between cell types. Spindle cells exhibit elongated nuclei that may contain eosinophilic nucleoli. In general, Ums containing spindle cells grow slowly and might be associated with better prognosis. On the other hand, UMs consisting of faster growing epithelioid cells, have a more aggressive behaviour, and are therefore associated with poor clinical outcome. Epithelioid cells have more polygonal cytoplasm and contain eccentric placed large pleomorphic nuclei and prominent eosinophilic nucleoli (figure 6). The mixed-cell type melanoma has variable proportion of spindle and epithelioid cells with a minimum of 10% of any one type (Edge & American Joint Committee on Cancer, 2010). Other inter-tumour factors, like the presence of certain extracellular matrix patterns (three closed loops located back to back identified by Periodic-acid Schiff (PAS) staining) and increased mitotic figures (number of mitoses per 50 high-power fields equal to 8mm2) can both provide additional adverse prognostic information (Folberg et al, 1993; Mooy et al, 1995). Other histological features associated with mortality and metastases are mean diameter of ten largest nucleoli, degree of pigmentation, presence of inflammation and tumour necrosis (Gill & Char, 2012). Extrascleral extension by perineural, perivascular, intravascular or direct scleral invasion is correlated with a worse prognosis, especially when the orbital fat resection margin is positive (Collaborative Ocular Melanoma Study Group, 1998).

Immunohistochemistry may be of diagnostic value. S-100 is expressed by cells of neuroectodermal origin. HMB-45 binds to gp100, an antigen expressed by melanocytes that can be useful in differentiating UM from nonmelanocytic tumours (Burnier et al, 1991).

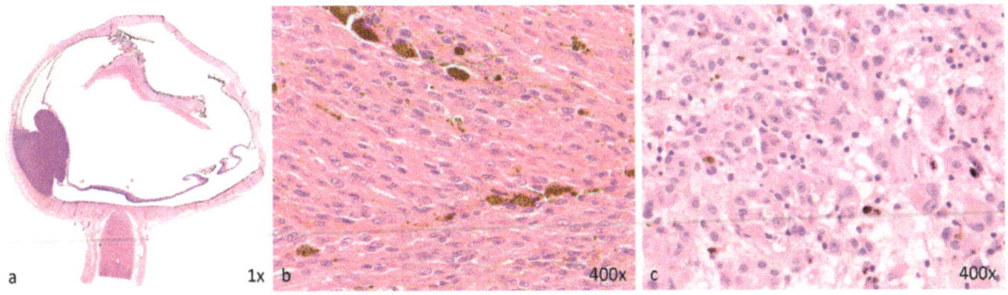

Figure 6. a: Haematoxylin and eosin staining of formalin fixed and paraffin embedded eye sample with a typical mushroom shaped melanoma.; 6b: Uveal melanoma tissue with spindle cell type characterised by elongated nuclei; 6c: Uveal melanoma tissue with epithelioid cells containing large pleomorphic nuclei and prominent eosinophilic nucleoli.

7. Genetic classification

Cytogenetic studies in solid tumours have been a greater challenge than in haematological malignancies since metaphase chromosome spreads of good quality are more difficult to obtain. Solid tumours frequently have highly complex chromosome alterations and are more heterogeneous. Despite this, UM has been well studied since the late eighties with different techniques, such as cytogenetic and fluorescent in situ hybridization (FISH) analysis. Over the years, we have learned that the majority of UMs contain non-random chromosomal anomalies on either the short arm (p) and or long arm (q) of chromosomes 1, 3, 6 and 8, which can serve as prognostic markers.

7.1. Cytogenetic and molecular techniques in UM research

To examine chromosomal changes in UM tissue several cytogenetic and molecular techniques are available. UMs are quite suitable for cytogenetic analysis because of their relatively simply karyotype. Large chromosomal gains, deletions and translocations can be visualized with conventional karyotyping and spectral karyotyping (SKY) (figure 7a). However, for the detection of smaller abnormalities other techniques are necessary, such as FISH (figure 7b), comparative genomic hybridization (CGH) or quantitative polymerase chain reaction (qPCR) based techniques. An approach is the multiplex ligation probe amplification (MLPA) which allows the relative quantification of multiple loci in one single reaction. MLPA can detect patients at risk for metastatic disease using the results for chromosome 3 and 8 with similar accuracy as FISH (Damato et al, 2009; Vaarwater et al, 2012). MLPA and other qPCR-based techniques as Multiplex Amplicon Quantification (MAQ) fill the gap between more expensive genome-wide screening assays and cheaper methods that only provide information on a single locus (Kumps et al, 2010). A different technique is microsatellite analysis (MSA). Microsatellites are tandem repeats of polymorphic sequences located in the non-coding regions of DNA. An extreme form of microsatellite instability was first described in hereditary nonpolyposis colorectal cancer syndrome (Thibodeau et al, 1993). This technique is used to study loss of heterozygosity (LOH) as an indicator of chromosomal loss. A drawback of MSA is that only a limited number of markers can be analyzed in one experiment.

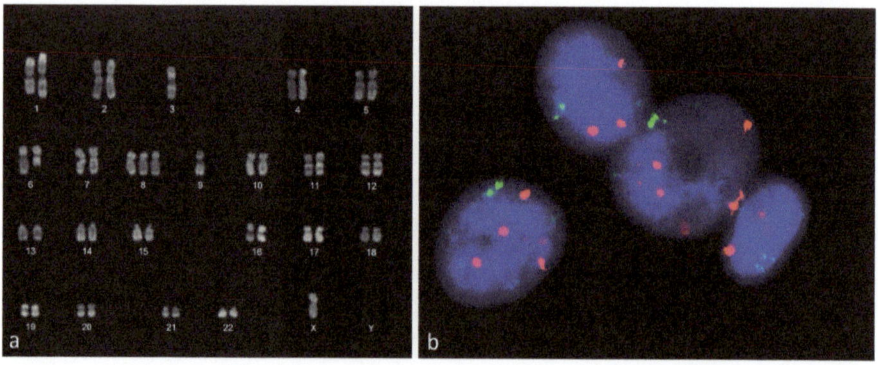

Figure 7. a: Example of a karyogram showing monosomy 3 and trisomy of chromosome 8; 7b: FISH analysis of a tumour demonstrates 1 signal for the probe on centromere 3 (green signals) and 3 to 4 signals of the probe on centromere 8 (red signals).

After completion of the human genome project, genome-wide DNA assays became available. Micro-assay based CGH, single nucleotide polymorphism (SNP) analysis and gene expression profiling (GEP) analysis are the frequently applied techniques. With the development of Next Generation Sequencing (NGS) technologies, the genome can be analyzed at base pair level. Genome-wide mutation analysis of tumour samples led to the discovery of a subset of genes in UM such as *GNAQ* and *BAP1*.

7.2. Chromosomal anomalies

7.2.1. Monosomy 3

Monosomy of chromosome 3 is observed in approximately 50% of the cases of UM and is strongly associated with clinical and histopathological prognostic factors and with metastatic death (Horsman et al, 1990; Prescher et al, 1990; Sisley et al, 1990). Prescher and associates were the first to find a strong correlation between loss of chromosome 3 and a poor prognosis of the patient (Prescher et al, 1996). Since then several groups have confirmed the prognostic value of monosomy 3 (Kilic et al, 2006; Sisley et al, 2000; Sisley et al, 1997; White et al, 1998). It is assumed that loss of chromosome 3 is a primary event, as it often occurs with other chromosomal aberrations in UM such as 1p loss, and gain of 6p and 8q (Prescher et al, 1995). Kiliç and colleagues established that tumours with concurrent loss of chromosome 1p and 3 are at higher risk of metastasizing than the tumours with other aberrations (Kilic et al, 2005). Mostly one entire copy of chromosome 3 is lost, although in some cases, isodisomy of chromosome 3 is acquired (Aalto et al, 2001; Scholes et al, 2001; White et al, 1998). Partial deletions or translocations have rarely been described on this chromosome making it difficult to map putative tumour suppressor genes. However, recently a mutation in the *BAP1* gene, located on chromosome 3, has been identified in UMs and this gene seems to play an important role in the tumour progression (Harbour et al, 2010). This gene will be discussed in more detail later in this chapter.

7.2.2. Chromosome 8

Abnormalities in chromosome 8, and in particular gain of 8q or an isochromosome 8q, are thought to be a secondary event in UM as variable copy numbers can be present in one melanoma (Horsman & White, 1993; Prescher et al, 1994). Gain of chromosome 8q is frequently found in tumours that also have loss of chromosome 3, and this is associated with a poor patient outcome (Aalto et al, 2001; Prescher et al, 1995; White et al, 1998). A SNP array analysis with this chromosome status is depicted in figure 8. The relationship between the percentages of aberrant copy numbers within UM cells and patient outcome has been investigated. A higher percentage of monosomy 3 and chromosome 8q gain in primary UM cells shows a strong relation with poor disease-free survival compared to low percentage aberrations (van den Bosch et al, 2012).

7.2.3. Chromosome 6

Rearrangements on chromosome 6 affect both arms of the chromosome, resulting in deletions of 6q and gains of 6p. The relative gain of chromosome 6p can occur either through an isochromosome of 6p or a deletion of 6q. Tumours with gain of 6p are thought to be a separate group within UM with an alternative genetic pathway in carcinogenesis, since gain of

6p is frequently found in tumours with disomy 3 (Ehlers et al, 2008; Hoglund et al, 2004; Sisley et al, 1997). However, this combination of gain of 6p with disomy 3 could not be confirmed by others (Mensink et al, 2009). Aberrations resulting in a relative increase of 6p have been found to be related with both a longer survival (White et al, 1998) or a decreased survival (Aalto et al, 2001). The effect of chromosome 6 aberrations on patient outcome is not conclusive.

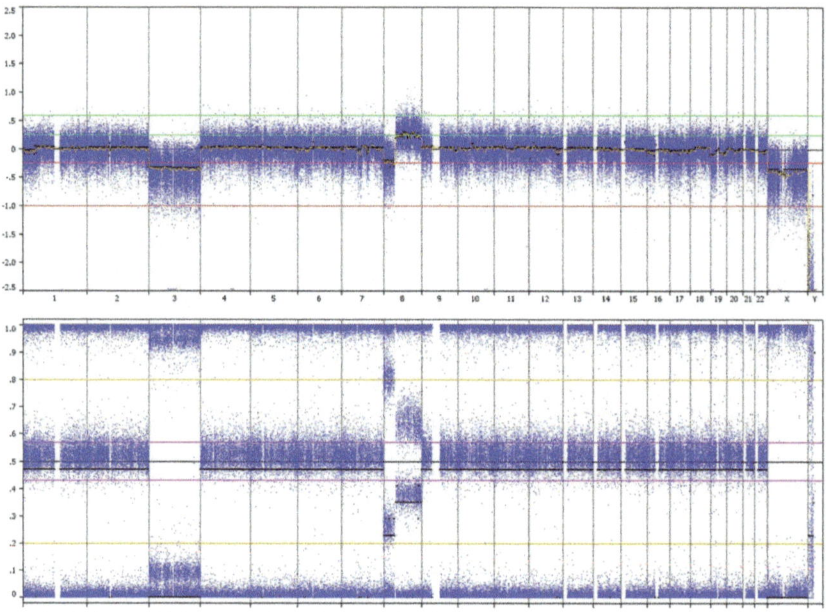

Figure 8. Single nucleotide polymorphism (SNP) array of an uveal melanoma. The upper panel (LogR ratio) shows loss of chromosome 3, partial loss of chromosome 8p and gain of chromosome 8q. The lower panel depicts the B-allele frequency representing allelic imbalance at these chromosomes.

7.2.4. Chromosome 1

In cutaneous melanoma rearrangements on the short arm of chromosome 1 are a common abnormality, occurring in about 80% of all cases (Fountain et al, 1990; Zhang et al, 1999). In UM this region on 1p is also frequently affected, giving rise to a deletion of 1p. However, these anomalies on chromosome 1 are less common than those in skin melanomas with a frequency of approximately 30% (Horsman & White, 1993; Parrella et al, 1999; Prescher et al, 1990; Prescher et al, 1995; Sisley et al, 2000).

Aberrations on other chromosomes have been explored, such as chromosome 9p21 (Scholes et al, 2001), chromosome 11q23 (Sisley et al, 2000), chromosome 18q22 (Mensink et al, 2008;

White et al, 2006), and chromosome 16q (Kilic et al, 2006; Vajdic et al, 2003). The impact on the prognosis, however, remains unclear due to contradictory findings.

7.2.5. Gene expression profiling

Using GEP UMs can be classified into two classes of tumours that correspond remarkably well with the ability of the tumour to metastasize. In a study of 25 UMs, class 1 tumours had a low risk of metastasizing and class 2 tumours had a high risk of developing metastasis (Onken et al, 2004). This molecular classification strongly predicts metastatic death and outperforms other clinical, histopathological and cytogenetic prognostic indicators (Petrausch et al, 2008; van Gils et al, 2008; Worley et al, 2007). Class 1 tumours predominantly show disomy of chromosome 3, whereas class 2 tumours consist mostly of monosomy 3 (Worley et al, 2007).

7.3. Candidate genes

After identifying the non-random chromosomal alterations in UM, the search for potential oncogenes and tumour suppressor genes followed. By narrowing down altered regions on chromosomes, researchers have tried to identify genes involved in tumourigenesis or progression towards metastasis. This way, studies have been conducted on chromosome 8q revealing potential oncogenes such as *MYC*, which is amplified in about 30% of the UMs (Parrella et al, 2001). Other oncogenes on chromosome 8q have been described, such as *DDEF1* and *NBS1* (now referred to as *ASAP1* and *NBN*, respectively) (Ehlers & Harbour, 2005; Ehlers et al, 2005). Yet, no specific oncogenic mutations on this region have been reported thus far. Other candidate genes were proposed, such as *HDM2*, *BCL-2* and *CCND1*. However, the pathogenic significance for any of these genes has not been established.

Mutations in certain genes have been well described for cutaneous melanoma. Examples of such genes are the oncogenes *NRAS*, *BRAF* and *AKT3*, and the tumour suppressors *CDKN2A*, *PTEN* and *TP53*. In contrast to skin melanomas, *PTEN* mutations were not observed in a study of nine cell lines (Naus et al, 2000). Nevertheless, in 15% of the UM cases mutations in *PTEN* were found resulting in activation of *AKT* and overexpression of the PI3K-PTEN-AKT pathway preventing apoptosis (Abdel-Rahman et al, 2006; Ehlers et al, 2008; Ibrahim & Haluska, 2009).

7.3.1. The RAS-RAF-MEK-ERK pathway

In a large proportion of the UMs the RAS-RAF-MEK-ERK pathway or mitogen-activated protein kinase (MAPK) pathway is constitutionally activated, leading to excessive cell proliferation and suggesting the presence of activating mutations upstream in the pathway (Weber et al, 2003; Zuidervaart et al, 2005). Mutation analysis on potential mutation sites in the *BRAF* gene were performed, since a single substitution (p.V600E) in *BRAF* occurs frequently in benign and premalignant cutaneous nevi (Davies et al, 2002; Pollock et al, 2003). However, *NRAS* and *BRAF* mutations have been reported in a few UMs but overall these mutations are rare (Cohen et al, 2003; Kilic et al, 2004; Mooy et al, 1991; Saldanha et al, 2004).

7.3.2. GNAQ and GNA11 gene

With the recent discovery of activating *GNAQ* and *GNA11* mutations new light has been shed on the MAPK pathway. Van Raamsdonk and co-workers demonstrated an alternative route to MAPK activation through G-protein signalling in melanocytic neoplasia including UMs. They reported a *GNAQ* mutation in 83% of blue naevi and in 46% of UM cases (Van Raamsdonk et al, 2009). Other studies confirmed these results, *GNAQ* mutations were found in half of the UM cases (Bauer et al, 2009; Onken et al, 2008). *GNAQ* and its paralog *GNA11* encode the heterotrimeric guanine nucleotide-binding protein G subunit alpha q and 11, respectively. Through mutations these subunits become activated and abrogate their intrinsic GTPase activity, which is required to return them to an inactive state. This oncogenic conversion is suggested to be the cause of constitutive MAPK pathway activation. A subsequent study reported that 83% of UM samples harboured Gα-protein mutations (*GNAQ* or *GNA11* mutations) affecting specific regions on either exon 4 or 5 (codon R183 or Q209, respectively) in a mutually exclusive pattern (Van Raamsdonk et al, 2010). There is no relation between *GNAQ* mutations and prognosis (Bauer et al, 2009). Hence, the presence of Gα-protein mutations in tumours at all stages of malignant progression and in melanocytic lesions of the choroid, suggests that they are early events in UM (Onken et al, 2008; Van Raamsdonk et al, 2009).

7.3.3. BAP1 gene

Exome genome sequencing led to the discovery of the BRCA1 associated protein 1 (*BAP1*) gene in UM (Harbour et al, 2010). *BAP1,* a nuclearly localized enzyme, was originally identified as an ubiquitin hydrolase that binds to the RING finger domain of BRCA1 (Farmer et al, 2005; Jensen et al, 1998). It has de-ubiquitinating activity and is involved in several biological processes, including regulation of cell cycle and cell growth, chromatin dynamics and DNA damage response (Farmer et al, 2005). *BAP1* is located on chromosome 3p21.1 and is thought to be a tumour suppressor gene (Ventii et al, 2008). Mutations in this gene first have been reported in a small number of breast and lung cancer cell lines (Jensen et al, 1998). Recently, inactivating somatic mutations were found in 84% of the metastasizing UMs. These mutations were only found in 1 out of 26 investigated class 1 tumours against 26 out of 31 class 2 tumours, implicating that *BAP1* mutations occur late in the UM progression (Harbour et al, 2010). In addition, co-segregating germline *BAP1* mutations have been described in several families with different range of diseases, such as cutaneous melanomas (Wiesner et al, 2011), malignant pleural mesotheliomas (Testa et al, 2011), and other cancers such as meningioma (Abdel-Rahman et al, 2011). Given the functional complexity of *BAP1*, different germline mutations in *BAP1* may predispose to divergent tumour types. To understand more about the impact of *BAP1* mutations on UM and other types of cancers, more extensive clinical, molecular genetic, and functional studies are ongoing.

8. Metastases

Irrespective of primary treatment of the UM nearly half of the patients develop metastases (Gilissen et al, 2011). UM spreads haematogenous, with a high tendency to metastasize to the liver in 90-95% of the patients. One explanation for the development of new distant metastasis years after the control of primary tumour is the presence of circulating tumour cells at time of the initial diagnosis (Manschot et al, 1995). In other words, the disease is often already disseminated at time of tumour diagnosis. Several pathways have been implicated in the preferential homing of tumour cells to the liver, such as hepatocyte growth factor (HGF) and it's corresponding receptor c-Met, insulin-like growth factor 1 (IGF-1), and chemokine CXCL12 (Bakalian et al, 2008). In case of liver metastasis prognosis is poor with a median survival of approximately 8 months (Eskelin et al, 2003).

Despite the fact that there a no therapeutic options for metastatic UM that improve survival or quality of life, the following methods can be used for screening of liver metastasis: liver function tests (gamma-glutamyl transpeptidase (γGT) and lactate dehydrogenase (LDH) from blood), liver imaging with US, CT and MRI. Although screening annually or semi-annually for liver metastasis by liver function tests are being widely used, there are reports of disseminated liver metastases and normal liver function tests (Donoso et al, 1985; Eskelin et al, 1999).

Patients have 97.5% chance or more of having no metastasis in the case of normal liver function tests, because of the high negative predictive value. However, isolated or combined liver function tests for aspartate aminotransferase (AST), alanine transaminase (ALT), yGT, LDH and phosphatidic acid (PA) are not indicated for detection of early liver metastasis (Mouriaux et al, 2012). Other upcoming screening options make use of serum markers, Among which S-100β (neural crest marker), melanoma inhibitory activity (MIA), tissue polypeptide specific antigen (TPS) and osteopontin (OPN). MIA and S-100β showed significant increase in levels before clinical diagnosis of metastasis (Barak et al, 2011). In a lead time of more than 6 months before clinical metastasis a significant increase in OPN and steeper trendlines in MIA and S-100β levels were demonstrated (Hendler et al, 2011).

9. Treatment of primary UM

Conservation of the eye in UM with useful vision has improved with advances in local irradiation (brachytherapy), heavy particle radiation techniques (proton and helium ion beam), stereotactic radiotherapy (SRT), endoresection, exoresection, transpupillary thermotherapy and photodynamic therapy (Spagnolo et al, 2012). If the tumours are larger, advanced and, in particular, if there is evidence of extraocular extension enucleation is advised (Spagnolo et al, 2012). In addition, enucleation is also performed after serious treatment induced complications (Hungerford, 1993; Shields et al, 1991). Choice of treatment depends on the location and size of the tumour and goals of therapy. Even though enucleation is sometimes required, eye-preserving approaches have shown to be equally successful regarding overall survival and metastasis-free survival (Seddon et al, 1985; Seddon et al, 1990). Brachytherapy is the most common method for treating UM, and currently the ruthenium-106 (Ru-106) and iodine-125 (I-125) applicators are the most frequently used. Brachytherapy can be used in combination with other methods of treatment of UM, such as local resection or transpupillary thermotherapy (Pe'er, 2012). Local control with plaque radiotherapy has provided overall survival comparable to enucleation. Radiation-induced side effects have necessitated secondary enucleation in 10-22% of the patients (Bell & Wilson, 2004; Char et al, 1993; Finger, 1997; Garretson et al, 1987; Gunduz et al, 1999; Lommatzsch et al, 2000; Packer et al, 1992; Shields et al, 1991; Tjho-Heslinga et al, 1999; Vrabec et al, 1991). Local recurrences after brachytherapy are reported between 4 - 28%, depending on the size of the tumour and the follow up time (Damato & Foulds, 1996; Gragoudas, 1997; Karlsson et al, 1989; Seregard et al, 1997; Tjho-Heslinga et al, 1999; Wilson & Hungerford, 1999; Zografos et al, 1992). Radiation-induced complications include radiation retinopathy, radiation maculopathy, radiation opticopathy as well as recurrences (Gragoudas et al, 1999; Kinyoun et al, 1996; Summanen et al, 1996). Heavy particle radiation with positive charged particles (protons or helium-ions) enables treatment of small, medium- and large-choroidal melanomas. The local recurrence rate for proton beam irradiation is similar to brachytherapy and at 10 years is usually around 5% (Gragoudas, 1997; Zografos et al, 1992). Secondary enucleation is performed in 10 - 15% of patients either due to complications or local recurrence. Other complications, such as maculopathy, opticopathy, cataract, glaucoma, vitreous haemorrhage, retinal detachment and dryness have also been described (Desjardins et al, 2012). In concordance with proton beam irradiation radiogenic side effects are also reported after SRT. Side effects, such as radiation retinopathy, opticopathy and neovascular glaucoma are responsible for the majority of secondary visual loss and secondary enucleations after SRT (Mueller et al, 2000; Zehetmayer et al, 2000). The efficacy of SRT for UM has been proven in different studies with local tumour control rates reported over 90%, 5 and 10 years after treatment (Zehetmayer, 2012). Local resection (endoresection and exoresection) of UM aims to conserve the eye and remain a useful vision. The tumour can be removed in several manners, through the vitrous and retinal with a vitreous cutter, endoresection, or through a scleral opening exoresection. Variations of exoresection include iridectomy, iridocyclectomy, cyclochoroidectomy, and choroidectomy. Endoresection as well as exoresection can be used as a primary procedure, after another conservative therapy as a treatment option for recurrences or toxic tumour syndrome. An advantage of local resection is that eyes that would otherwise be inoperable can be preserved, while relative large tumour samples are available for prognostication and research (Damato & Foulds, 1996; Damato, 2012; Robertson, 2001).

10. Treatment of liver metastases

Although treatment options for small to medium sized melanoma improves visual outcome, there has not been any standardized therapy that improves survival in metastatic disease. Systemic treatment options, such as intravenous chemotherapy and immunotherapy do not seem to give promising results or survival benefit (Augsburger et al, 2009).

Several locoregional techniques are available, for example immunoembolization, chemoembolization, isolated liver perfusion and hepatic intra-arterial chemotherapy. In highly selected patients, surgical resection of liver metastases can be beneficial. Operating on patients with a time from diagnosis of the primary tumour to liver metastases of > 24 months, ≤ 4 liver metastatic lesions and absence of 'miliary' disease (multiple, diffuse, millimetre-sized, dark punctuate lesions on CT) is associated with prolonged survival. A median survival of 27 months has been described in patients with microscopically complete liver resection versus 14 months in patients with microscopically or macroscopically incomplete liver resection (Mariani et al, 2009).

11. Future prospects

With the discovery of *GNAQ* and *BAP1* mutations, new therapeutic strategies based on the specific mutated gene content seem promising. For tumours with Gα-protein mutations, the therapeutic goal is to inhibit downstream signalling molecules in the MAPK pathway that are activated. Preclinical studies show that inhibition of MAPK pathway in UM cell lines results in decreased cell proliferation (Van Raamsdonk et al, 2009). There are several key molecules in the MAPK pathway, which have been explored as potential therapeutic targets. One of such is MEK, and Gα-protein mutant UM cells showed to be mildly sensitive to the MEK inhibitor AZD6244 (Gill & Char, 2012). Another recent preclinical study proposed to target both the MAPK and PI3K/AKT pathway since both pathways are activated in UM. A combination of MEK and PI3K inhibition treatment resulted in induction of apoptosis in a Gα-mutant UM cells (Khalili et al, 2012). Other potential targets in the MAPK pathway are currently being investigated, including protein kinase C, which is a component of signalling from *GNAQ* to Erk1/2 (Wu et al, 2012).

Therapeutically targeting UMs with a *BAP1* mutation works in a different manner than the Gα-protein mutations, since *BAP1* acts as a tumour suppressor gene. Regaining lost functions of suppressor genes are in general more challenging than inhibiting an overactive oncogene. Nevertheless, ongoing studies show that histone deacetylase (HDAC) inhibitors may have therapeutic potential in UM. Landreville and colleagues established that HDAC inhibitors can reverse the histone H2A hyperubiquitination that occurs in cultured UM cells depleted of *BAP1*, and it induces morphologic differentiation, cell-cycle exit, and shifts to a differentiated, melanocytic GEP (Landreville et al, 2012). Examples of HDAC inhibitors are valproic acid, trichostatin A, LBH-589, and suberoylanilide hydroxamic acid. Clinical trials are needed to evaluate the effect of these compounds in UM patients, and hopefully UM specific treatment based on mutational content will lead to improved patient survival.

Abbreviations

UM: uveal melanoma

RPE: retina pigment epithelia

FAMM: familial atypical mole and melanoma syndrome

US: ultrasonography

OCT: optical coherence tomography

MRI: magnetic resonance imaging

CT: computed tomography

CHRPE: congenital hypertrophy of the retinal pigment epithelium

PEHC: peripheral exudative hemorrhagic chorioretinopathy

H&E: haematoxylin and eosin

PAS: Periodic-acid Schiff

FISH: fluorescent in situ hybridization

SKY: spectral karyotyping

CGH: comparative genomic hybridization

qPCR: quantitative polymerase chain reaction

MLPA: multiplex ligation probe amplification

MAQ: multiplex amplicon quantification

MSA: microsatellite analysis

LOH: loss of heterozygosity

SNP: single nucleotide polymorphism

GEP: gene expression profiling

NGS: next generation sequencing

MAPK: mitogen-activated protein kinase

HGF: hepatocyte growth factor

IGF-1: insulin-like growth factor 1

γGT: gamma-glutamyl transpeptidase

LDH: lactate dehydrogenase

AST: aspartate aminotransferase

ALT : alanine transaminase

PA: phosphatidic acid

MIA: melanoma inhibitory activity

TPS: tissue polypeptide specific antigen

OPN: osteopontin

SRT: stereotactic radiotherapy

Ru-106: ruthenium-106

I-125: iodine-125

HDAC: histone deacetylase

Author details

J.G.M. van Beek[1], A.E. Koopmans[1,2], R.M. Verdijk[3], N.C. Naus[1], A. de Klein[2] and E. Kilic[1]

1 Department of Ophthalmology, Erasmus MC, Rotterdam, The Netherlands

2 Department of Clinical Genetics, The Netherlands

3 Department of Pathology, The Netherlands

References

[1] Collaborative Ocular Melanoma Study Group (1997). Factors predictive of growth and treatment of small choroidal melanoma: COMS Report No. 5. *Arch Ophthalmol* 115: 1537-1544.

[2] Collaborative Ocular Melanoma Study Group (1998). Histopathologic characteristics of uveal melanomas in eyes enucleated from the Collaborative Ocular Melanoma Study. COMS report no. 6. *Am J Ophthalmol* 125: 745-766.

[3] Aalto Y, Eriksson L, Seregard S, Larsson O & Knuutila S (2001) Concomitant loss of chromosome 3 and whole arm losses and gains of chromosome 1, 6, or 8 in metastasizing primary uveal melanoma. *Invest Ophthalmol Vis Sci* 42: 313-317.

[4] Abdel-Rahman MH, Pilarski R, Cebulla CM, Massengill JB, Christopher BN, Boru G, Hovland P & Davidorf FH (2011) Germline BAP1 mutation predisposes to uveal melanoma, lung adenocarcinoma, meningioma, and other cancers. *J Med Genet* 48: 856-859.

[5] Abdel-Rahman MH, Yang Y, Zhou XP, Craig EL, Davidorf FH & Eng C (2006) High frequency of submicroscopic hemizygous deletion is a major mechanism of loss of expression of PTEN in uveal melanoma. *J Clin Oncol* 24: 288-295.

[6] Amer R, Pe'er J, Chowers I & Anteby I (2004) Treatment options in the management of choroidal metastases. *Ophthalmologica* 218: 372-377.

[7] Atmaca LS, Batioğlu F & Atmaca P. (1999). Fluorescein and indocyanine green videoangiography of choroidal melanomas. In *Jpn J Ophthalmol*, Vol. 43. pp. 25-30.

[8] Augsburger JJ, Corrêa ZM & Shaikh AH. (2009). Effectiveness of treatments for metastatic uveal melanoma. In *Am J Ophthalmol*, Vol. 148. pp. 119-127.

[9] Augsburger JJ, Schroeder RP, Territo C, Gamel JW & Shields JA. (1989). Clinical parameters predictive of enlargement of melanocytic choroidal lesions. In *Br J Ophthalmol*, Vol. 73. pp. 911-917.

[10] Bakalian S, Marshall JC, Logan P, Faingold D, Maloney S, Di Cesare S, Martins C, Fernandes BF & Burnier MN, Jr. (2008) Molecular pathways mediating liver metastasis in patients with uveal melanoma. *Clin Cancer Res* 14: 951-956.

[11] Barak V, Kaiserman I, Frenkel S, Hendler K, Kalickman I & Pe'er J (2011) The dynamics of serum tumor markers in predicting metastatic uveal melanoma (part 1). *Anticancer Res* 31: 345-349.

[12] Bauer J, Kilic E, Vaarwater J, Bastian BC, Garbe C & de Klein A (2009) Oncogenic GNAQ mutations are not correlated with disease-free survival in uveal melanoma. *Br J Cancer* 101: 813-815.

[13] Bell DJ & Wilson MW (2004) Choroidal melanoma: natural history and management options. *Cancer Control* 11: 296-303.

[14] Biswas J, Krishnakumar S & Shanmugam MP. (2002). Uveal melanoma in Asian Indians: a clinicopathological study. In *Arch Ophthalmol*, Vol. 120. pp. 522-523.

[15] Boldt HC, Byrne SF, Gilson MM, Finger PT, Green RL, Straatsma BR, Simpson ER & Hawkins BS (2008) Baseline echographic characteristics of tumors in eyes of patients enrolled in the Collaborative Ocular Melanoma Study: COMS report no. 29. *Ophthalmology* 115: 1390-1397, 1397 e1391-1392.

[16] Burnier MN, Jr., McLean IW & Gamel JW (1991) Immunohistochemical evaluation of uveal melanocytic tumors. Expression of HMB-45, S-100 protein, and neuron-specific enolase. *Cancer* 68: 809-814.

[17] Callender GR (1931) Malignant melanotic tumors of the eye: a study of histologic types in 111 cases. *Trans Am Acad Ophthalmol Otolaryngol* 36: 131-142.

[18] Campbell RJ, Sobin LH, Zimmerman LE & World Health Organization. (1998). *Histological typing of tumours of the eye and its adnexa*. International histological classification of tumours. Springer: Berlin ; London.

[19] Carreno E, Saornil MA, Garcia-Alvarez C, Lopez-Lara F, De Frutos-Baraja JM & Almaraz A (2012) Prevalence of ocular and oculodermal melanocytosis in Spanish population with uveal melanoma. *Eye (Lond)* 26: 159-162.

[20] Char DH, Kroll S, Stone RD, Harrie R & Kerman B. (1990). Ultrasonographic measurement of uveal melanoma thickness: interobserver variability. In *Br J Ophthalmol*, Vol. 74. pp. 183-185.

[21] Char DH & Miller T. (1995). Accuracy of presumed uveal melanoma diagnosis before alternative therapy. In *Br J Ophthalmol*, Vol. 79. pp. 692-696.

[22] Char DH, Quivey JM, Castro JR, Kroll S & Phillips T (1993) Helium ions versus iodine 125 brachytherapy in the management of uveal melanoma. A prospective, randomized, dynamically balanced trial. *Ophthalmology* 100: 1547-1554.

[23] Char DH, Stone RD, Irvine AR, Crawford JB, Hilton GF, Lonn LI & Schwartz A (1980) Diagnostic modalities in choroidal melanoma. *Am J Ophthalmol* 89: 223-230.

[24] Cohen Y, Goldenberg-Cohen N, Parrella P, Chowers I, Merbs SL, Pe'er J & Sidransky D (2003) Lack of BRAF mutation in primary uveal melanoma. *Invest Ophthalmol Vis Sci* 44: 2876-2878.

[25] Coleman DJ, Abramson DH, Jack RL & Franzen LA (1974) Ultrasonic diagnosis of tumors of the choroid. *Arch Ophthalmol* 91: 344-354.

[26] Collaborative Ocular Melanoma Study Group (2003) Comparison of clinical, echographic, and histopathological measurements from eyes with medium-sized choroidal melanoma in the collaborative ocular melanoma study: COMS report no. 21. *Arch Ophthalmol* 121: 1163-1171.

[27] Damato B (2010) Does ocular treatment of uveal melanoma influence survival? *Br J Cancer* 103: 285-290.

[28] Damato B, Dopierala J, Klaasen A, van Dijk M, Sibbring J & Coupland SE (2009) Multiplex ligation-dependent probe amplification of uveal melanoma: correlation with metastatic death. *Invest Ophthalmol Vis Sci* 50: 3048-3055.

[29] Damato B & Foulds WS (1996) Indications for trans-scleral local resection of uveal melanoma. *Br J Ophthalmol* 80: 1029-1030.

[30] Damato BE (2012) Local resection of uveal melanoma. *Dev Ophthalmol* 49: 66-80.

[31] Damato BE & Coupland SE (2012) Differences in uveal melanomas between men and women from the British Isles. *Eye (Lond)* 26: 292-299.

[32] Davies H, Bignell GR, Cox C, Stephens P, Edkins S, Clegg S, Teague J, Woffendin H, Garnett MJ, Bottomley W, Davis N, Dicks E, Ewing R, Floyd Y, Gray K, Hall S, Hawes R, Hughes J, Kosmidou V, Menzies A, Mould C, Parker A, Stevens C, Watt S, Hooper S, Wilson R, Jayatilake H, Gusterson BA, Cooper C, Shipley J, Hargrave D, Pritchard-Jones K, Maitland N, Chenevix-Trench G, Riggins GJ, Bigner DD, Palmieri G, Cossu A, Flanagan A, Nicholson A, Ho JW, Leung SY, Yuen ST, Weber BL, Seigler HF, Darrow TL, Paterson H, Marais R, Marshall CJ, Wooster R, Stratton MR & Futreal PA (2002) Mutations of the BRAF gene in human cancer. *Nature* 417: 949-954.

[33] Demirci H, Shields CL, Chao A-N & Shields JA. (2003). Uveal metastasis from breast cancer in 264 patients. In *Am J Ophthalmol*, Vol. 136. pp. 264-271.

[34] Desjardins L, Lumbroso-Le Rouic L, Levy-Gabriel C, Cassoux N, Dendale R, Mazal A, Delacroix S, Sastre X, Plancher C & Asselain B (2012) Treatment of uveal melanoma by accelerated proton beam. *Dev Ophthalmol* 49: 41-57.

[35] Diener-West M, Hawkins BS, Markowitz JA & Schachat AP. (1992). A review of mortality from choroidal melanoma. II. A meta-analysis of 5-year mortality rates following enucleation, 1966 through 1988. In *Arch Ophthalmol,* Vol. 110. pp. 245-250.

[36] Donoso LA, Shields JA, Augsburger JJ, Orth DH & Johnson P (1985) Metastatic uveal melanoma: diffuse hepatic metastasis in a patient with concurrent normal serum liver enzyme levels and liver scan. *Arch Ophthalmol* 103: 758.

[37] Edge SB & American Joint Committee on Cancer. (2010). *AJCC cancer staging manual.* Springer: New York ; London.

[38] Ehlers JP & Harbour JW (2005) NBS1 expression as a prognostic marker in uveal melanoma. *Clin Cancer Res* 11: 1849-1853.

[39] Ehlers JP, Worley L, Onken MD & Harbour JW (2005) DDEF1 is located in an amplified region of chromosome 8q and is overexpressed in uveal melanoma. *Clin Cancer Res* 11: 3609-3613.

[40] Ehlers JP, Worley L, Onken MD & Harbour JW (2008) Integrative genomic analysis of aneuploidy in uveal melanoma. *Clin Cancer Res* 14: 115-122.

[41] Eskelin S & Kivelä T. (2002). Mode of presentation and time to treatment of uveal melanoma in Finland. In *Br J Ophthalmol,* Vol. 86. pp. 333-338.

[42] Eskelin S, Pyrhonen S, Hahka-Kemppinen M, Tuomaala S & Kivela T (2003) A prognostic model and staging for metastatic uveal melanoma. *Cancer* 97: 465-475.

[43] Eskelin S, Pyrhönen S, Summanen P, Hahka-Kemppinen M & Kivelä T. (2000). Tumor doubling times in metastatic malignant melanoma of the uvea: tumor progression before and after treatment. In *Ophthalmology,* Vol. 107. pp. 1443-1449.

[44] Eskelin S, Pyrhonen S, Summanen P, Prause JU & Kivela T (1999) Screening for metastatic malignant melanoma of the uvea revisited. *Cancer* 85: 1151-1159.

[45] Farmer H, McCabe N, Lord CJ, Tutt AN, Johnson DA, Richardson TB, Santarosa M, Dillon KJ, Hickson I, Knights C, Martin NM, Jackson SP, Smith GC & Ashworth A (2005) Targeting the DNA repair defect in BRCA mutant cells as a therapeutic strategy. *Nature* 434: 917-921.

[46] Ferry AP (1964) Lesions Mistaken for Malignant Melanoma of the Posterior Uvea. A Clinicopathologic Analysis of 100 Cases with Ophthalmoscopically Visible Lesions. *Arch Ophthalmol* 72: 463-469.

[47] Finger PT (1997) Radiation therapy for choroidal melanoma. *Surv Ophthalmol* 42: 215-232.

[48] Folberg R, Rummelt V, Parys-Van Ginderdeuren R, Hwang T, Woolson RF, Pe'er J & Gruman LM (1993) The prognostic value of tumor blood vessel morphology in primary uveal melanoma. *Ophthalmology* 100: 1389-1398.

[49] Fountain JW, Bale SJ, Housman DE & Dracopoli NC (1990) Genetics of melanoma. *Cancer Surv* 9: 645-671.

[50] Frenkel S, Barzel I, Levy J, Lin AY, Bartsch DU, Majumdar D, Folberg R & Pe'er J (2008) Demonstrating circulation in vasculogenic mimicry patterns of uveal melanoma by confocal indocyanine green angiography. *Eye (Lond)* 22: 948-952.

[51] Garretson BR, Robertson DM & Earle JD (1987) Choroidal melanoma treatment with iodine 125 brachytherapy. *Arch Ophthalmol* 105: 1394-1397.

[52] Gass JD (1977) Problems in the differential diagnosis of choroidal nevi and malignant melanomas. The XXXIII Edward Jackson Memorial Lecture. *Am J Ophthalmol* 83: 299-323.

[53] Gilissen C, Hoischen A, Brunner HG & Veltman JA (2011) Unlocking Mendelian disease using exome sequencing. *Genome Biol* 12: 228.

[54] Gill HS & Char DH (2012) Uveal melanoma prognostication: from lesion size and cell type to molecular class. *Can J Ophthalmol* 47: 246-253.

[55] Gonder JR, Shields JA, Albert DM, Augsburger JJ & Lavin PT (1982) Uveal malignant melanoma associated with ocular and oculodermal melanocytosis. *Ophthalmology* 89: 953-960.

[56] Gragoudas ES (1997) 1996 Jules Gonin Lecture of the Retina Research Foundation. Long-term results after proton irradiation of uveal melanomas. *Graefes Arch Clin Exp Ophthalmol* 235: 265-267.

[57] Gragoudas ES, Li W, Lane AM, Munzenrider J & Egan KM (1999) Risk factors for radiation maculopathy and papillopathy after intraocular irradiation. *Ophthalmology* 106: 1571-1577; discussion 1577-1578.

[58] Collaborative Ocular Melanoma Study Group (1990). Accuracy of diagnosis of choroidal melanomas in the Collaborative Ocular Melanoma Study. COMS report no. 1. In *Arch Ophthalmol*, Vol. 108. pp. 1268-1273.

[59] Guenel P, Laforest L, Cyr D, Fevotte J, Sabroe S, Dufour C, Lutz JM & Lynge E (2001) Occupational risk factors, ultraviolet radiation, and ocular melanoma: a case-control study in France. *Cancer Causes Control* 12: 451-459.

[60] Gunduz K, Shields CL, Shields JA, Cater J, Freire JE & Brady LW (1999) Radiation complications and tumor control after plaque radiotherapy of choroidal melanoma with macular involvement. *Am J Ophthalmol* 127: 579-589.

[61] Guyer DR, Yannuzzi LA, Krupsky S, Slakter JS, Sorenson JA, Orlock D, Friedman E & Gragoudas ES (1993) Digital indocyanine-green videoangiography of intraocular tumors. *Semin Ophthalmol* 8: 224-229.

[62] Hammer H, Tóth-Molńar E, Oláh J & Dobozy A. (1995). Cutaneous dysplastic naevi: risk factor for uveal melanoma. In *Lancet*, Vol. 346. pp. 255-256.

[63] Harbour JW, Onken MD, Roberson ED, Duan S, Cao L, Worley LA, Council ML, Matatall KA, Helms C & Bowcock AM (2010) Frequent mutation of BAP1 in metastasizing uveal melanomas. *Science* 330: 1410-1413.

[64] Heindl LM, Mardin CY, Holbach LM, Naumann GO, Kruse FE & Knorr HL (2009) Vitreal seeding from uveal melanoma detected by high-resolution spectral-domain optical coherence tomography. *Arch Ophthalmol* 127: 1062-1064.

[65] Hendler K, Pe'er J, Kaiserman I, Baruch R, Kalickman I, Barak V & Frenkel S (2011) Trends in liver function tests: a comparison with serum tumor markers in metastatic uveal melanoma (part 2). *Anticancer Res* 31: 351-357.

[66] Hoglund M, Gisselsson D, Hansen GB, White VA, Sall T, Mitelman F & Horsman D (2004) Dissecting karyotypic patterns in malignant melanomas: temporal clustering of losses and gains in melanoma karyotypic evolution. *Int J Cancer* 108: 57-65.

[67] Holly EA, Aston DA, Char DH, Kristiansen JJ & Ahn DK. (1990). Uveal melanoma in relation to ultraviolet light exposure and host factors. In *Cancer Res.*, Vol. 50. pp. 5773-5777.

[68] Honavar SG, Singh AD, Shields CL, Shields JA & Eagle RC. (2000). Iris melanoma in a patient with neurofibromatosis. In *Surv Ophthalmol*, Vol. 45. pp. 231-236.

[69] Horsman DE, Sroka H, Rootman J & White VA (1990) Monosomy 3 and isochromosome 8q in a uveal melanoma. *Cancer Genet Cytogenet* 45: 249-253.

[70] Horsman DE & White VA (1993) Cytogenetic analysis of uveal melanoma. Consistent occurrence of monosomy 3 and trisomy 8q. *Cancer* 71: 811-819.

[71] Hosten N, Bornfeld N, Wassmuth R, Lemke AJ, Sander B, Bechrakis NE & Felix R (1997) Uveal melanoma: detection of extraocular growth with MR imaging and US. *Radiology* 202: 61-67.

[72] Hungerford JL (1993) Surgical treatment of ocular melanoma. *Melanoma Res* 3: 305-312.

[73] Ibrahim N & Haluska FG (2009) Molecular pathogenesis of cutaneous melanocytic neoplasms. *Annu Rev Pathol* 4: 551-579.

[74] Jensen DE, Proctor M, Marquis ST, Gardner HP, Ha SI, Chodosh LA, Ishov AM, Tommerup N, Vissing H, Sekido Y, Minna J, Borodovsky A, Schultz DC, Wilkinson KD, Maul GG, Barlev N, Berger SL, Prendergast GC & Rauscher FJ, 3rd (1998) BAP1: a novel ubiquitin hydrolase which binds to the BRCA1 RING finger and enhances BRCA1-mediated cell growth suppression. *Oncogene* 16: 1097-1112.

[75] Kanthan GL, Jayamohan J, Yip D & Conway RM. (2007). Management of metastatic carcinoma of the uveal tract: an evidence-based analysis. In *Clin Experiment Ophthalmol*, Vol. 35. pp. 553-565.

[76] Karlsson UL, Augsburger JJ, Shields JA, Markoe AM, Brady LW & Woodleigh R (1989) Recurrence of posterior uveal melanoma after 60Co episcleral plaque therapy. *Ophthalmology* 96: 382-388.

[77] Khalili JS, Yu X, Wang J, Hayes BC, Davies MA, Lizee G, Esmaeli B & Woodman SE (2012) Combination Small Molecule MEK and PI3K Inhibition Enhances Uveal Melanoma Cell Death in a Mutant GNAQ- and GNA11-Dependent Manner. *Clin Cancer Res* 18: 4345-4355.

[78] Khan J & Damato BE (2007) Accuracy of choroidal melanoma diagnosis by general ophthalmologists: a prospective study. *Eye (Lond)* 21: 595-597.

[79] Kilic E, Bruggenwirth HT, Verbiest MM, Zwarthoff EC, Mooy NM, Luyten GP & de Klein A (2004) The RAS-BRAF kinase pathway is not involved in uveal melanoma. *Melanoma Res* 14: 203-205.

[80] Kilic E, Naus NC, van Gils W, Klaver CC, van Til ME, Verbiest MM, Stijnen T, Mooy CM, Paridaens D, Beverloo HB, Luyten GP & de Klein A (2005) Concurrent loss of chromosome arm 1p and chromosome 3 predicts a decreased disease-free survival in uveal melanoma patients. *Invest Ophthalmol Vis Sci* 46: 2253-2257.

[81] Kilic E, van Gils W, Lodder E, Beverloo HB, van Til ME, Mooy CM, Paridaens D, de Klein A & Luyten GP (2006) Clinical and cytogenetic analyses in uveal melanoma. *Invest Ophthalmol Vis Sci* 47: 3703-3707.

[82] Kinyoun JL, Lawrence BS & Barlow WE (1996) Proliferative radiation retinopathy. *Arch Ophthalmol* 114: 1097-1100.

[83] Krohn J, Froystein T & Dahl O. (2008). Posterior uveal melanoma. Distribution of the sites of origin and patterns of tumour extent in the ocular fundus. In *Br J Ophthalmol,* Vol. 92. pp. 751-756.

[84] Kumps C, Van Roy N, Heyrman L, Goossens D, Del-Favero J, Noguera R, Vandesompele J, Speleman F & De Preter K (2010) Multiplex Amplicon Quantification (MAQ), a fast and efficient method for the simultaneous detection of copy number alterations in neuroblastoma. *BMC Genomics* 11: 298.

[85] Landreville S, Agapova OA, Matatall KA, Kneass ZT, Onken MD, Lee RS, Bowcock AM & Harbour JW (2012) Histone deacetylase inhibitors induce growth arrest and differentiation in uveal melanoma. *Clin Cancer Res* 18: 408-416.

[86] Lavinsky D, Belfort RN, Navajas E, Torres V, Martins MC & Belfort R, Jr. (2007) Fundus autofluorescence of choroidal nevus and melanoma. *Br J Ophthalmol* 91: 1299-1302.

[87] Lee CS, Bae JH, Jeon IH, Byeon SH, Koh HJ & Lee SC. (2010). Melanocytoma of the optic disk in the Korean population. In *Retina (Philadelphia, Pa),* Vol. 30. pp. 1714-1720.

[88] Li W, Judge H, Gragoudas ES, Seddon JM & Egan KM. (2000). Patterns of tumor initiation in choroidal melanoma. In *Cancer Res.*, Vol. 60. pp. 3757-3760.

[89] Lommatzsch PK, Werschnik C & Schuster E (2000) Long-term follow-up of Ru-106/Rh-106 brachytherapy for posterior uveal melanoma. *Graefes Arch Clin Exp Ophthalmol* 238: 129-137.

[90] Mafee MF, Peyman GA, Grisolano JE, Fletcher ME, Spigos DG, Wehrli FW, Rasouli F & Capek V (1986) Malignant uveal melanoma and simulating lesions: MR imaging evaluation. *Radiology* 160: 773-780.

[91] Manschot WA, Lee WR & van Strik R (1995) Uveal melanoma: updated considerations on current management modalities. *Int Ophthalmol* 19: 203-209.

[92] Mantel I, Uffer S & Zografos L (2009) Peripheral exudative hemorrhagic chorioretinopathy: a clinical, angiographic, and histologic study. *Am J Ophthalmol* 148: 932-938 e931.

[93] Margo CE, Mulla Z & Billiris K. (1998). Incidence of surgically treated uveal melanoma by race and ethnicity. In *Ophthalmology*, Vol. 105. pp. 1087-1090.

[94] Mariani P, Piperno-Neumann S, Servois V, Berry MG, Dorval T, Plancher C, Couturier J, Levy-Gabriel C, Lumbroso-Le Rouic L, Desjardins L & Salmon RJ (2009) Surgical management of liver metastases from uveal melanoma: 16 years' experience at the Institut Curie. *Eur J Surg Oncol* 35: 1192-1197.

[95] Mashayekhi A, Siu S, Shields CL & Shields JA (2011) Slow enlargement of choroidal nevi: a long-term follow-up study. *Ophthalmology* 118: 382-388.

[96] McCluskey PJ, Watson PG, Lightman S, Haybittle J, Restori M & Branley M. (1999). Posterior scleritis: clinical features, systemic associations, and outcome in a large series of patients. In *Ophthalmology*, Vol. 106. pp. 2380-2386.

[97] Mensink HW, Kilic E, Vaarwater J, Douben H, Paridaens D & de Klein A (2008) Molecular cytogenetic analysis of archival uveal melanoma with known clinical outcome. *Cancer Genet Cytogenet* 181: 108-111.

[98] Mensink HW, Vaarwater J, Kilic E, Naus NC, Mooy N, Luyten G, Bruggenwirth HT, Paridaens D & de Klein A (2009) Chromosome 3 intratumor heterogeneity in uveal melanoma. *Invest Ophthalmol Vis Sci* 50: 500-504.

[99] Meyer D, Ge J, Blinder KJ, Sinard J & Xu S. (1999). Malignant transformation of an optic disk melanocytoma. In *Am J Ophthalmol*, Vol. 127. pp. 710-714.

[100] Mooy CM, Luyten GP, de Jong PT, Luider TM, Stijnen T, van de Ham F, van Vroonhoven CC & Bosman FT (1995) Immunohistochemical and prognostic analysis of apoptosis and proliferation in uveal melanoma. *Am J Pathol* 147: 1097-1104.

[101] Mooy CM, Van der Helm MJ, Van der Kwast TH, De Jong PT, Ruiter DJ & Zwarthoff EC (1991) No N-ras mutations in human uveal melanoma: the role of ultraviolet light revisited. *Br J Cancer* 64: 411-413.

[102] Mouriaux F, Diorio C, Bergeron D, Berchi C & Rousseau A (2012) Liver function testing is not helpful for early diagnosis of metastatic uveal melanoma. *Ophthalmology* 119: 1590-1595.

[103] Mueller AJ, Talies S, Schaller UC, Hoops JP, Schriever S, Kampik A, Wowra B, Horstmann G & Mack A (2000) [Stereotaxic precision irradiation of large uveal melanomas with the gamma knife]

[104] Die stereotaktische Prazisionsbestrahlung grosser uvealer Melanome mit dem Gamma-Knife. *Ophthalmologe* 97: 537-545.

[105] Muscat S, Parks S, Kemp E & Keating D (2004) Secondary retinal changes associated with choroidal naevi and melanomas documented by optical coherence tomography. *Br J Ophthalmol* 88: 120-124.

[106] Muscat S, Srinivasan S, Sampat V, Kemp E, Parks S & Keating D (2001) Optical coherence tomography in the diagnosis of subclinical serous detachment of the macula secondary to a choroidal nevus. *Ophthalmic Surg Lasers* 32: 474-476.

[107] Nakamura S, Hikita, Yamakawa, Moriya, Yano, Furusato, Cameron & Rushing. (2012). A clinically challenging diagnosis of adenoma of the retinal pigment epithelium presenting with clinical features of choroidal hemangioma. In *OPTH* pp. 497.

[108] Naus NC, Zuidervaart W, Rayman N, Slater R, van Drunen E, Ksander B, Luyten GP & Klein A (2000) Mutation analysis of the PTEN gene in uveal melanoma cell lines. *Int J Cancer* 87: 151-153.

[109] Onken MD, Worley LA, Ehlers JP & Harbour JW (2004) Gene expression profiling in uveal melanoma reveals two molecular classes and predicts metastatic death. *Cancer Res* 64: 7205-7209.

[110] Onken MD, Worley LA, Long MD, Duan S, Council ML, Bowcock AM & Harbour JW (2008) Oncogenic mutations in GNAQ occur early in uveal melanoma. *Invest Ophthalmol Vis Sci* 49: 5230-5234.

[111] Packer S, Stoller S, Lesser ML, Mandel FS & Finger PT (1992) Long-term results of iodine 125 irradiation of uveal melanoma. *Ophthalmology* 99: 767-773; discussion 774.

[112] Pane AR & Hirst LW (2000) Ultraviolet light exposure as a risk factor for ocular melanoma in Queensland, Australia. *Ophthalmic Epidemiol* 7: 159-167.

[113] Parrella P, Caballero OL, Sidransky D & Merbs SL (2001) Detection of c-myc amplification in uveal melanoma by fluorescent in situ hybridization. *Invest Ophthalmol Vis Sci* 42: 1679-1684.

[114] Parrella P, Sidransky D & Merbs SL (1999) Allelotype of posterior uveal melanoma: implications for a bifurcated tumor progression pathway. *Cancer Res* 59: 3032-3037.

[115] Pe'er J (2012) Ruthenium-106 brachytherapy. *Dev Ophthalmol* 49: 27-40.

[116] Petrausch U, Martus P, Tonnies H, Bechrakis NE, Lenze D, Wansel S, Hummel M, Bornfeld N, Thiel E, Foerster MH & Keilholz U (2008) Significance of gene expression

analysis in uveal melanoma in comparison to standard risk factors for risk assessment of subsequent metastases. *Eye (Lond)* 22: 997-1007.

[117] Peyster RG, Augsburger JJ, Shields JA, Satchell TV, Markoe AM, Clarke K & Haskin ME (1985) Choroidal melanoma: comparison of CT, fundoscopy, and US. *Radiology* 156: 675-680.

[118] Pollock PM, Harper UL, Hansen KS, Yudt LM, Stark M, Robbins CM, Moses TY, Hostetter G, Wagner U, Kakareka J, Salem G, Pohida T, Heenan P, Duray P, Kallioniemi O, Hayward NK, Trent JM & Meltzer PS (2003) High frequency of BRAF mutations in nevi. *Nat Genet* 33: 19-20.

[119] Prescher G, Bornfeld N & Becher R (1990) Nonrandom chromosomal abnormalities in primary uveal melanoma. *J Natl Cancer Inst* 82: 1765-1769.

[120] Prescher G, Bornfeld N & Becher R (1994) Two subclones in a case of uveal melanoma. Relevance of monosomy 3 and multiplication of chromosome 8q. *Cancer Genet Cytogenet* 77: 144-146.

[121] Prescher G, Bornfeld N, Friedrichs W, Seeber S & Becher R (1995) Cytogenetics of twelve cases of uveal melanoma and patterns of nonrandom anomalies and isochromosome formation. *Cancer Genet Cytogenet* 80: 40-46.

[122] Prescher G, Bornfeld N, Hirche H, Horsthemke B, Jockel KH & Becher R (1996) Prognostic implications of monosomy 3 in uveal melanoma. *Lancet* 347: 1222-1225.

[123] Ratanatharathorn V, Powers WE, Grimm J, Steverson N, Han I, Ahmad K & Lattin PB (1991) Eye metastasis from carcinoma of the breast: diagnosis, radiation treatment and results. *Cancer Treat Rev* 18: 261-276.

[124] Richter MN, Bechrakis NE, Stoltenburg-Didinger G & Foerster MH. (2003). Transscleral resection of a ciliary body leiomyoma in a child: case report and review of the literature. In *Graefes Arch Clin Exp Ophthalmol*, Vol. 241. pp. 953-957.

[125] Richtig E, Langmann G, M uuml llner K & Smolle J. (2004). Ocular Melanoma: Epidemiology, Clinical Presentation and Relationship with Dysplastic Nevi. In *Neuropsychobiology*, Vol. 218. pp. 111-114.

[126] Robertson DM (2001) Melanoma endoresection: a perspective. *Retina* 21: 403-407.

[127] Ross JJ & Kemp EG (2009) Large choroidal osteoma with macular decalcification. *Retina* 29: 413-414.

[128] Rosset A, Zografos L, Coucke P, Monney M & Mirimanoff RO (1998) Radiotherapy of choroidal metastases. *Radiother Oncol* 46: 263-268.

[129] Rottinger EM, Heckemann R, Scherer E, Vogel M & Meyer-Schwickerath G (1976) Radiation therapy of choroidal metastases from breast cancer. *Albrecht Von Graefes Arch Klin Exp Ophthalmol* 200: 243-250.

[130] Saldanha G, Purnell D, Fletcher A, Potter L, Gillies A & Pringle JH (2004) High BRAF mutation frequency does not characterize all melanocytic tumor types. *Int J Cancer* 111: 705-710.

[131] Schaudig U, Hassenstein A, Bernd A, Walter A & Richard G (1998) Limitations of imaging choroidal tumors in vivo by optical coherence tomography. *Graefes Arch Clin Exp Ophthalmol* 236: 588-592.

[132] Schmidt-Pokrzywniak A, Jöckel K-H, Bornfeld N, Sauerwein W & Stang A. (2009). Positive interaction between light iris color and ultraviolet radiation in relation to the risk of uveal melanoma: a case-control study. In *Ophthalmology*, Vol. 116. pp. 340-348.

[133] Scholes AG, Liloglou T, Maloney P, Hagan S, Nunn J, Hiscott P, Damato BE, Grierson I & Field JK (2001) Loss of heterozygosity on chromosomes 3, 9, 13, and 17, including the retinoblastoma locus, in uveal melanoma. *Invest Ophthalmol Vis Sci* 42: 2472-2477.

[134] Scott IU, Murray TG & Hughes JR (1998) Evaluation of imaging techniques for detection of extraocular extension of choroidal melanoma. *Arch Ophthalmol* 116: 897-899.

[135] Seddon JM, Gragoudas ES, Albert DM, Hsieh CC, Polivogianis L & Friedenberg GR (1985) Comparison of survival rates for patients with uveal melanoma after treatment with proton beam irradiation or enucleation. *Am J Ophthalmol* 99: 282-290.

[136] Seddon JM, Gragoudas ES, Egan KM, Glynn RJ, Howard S, Fante RG & Albert DM (1990) Relative survival rates after alternative therapies for uveal melanoma. *Ophthalmology* 97: 769-777.

[137] Seregard S, aft Trampe E, Lax I, Kock E & Lundell G (1997) Results following episcleral ruthenium plaque radiotherapy for posterior uveal melanoma. The Swedish experience. *Acta Ophthalmol Scand* 75: 11-16.

[138] Shah CP, Weis E, Lajous M, Shields JA & Shields CL. (2005). Intermittent and Chronic Ultraviolet Light Exposure and Uveal Melanoma. In *Ophthalmology*, Vol. 112. pp. 1599-1607.

[139] Shields CL, Bianciotto C, Pirondini C, Materin MA, Harmon SA & Shields JA. (2008). Autofluorescence of choroidal melanoma in 51 cases. In *Br J Ophthalmol*, Vol. 92. pp. 617-622.

[140] Shields CL, Cater J, Shields JA, Singh AD, Santos MC & Carvalho C (2000) Combination of clinical factors predictive of growth of small choroidal melanocytic tumors. *Arch Ophthalmol* 118: 360-364.

[141] Shields CL, Furuta M, Berman EL, Zahler JD, Hoberman DM, Dinh DH, Mashayekhi A & Shields JA (2009a) Choroidal nevus transformation into melanoma: analysis of 2514 consecutive cases. *Arch Ophthalmol* 127: 981-987.

[142] Shields CL, Furuta M, Thangappan A, Nagori S, Mashayekhi A, Lally DR, Kelly CC, Rudich DS, Nagori AV, Wakade OA, Mehta S, Forte L, Long A, Dellacava EF, Kaplan

B & Shields JA. (2009b). Metastasis of uveal melanoma millimeter-by-millimeter in 8033 consecutive eyes. In *Arch Ophthalmol*, Vol. 127. pp. 989-998.

[143] Shields CL, Kaliki S, Furuta M, Mashayekhi A & Shields JA (2012) Clinical spectrum and prognosis of uveal melanoma based on age at presentation in 8,033 cases. *Retina* 32: 1363-1372.

[144] Shields CL, Salazar PF, Mashayekhi A & Shields JA. (2009c). Peripheral Exudative Hemorrhagic Chorioretinopathy Simulating Choroidal Melanoma in 173 Eyes. In *Ophthalmology*, Vol. 116. pp. 529-535. American Academy of Ophthalmology.

[145] Shields CL, Salazar PF, Mashayekhi A & Shields JA (2009d) Peripheral exudative hemorrhagic chorioretinopathy simulating choroidal melanoma in 173 eyes. *Ophthalmology* 116: 529-535.

[146] Shields CL, Shields JA, Gross NE, Schwartz GP & Lally SE (1997) Survey of 520 eyes with uveal metastases. *Ophthalmology* 104: 1265-1276.

[147] Shields CL, Shields JA, Kiratli H, De Potter P & Cater JR. (1995). Risk factors for growth and metastasis of small choroidal melanocytic lesions. In *Trans Am Ophthalmol Soc*, Vol. 93. pp. 259-275- discussion 275-259.

[148] Shields CL, Sun H, Demirci H & Shields JA. (2005a). Factors predictive of tumor growth, tumor decalcification, choroidal neovascularization, and visual outcome in 74 eyes with choroidal osteoma. In *Arch Ophthalmol*, Vol. 123. pp. 1658-1666.

[149] Shields JA. (1973). Lesions simulating malignant melanoma of the posterior uvea. In *Arch Ophthalmol*, Vol. 89. pp. 466-471.

[150] Shields JA, Demirci H, Mashayekhi A, Eagle Jr. RC & Shields CL. (2006). Melanocytoma of the optic disk: a review. In *Surv Ophthalmol*, Vol. 51. pp. 93-104.

[151] Shields JA, Demirci H, Mashayekhi A & Shields CL. (2004). Melanocytoma of optic disc in 115 cases. In *Ophthalmology*, Vol. 111. pp. 1739-1746.

[152] Shields JA, Eagle RC, Shields CL, Brown GC & Lally SE. (2009e). Malignant Transformation of Congenital Hypertrophy of the Retinal Pigment Epithelium. In *OPHTHA*, Vol. 116. pp. 2213-2216. Elsevier Inc.

[153] Shields JA, Mashayekhi A, Ra S & Shields CL (2005b) Pseudomelanomas of the posterior uveal tract: the 2006 Taylor R. Smith Lecture. *Retina* 25: 767-771.

[154] Shields JA, Shields CL & Donoso LA (1991) Management of posterior uveal melanoma. *Surv Ophthalmol* 36: 161-195.

[155] Shields JA, Shields CL, Eagle RC & De Potter P. (1994). Observations on seven cases of intraocular leiomyoma. The 1993 Byron Demorest Lecture. In *Arch Ophthalmol*, Vol. 112. pp. 521-528.

[156] Singh AD, Bergman L & Seregard S. (2005a). Uveal melanoma: epidemiologic aspects. In *Ophthalmol Clin North Am*, Vol. 18. pp. 75-84- viii.

[157] Singh AD, Damato BE, Pe'er J, Murphee AL & Perry JD. (2009). Essentials of Ophthalmic Oncology pp. 288. Slack Incorporated.

[158] Singh AD, De Potter P, Fijal BA, Shields CL, Shields JA & Elston RC (1998) Lifetime prevalence of uveal melanoma in white patients with oculo(dermal) melanocytosis. *Ophthalmology* 105: 195-198.

[159] Singh AD, Kalyani P & Topham A (2005b) Estimating the risk of malignant transformation of a choroidal nevus. *Ophthalmology* 112: 1784-1789.

[160] Singh AD, Rennie IG, Seregard S, Giblin M & McKenzie J. (2004). Sunlight exposure and pathogenesis of uveal melanoma. In *Surv Ophthalmol*, Vol. 49. pp. 419-428.

[161] Singh AD, Shields CL, De Potter P, Shields JA, Trock B, Cater J & Pastore D. (1996). Familial uveal melanoma. Clinical observations on 56 patients. In *Arch Ophthalmol*, Vol. 114. pp. 392-399.

[162] Singh AD, Shields CL, Shields JA, Eagle RC & De Potter P. (1995). Uveal melanoma and familial atypical mole and melanoma (FAM-M) syndrome. In *Ophthalmic Genet.*, Vol. 16. pp. 53-61.

[163] Singh AD & Topham A (2003) Incidence of uveal melanoma in the United States: 1973-1997. *Ophthalmology* 110: 956-961.

[164] Singh AD, Turell ME & Topham AK. (2011). Uveal Melanoma: Trends in Incidence, Treatment, and Survival. In *Ophthalmology*, Vol. 118. pp. 1881-1885. Elsevier Inc.

[165] Singh N, Kulkarni P, Aggarwal AN, Mittal BR, Gupta N, Behera D & Gupta A. (2012). Choroidal Metastasis as a Presenting Manifestation of Lung Cancer. In *Medicine*, Vol. 91. pp. 179-194.

[166] Sisley K, Parsons MA, Garnham J, Potter AM, Curtis D, Rees RC & Rennie IG (2000) Association of specific chromosome alterations with tumour phenotype in posterior uveal melanoma. *Br J Cancer* 82: 330-338.

[167] Sisley K, Rennie IG, Cottam DW, Potter AM, Potter CW & Rees RC (1990) Cytogenetic findings in six posterior uveal melanomas: involvement of chromosomes 3, 6, and 8. *Genes Chromosomes Cancer* 2: 205-209.

[168] Sisley K, Rennie IG, Parsons MA, Jacques R, Hammond DW, Bell SM, Potter AM & Rees RC (1997) Abnormalities of chromosomes 3 and 8 in posterior uveal melanoma correlate with prognosis. *Genes Chromosomes Cancer* 19: 22-28.

[169] Sobottka B, Schlote T, Krumpaszky HG & Kreissig I. (1998). Choroidal metastases and choroidal melanomas: comparison of ultrasonographic findings. In *Br J Ophthalmol*, Vol. 82. pp. 159-161.

[170] Spagnolo F, Caltabiano G & Queirolo P. (2012). Uveal melanoma. In *Cancer Treatment Reviews*, Vol. 38. pp. 549-553. Elsevier Ltd.

[171] Stanga PE, Lim JI & Hamilton P (2003) Indocyanine green angiography in chorioretinal diseases: indications and interpretation: an evidence-based update. *Ophthalmology* 110: 15-21; quiz 22-13.

[172] Sumich P, Mitchell P & Wang JJ. (1998). Choroidal nevi in a white population: the Blue Mountains Eye Study. In *Arch Ophthalmol*, Vol. 116. pp. 645-650.

[173] Summanen P, Immonen I, Kivela T, Tommila P, Heikkonen J & Tarkkanen A (1996) Radiation related complications after ruthenium plaque radiotherapy of uveal melanoma. *Br J Ophthalmol* 80: 732-739.

[174] Testa JR, Cheung M, Pei J, Below JE, Tan Y, Sementino E, Cox NJ, Dogan AU, Pass HI, Trusa S, Hesdorffer M, Nasu M, Powers A, Rivera Z, Comertpay S, Tanji M, Gaudino G, Yang H & Carbone M (2011) Germline BAP1 mutations predispose to malignant mesothelioma. *Nat Genet* 43: 1022-1025.

[175] Thibodeau SN, Bren G & Schaid D (1993) Microsatellite instability in cancer of the proximal colon. *Science* 260: 816-819.

[176] Tjho-Heslinga RE, Davelaar J, Kemme HM, de Vroome H, Oosterhuis JA, Bleeker JC & Leer JW (1999) Results of ruthenium irradiation of uveal melanomas: the Dutch experience. *Radiother Oncol* 53: 133-137.

[177] Toth-Molnar E, Hammer H & Olah J (2000) Cutaneous dysplastic naevi in uveal melanoma patients: markers for prognosis? *Melanoma Res* 10: 36-39.

[178] Tsina EK, Lane AM, Zacks DN, Munzenrider JE, Collier JM & Gragoudas ES (2005) Treatment of metastatic tumors of the choroid with proton beam irradiation. *Ophthalmology* 112: 337-343.

[179] Vaarwater J, van den Bosch T, Mensink HW, van Kempen C, Verdijk RM, Naus NC, Paridaens D, Bruggenwirth HT, Kilic E & de Klein A (2012) Multiplex ligation-dependent probe amplification equals fluorescence in-situ hybridization for the identification of patients at risk for metastatic disease in uveal melanoma. *Melanoma Res* 22: 30-37.

[180] Vajdic CM, Hutchins AM, Kricker A, Aitken JF, Armstrong BK, Hayward NK & Armes JE (2003) Chromosomal gains and losses in ocular melanoma detected by comparative genomic hybridization in an Australian population-based study. *Cancer Genet Cytogenet* 144: 12-17.

[181] Vajdic CM, Kricker A, Giblin M, McKenzie J, Aitken J, Giles GG & Armstrong BK (2002) Sun exposure predicts risk of ocular melanoma in Australia. *Int J Cancer* 101: 175-182.

[182] van den Bosch T, van Beek JG, Vaarwater J, Verdijk RM, Naus NC, Paridaens D, de Klein A & Kilic E (2012) Higher percentage of FISH-determined monosomy 3 and 8q amplification in uveal melanoma cells relate to poor patient prognosis. *Invest Ophthalmol Vis Sci* 53: 2668-2674.

[183] van Gils W, Lodder EM, Mensink HW, Kilic E, Naus NC, Bruggenwirth HT, van Ijcken W, Paridaens D, Luyten GP & de Klein A (2008) Gene expression profiling in uveal melanoma: two regions on 3p related to prognosis. *Invest Ophthalmol Vis Sci* 49: 4254-4262.

[184] van Hees CL, de Boer A, Jager MJ, Bleeker JC, Kakebeeke HM, Crijns MB, Vandenbroucke JP & Bergman W (1994) Are atypical nevi a risk factor for uveal melanoma? A case-control study. *J Invest Dermatol* 103: 202-205.

[185] Van Raamsdonk CD, Bezrookove V, Green G, Bauer J, Gaugler L, O'Brien JM, Simpson EM, Barsh GS & Bastian BC (2009) Frequent somatic mutations of GNAQ in uveal melanoma and blue naevi. *Nature* 457: 599-602.

[186] Van Raamsdonk CD, Griewank KG, Crosby MB, Garrido MC, Vemula S, Wiesner T, Obenauf AC, Wackernagel W, Green G, Bouvier N, Sozen MM, Baimukanova G, Roy R, Heguy A, Dolgalev I, Khanin R, Busam K, Speicher MR, O'Brien J & Bastian BC (2010) Mutations in GNA11 in uveal melanoma. *N Engl J Med* 363: 2191-2199.

[187] Ventii KH, Devi NS, Friedrich KL, Chernova TA, Tighiouart M, Van Meir EG & Wilkinson KD (2008) BRCA1-associated protein-1 is a tumor suppressor that requires deubiquitinating activity and nuclear localization. *Cancer Res* 68: 6953-6962.

[188] Verbeek AM (1985) Differential diagnosis of intraocular neoplasms with ultrasonography. *Ultrasound Med Biol* 11: 163-170.

[189] Virgili G, Gatta G, Ciccolallo L, Capocaccia R, Biggeri A, Crocetti E, Lutz J-M & Paci E. (2007). Incidence of Uveal Melanoma in Europe. In *Ophthalmology*, Vol. 114. pp. 2309-2315.e2302.

[190] Vrabec TR, Augsburger JJ, Gamel JW, Brady LW, Hernandez C & Woodleigh R (1991) Impact of local tumor relapse on patient survival after cobalt 60 plaque radiotherapy. *Ophthalmology* 98: 984-988.

[191] Weber A, Hengge UR, Urbanik D, Markwart A, Mirmohammadsaegh A, Reichel MB, Wittekind C, Wiedemann P & Tannapfel A (2003) Absence of mutations of the BRAF gene and constitutive activation of extracellular-regulated kinase in malignant melanomas of the uvea. *Lab Invest* 83: 1771-1776.

[192] Wei W, Mo J, Jie Y & Li B (2010) Adenoma of the retinal pigment epithelium: a report of 3 cases. *Can J Ophthalmol* 45: 166-170.

[193] White JS, McLean IW, Becker RL, Director-Myska AE & Nath J (2006) Correlation of comparative genomic hybridization results of 100 archival uveal melanomas with patient survival. *Cancer Genet Cytogenet* 170: 29-39.

[194] White VA, Chambers JD, Courtright PD, Chang WY & Horsman DE (1998) Correlation of cytogenetic abnormalities with the outcome of patients with uveal melanoma. *Cancer* 83: 354-359.

[195] Wiesner T, Obenauf AC, Murali R, Fried I, Griewank KG, Ulz P, Windpassinger C, Wackernagel W, Loy S, Wolf I, Viale A, Lash AE, Pirun M, Socci ND, Rutten A, Pal-

medo G, Abramson D, Offit K, Ott A, Becker JC, Cerroni L, Kutzner H, Bastian BC & Speicher MR (2011) Germline mutations in BAP1 predispose to melanocytic tumors. *Nat Genet* 43: 1018-1021.

[196] Wilder HC (1946) Intra-ocular tumors in soldiers, World War II. *Mil Surg* 99: 459-490.

[197] Wilson MW & Hungerford JL (1999) Comparison of episcleral plaque and proton beam radiation therapy for the treatment of choroidal melanoma. *Ophthalmology* 106: 1579-1587.

[198] Worley LA, Onken MD, Person E, Robirds D, Branson J, Char DH, Perry A & Harbour JW (2007) Transcriptomic versus chromosomal prognostic markers and clinical outcome in uveal melanoma. *Clin Cancer Res* 13: 1466-1471.

[199] Wu X, Zhu M, Fletcher JA, Giobbie-Hurder A & Hodi FS (2012) The protein kinase C inhibitor enzastaurin exhibits antitumor activity against uveal melanoma. *PLoS One* 7: e29622.

[200] Yang SS, Fu AD, McDonald HR, Johnson RN, Ai E & Jumper JM (2003) Massive spontaneous choroidal hemorrhage. *Retina* 23: 139-144.

[201] Zehetmayer M (2012) Stereotactic photon beam irradiation of uveal melanoma. *Dev Ophthalmol* 49: 58-65.

[202] Zehetmayer M, Kitz K, Menapace R, Ertl A, Heinzl H, Ruhswurm I, Georgopoulos M, Dieckmann K & Potter R (2000) Local tumor control and morbidity after one to three fractions of stereotactic external beam irradiation for uveal melanoma. *Radiother Oncol* 55: 135-144.

[203] Zhang J, Glatfelter AA, Taetle R & Trent JM (1999) Frequent alterations of evolutionarily conserved regions of chromosome 1 in human malignant melanoma. *Cancer Genet Cytogenet* 111: 119-123.

[204] Zografos L, Bercher L, Egger E, Chamot L, Gailloud C, Uffer S, Perret C & Markovits C (1992) [Treatment of eye tumors by accelerated proton beams. 7 years experience]

[205] Le traitement des tumeurs oculaires par faisceau de protons acceleres. 7 ans d'experience. *Klin Monbl Augenheilkd* 200: 431-435.

[206] Zuidervaart W, van Nieuwpoort F, Stark M, Dijkman R, Packer L, Borgstein AM, Pavey S, van der Velden P, Out C, Jager MJ, Hayward NK & Gruis NA (2005) Activation of the MAPK pathway is a common event in uveal melanomas although it rarely occurs through mutation of BRAF or RAS. *Br J Cancer* 92: 2032-2038.

Chapter 7

Pars Plana Vitrectomy Associated with or Following Plaque Brachytherapy for Choroidal Melanoma

John O. Mason and Sara Mullins

Additional information is available at the end of the chapter

1. Introduction

There are underlying concerns regarding the safety of vitrectomy surgery in eyes with intraocular malignancy. These concerns are associated with vitrectomy, both with or without plaque brachytherapy for choroidal melanoma. These include the possibility of local tumor dissemination, extension of malignant cells to the ocular surface and orbit, and remote metastasis. The purpose of this chapter is to discuss the safety and efficacy of employing pars plana vitrectomy in the setting of choroidal melanoma, whether concurrent with treatment or post radiation treatment.

Uveal melanomas are the most common primary intraocular malignancy and, besides the skin, the uvea is the area most commonly affected by melanoma. The incidence of ocular melanoma in the United States is approximately six cases per one million population each year with a median age of onset of 55 years. [1,2] Distant metastasis peaks two to three years after enucleation with uveal melanomas, and patients with remote metastasis seldom survive longer than one year. [3]

Currently, treatments for remote metastasis include immunotherapy, hepatic chemoembolization, as well as experimental treatment modalities. Unfortunately, survival has not dramatically increased with any of the current treatment modalities for metastatic choroidal melanoma. Many factors have been suggested as being of prognostic value including larger tumor size, anterior tumor margin, cellular pleomorphism, extrascleral extension, and genetics including monosomy 3 and genetic expression profiling. These will be discussed in later paragraphs.

The indications for pars plana vitrectomy (PPV) have increased exponentially since its inception in the 1970s. Traditionally, 20-gauge PPV has caused delayed wound healing, requirement of sclerotomy sutures, postoperative astigmatism, and patient discomfort. Recently, small gauge PPV has been introduced. The 25-gauge transconjunctival sutureless PPV system enables sutureless three-port PPV without the need for conjunctival peritomies, decreases mean operative times, reduces post surgical patient discomfort, and decreases surgically-induced trauma at sclerotomy sites. [4] Decreased traumatic conjunctival and scleral manipulation with less postop inflammation, as well as less induced astigmatism, allows for more rapid postoperative visual recovery. The self-sealing nature of the incisions in sutureless PPV, however, does pose potential concerns for the possibility of vitreous incarceration, postoperative endophthalmitis, and hypotony. [5-7]

Posterior uveal melanomas can cause visual disturbances secondary to vitreous hemorrhage, exudative retinal detachments, and radiation-related complications. Treatment consisted of enucleation prior to the Collaborative Ocular Melanoma Study (COMS), which found that at twelve years, there were no significant differences in survival between enucleation and plaque brachytherapy with regards to medium size choroidal melanomas. [8] Radiation has resulted in a new set of complications, some of which are amenable to the use of vitrectomy surgery in the setting of a treated choroidal melanoma. This chapter will discuss the safety and efficacy of vitrectomy regarding diagnosis and biopsy, endoresection, and radiation-induced complications.

2. Pars plana vitrectomy for diagnostic biopsy as well as molecular genetic testing

The diagnosis of posterior choroidal melanoma is often made clinically, as well as aided by ancillary testing, such as ultrasonography, optical coherence tomography, transillumination, and angiography. Choroidal melanoma rarely requires a biopsy to make the diagnosis. With the advent of cytogenetic and molecular genetic studies, there has been a recent effort to obtain fresh tumor tissue. Early cytogenetic studies suggested that certain chromosomes (chromosome 3, 6, and 8) abnormalities were associated with a higher likelihood for metastatic disease. In the early 1990s, it was recognized that a chromosomal 3 alteration was closely associated with metastatic disease. The most important was monosomy 3 (loss of one copy of chromosome 3), which is closely associated with metastatic disease. [9,10]

Other chromosomal changes have been associated with metastatic disease including loss of 1p and 8p as well as gain of 8q, loss of 6q, and gain of 6p. These have been linked statistically to metastatic death in choroidal melanoma. [11]

This cytogenetic information has become increasingly accessible to physicians, and the risk of misinterpreting this information has also increased. Cytogenetic analysis for choroidal melanoma was first performed with standard karyotyping, in which direct visualization was used and chromosomal abnormalities identified by morphologic changes and chromosome banding pattern and size. However, this technique required the need for a highly trained cytogeneticist, led to sampling error due to analysis of only a few tumor cells, and had an inability to detect small changes. There are other techniques that rely on direct analysis of chromosomes including spectral karyotyping (SKY), fluorescence in situ hybridization (FISH), and comparative genomic hybridization (CGH).

The above techniques were superior to clinical and histopathologic variables alone in predicting which patients will develop metastatic disease. However, these techniques had limitations including false positives and negatives, a high rate of failure due to the amount of tissue required, the variability of technique from center to center, and intratumoral heterogeneity. Perhaps the most limiting factor in the accuracy of monosomy 3 analysis is due to heterogeneity. A single choroidal melanoma can be comprised of a mixture of cells, some of which contain one copy of chromosome 3 and others that contain the normal two copies. Sampling one portion of the tumor can often produce the wrong test result.

Recently, thousands of genes could be monitored simultaneously for micro-RNA (mRNA) expression. [12] With the advent of newer software, massive amounts of data could be analyzed and multidimensional analysis could provide new heights of biologic information that were previously unobtainable. This was seen in cancer, where gene expression profiling (GEP) revealed many types of cancer that were thought to be uniform based on their common tissue source, but were instead composed of multiple subtypes of molecularly distinct cancers. This was the case with choroidal melanoma. GEP has helped to simplify our molecular understanding of choroidal melanoma. Rather than many different molecular subtypes, there are only two major choroidal melanoma subtypes, class 1 and class 2. GEP is extremely accurate for predicting patient metastatic rates. Class 1 tumors have a very low risk and class 2 have a very high risk of metastatic disease. [12]

The superiority of GEP over monosomy 3 has been verified by multiple groups. [12] In the past, the major disadvantage of GEP was the expense and limited availability. [13] However, once the value of GEP became clear, considerable effort was devoted to optimizing it for application and use. With regards to choroidal melanoma, GEP evaluates 15 different genetic abnormalities resulting in a class 1 or class 2 classification. This small number of genes has allowed a commercially available, relatively inexpensive assay. This is a polymerase chain reaction based assay, which requires a much smaller biopsy sample and has a very low failure rate. With this technology, we can now identify uveal melanoma patients who are likely to develop metastatic disease. But the question remains, what is the role of vitrectomy with regards to biopsying choroidal melanoma?

Obtaining cells for analysis requires a fine-needle aspiration biopsy (FNAB). Techniques for performing biopsy may be transvitreal or transscleral. Newer techniques even involve the use of small gauge vitrectomy. Transscleral biopsy involves the use of a 27- or 30-gauge needle that is inserted tangentially through the sclera at the base of the tumor. Traditionally following transscleral biopsy, a radioactive plaque is then placed. Transvitreal biopsy may also be performed with a 25- or 27-gauge needle via a pars plana approach. The needle is inserted into the tumor and tumor cells are aspirated. [14] Paul Finger, M.D. was a pioneer in introducing the 25-gauge vitrector to biopsy ocular melanomas. He first used the technique to aspirate cells from an iris melanoma. [13] More recently with the advent of sutureless vitrectomy, newer techniques include performing a 25-gauge vitrectomy followed by inserting a

25- or 27-gauge needle through the 25-gauge cannula and into the center of the tumor, followed by aspiration of tumor cells. [15]

Potential complications of biopsy include vitreous hemorrhage, retinal detachment, and the potential for intraocular or extraocular tumor dissemination. In a series of 500 fine needle biopsy procedures, there were no cases of local recurrence or intraocular dissemination. [16] However, follow up was only three years. There were no cases of extrascleral extension due to FNAB. In another publication by Shields et al, they focused on the outcome of each patient after FNAB. [17] Each patient was treated with plaque brachytherapy at the time of FNAB, and there were no enucleations as all biopsy specimens were obtained by needle sampling. There were no complications in this study as well. Twenty-five-gauge PPV using the vitrector to obtain cells has also resulted in no intraocular dissemination or increased metastasis to date. [13,15]

Most recently, investigators at the Jules Stein Eye Institute performed an Institutional Review Board approved retrospective study to evaluate local and systemic outcomes in patients undergoing FNAB at the time of plaque surgery for choroidal melanoma. Included were all patients with choroidal melanoma treated with Iodine-125 brachytherapy and intraoperative transscleral FNAB from 2005 to 2010. [18] The study included 170 consecutive patients. The technique used for FNAB involved transscleral approach using a 30-gauge needle. They found no cases of treatment failure and there were no cases of orbital dissemination. Metastatic disease developed in 14 of the 170 patients. The metastatic rate in their study was similar to the metastatic rate in the COMS. The COMS did not include FNAB of tumors. In this study, when compared with the largest multicenter prospective study ever performed in ocular oncology, performing FNAB did not increase the risk of developing metastatic disease from choroidal melanoma.

3. Pars plana vitrectomy for treatment of choroidal melanoma using endoresection

Removal of a tumor using an internal approach (endoresection) was first investigated for posterior choroidal melanomas in the 1980s, primarily for small juxtapapillary melanomas that were not amenable to other forms of treatment including brachytherapy at that time. Endoresection has never gained widespread popularity. However, studies have investigated the use of endoresection as an alternative to plaque brachytherapy to avoid radiation related complications such as radiation retinopathy, optic neuropathy, and retinal ischemia. Surgical techniques vary dependent upon surgeon, however the basic principles remain. A three-port PPV is performed with posterior hyaloid dissection. Diathermy or endolaser is used around the periphery of the tumor, followed by creation of a retinotomy. The vitreous cutter is used to excise the tumor to bare sclera. Photocoagulation is then used followed by gas or silicone oil tamponade to flatten the retina. This surgical technique has many complications including retinal detachment, proliferative vitreoretinopathy, severe bleeding, and cataract. The results for local tumor control and metastasis have been favorable, with complications ranging from 2% to 9.4%. [19-22] A very large risk and potential drawback has been the question of whether this procedure results in liberating active tumor causing a potential increase in orbital recurrence and metastatic disease. This question will be answered by the studies cited below.

Kertes et al, in the *British Journal of Ophthalmology*, followed 32 consecutive patients that were treated with endoresection. The patient's choroidal melanoma was pathologically confirmed and all patients were followed for a mean of 40.1 months. At the time, this was the longest follow up and largest series reporting on endoresection for posterior uveal melanoma. [19] The authors found that only three patients developed distant metastasis and died of malignant melanoma. In one case, distant metastasis developed in association with an intraocular recurrence. The most common complications the authors encountered were vitreous hemorrhage in 37.5% of patients, cataract in eight of 32 eyes, and three cases of retinal detachment. With an average of almost three and one-half years follow up, the authors concluded that their results, with regards to metastatic disease, were no worse than patients treated with plaque brachytherapy. They stated that their experience did not support the contention that surgical manipulation of malignant choroidal melanoma promotes metastasis. Furthermore, endoresection is a reasonable and safe alternative to the management of posterior uveal melanoma. Approximately 50% of uveal melanomas occur less than 3mm from the optic nerve or fovea, and the authors felt that their technique was particularly well suited to the treatment of choroidal melanomas that are in close proximity to the optic nerve and fovea.

Damato and associates, in a 1998 *British Journal of Ophthalmology* article, reported on 52 patients undergoing endoresection for choridal melanoma. Their technique involved vitrectomy, retinal incision, hemostasis by raising intraocular pressure and by moderate hypotensive anesthesia, endoresection using the vitrector, endodiathermy, endolaser, and fluid-air exchange to reattach the retina. [20] They used adjunctive ruthenium plaque radiotherapy in selected cases. Their patients had a mean tumor thickness of 3.9 mm. Most of the choroidal melanomas extended to within two disc diameters of the optic nerve. Follow up was a median of 20 months. The main complications included retinal detachment in 16 of 52 patients and cataract in 25 of 52 patients. Twenty-three of the 52 patients had 20/200 or better vision postoperatively. No patients developed local tumor recurrence. Only one of the 52 patients undergoing endoresection developed metastatic disease, 41 months postoperatively. The authors concluded that endoresection did not increase the rate of metastatic disease.

Garcia-Arumi and associates reported on 25 consecutive patients undergoing vitreoretinal surgery with endoresection for high posterior choroidal melanomas. [21] The tumor thickness ranged from 9.1 mm to 12.8 mm. The authors employed standard endoresection technique, but did use a 120-degree anterior retinotomy prior to endoresecting the melanoma and reattaching the retina. The postoperative complications included cataract in 40%, retinal detachment in 16%, epiretinal macular proliferation in 8%, and submacular hemorrhage in 4%. The final visual acuity postoperatively ranged from hand motion to 20/30, with a mean of 20/100. Remarkably, no tumors recurred, and there was no evidence of metastatic disease in follow up, which ranged from 12 to 72 months. The authors state that the reason for having such a low rate of retinal detachment was due to modifying their technique, including trimming the vitreous base, examining the peripheral retina carefully for breaks, and avoiding high infusion pressure. These authors also concluded that endoresection was efficacious and did not increase the rate of metastatic disease.

Most recently, Karkhaneh and associates reported on 20 patients undergoing endoresection for medium size posterior choroidal melanoma. [22] Tumor thickness ranged from 5.5 mm to 11 mm. Preoperative visual acuity ranged from hand motion to 20/40, while postoperative visual acuity ranged from no light perception to 20/30. The authors stated that for tumors with thickness less than 9 mm in their study, they could have been treated with radiotherapy, but endoresection of the tumor may be an alternative approach in some parts of the world where radiotherapy is not readily available. Of the authors' patients, 6.7% had 20/40 or better vision at three years, while 73% had 20/200 or less. Only one in 20 patients died of metastatic disease in a mean follow up of 89.5 months. This is the longest follow up of all case series of patients undergoing endoresection for choroidal melanoma. This rate of metastatic disease is certainly lower than the metastatic rate seen in the COMS.

In contrast to enucleation, endoresection of posterior choroidal melanoma is designed to preserve vision and maintain a cosmetically acceptable eye. In contrast to brachytherapy, endoresection has fewer long-term complications such as radiation optic neuropathy or radiation retinopathy. Immediate complications of endoresection can be severe, including vitreous hemorrhage, retinal detachment, cataract, and proliferative vitreoretinopathy. [19-22] The primary goal of endoresection is to eradicate the tumor while preserving vision. However, the question of cutting into a malignant tumor and liberating cells, some of which may lead to local tumor recurrence or orbital tumor recurrence and/or distant metastasis, needed to be answered. There is no current evidence that endoresection of posterior choroidal melanoma is different from enucleation or brachytherapy with regard to patient survival and metastatic disease, seen in the above detailed literature. [19-22]

4. Pars plana vitrectomy for exudative retinal detachment secondary to choroidal melanoma

Exudative retinal detachment is the most common etiology of vision loss from untreated, recently diagnosed choroidal melanoma. Historically, management has been conservative, as the exudative retinal detachment will often resolve following brachytherapy for choroidal melanoma. However, large exudative retinal detachments secondary to choroidal melanoma often will not resolve and can lead to irreversible vision loss from photoreceptor damage during the several months needed for post brachytherapy resolution. The consistency of subretinal fluid associated with exudative retinal detachment from choroidal melanoma is found to be more viscous compared to subretinal fluid in rhegmatogenous retinal detachments, which can explain the longer duration of reabsorption leading to limited visual recovery. [23]

Gibran and Kapoor reported on six consecutive patients with choroidal melanoma and secondary exudative retinal detachment that underwent radiation therapy, transretinal biopsy with the 25-gauge vitrector, and surgical treatment of the exudative retinal detachment, including vitrectomy and drainage of subretinal fluid with retinal tamponade. [23] All patients had a successful reattachment of the retina with significant restoration of vision. There were no recurrences of exudative retinal detachment. Five of the six patients had 20/40 or better vision postoperatively. More importantly, there were no cases of extrascleral extension or metastatic disease.

5. Pars plana vitrectomy for complications after brachytherapy for choroidal melanoma

Posterior choroidal melanoma treated by brachytherapy can often result in decreased visual acuity due to retinal detachment, vitreous hemorrhage, radiation retinopathy, radiation optic neuropathy, radiation macular ischemia, epimacular proliferation, vitreous debris, and cataract. Potential indications for vitrectomy following melanoma brachytherapy include exudative retinal detachment, tractional and rhegmatogenous retinal detachment, vitreous hemorrhage, vitreous debris, and epimacular proliferation.

There is controversy regarding surgical treatment of eyes harboring a melanoma, whether treated or untreated, and whether there are viable tumor cells that may increase intraocular recurrence, extraocular recurrence, and metastatic disease. This question will be answered by the articles discussed below, as well as our data at Retina Consultants of Alabama/The University of Alabama at Birmingham School of Medicine, Department of Ophthalmology.

Foster and associates reported on nine patients undergoing 20-gauge PPV in eyes containing a treated posterior uveal melanoma. [24] In their series, vitrectomy was performed for vitreous hemorrhage in five patients, macular pucker in two patients, macular hole in one patient, and rhegmatogenous retinal detachment in one patient. Vitrectomy was performed at a mean 24.7 months after melanoma radiation treatment. Dispersion of tumor cells during vitrectomy was not observed in any patient. One patient had melanoma cells detected in the vitreous aspirate. This patient had intratumoral and vitreous hemorrhage before plaque brachytherapy, underwent combined cataract extraction and vitrectomy, and developed intraocular tumor dissemination 56 months after vitrectomy. No other patients developed intraocular tumor dissemination. None of the nine patients developed systemic metastatic disease.

More recently, Bansal et al reported on the author's experience with vitrectomy for vitreous hemorrhage in eyes with posterior choroidal melanoma. [25] They reviewed the medical records of 47 patients who underwent vitrectomy for vitreous hemorrhage following Iodine-125 brachytherapy for posterior choroidal melanoma. The primary outcome of their analysis included rates of intraocular tumor dissemination, extrascleral extension, local tumor recurrence, and systemic metastasis. The average time to develop vitreous hemorrhage was 22 months following brachytherapy. With a mean follow up of five years, only four of the 47 patients (8%) developed metastatic disease, and no cases had intraocular tumor dissemination or extraocular extension.

In 2012, Sisk and Murray reported on combined phacoemulsification and sutureless vitrectomy for complex vitreoretinal diseases. [26] In their retrospective review of 114 eyes that had vitrectomy and cataract extraction, 72 of these eyes had a diagnosis of melanoma post radiation treatment. The authors' primary outcome measures were visual acuity and perioperative complications. They did not report on tumor recurrence or metastatic disease.

We at Retina Consultants of Alabama/The University of Alabama at Birmingham School of Medicine, Department of Ophthalmology reviewed the medical records of 155 consecutive patients with choroidal melanoma treated with Iodine-125 brachytherapy. [15] We identified 20 patients that subsequently underwent 25-gauge PPV following brachytherapy. The average age was 64. The etiology for 25-gauge PPV was epimacular proliferation in one patient, vitreous debris in two patients, rhegmatogenous retinal detachment in three patients, exudative retinal detachment in one patient, and vitreous hemorrhage in 13 patients. The average interval from plaque brachytherapy to 25-gauge vitrectomy was 59 months (range 16 to 98 months). Patients were followed after their 25-gauge PPV an average of 36 months (range nine to 100 months). We found one of 20 patients to have local intraocular recurrence. One patient subsequently was enucleated for a blind painful eye secondary to neovascular glaucoma. Sixteen of the 20 patients had improvement in vision following PPV. Most importantly, no systemic metastatic disease was reported in any of the 20 patients at their last visit, which was a mean of 36 months following their 25-gauge PPV.

In summary, the reports by Foster et al, [24] Bansal et al, [25] and Mason and Mullins [15] reveal the safety of performing vitrectomy in patients who have been treated with brachytherapy for choroidal melanoma. The combined reports by Foster and Mason found zero of 29 patients developed metastatic disease following vitrectomy, while Bansal found only four of 47 patients to have developed metastatic disease following vitrectomy in patients with treated choroidal melanoma. This meta-analysis certainly reveals a much lower incidence of metastatic disease than previous reports, including the COMS (which did not include PPV following brachytherapy). [8] Our current findings based on the above literature, are the following: sutureless vitrectomy may be performed safely in patients having post brachytherapy complications, sutureless vitrectomy does not increase the rate of metastatic disease, and, patients may take comfort that vitrectomy following brachytherapy for choroidal melanoma may result in an increase in vision with no threat of increasing metastatic disease.

6. Conclusion

With the advent of globe salvaging techniques regarding management of choroidal melanoma, ocular oncologists face challenges in the care of these patients. Tumor biopsy is gaining widespread acceptance to obtain tissue for genetic analyses, allowing for more precise determination of metastatic disease prognosis. The use of vitrectomy with regards to tumor biopsy, endoresection, and post radiation complications has expanded rapidly.

Fortunately, all literature to date has shown PPV to be very efficacious and safe in the setting of a patient with choroidal melanoma. Furthermore, there has been no increased rate of metastasis of choroidal melanoma when vitrectomy has been employed prior to or following treatment of the tumor.

Author details

John O. Mason[1*] and Sara Mullins[2]

*Address all correspondence to: masonallmason@yahoo.com

1 Retina Consultants of Alabama, P.C. and the University of Alabama at Birmingham School of Medicine, Department of Ophthalmology, Birmingham, Alabama, USA

2 University of Alabama at Birmingham School of Medicine, Department of Ophthalmology, Birmingham, Alabama, USA

References

[1] Scotto J, Fraumeni JF Jr, Lee JAH. Melanomas of the Eye and Other Noncutaneous Sites: Epidemiologic Aspects. Journal of National Cancer Institute 1976;56 489-491.

[2] Seddon JM, Egan KM, Gragoudas ES. Epidemiology of Uveal Melanoma. In: Ryan SJ. (ed.) Retina. Volume 1. Second Edition. St. Louis: CV Mosby; 1994. p717-724.

[3] Zimmerman LE, McLean IW. An Evaluation of Enucleation in the Management of Uveal Melanomas. American Journal of Ophthalmology 1979;87 741-760.

[4] Fujii GY, de Juan E Jr, Humayun MS, et al. Initial Experience Using the Transconjuctival Sutureless Vitrectomy System for Vitreoretinal Surgery. Ophthalmology 2002;109 1814-1820.

[5] Taylor SR, Aylward GW. Endophthalmitis Following 25-Gauge Vitrectomy. Eye 2005;19 1228-1229.

[6] Taban M, Ufret-Vincenty RL, Sears JE. Endophthalmitis After 25-Gauge Transconjunctival Sutureless Vitrectomy. Retina 2006;26 830-831.

[7] Magasso L, Maia A, Maia Mauricio, et al. Endophthalmitis After 25-Gauge Pars Plana Vitrectomy. Retinal Cases and Brief Reports 2007;1 185-187.

[8] The Collaborative Ocular Melanoma Study Randomized Trial of Iodine 125 Brachytherapy for Choroidal Melanoma: V. Twelve-Year Mortality Rates and Prognostic Factors: COMS Report No. 28. Archives of Ophthalmology 2006;124 1684-1693.

[9] Kilic E, Naus NC, van Gils W, et al. Concurrent Loss of Chromosome Arm 1p and Chromosome 3 Predicts a Decreased Disease-Free Survival in Uveal Melanoma Patients. Investigative Ophthalmology and Visual Science 2005;46(7) 2253-2257.

[10] Maat W, Jordanova ES, van Zelderen-Bhola SL, et al. The Heterogeneous Distribution of Monosomy 3 in Uveal Melanomas: Implications for Prognostication Based on Fine-Needle Aspiration Biopsies. Archives of Pathology and Laboratory Medicine 2007;131(1) 91-96.

[11] Sisley K, Rennie IG, Cottam DW, Potter AM, Potter CW, Rees RC. Cytogenetic Findings in Six Posterior Uveal Melanomas: Involvement of Chromosomes 3, 6, and 8. Genes Chromosomes and Cancer 1990;2(3) 205-209.

[12] Harbour JW, Onken MD, Roberson ED, et al. Frequent Mutation of BAP1 in Metastasizing Uveal Melanomas. Science 2010;330 1410-1413.

[13] Finger PT. A New Technique for 25-Gauge Iridotomy, Iridectomy, and Tumor Biopsy: The Finger Iridectomy Technique May be a Flexible and Safe Way to Biopsy Tumors. Retinal Physician 2006;May/Jun 73-76, 95.

[14] Faulkner-Jones BE, Foster WJ, Harbour JW, Smith ME, Davila RM. Fine Needle Aspiration Biopsy with Adjunct Immunohistochemistry in Intraocular Tumor Management. Acta Cytologica 2005;49 297-308.

[15] Mason JO III, Mullins S. Risk and Benefit of Pars Plana Vitrectomy in Eyes Treated with Plaque Therapy for Choroidal Melanoma: Proceedings of the University of Alabama at Birmingham School of Medicine, Department of Ophthalmology Annual Clinical and Research Symposium 2012, 27-28 April 2012, Birmingham, Alabama, United States of America.

[16] Shields CL, Ganguly A, Bianciotto CG, Turaka K, Tavallali A, Shields JA. Prognosis of Uveal Melanoma in 500 Cases Using Genetic Testing of Fine-Needle Aspiration Biopsy Specimens. Ophthalmology 2011;118 396-401.

[17] Shields CL, Ganguly A, Materin MA, Teixeira L, Mashayekhi A, Swanson LA, Marr BP, Shields JA. Chromosome 3 Analysis of Uveal Melanoma Using Fine-Needle Aspiration Biopsy at the Time of Plaque Radiotherapy in 140 Consecutive Cases. Transamerican Ophthalmological Society 2007;105 43-52.

[18] Johansson CC, Mougiakakos D, Trocme E, et al. Expression and Prognostic Significance of iNO8 in Uveal Melanoma. International Journal of Cancer 2010;126 2682-2689.

[19] Kertes PJ, Johnson JC, Peyman GA. Internal Resection of Posterior Uveal Melanomas. British Journal of Ophthalmology 1998;82 1147-1153.

[20] Damato B, Groenewald C, McGalliard J, Wong D. Endoresection of Choroidal Melanoma. British Journal of Ophthalmology 1998;82 213-218.

[21] Garcia-Arumi J, Sararols L, Martinez V, Corcostegui B. Vitreoretinal Surgery and Endoresection in High Posterior Choroidal Melanomas. Retina 2001;21(5) 445-452.

[22] Karkhaneh R, Chams H, Amoli FA, Riazi-Esfahani M, et al. Long-Term Surgical Outcome of Posterior Choroidal Melanoma Treated by Endoresection. Retina 2007;27(7) 908-914.

[23] Gibran SK, Kapoor KG. Management of Exudative Retinal Detachment in Choroidal Melanoma. Clinical and Experimental Ophthalmology 2009;37 654-659.

[24] Foster WJ, Harbour W, Holekamp NM, Shah GK, Thomas MA. Pars Plana Vitrectomy in Eyes Containing a Treated Posterior Uveal Melanoma. American Journal of Ophthalmology 2003;136 471-476.

[25] Bansal AS, Bianciotto C, Maguire JI, Regillo CD, Shields JA, Shields CA. Pars Plana Vitrectomy in Eyes with Treated Posterior Uveal Melanoma. Retina Today 2011;Nov/Dec 54-56.

[26] Sisk RA, Murray TG. Combined Phacoemulsification and Sutureless 23-Gauge Pars Plana Vitrectomy for Complex Vitreoretinal Diseases. British Journal of Ophthalmology 2010;94 1028-1032.

Chapter 8

Acquired Resistance to Targeted MAPK Inhibition in Melanoma

Kavitha Gowrishankar, Matteo S. Carlino and Helen Rizos

Additional information is available at the end of the chapter

1. Introduction

The worldwide incidence of cutaneous melanoma has steadily increased in fair-skinned individuals over recent decades with estimates suggesting a doubling of melanoma incidence every 10-20 years [1]. Melanoma remains the major cause of skin cancer related deaths [2], with survival rates averaging less than six months for patients with metastases in visceral organs [3]. Conventional systemic therapies, including single agent dacarbazine and temozolamide, produce response rates of less than 10%, and are not proven to improve survival (reviewed in [4]). Recently, however, the treatment of melanoma has been revolutionized by therapies targeting the RAF-MEK-ERK mitogen activated protein kinase (MAPK) pathway. This pathway is constitutively activated in the majority of melanomas via oncogenic mutations in the BRAF kinase or its upstream regulator, N-RAS [5, 6].

Most BRAF mutations produce a single amino acid substitution of valine by glutamic acid at amino acid 600 (V600E), and this leads to a 500-fold increase in kinase activity [5, 7]. Targeting this mutant BRAF with the highly specific inhibitors, vemurafenib (PLX4032) and dabrafenib (GSK2118436) has produced response rates above 50% and improved progression-free survival in patients with BRAF-mutant metastatic melanoma [8-12]. Both BRAF inhibitors are active against melanoma brain metastases [13, 14] and vemurafenib treatment prolongs overall survival compared with dacarbazine [11]. Despite the marked initial responses to BRAF inhibitors, tumor re-growth occurs in most patients with a median progression-free survival of 5 to 6 months [8, 11, 15].

The U.S Food and Drug Administration (FDA) approved the use of vemurafenib for the treatment of BRAF-mutant melanoma in 2011, and submissions for the use of dabrafenib in the treatment of BRAF-mutant melanoma were made in late 2012. We are now beginning to understand the complex pathways regulating the response and side-effect profiles of these targeted inhibitors. The challenge is to define the molecular drivers and pathways of resistance and response and to translate these molecular findings into rational strategies for clinical testing and improved therapies. In the following chapter we describe the molecular mechanisms that contribute to BRAF inhibitor resistance *in vitro* and *in vivo*. We also highlight the current strategies employed to dissect resistance drivers and explore the future of targeted therapies in the long-term treatment of melanoma.

2. The BRAF kinase and the MAPK pathway

Aberrant activation of the MAPK pathway is present in over 80% of primary cutaneous melanomas [16]. MAPK signalling is driven by mutated N-RAS and activating mutations in the downstream RAS effector, BRAF, in 20% and 60% of melanomas, respectively (Figure 1) [16]. Of cutaneous melanomas with no mutations in BRAF or N-RAS, many activate MAPK signalling via oncogenic mutations in the receptor tyrosine kinase, c-Kit [17], activating mutations in the Rac1 GTPase or inactivating mutations in the N-RAS inhibitor NF1 [18].

Among the BRAF mutations identified in melanoma, over 80% involve a single nucleotide mutation resulting in the substitution of valine for glutamic acid at amino acid 600. This mutation is also present in up to 80% of benign, growth-arrested nevi [19], implicating BRAF as an initiating event that co-operates with additional genetic lesions to promote melanoma. Over 60 other mutations in BRAF have been described in melanoma; most affect codon 600 (V600E, V600K, V600R and V600D), lie within the kinase domain and show elevated kinase activity. In particular, alterations affecting codon 600 show 150- ($BRAF^{V600K}$) to 700- ($BRAF^{V600D}$) fold more kinase activity than the wild type BRAF protein [7].

A wealth of preclinical data has demonstrated the critical role of $BRAF^{V600E}$ as an oncogene in melanoma. The specific silencing of BRAF with short interfering (si)RNA resulted in decreased ERK signalling, diminished proliferation and regression of BRAF mutant melanomas [20-23]. More importantly, class I RAF inhibitors, which target the activated form of RAF kinases, show remarkable antitumor activity; both vemurafenib and dabrafenib have shown response rates of 50% in patients with BRAF-mutant melanoma [8-12]. In addition, the selective inhibition of the BRAF target proteins, MEK1/2, with trametinib (GSK11202212) improved rates of progression-free and overall survival amongst patients with BRAF mutant melanoma when compared to dacarbazine [9, 15, 24, 25].

3. Mechanisms of acquired BRAF inhibitor resistance in melanoma

Despite the marked initial responses to single-agent BRAF inhibitors, tumor re-growth occurs in most patients and 5-20% of individuals fail to respond early during treatment [8, 10, 11, 26]. The acquisition of resistance to targeted therapy is common and resistance has been observed with trastuzumab in HER2-amplified breast cancer, imatinib in gastrointestinal stromal tumors (GISTs) and chronic myelogenous leukemia (CML), epidermal growth factor receptor (EGFR) inhibitors in lung cancer and hedgehog inhibitors in medulloblastoma [27]. Resistance mechanisms to these drugs are complex but include the acquisition of secondary mutations in the target oncogene that prevent drug binding, up-regulation of signalling pathways downstream of the target and the induction of alternate, secondary survival pathways. Defining the mechanisms of melanoma resistance to targeted inhibitors is a high priority, as it can guide the selection of appropriate drug combinations and advance the development of new and improved drugs. This is best demonstrated for imatinib-resistant leukemias. The identification of secondary Bcr-Abl mutations in these resistant cancers promoted the development of the potent, next-generation receptor tyrosine kinase inhibitors dasatanib and nilotinib [28].

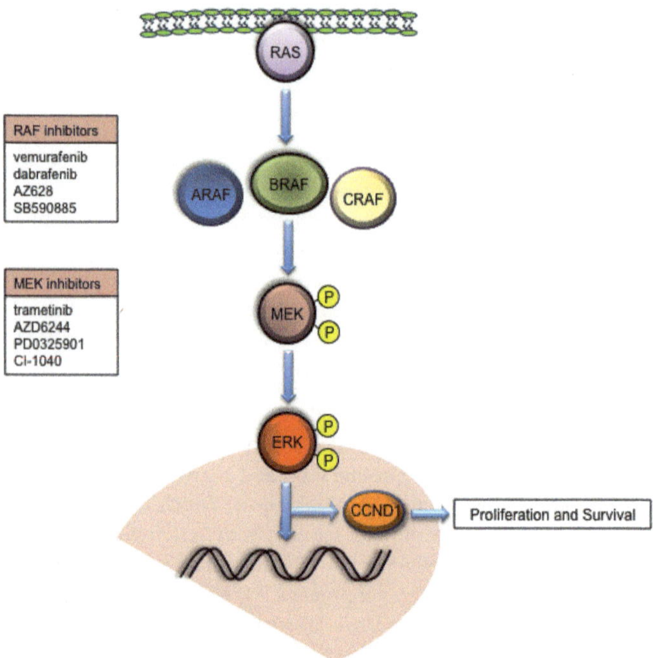

Figure 1. MAPK signalling cascade. Activation of the RAS GTPase promotes the kinase activity of the RAF serine/threonine protein kinases, ARAF, BRAF and CRAF. Activated RAF kinases promote the sequential phosphorylation and activation of the MEK1/2 and ERK1/2 kinases. The ERK proteins translocate into the nucleus and stimulate the translation of proteins and the activities of many transcription factors. This leads to a series of gene expression changes, including elevated CCND1 that promotes cell proliferation and survival. Specific inhibitors to RAF and MEK kinases are indicated. ARAF, v-raf murine sarcoma 3611 viral oncogene homolog; BRAF, v-raf murine sarcoma viral oncogene B1; CCND1, cyclin D1; CRAF, v-raf-1 murine leukemia viral oncogene homolog 1; ERK, extracellular signal-regulated kinase; MEK mitogen-activated protein kinase kinase.

4. Alterations affecting BRAF

Drug resistance is often associated with the acquisition of so-called gatekeeper mutations in the target oncogene that prevent drug binding. In a series of detailed reports, deep sequencing of melanoma biopsies derived from patients progressing on vemurafenib treatment did not find any secondary BRAF mutations. Moreover, immunoprecipitated BRAF from vemurafenib-resistant melanomas retained drug sensitivity in an *in vitro* kinase assay, confirming drug-target binding was maintained [29].

4.1. BRAF copy number gain

The amplification and overexpression of $BRAF^{V600E}$ is associated with BRAF inhibitor resistance in melanoma [30] (Figure 2). In a sequencing screen of 20 pairs of patient-matched baseline (before BRAF inhibitor therapy) and progressing (acquired resistance to BRAF inhibition) melanoma tissue, 20% showed $BRAF^{V600E}$ copy-number gains, ranging from 2- to 14- fold. These copy-number gains, which are likely underestimates due to non-tumor cell contamination, correlated with increased BRAF protein expression in tumor specimens. Moreover, preclinical melanoma cell models with ectopically expressed $BRAF^{V600E}$ confirmed that cells overexpressing mutant BRAF developed resistance to vemurafenib and that this resistance could be overcome by increasing the dose of vemurafenib, applying MEK inhibitors (AZD6244) or concurrently inhibiting both MEK and BRAF (Figure 1) [30].

Unlike melanoma cell models [30], BRAF-mutant colorectal cancer cells with amplification of the BRAF gene (2- to 7- fold) were resistance to the MEK inhibitor AZD6244 [31]. In these colon cancer cells, the increased expression of mutant BRAF resulted in excess activation of MEK and ERK, rendering cells unresponsive to MEK inhibition. In the presence of the BRAF inhibitor, AZ628, however, the abundance of activated MEK was reduced and the allosteric MEK inhibitor AZD6244 prevented ERK phosphorylation [31]. Thus, the concurrent inhibition of MEK and BRAF overcomes resistance mediated by BRAF amplification in both melanoma and colorectal cancers.

Intriguingly, BRAF copy-number gains (3- to 4-fold) were also identified in baseline (drug-naive) melanoma and colorectal tumor samples. In one such colorectal tumor only 28% of cells showed BRAF amplification and 10% of these tumor cells had more than 10 copies of BRAF [30, 31]. These data indicate that cell sensitivity to MEK and BRAF inhibition is likely to reflect the level of BRAF amplification and resistance may arise from the expansion of a limited number of cells with pre-existing BRAF gains. This notion is consistent with a recent study showing that K-RAS mutations conferring resistance to EGFR inhibitors were likely to be present in a clonal subpopulation of the colorectal tumor cells prior to the initiation of targeted therapy. These results may explain resistance to RAF inhibitors and other targeted therapies occurs in a highly reproducible fashion within 5 to 6 months [32].

4.2. BRAF splicing variants

In other melanomas, resistance to vemurafenib was acquired via the expression of splice variant isoforms of $BRAF^{V600E}$. Three of five vemurafenib-resistant clones of the SKMEL-238 melanoma cells expressed a novel 61kDa variant of $BRAF^{V600E}$. This $p61BRAF^{V600E}$ splice variant, lacked exons 4-8, a region encoding the RAS binding domain, and was sufficient to render MEK activation resistant to vemurafenib (Figure 3). The variant appears to arise from a splicing defect as no intragenic somatic deletions within the BRAF gene were detected [33].

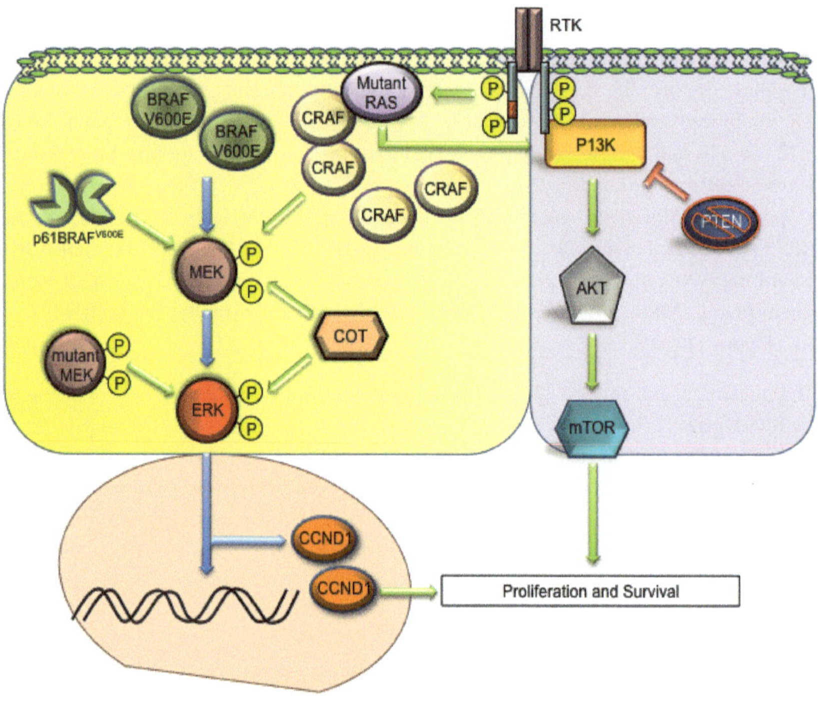

Figure 2. Mechanisms of resistance to BRAF inhibition. MAPK re-activation, in the presence of RAF inhibitors, can occur via A. the mutational activation and amplification of RAS, B. the upregulation of RTKs such as PDGFRß and IGF-1R, C. elevated expression of CRAF, COT or CCND1, D. MEK mutations, or E. the expression and dimerization of $BRAF^{V600E}$ splice variants, such as p61BRAFV600E. Mutant RAS and upregulated RTKs also activate the PI3K/mTOR survival pathway, which is further activated by the loss of PTEN (adapted from [87]). AKT, v-akt murine thymoma viral oncogene; BRAF, v-raf murine sarcoma viral oncogene B1; CCND1, cyclin D1; CRAF, v-raf-1 murine leukemia viral oncogene homolog 1; ERK, extracellular signal-regulated kinase; COT, mitogen-activated protein kinase kinase kinase 8; MEK mitogen-activated protein kinase kinase; mTOR, mechanistic target of rapamycin; PI3K, phosphoinositide-3-kinase PTEN, phosphatase and tensin homolog; RTK, receptor tyrosine kinase.

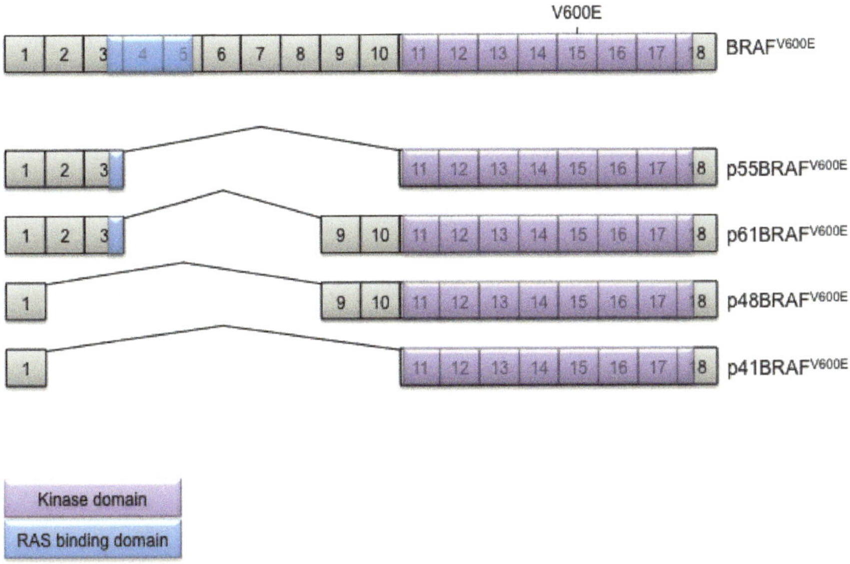

Figure 3. Aberrant splicing of BRAF^{V600E} confers RAF inhibitor resistance. Several in frame BRAF^{V600E} splice variants lacking the RAS binding domain have been detected in vemurafenib-resistant melanoma tumor specimens. The exon structure of full-length and spice variant forms of BRAF are shown. The location of the activating V600E mutation, the RAS binding and kinase domains are highlighted (adapted from [33]).

It is known that the amino terminus of BRAF negatively regulates its kinase activity by masking the carboxy-terminal catalytic domain. Upon binding to activated RAS, the amino-terminal regulatory domain of RAF proteins unfolds to expose the carboxy terminal sites that are required for dimerization and full kinase activity. The in-frame deletion in the p61BRAF^{V600E} variant leads to the constitutive dimerization of BRAF in the absence of activated RAS [34]. Dimerization of p61BRAF^{V600E} was shown to be critical for mediating BRAF-inhibitor resistance, as the R509H dimerization-deficient mutant form of p61BRAF^{V600E} was sensitive to vemurafenib and monomeric p61BRAF^{V600E} was inhibited by vemurafenib *in vitro*. Thus, it has been proposed that binding of vemurafenib to one p61BRAF^{V600E} protomer elicits an allosteric change in the other, drug-free protomer, thereby decreasing its affinity for the drug (Figure 4). Four independent BRAF splicing variants were also detected in tumors derived from six of nineteen patients with acquired resistance to vemurafenib (Figure 3). In each case, the alternative splice variants were in frame, lacked the RAS binding domain and were confined to the mutant allele [33]. This indicates that BRAF missplicing is likely due to a mutation or epigenetic change that specifically impacts the BRAF^{V600E} allele. Importantly, no splice BRAF variants were detected in 27 melanomas resected from vemurafenib-naive patients [33].

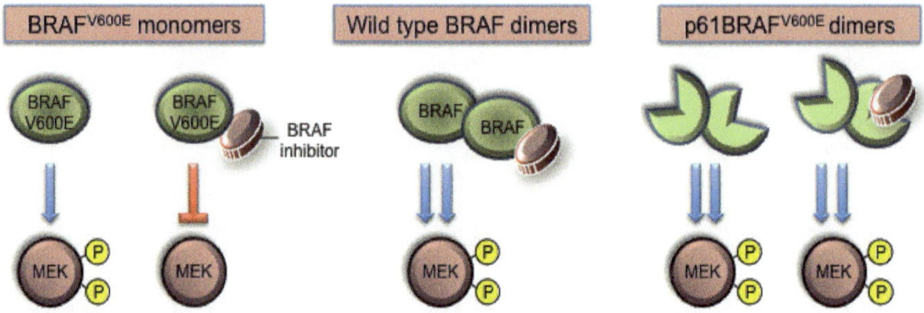

Figure 4. BRAF dimerization, RAF inhibitor binding and MAPK signalling. Mutant BRAF functions as a monomer and is effectively inhibited at low RAF inhibitor concentrations. In cells with activated RAS, the binding of RAS to RAF kinases promotes the homo- and heterodimerization (not shown) of wild type RAF proteins. In the presence of low BRAF inhibitor concentrations, one protomer of the RAF dimer binds inhibitor and this promotes the transactivation of the second, inhibitor-free RAF protomer. Thus in RAS-activated cells, BRAF inhibitor can induce the activation of RAF dimers and promote elevated MAPK signalling. Similarly, dimers of p61BRAF^{V600E} splicing variant are resistant to BRAF inhibition because binding of the drug to one protomer, allosterically alters the second protomer and diminishes its affinity for the RAF inhibitor. Much higher concentrations of RAF inhibitor are required to bind both protomers in a RAF dimer and inhibit ERK signalling.

5. N-RAS mutations

In the normal physiological setting, activated RAS signalling promotes the dimerization and activation of RAF proteins. In the presence of BRAF inhibitors and RAS signalling, the binding of drug to one molecule in a non-mutated RAF dimer can promote activation of the second RAF molecule (Figure 4). Thus, in the presence of RAS activation, the activity of homo- and heterodimeric RAF complexes can be paradoxically activated by RAF inhibitors [35-37].

In melanomas with BRAF^{V600E}, any alterations promoting RAF dimerization are predicted to confer resistance to RAF inhibitors. As expected, activating N-RAS mutations mediate resistance to vemurafenib [29] and dabrafenib [38]. Oncogenic N-RAS^{Q61K} was detected in a single vemurafenib-resistant clone derived from the M249 melanoma cells. This resistant subclone maintained ERK activation in the presence of vemurafenib, presumably via a kinase switch from BRAF to CRAF (Figure 1) [39, 40]. These cells were also sensitive to inhibition with the MEK inhibitor, AZD6244 in the presence or absence of vemurafenib, suggesting that in this cell clone oncogenic N-RAS confers resistance by principally engaging the MAPK cascade. Oncogenic N-RAS mutations were also detected in a patient with acquired resistance to vemurafenib; separate N-RAS mutations (Q61K and Q61R) were detected in two melanoma biopsies taken on initial progression and six months after initial progression. Both mutations were associated with copy-number amplification and N-RAS overexpression [29].

In a second study, oncogenic N-RAS^{Q61H} was detected in two of six dabrafenib resistant subclones, generated from the MelRMu cell line. In contrast to the initial report [29], these two N-RAS mutant, MelRMu sublines showed diminished sensitivity to MEK inhibitor, trametinib and to the combined inhibition of BRAF and MEK, when compared to the parental cells. Moreover, ectopic expression of N-RAS^{Q61K} in the MelRMu cells diminished the efficacy of combined MEK and BRAF inhibition [38]. A third report also identified N-RAS mutations (N-RAS^{Q61K} and N-RAS^{A146T}) in two melanoma sublines with acquired resistance to dabrafenib. These mutations were shown to confer dabrafenib resistance, and induced the heterodimerization of BRAF^{V600E} with C-RAF in the presence of drug [41]. These N-RAS mutant clones showed partial sensitivity to trametinib and to the concurrent inhibition of BRAF and MEK proteins [41]. It is known that mutant N-RAS can signal via multiple pathways including the PI3K/AKT/mTOR survival cascade [42] and consequently, N-RAS mutant dabrafenib-resistant melanoma cells were responsive to the simultaneous inhibition of MEK and the PI3K/mTOR pathway [41].

There are some discrepancies in the literature regarding the role of activated RAS in selectively sensitizing cancer cells to MEK inhibition. Certainly, N-RAS mutation status did not predict MEK inhibitor sensitivity in melanoma cell lines [43], and MEK inhibitors show only modest clinical activity in patients with RAS-mutant tumors [9, 44]. It seems likely that the impact of mutant N-RAS on MEK inhibitor responses reflects its expression and activity and ultimately the network of activated N-RAS-dependent effectors. This is in agreement with a recent report demonstrating that K-RAS^{13D}-mutant HCT116 colorectal cancer cells became resistant to MEK inhibition upon amplification of the driving K-RAS^{13D} oncogene [45].

6. CRAF overexpression

Increased expression of the CRAF kinase has also been associated with BRAF inhibitor resistance (Figure 2). Villanueva et al. (2010) observed increased CRAF protein levels in melanoma cells chronically treated with the BRAF inhibitor SB-590885. In this cell model MAPK signalling driven by persistent insulin growth factor receptor (IGF-1R) activity, was rewired to utilise both CRAF and ARAF (Figure 1), and the inhibition of all three RAF isoforms was required to inhibit the proliferation of these 885-resistant cells [46]. This is in contrast to melanoma sublines rendered resistant to the pan-RAF inhibitor AZ628. These AZ628-resistant cells showed elevated basal levels of CRAF protein, but the knockdown of CRAF alone strongly inhibited cell proliferation, in the absence of AZ628 treatment [47]. These cells switched from BRAF to CRAF dependence, and the precise mechanism of CRAF-mediated AZ628 resistance remains unclear, as this inhibitor strongly suppresses both BRAF^{V600E} and CRAF [48]. The role of CRAF in conferring RAF-inhibitor resistance may reflect the distinct genetic profiles of the melanoma cells used, the pathway rewiring involved in resistance, the mechanism of drug action and its impact on the RAF protein dimerization.

7. MEK mutations

Mutations in mitogen activated protein kinase, MEK1 have also been shown to confer resistance to MAPK inhibitors. A random mutagenesis screen of MEK1 revealed that mutations interfering with target-drug binding (e.g. I99T, G128D, L215P) and mutations that upregulate MEK1 intrinsic activity (e.g. Q56P, P124S) conferred resistance to the allosteric MEK inhibitor AZD6244 [49]. The G128D MEK1 mutation also conferred resistance to the BRAF inhibitor PLX4720 [50] (Figure 5).

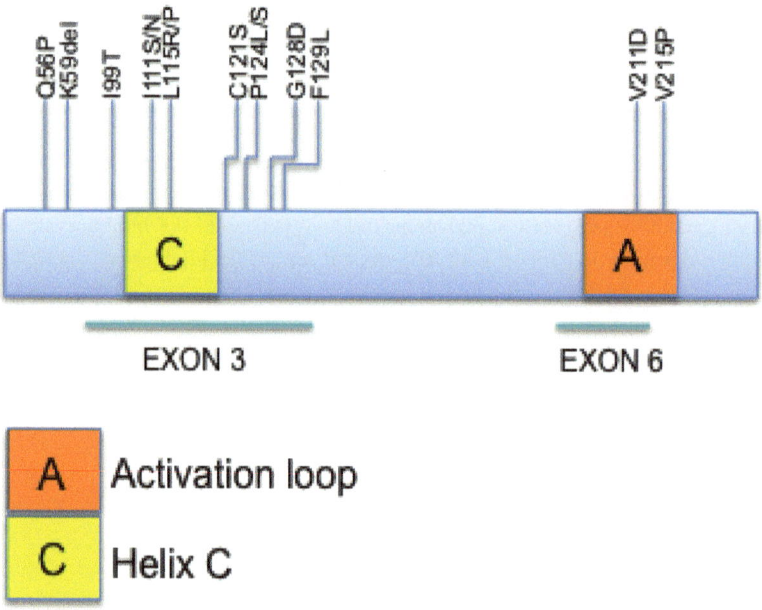

Figure 5. MEK1 mutations associated with MAPK inhibitor resistance. Allosteric MEK inhibitors binds to the MEK1 hydrophobic pocket that includes residues from helix C and the activation loop. Primary MEK1 mutations affect this drug-binding pocket (e.g. I99T, I111N/S, L115P/R, G128D, F129L, V211D and L215P) and can directly perturb the allosteric binding of the MEK inhibitor. Secondary MEK1 mutations reside outside the drug-binding region and include mutations near the amino terminus (e.g. Q56P) and proximal to the helix C (C121S, P124S/L). These secondary MEK1 mutations increase MEK1 kinase activity. The C121S and P124L MEK1 mutation have been detected in MEK inhibitor resistant patient tumors [50], whereas P124S and I111S MEK1 mutations were identified in pre-treatment melanomas [54]. Shi et al. found that of the P124S, I111S and C121S, only C121S conferred vemurafenib resistance in melanoma cells.

Deep sequencing of tumors from five patients progressing on AZD6244 treatment, identified the $MEK1^{P124L}$ mutation in the progressing, but not pre-treatment tumor sample from one patient. The existence of this MEK1 mutation was independently verified in *ex vivo* cell lines established from tumor material, and its activity in conferring MEK- and BRAF-inhibitor resistance validated in transfected melanoma cells. As with BRAF truncation and amplification, alterations in MEK1 protein did not alter the sensitivity of melanoma cells to the combined inhibition of BRAF and MEK inhibitors. A $MEK1^{C121S}$ mutation was detected via mutational profiling in a melanoma sample from a patient with acquired resistance to vemurafenib. This mutation was not detected in the pre-treatment biopsy, showed increased intrinsic kinase activity and conferred resistance to BRAF and MEK inhibition *in vitro* [50]. BRAFi-resistant YUSIT1 melanoma cells also acquired a MEK1 mutation with increased kinase activity (K59del). These cells were dependent on MEK1 for proliferation and displayed higher ERK phosphorylation following treatment with dabrafenib [41].

Resistance to the allosteric MEK inhibitor PD0325901 in breast and colorectal cancer cell lines was also consistently associated with MEK mutations in the allosteric binding domain. MEK-inhibitor resistant sublines derived from the MDA-MB-231 breast and HCT-116 colon cancer cells gained the $MEK1^{L115P}$ and $MEK1^{F129L}$ mutations, respectively and the MEK-inhibitor resistant LoVo colorectal cells acquired a $MEK2^{V215E}$ mutation (homologous to V211D mutations in MEK1) (Figure 5). The L115P and V211D mutations abrogated MEK inhibitor binding, while F129L increased the intrinsic activity of MEK and showed enhanced interaction with CRAF [51, 52]. Cell lines expressing mutant $MEK1^{K57N}$, which was identified in two lung adenocarcinomas, also showed decreased sensitivity to MEK inhibition [53].

A recent study found that MEK1 mutations identified in resistant melanoma lesions might not predict BRAF-inhibitor sensitivity. Shi *et al* found that five of 31 melanomas excised pre-BRAF inhibitor treatment carried concurrent somatic BRAF and MEK1 ($MEK1^{P124S}$ and MEK^{I111S}) activating mutations and that three of these five patients showed objective tumor responses. When the P124S, I111S and C121S MEK1 mutants were stably introduced into a series of melanoma cell lines, only the $MEK1^{C121S}$ mutant restored p-ERK levels in the presence of vemurafenib, even though all mutants showed intrinsically enhanced kinase activity [54] (Figure 5). Thus, the relative impact of MEK1 mutations may vary depending on the type of mutation, tumor genetic background and the dependence on BRAF. For instance, YUSIT1 cells were dependent on the $MEK1^{K59del}$ for proliferation, and the $MEK1^{F129L}$ mutant may induce a BRAF to CRAF kinase switch [41, 51]. Finally, a more detailed tumor profile, correlating tumor response with the relative proportion of double-BRAF/MEK1 mutant cells within metastases, will help clarify the precise role of MEK1 in mediating BRAF-inhibitor resistance.

8. COT overexpression

A recent gain of function screen tested the activity of 597 kinases (75% of the annotated human kinases) in conferring vemurafenib resistance in the A375 melanoma cell line. Nine candidates, including receptor tyrosine kinases (Axl, ERBB2), conferred significant resistance with the mitogen activated protein kinase kinase kinase 8 (the gene encoding COT/Tpl2) emerging as the top candidate. Overexpression of COT resulted in constitutive ERK activation in the presence of vemurafenib (Figure 2). COT activated ERK via MEK-dependent and

-independent mechanisms and ectopic COT expression conferred decreased sensitivity to the MEK inhibitors CI-1040 and AZD6244. COT expression was also elevated in two of three patient samples obtained early in the course of treatment and further increased in a relapsing specimen relative to its pre-treatment and on-treatment controls. Considering that inhibition of $BRAF^{V600E}$ increases COT expression, it is possible that COT accumulation may reflect secondary responses to BRAF inhibition and resistance. Nevertheless, the silencing and inhibition of COT in the RPMI-7951 melanoma cells, which express increased COT, decreased ERK phosphorylation and suppressed cell viability [55].

9. Activation of receptor tyrosine kinases

An emerging theme in BRAF inhibitor resistance is the upregulation and activation of receptor tyrosine kinases. Garraway and co-workers demonstrated that ectopically expressed receptor tyrosine kinases Axl and ERBB2, circumvented vemurafenib activity [55], and two independent reports detected increased expression and activity of the platelet derived growth factor (PDGFRß) and IGF-1R in vemurafenib-resistant melanoma sublines [29, 46] (Figure 2). Vemurafenib-resistant tumor biopsies derived from patients also showed overexpression of PDGFRß (4 of 11 patients) and IGF-1R (2 of 5 patients) compared to the corresponding pre-treatment tumor specimens [29, 46]. The knockdown or inhibition of PDGFRß and IGF-1R overcame vemurafenib resistance in cell lines, but resistance was not due to activation of ERK alone [29, 46]. Instead, receptor tyrosine kinase-upregulated, vemurafenib resistant melanoma cell lines, showed phosphorylation of both ERK and PI3K/AKT (Figure 2), and the concurrent and sustained inhibition of the MAPK and PI3K/AKT/mTOR pathways was required to overcome PDGFRß- and IGF-1R-mediated vemurafenib resistance [46, 56]. The upregulation and activation of these receptors was not due to gene amplification or genetic alterations within the coding sequence [29, 46].

These studies predict that RTK activation via increased autocrine tumor cell ligand secretion, or paracrine ligand production from stromal cells may confer resistance to MAPK inhibition. A recent report found increased activation of the fibroblast growth factor (FGF) receptor 3 was associated with elevated levels of autocrine secreted FGF2 ligand in vemurafenib resistant melanoma sublines [57]. Moreover the secretion of growth factors from co-cultured fibroblast cells conferred vemurafenib resistance to BRAF-mutant melanoma cell lines. Stromal cell secretion of the hepatocyte growth factor (HGF) correlated best with vemurafenib resistance in this cell screen, and HGF was detected in tumor-associated stromal cells in 23 of 34 melanoma tumors resected from patients prior to MAPK inhibitor treatment. Critically, these 23 patients also showed activation of the HGF receptor MET in their tumor biopsies, and had a poorer response to MAPK-inhibitor treatment compared to patients whose stromal cells lacked HGF expression [58]. Increased plasma HGF levels in 126 metastatic melanoma patients, prior to treatment with vemurafenib, was also associated with a reduction in the progression-free and overall survival rates [59]. The stromal cell secretion of HGF resulted in reactivation of the MAPK and PI3K/mTOR signalling pathways and immediate (innate) resistance to RAF inhibition. Whether activation of MET also has a role in acquired resistance to RAF inhibitors remains to be determined, but activating somatic MET mutations and amplifications have been detected in human cancers [60-62]. Regardless, of the mechanism of MET activation, the sensitivity of MET-activated melanoma cells can be restored by the simultaneous inhibition of RAF and either HGF or MET [58]. Finally, it is worth noting that although activation of PDGFRß and IGF-1R are associated with vemurafenib resistance [29, 46], the ligand activation of these two receptors appears insufficient to drive sustained pathway activation or vemurafenib resistance [58, 59].

10. Other regulators of response to MAPK inhibitors

Typically, the suppression of MAPK signalling promotes cell cycle arrest that is associated with increased expression of the CDK inhibitor $p27^{Kip1}$ and inhibition of cyclin D1 expression (Figure 1). Cyclin D1 is a regulator of the cyclin dependent kinases (CDKs) 4 and 6 and the formation of binary cyclin D-CDK4/6 complexes promote the phosphorylation of the retinoblastoma protein (pRb) and cell cycle progression [63-65]. Cyclin D1 is commonly amplified in melanoma and often in conjunction with mutated BRAF [66, 67]. The clinical significance of this genotype was demonstrated in BRAF-mutant melanoma cell lines with increased cyclin D1 protein expression. These cells showed intrinsic resistance to the growth-arresting effects of the RAF inhibitor, SB590885 and the ectopic expression of cyclin D1 conferred RAF-inhibitor resistance, which was enhanced by the dual overexpression of CDK4 and cyclin D1 [67]. These data confirm that the MAPK-independent expression of critical MAPK downstream targets will regulate RAF-inhibitor response and may diminish the dependence of cells to oncogenic BRAF.

Several independent studies have shown that loss of the phosphatase and tensin homolog (PTEN) tumor suppressor, which occurs in over 10% of melanoma tumors, is predictive of attenuated RAF-inhibitor mediated cytotoxicity [68, 69]. Cells lacking PTEN remain dependent on MAPK for proliferation but utilise increased AKT signalling for survival (Figure 2). Elevated AKT promotes the nuclear exclusion of the FOXO3a transcription factor, which leads to the downstream suppression of the FOXO3a pro-apoptotic target BIM [69, 70]. Predictably, ectopic expression of activated AKT3 also prevented BRAF inhibitor induced BIM and apoptosis [71] and MEK inhibitor-sensitive cancer cell lines show significantly higher FOXO3a and BIM protein levels compared to resistant cell lines [70]. Similar to RTK-induced resistance, the simultaneous inhibition of the MAPK and AKT pathways is required to restore PTEN-null cell sensitivity to MAPK inhibitors [68]. Finally, homozygous PTEN loss and increased pAKT levels were associated with vemurafenib resistance in a progressing biopsy derived from a single patient [46].

Considering the independent roles of cyclin D and PTEN in diminishing dependence on MAPK signalling and engaging the AKT survival cascade, it is anticipated that the concurrent alteration of these cell cycle regulators would confer increased levels of resistance to MAPK inhibitors. In a recent study, vemurafenib was shown to have purely cytostatic effects in melanoma cells with either PTEN or pRb loss; pRb deleted cells should behave as cells with elevated cyclinD1/CDK4 overexpression. $BRAF^{V600E}$ cells with concurrent loss of both pRb and PTEN were completely resistant to RAF inhibition, and these cells continued proliferating in the presence of this RAF inhibitor [68]. The clinical significance of pRb loss in conferring MAPK inhibitor resistance is uncertain, however, as pRb loss is uncommon in melanoma [72].

Finally, activation of the STAT3 pathway was found to be associated with AZD6244 resistance in a panel of lung cancer cell lines. STAT3 activity was shown to decrease BIM accumulation through the upregulation of miR-17, and the inhibition of STAT3 or miR-17 upregulated BIM and sensitized resistant cells to MEK inhibition [73].

11. Therapies to overcome MAPK inhibitor resistance

Irrespective of the precise mechanisms of resistance to class I RAF inhibitors, tumors that acquire resistance or are inherently insensitive to these inhibitors often maintain some dependency on the MAPK pathway [29, 33, 38, 55, 57, 74]. These data suggest that further inhibition of the MAPK cascade at the downstream MEK or ERK nodes may be effective in treating resistance to single agent BRAF inhibitors. Despite the preclinical evidence of MEK-inhibitor sensitivity in cells with acquired resistance to BRAF inhibitors [38], clinical trials applying this strategy have been disappointing. The MEK inhibitor trametinib showed minimal activity (response rates of 3%) in patients previously treated with a BRAF inhibitor [75]. Clinical benefit was observed, however, when patients who progressed on prior BRAF inhibitor were treated with a combination of BRAF and MEK inhibitors. Partial responses were observed in 17% of patients, suggesting that dual MAPK blockade can abrogate some BRAF inhibitor resistance mechanisms [76]. The triaging of patients, based on BRAF inhibitor resistance drivers, may also improve the clinical benefit of second line MAPK inhibitor therapies. For instance, melanoma cells expressing BRAF splice variants are sensitive to MEK inhibition [33], whereas cells with BRAF copy number gains respond to the concurrent inhibition of BRAF and MEK [30, 31]. Finally, specific inhibitors of ERK have recently become available, and these show anti-proliferative activity in MEK-inhibitor resistant cells and synergise with MEK inhibitors to prevent or delay the emergence of acquired resistance [52].

Sustained and significant responses have also been observed when RAF-inhibitor resistant cell lines are treated with combination MAPK and PI3K/mTOR inhibitors. For instance, in RTK-expressing vemurafenib-resistant cells, inhibition of PI3K/mTOR activity in combination with vemurafenib showed potent synergy. Compensatory signalling via MEK permitted survival in the presence of PI3K/mTOR/MAPK inhibition, but cytotoxicity was restored using a combination of MEK inhibitor with the dual PI3K/mTOR inhibitor BEZ235 [56]. A number of combinations of MEK and PI3K/mTOR pathway inhibitors combinations have entered early phase clinical trials, however their benefit in the setting of BRAF/MEK inhibitor resistance remains untested.

Many of the proteins involved in melanoma development and RAF-inhibitor resistance are targets of the heat shock protein (Hsp)-90 family of chaperones. Hsp90 proteins regulate the conformation, stability and function of many RTKs and kinases, including IGF-1R, BRAF, CRAF, CDK4, AKT and cyclin D1 [77, 78]. The pharmacological inhibition of Hsp90 using the selective inhibitor, XL888 abrogated acquired and intrinsic vemurafenib resistance. XL888 induced apoptosis in melanoma cells with mutant N-RAS, elevated PDGFRß, COT, IGF-1R, CRAF and cyclin D1. Apoptosis was associated with diminished accumulation of the resistance driver, nuclear accumulation of FOXO3a and an increase in BIM expression. Moreover, Hsp90 inhibition was a more effective apoptotic inducer when combined with MEK and PI3K inhibition [79]. Hsp90 inhibitors have shown promising results in ERBB2-amplified breast cancers [80], but lacked clinical activity in vemurafenib-naive melanoma patients [81]. Evaluation of pre- and post treatment melanoma biopsies confirmed incomplete degradation of $BRAF^{V600E}$, when the inhibitor was given on a weekly schedule. Whether Hsp90 inhibition will prove effective when administered more frequently, in RAF-inhibitor resistant melanoma patients, or in combination with MAPK inhibitors remains to be tested.

12. Conclusions

BRAF-targeted therapy has recently emerged as the standard treatment for patients with BRAF-mutant melanoma. Responses are not durable, however and studies of acquired resistance to BRAF inhibition reveal a diversity of resistance mechanism but a common resistance theme. Melanoma cells adapt by re-engaging MAPK signalling and activating parallel survival networks. The management and prevention of BRAF inhibitor resistance is likely to be achieved through combination therapies. The combination of BRAF and MEK inhibitors has shown better response than single agent therapy [25] and is currently being evaluated in phase III clinical trials compared to vemurafenib (NCT01597908) or dabrafenib (NCT01584648) in treatment naive patients with $BRAF^{V600E}$ mutant melanoma. Trials combining MEK with AKT inhibitors (NCT01021748), the pan-RAF inhibitor sorafenib and MEK inhibition (NCT0034999206), testing HDAC inhibition with vorinostat (NCT006670820) are also under way. Further, Phase I trials for inhibition of PDGFRβ, FGFR and other tyrosine kinases using Dovitinib in patients with advanced melanoma has shown promising results [82]. Finally, rechallenging patients with selective BRAF inhibitors after a treatment-free interval provided clinical benefit to two patients who had previously progressed on MAPK inhibitors [83]. Additional studies are required to determine the significance of rechallenging patients after treatment interruption.

It has been suggested that a detailed catalogue of resistance mechanism in an individual's tumor should inform effective second line therapy [84]. This strategy may not prove sufficient, as it does not account for stromal-mediated resistance drivers, the heterogeneous nature of melanoma and the fact that melanoma tumors from a single patient may develop multiple mechanisms of resistance. For instance, two independent vemurafenib-resistant nodal metastases derived from a single patient, harboured distinct N-RAS activating mutations

[29] and intra-tumoral heterogeneity has been observed in a progressing BRAF-mutant melanoma metastases from patients treated with BRAF inhibitors [85, 86].

Nevertheless, defining the mechanisms of RAF-inhibitor resistance is a critical step in understanding the signalling pathways required to circumvent therapy. At present, up to 40% of RAF-inhibitor resistant melanomas have undefined resistance drivers, and the role of MAPK and PI3K signalling needs to be assessed in this subgroup. The fact that half of all melanoma patients have wild type BRAF melanoma, further highlights the need for an integrated preclinical and clinical approach to guide rational design of effective initial and second-line treatment options.

Acknowledgements

This work is supported by Program Grant 633004 and project grants of the National Health and Medical Research Council of Australia (NHMRC) and an infrastructure grant to Westmead Millennium Institute by the Health Department of NSW through Sydney West Area Health Service. HR is a recipient of a Cancer Institute New South Wales, Research Fellowship and a NHMRC Senior Research Fellowship. MSC is supported by a Rotary Health Australia scholarship

Author details

Kavitha Gowrishankar, Matteo S. Carlino and Helen Rizos

*Address all correspondence to: helen.rizos@sydney.edu.au

Westmead Institute for Cancer Research, University of Sydney at Westmead Millennium Institute and Melanoma Institute Australia, Westmead Hospital, Westmead, Australia

References

[1] Jemal A, Siegel R, Xu J, Ward E. Cancer statistics, 2010. CA Cancer J Clin. 2010;60(5): 277-300.

[2] Cummins DL, Cummins JM, Pantle H, Silverman MA, Leonard AL, Chanmugam A. Cutaneous malignant melanoma. Mayo Clin Proc. 2006;81(4):500-7.

[3] Balch CM, Gershenwald JE, Soong SJ, Thompson JF, Atkins MB, Byrd DR, et al. Final version of 2009 AJCC melanoma staging and classification. J Clin Oncol. 2009;27(36): 6199-206..

[4] Thompson JF, Scolyer RA, Kefford RF. Cutaneous melanoma. Lancet. 2005;365:687-701.

[5] Davies H, Bignell GR, Cox C, Stephens P, Edkins S, Clegg S, et al. Mutations of the BRAF gene in human cancer. Nature. 2002;417(6892):949-54.

[6] Lee JH, Choi JW, Kim YS. Frequencies of BRAF and NRAS mutations are different in histological types and sites of origin of cutaneous melanoma: a meta-analysis. Br J Dermatol. 2011;164(4):776-84.

[7] Wan PT, Garnett MJ, Roe SM, Lee S, Niculescu-Duvaz D, Good VM, et al. Mechanism of activation of the RAF-ERK signaling pathway by oncogenic mutations of B-RAF. Cell. 2004;116(6):855-67.

[8] Flaherty KT, Puzanov I, Kim KB, Ribas A, McArthur GA, Sosman JA, et al. Inhibition of mutated, activated BRAF in metastatic melanoma. N Engl J Med. 2010;363(9): 809-19.

[9] Falchook GS, Lewis KD, Infante JR, Gordon MS, Vogelzang NJ, Demarini DJ, et al. Activity of the oral MEK inhibitor trametinib in patients with advanced melanoma: a phase 1 dose-escalation trial. Lancet Oncol. 2012;13(8):782-9.

[10] Hauschild A, Grob JJ, Demidov LV, Jouary T, Gutzmer R, Millward M, et al. Dabrafenib in BRAF-mutated metastatic melanoma: a multicentre, open-label, phase 3 randomised controlled trial. Lancet. 2012;380(9839):358-65.

[11] Chapman PB, Hauschild A, Robert C, Haanen JB, Ascierto P, Larkin J, et al. Improved Survival with Vemurafenib in Melanoma with BRAF V600E Mutation. N Engl J Med. 2011;364:2507-16.

[12] Sosman JA, Kim KB, Schuchter L, Gonzalez R, Pavlick AC, Weber JS, et al. Survival in BRAF V600-mutant advanced melanoma treated with vemurafenib. N Engl J Med. 2012;366(8):707-14.

[13] Long GV, Trefzer U, Davies MA, Kefford RF, Ascierto PA, Chapman PB, et al. Dabrafenib in patients with Val600Glu or Val600Lys BRAF-mutant melanoma metastatic to the brain (BREAK-MB): a multicentre, open-label, phase 2 trial. Lancet Oncol. 2012 (in press).

[14] Dummer R, Rinderknecht J, Goldinger S, Wagner I, Mitchell L, Veronese M, et al. An open-label pilot study of vemurafenib in previously treated metastatic melanoma patients with brain metastases. J Clin Oncol. 2011;29:(suppl; abstr 8548).

[15] Falchook GS, Long GV, Kurzrock R, Kim KB, Arkenau TH, Brown MP, et al. Dabrafenib in patients with melanoma, untreated brain metastases, and other solid tumours: a phase 1 dose-escalation trial. Lancet. 2012;379:1893-901.

[16] Platz A, Egyhazi S, Ringborg U, Hansson J. Human cutaneous melanoma; a review of NRAS and BRAF mutation frequencies in relation to histogenetic subclass and body site. Mol Oncol. 2008;1(4):395-405.

[17] Curtin JA, Busam K, Pinkel D, Bastian BC. Somatic activation of KIT in distinct subtypes of melanoma. Journal of clinical oncology : official journal of the American Society of Clinical Oncology. 2006;24(26):4340-6.

[18] Krauthammer M, Kong Y, Ha BH, Evans P, Bacchiocchi A, McCusker JP, et al. Exome sequencing identifies recurrent somatic RAC1 mutations in melanoma. Nat Genet. 2012;29(10).

[19] Pollock PM, Harper UL, Hansen KS, Yudt LM, Stark M, Robbins CM, et al. High frequency of BRAF mutations in nevi. Nat Genet. 2003;33(1):19-20.

[20] Hingorani SR, Jacobetz MA, Robertson GP, Herlyn M, Tuveson DA. Suppression of BRAF(V599E) in human melanoma abrogates transformation. Cancer Res. 2003;63:5198-202.

[21] Karasarides M, Chiloeches A, Hayward R, Niculescu-Duvaz D, Scanlon I, Friedlos F, et al. B-RAF is a therapeutic target in melanoma. Oncogene. 2004;23(37):6292-8.

[22] Hoeflich KP, Gray DC, Eby MT, Tien JY, Wong L, Bower J, et al. Oncogenic BRAF is required for tumor growth and maintenance in melanoma models. Cancer Res. 2006;66(2):999-1006.

[23] Sumimoto H, Miyagishi M, Miyoshi H, Yamagata S, Shimizu A, Taira K, et al. Inhibition of growth and invasive ability of melanoma by inactivation of mutated BRAF with lentivirus-mediated RNA interference. Oncogene. 2004;23(36):6031-9.

[24] Flaherty KT, Robert C, Hersey P, Nathan P, Garbe C, Milhem M, et al. Improved survival with MEK inhibition in BRAF-mutated melanoma. N Engl J Med. 2012;367(2): 107-14.

[25] Flaherty KT, Infante JR, Daud A, Gonzalez R, Kefford RF, Sosman J, et al. Combined BRAF and MEK Inhibition in Melanoma with BRAF V600 Mutations. N Engl J Med. 2012 (in press)

[26] Kefford R, Arkenau H-T, Brown MP, Millward M, Infante J, Long G, et al., editors. Selective inhibition of oncogenic BRAF V600E/K/D by GSK2118436: Evidence of clinical activity in subjects with metastatic melanoma. 7th International Melanoma Research Congress; 2010; Sydney, Australia.

[27] Ellis LM, Hicklin DJ. Resistance to Targeted Therapies: Refining Anticancer Therapy in the Era of Molecular Oncology. Clin Cancer Res. 2009;15(24):7471-8.

[28] Bixby D, Talpaz M. Seeking the causes and solutions to imatinib-resistance in chronic myeloid leukemia. Leukemia. 2011;25(1):7-22.

[29] Nazarian R, Shi H, Wang Q, Kong X, Koya RC, Lee H, et al. Melanomas acquire resistance to B-RAF(V600E) inhibition by RTK or N-RAS upregulation. Nature. 2010;468(7326):973-7.

[30] Shi H, Moriceau G, Kong X, Lee MK, Lee H, Koya RC, et al. Melanoma whole-exome sequencing identifies (V600E)B-RAF amplification-mediated acquired B-RAF inhibitor resistance. Nat Commun. 2012;3(724):724.

[31] Corcoran RB, Dias-Santagata D, Bergethon K, Iafrate AJ, Settleman J, Engelman JA. BRAF Gene Amplification Can Promote Acquired Resistance to MEK Inhibitors in Cancer Cells Harboring the BRAF V600E Mutation. Sci Signal. 2010;3(149):ra84.

[32] Diaz LA, Jr., Williams RT, Wu J, Kinde I, Hecht JR, Berlin J, et al. The molecular evolution of acquired resistance to targeted EGFR blockade in colorectal cancers. Nature. 2012;486(7404):537-40.

[33] Poulikakos PI, Persaud Y, Janakiraman M, Kong X, Ng C, Moriceau G, et al. RAF inhibitor resistance is mediated by dimerization of aberrantly spliced BRAF(V600E). Nature. 2011;480:387-90.

[34] Weber CK, Slupsky JR, Kalmes HA, Rapp UR. Active Ras induces heterodimerization of cRaf and BRaf. Cancer Res. 2001;61(9):3595-8.

[35] Heidorn SJ, Milagre C, Whittaker S, Nourry A, Niculescu-Duvas I, Dhomen N, et al. Kinase-dead BRAF and oncogenic RAS cooperate to drive tumor progression through CRAF. Cell. 2010;140(2):209-21.

[36] Poulikakos PI, Zhang C, Bollag G, Shokat KM, Rosen N. RAF inhibitors transactivate RAF dimers and ERK signalling in cells with wild-type BRAF. Nature. 2010;464(7287):427-30.

[37] Hatzivassiliou G, Song K, Yen I, Brandhuber BJ, Anderson DJ, Alvarado R, et al. RAF inhibitors prime wild-type RAF to activate the MAPK pathway and enhance growth. Nature. 2010;464(7287):431-5.

[38] Gowrishankar K, Snoyman S, Pupo GM, Becker TM, Kefford RF, Rizos H. Acquired Resistance to BRAF Inhibition Can Confer Cross-Resistance to Combined BRAF/MEK Inhibition. J Invest Dermatol. 2012;132(7):1850-9.

[39] Dumaz N, Hayward R, Martin J, Ogilvie L, Hedley D, Curtin JA, et al. In melanoma, RAS mutations are accompanied by switching signaling from BRAF to CRAF and disrupted cyclic AMP signaling. Cancer Res. 2006;66(19):9483-91.

[40] Jaiswal BS, Janakiraman V, Kljavin NM, Eastham-Anderson J, Cupp JE, Liang Y, et al. Combined targeting of BRAF and CRAF or BRAF and PI3K effector pathways is required for efficacy in NRAS mutant tumors. PLoS ONE. 2009;4(5):e5717.

[41] Greger J, Eastman S, Zhang V, Bleam MR, Hughes A, Smitheman KN, et al. Combinations of BRAF, MEK, and PI3K/mTOR inhibitors overcome acquired resistance to the BRAF inhibitor GSK2118436 dabrafenib, mediated by NRAS or MEK mutations. Mol Cancer Ther. 2012;11(4):909-20.

[42] Smalley KS. Understanding melanoma signaling networks as the basis for molecular targeted therapy. J Invest Dermatol. 2010;130(1):28-37.

[43] Solit DB, Garraway LA, Pratilas CA, Sawai A, Getz G, Basso A, et al. BRAF mutation predicts sensitivity to MEK inhibition. Nature. 2006;439(7074):358-62.

[44] Nissan MH, Solit DB. The "SWOT" of BRAF Inhibition in Melanoma: RAF Inhibitors, MEK Inhibitors or Both? Curr Oncol Rep. 2011;13(6):479-87.

[45] Little AS, Balmanno K, Sale MJ, Newman S, Dry JR, Hampson M, et al. Amplification of the Driving Oncogene, KRAS or BRAF, Underpins Acquired Resistance to MEK1/2 Inhibitors in Colorectal Cancer Cells. Sci Signal. 2011;4(166):ra17.

[46] Villanueva J, Vultur A, Lee JT, Somasundaram R, Fukunaga-Kalabis M, Cipolla AK, et al. Acquired resistance to BRAF inhibitors mediated by a RAF kinase switch in melanoma can be overcome by cotargeting MEK and IGF-1R/PI3K. Cancer Cell. 2010;18(6):683-95.

[47] Montagut C, Sharma SV, Shioda T, McDermott U, Ulman M, Ulkus LE, et al. Elevated CRAF as a potential mechanism of acquired resistance to BRAF inhibition in melanoma. Cancer Res. 2008;68(12):4853-61.

[48] Shen M, Wu A, Aquila B, Lyne P, Drew L, editors. Linking molecular characteristics to the pharmacological response of a panel of cancer cell lines to the BRAF inhibitor, AZ628. AACR 98th Meeting; 2007 June 9, 2011; Los Angeles.

[49] Emery CM, Vijayendran KG, Zipser MC, Sawyer AM, Niu L, Kim JJ, et al. MEK1 mutations confer resistance to MEK and B-RAF inhibition. Proc Natl Acad Sci U S A. 2009;106(48):20411-6.

[50] Wagle N, Emery C, Berger MF, Davis MJ, Sawyer A, Pochanard P, et al. Dissecting Therapeutic Resistance to RAF Inhibition in Melanoma by Tumor Genomic Profiling. J Clin Oncol. 2011;29(22):3085-96.

[51] Wang H, Daouti S, Li WH, Wen Y, Rizzo C, Higgins B, et al. Identification of the MEK1(F129L) activating mutation as a potential mechanism of acquired resistance to MEK inhibition in human cancers carrying the B-RafV600E mutation. Cancer Res. 2011;71(16):5535-45.

[52] Hatzivassiliou G, Liu B, O'Brien C, Spoerke JM, Hoeflich KP, Haverty PM, et al. ERK inhibition overcomes acquired resistance to MEK inhibitors. Mol Cancer Ther. 2012;11(5):1143-54.

[53] Marks JL, Gong Y, Chitale D, Golas B, McLellan MD, Kasai Y, et al. Novel MEK1 mutation identified by mutational analysis of epidermal growth factor receptor signaling pathway genes in lung adenocarcinoma. Cancer Res. 2008;68(14):5524-8.

[54] Shi H, Moriceau G, Kong X, Koya RC, Nazarian R, Pupo GM, et al. Preexisting MEK1 Exon 3 Mutations in V600E/KBRAF Melanomas Do Not Confer Resistance to BRAF Inhibitors. Cancer Discov. 2012;2(5):414-24.

[55] Johannessen CM, Boehm JS, Kim SY, Thomas SR, Wardwell L, Johnson LA, et al. COT drives resistance to RAF inhibition through MAP kinase pathway reactivation. Nature. 2010;468:968-72.

[56] Shi H, Kong X, Ribas A, Lo RS. Combinatorial treatments that overcome PDGFRbeta-driven resistance of melanoma cells to V600EB-RAF inhibition. Cancer Res. 2011;71(15):5067-74.

[57] Yadav V, Zhang X, Liu J, Estrem S, Li S, Gong XQ, et al. Reactivation of Mitogen-Activated Protein Kinase (MAPK) Pathway by FGF Receptor 3 (FGFR3)/Ras Mediates Resistance to Vemurafenib in Human B-RAF V600E Mutant Melanoma. J Biol Chem. 2012;287(33):28087-98.

[58] Straussman R, Morikawa T, Shee K, Barzily-Rokni M, Qian ZR, Du J, et al. Tumour micro-environment elicits innate resistance to RAF inhibitors through HGF secretion. Nature. 2012;487(7408):500-4.

[59] Wilson TR, Fridlyand J, Yan Y, Penuel E, Burton L, Chan E, et al. Widespread potential for growth-factor-driven resistance to anticancer kinase inhibitors. Nature. 2012 Jul 4;487(7408):505-9.

[60] Puri N, Ahmed S, Janamanchi V, Tretiakova M, Zumba O, Krausz T, et al. c-Met is a potentially new therapeutic target for treatment of human melanoma. Clin Cancer Res. 2007;13(7):2246-53.

[61] Lorenzato A, Olivero M, Patane S, Rosso E, Oliaro A, Comoglio PM, et al. Novel somatic mutations of the MET oncogene in human carcinoma metastases activating cell motility and invasion. Cancer Res. 2002;62(23):7025-30.

[62] Engelman JA, Zejnullahu K, Mitsudomi T, Song Y, Hyland C, Park JO, et al. MET amplification leads to gefitinib resistance in lung cancer by activating ERBB3 signaling. Science. 2007;316(5827):1039-43.

[63] Sherr CJ, Roberts JM. CDK inhibitors: positive and negative regulators of G1-phase progression. Genes Dev. 1999;13(12):1501-12.

[64] Lavoie JN, L'Allemain G, Brunet A, Muller R, Pouyssegur J. Cyclin D1 expression is regulated positively by the p42/p44MAPK and negatively by the p38/HOGMAPK pathway. J Biol Chem. 1996;271(34):20608-16.

[65] Donovan JC, Milic A, Slingerland JM. Constitutive MEK/MAPK activation leads to p27(Kip1) deregulation and antiestrogen resistance in human breast cancer cells. J Biol Chem. 2001;276(44):40888-95.

[66] Lazar V, Ecsedi S, Szollosi AG, Toth R, Vizkeleti L, Rakosy Z, et al. Characterization of candidate gene copy number alterations in the 11q13 region along with BRAF and NRAS mutations in human melanoma. Mod Pathol. 2009;22(10):1367-78.

[67] Smalley KS, Lioni M, Dalla Palma M, Xiao M, Desai B, Egyhazi S, et al. Increased cyclin D1 expression can mediate BRAF inhibitor resistance in BRAF V600E-mutated melanomas. Mol Cancer Ther. 2008;7(9):2876-83.

[68] Xing F, Persaud Y, Pratilas CA, Taylor BS, Janakiraman M, She QB, et al. Concurrent loss of the PTEN and RB1 tumor suppressors attenuates RAF dependence in melanomas harboring (V600E)BRAF. Oncogene. 2012;31(4):446-57.

[69] Paraiso KH, Xiang Y, Rebecca VW, Abel EV, Chen A, Munko AC, et al. PTEN loss confers BRAF inhibitor resistance to melanoma cells through the suppression of BIM expression. Cancer Res. 2011;71:2750-60.

[70] Yang JY, Chang CJ, Xia W, Wang Y, Wong KK, Engelman JA, et al. Activation of FOXO3a is sufficient to reverse mitogen-activated protein/extracellular signal-regulated kinase kinase inhibitor chemoresistance in human cancer. Cancer Res. 2010;70(11):4709-18.

[71] Shao Y, Aplin AE. Akt3-mediated resistance to apoptosis in B-RAF-targeted melanoma cells. Cancer Res. 2010;70(16):6670-81.

[72] Saenz-Santamaria MC, McNutt NS, Shea CR. Immunohistochemical expression of retinoblastoma protein in cutaneous melanomas. Br J Dermatol. 1995;133(6):890-5.

[73] Dai B, Meng J, Peyton M, Girard L, Bornmann WG, Ji L, et al. STAT3 mediates resistance to MEK inhibitor through microRNA miR-17. Cancer Res. 2011;71(10):3658-68.

[74] Paraiso KH, Fedorenko IV, Cantini LP, Munko AC, Hall M, Sondak VK, et al. Recovery of phospho-ERK activity allows melanoma cells to escape from BRAF inhibitor therapy. Br J Cancer. 2010;102(12):1724-30.

[75] Kim KB, Lewis K, Pavlick AC, Infante JR, Ribas A, Sosman JA, et al., editors. A phase II study of the MEK1/MEK2 inhibitor GSK1120212 in metastatic BRAF-V600E or K mutant cutaneous melanoma patients previously treated with or without a BRAF inhibitor. International Melanoma Congress; 2011; Tampa, Florida, USA: Pigment Cell Res.

[76] Flaherty K, Infante JR, Falchook G, Weber JD, Daud A, Hamid O, et al., editors. Phase I/II expansion cohort of BRAF inhibitor GSK2118436 + MEK inhibitor GSK1120212 in patients with BRAF mutant metastatic melanoma who progressed on a prior BRAF inhibitor. International Melanoma Congress; 2011; Tampa, Florida, USA: Pigment Cell Res.

[77] Den RB, Lu B. Heat shock protein 90 inhibition: rationale and clinical potential. Ther Adv Med Oncol. 2012;4(4):211-8.

[78] Whitesell L, Santagata S, Lin NU. Inhibiting HSP90 to treat cancer: a strategy in evolution. Curr Mol Med. 2012;17:17.

[79] Paraiso KH, Haarberg E, Wood E, Rebecca VW, Chen YA, Xiang Y, et al. The heat shock protein-90 inhibitor XL888 overcomes BRAF inhibitor resistance mediated through diverse mechanisms. Clin Cancer Res. 2012;18(9):2502-14.

[80] Modi S, Stopeck A, Linden H, Solit D, Chandarlapaty S, Rosen N, et al. HSP90 inhibition is effective in breast cancer: a phase II trial of tanespimycin (17-AAG) plus trastuzumab in patients with HER2-positive metastatic breast cancer progressing on trastuzumab. Clin Cancer Res. 2011;17(15):5132-9.

[81] Solit DB, Osman I, Polsky D, Panageas KS, Daud A, Goydos JS, et al. Phase II trial of 17-allylamino-17-demethoxygeldanamycin in patients with metastatic melanoma. Clin Cancer Res. 2008 Dec 15;14(24):8302-7.

[82] Nikolaou VA, Stratigos AJ, Flaherty KT, Tsao H. Melanoma: new insights and new therapies. J Invest Dermatol. 2012;132(3 Pt 2):854-63.

[83] Neyns B, Seghers AC, Wilgenhof S, Lebbe C. Successful rechallenge in two patients with BRAF-V600-mutant melanoma who experienced previous progression during treatment with a selective BRAF inhibitor. Melanoma Res. 2012 (in press).

[84] Alcala AM, Flaherty KT. BRAF Inhibitors for the Treatment of Metastatic Melanoma: Clinical Trials and Mechanisms of Resistance. Clin Cancer Res. 2012;18(1):33-9.

[85] Wilmott JS, Tembe V, Howle JR, Sharma R, Thompson JF, Rizos H, et al. Intratumoral molecular heterogeneity in a BRAF-mutant, BRAF inhibitor-resistant melanoma: a case illustrating the challenges for personalized medicine. Molecular cancer therapeutics. 2012 (in press)

[86] Richtig E, Schrama D, Ugurel S, Fried I, Niederkorn A, Massone C, et al. BRAF mutation analysis of only one single metastatic lesion can restrict the treatment of melanoma - a case report. Br J Dermatol. 2012;7(10):1365-2133.

[87] Catalanotti F, Solit DB. Will Hsp90 inhibitors prove effective in BRAF-mutant melanomas? Clin Cancer Res. 2012;18(9):2420-2.

Chapter 9

Combination Therapies to Improve Delivery of Protective T Cells into the Melanoma Microenvironment

Devin B. Lowe, Jennifer L. Taylor and Walter J. Storkus

Additional information is available at the end of the chapter

1. Introduction

Incidence rates for melanoma continue to rise between 2-3% each year in the United States [1]. Although melanoma accounts for 5% of new cancer cases, the disease is responsible for most deaths resulting from skin cancer. Five-year survival rates for localized disease have historically been greater than 95% after successfully excising tumors that are less than 1 mm thick [2]. Yet, despite intense efforts in the field, the ability to improve patient survival with invasive forms of the disease has changed little over the past two decades. Current five-year prognostic rates for regional and metastatic melanoma are approximately 66% and 15%, respectfully [1].

FDA-approved agents dacarbazine (DTIC), interferon-α, and high-dose IL-2 have long been employed as palliative therapies in advanced-stage melanoma patients (albeit with significant adverse side effects) [3]. Recent exciting data from large multicenter clinical trials has helped usher in the FDA approval of two new therapies that significantly improve upon the efficacy of existing first-line treatments such as DTIC. Ipilimumab is a humanized monoclonal antibody that functionally blocks the CTLA-4 molecule involved in suppressing T cell activation. In a randomized, double-blind phase III study, metastatic melanoma patients with unresectable stage III or IV disease were administered ipilimumab, ipilimumab plus a peptide vaccine specific to the melanosomal antigen gp100, or gp100 vaccine alone [4]. Ipilimumab therapy resulted in at least a 10 month median overall survival compared to 6.4 months for the gp100 vaccine treatment arm, but no statistical differences were observed between the ipilimumab treatment groups. In a follow-up phase III trial, patients with treatment-naive stage III or IV melanoma received DTIC alone or combined ipilimumab and DTIC therapy [5]. Although there was an improvement to median overall survival (9.1 versus 11.2 months, respectively), treatment with ipilimumab/DTIC significantly improved survival rates in patients at 3 years of follow-up. Vemurafenib is a small molecule drug that inhibits the activity of mutant BRAF (BRAF V600E) molecules in melanoma cells that constitutively signal via the MAPK pathway, promoting tumor cell proliferation and preventing cancer cell apoptosis [6]. Patients with previously untreated metastatic melanoma were first screened for the BRAF V600E mutation and then randomized to receive vemurafenib or DTIC in a phase III clinical trial [7]. At 6 months post therapy, vemurafenib resulted in an improved overall survival rate of 84% relative to 64% for DTIC treatment. Objective responses were also observed in 48% of vemurafenib-treated patients compared to 5% confirmed responses in the DTIC treatment arm. Although these preliminary findings are promising, the follow-up time of the study was inadequate to address the final objective and evaluation of progression-free survival rates for these patients is currently ongoing [8]. In a similarly structured phase II trial, vemurafenib administration in previously-treated BRAF V600E-selected melanoma patients led to a median overall survival of 15.9 months, which exceeds that previously observed for standard first-line treatments in patients with metastatic melanoma [9]. Unfortunately, the current level of care for metastatic melanoma remains far below the general expectations of wide-spread durable responses since most patients relapse from the above mentioned therapeutic interventions and eventually succumb to disease.

2. Supposed barriers to effective treatment

Improving tumor stage classification, candidate drug/therapy selection, and prediction of a patient's outcome to treatment could result from defining molecular events involved in the transformation of normal melanocytes into melanomas [2]. The delineation of these molecular patterns has proven difficult, however, since melanoma contains high frequencies of dissimilar gene mutations, deletions, duplications, and translocations across the range of patients evaluated [10]. A number of inherited events have been illuminated (transmissible through genetic or epigenetic means) that appear directly involved in initiating a melanocyte's pathway to malignancy by first inducing the clonal selection and outgrowth of cells [11]. Examples include alterations in the kinases BRAF and KIT and the tumor suppressor protein PTEN. The activating BRAF (BRAF-V600E) point mutation occurs in approximately 50% of melanomas (more commonly in cutaneous melanomas) and constitutively drives the MAPK pathway - without upstream RAS activation - leading to cell proliferation and survival [12]. The frequency of BRAF mutations is also preserved among primary and metastatic melanoma lesions, supporting the hypothesis that genetic disruption of BRAF is an early event that does not drive metastasis alone [12, 13]. KIT alterations account for up to 25% of acral and mucosal melanoma subtypes [6, 14]. The most common genetic change in KIT is an activating point mutation that stimulates the MAPK and PI3K-AKT signaling pathways, promoting cell growth and migration and preventing apoptosis [15]. Additional common melanoma defects are cells disrupted/deficient in the gene encoding PTEN. Under normal physiologic conditions, growth factors bind their respective cell surface receptor tyrosine kinase (RTK) and induce PI3K activity. PTEN serves to block PI3K function by preventing phosphorylation of PIP2 to PIP3, which ultimately drives signaling events through the PI3K-AKT pathway. In the absence of the phosphatase activity of PTEN, the AKT signaling cascade is unrestrained, driving the cell into a pro-survival mode. Simultaneous PTEN and BRAF alterations are two of the more widely documented correlative markers in late-stage melanoma patients and highlight the importance of the overlapping and non-overlapping functions of the AKT and MAPK pathways, respectively, in maintaining a malignant state. The common melanoma genetic aberrations (e.g., BRAF, KIT, PTEN) are not currently utilized for clinical diagnosis or prognosis, though, considering the seemingly paradoxical instances where gene markers do not correlate with independent classifiers of tumorigenesis [2]. For example, PTEN expression profiles have been reported to predict more aggressive forms of melanoma in cases of PTEN gene disruption [16] or activation [17] alongside clinico-pathological results. Drug-candidate discovery and testing has instead flourished with the improved knowledge of recurring primary genetic aberrations that appear to induce melanoma, as highlighted above for the FDA-approved BRAF inhibitor vemurafenib. Many other potential therapies have entered into clinical trials and have been well-described in a recent review [6]. One such promising drug is the RTK inhibitor dasatinib. With regard to melanoma, dasatinib targets KIT (and a limited range of alternate RTKs), leading to the disruption of the MAPK and PI3K signaling pathways. In a recently completed phase I trial, unselected patients with stage III or IV metastatic melanoma were administered dasatinib along with DTIC [18]. Combined treatment resulted in an objective response rate of 13.8% and median progression free survival of 13.4 weeks and appeared to be more active than either agent applied alone based on historical controls. Although these results are promising and support follow-up studies with this TKI, clinical evidence suggests that dasatinib preferably inhibits mutated KIT (occurring at exon 11 or 13) versus overexpressed wild-type KIT in melanoma patients [19-21]. It will, therefore, be of interest to closely monitor the differential anti-tumor efficacy of dasatinib treatment in melanoma patients harboring KIT mutations in future trials in order to select the most suitable patient population for clinical trial accrual.

Monotherapeutic use of drugs specific to the more commonly disrupted signaling pathways in melanoma has several drawbacks. At best, known drug/molecular target combinations are available for no more than 50% of melanoma patients (as in the case with vemurafenib and mutated BRAF), which severely limits treatment options for excluded patients. Drug resistance also presents a major concern in melanoma patients treated under these regimes. Tumor cells are capable of thwarting the benefits of targeted molecular approaches based on a number of innate and acquired mechanisms that include utilizing compensatory cell signaling pathways [22] and survival signals provided by the supportive TME [23]. In the instance of vemurafenib treatment, most BRAF-V600E-selected patients respond to therapy in the short-term (~80%) but fail to maintain durable responses [24]. Such clinical observations are not specific to melanoma but describe a wider phenomenon of eventually developing resistance to molecularly-targeted approaches in solid tumors [25, 26]. It has been hypothesized that therapy administration actually promotes the natural selection of a resistant tumor mass in the host [27]. These problematic corollaries will have to be overcome through the prudent use of combinational strategies that coordinately attack tumor cells and/or the tumor stroma at multiple, non-redundant levels. As one example, tyrosine kinase inhibitor (TKI) drugs (e.g., sunitinib, axitinib, dasatinib) remain attractive front-line agents to improve the efficacy of other co-applied strategies such as immunotherapy since these small molecule inhibitors may enable heightened responses to immune intervention based on the removal of suppression pathways inherent in the TME (as discussed in subsequent sections).

The initial driver mutations occurring in a melanocyte (e.g., BRAF, KIT, PTEN) are directly implicated in arresting cell cycle control points and promoting the clonal selection and expansion of cells that may disseminate systemically [11]. These primary genetic aberrations also induce an array of secondary events – all of which may contribute to molecular intra- and inter-patient heterogeneity. The pattern of tumor growth typically follows a course, whereby, melanomas transition from a benign radial phase in the epidermis (i.e., nevus) to vertical growth into the dermis and eventual systemic spread [28]. Upon reaching a size of 1-2 mm, a primary tumor nodule is growth-limited based on the need to develop a blood supply capable of providing sufficient nutrients to cells and effectively discharging metabolic waste [29]. To progress beyond this 1-2 mm limit, molecular signals in the tumor must be initiated to promote neovascularization. Hypoxia serves as one stimulus to initiate the expression of vascular endothelial growth factor (VEGF) by melanoma cells [30]. VEGF secretion by tumor cells can also result from inflammatory cytokines derived from infiltrating immunosuppressive cell populations such as tumor-associated macrophages (TAMs) and myeloid-derived suppressor cells (MDSCs). In general terms, locoregional VEGF production recruits endothelial precursor cells by binding its cognate high affinity receptor VEGFR2 [29, 30]. Endothelial cells in turn promote pericyte trafficking and coverage via elaboration of platelet-derived growth factor (PDGF). The effects of angiogenic pathways induced under conditions of tumor growth, however, do not resemble normal physiologic conditions. There is no hierarchical structure of arterioles to venules to capillaries. Instead, the tumor blood supply consists of a chaotic distribution of immature and mature endothelial cells, which are partly due to continued VEGF signaling by melanoma and endothelial cells and pericytes. Chronic VEGF expression serves to antagonize the interaction of endothelial cells and pericytes (by inhibiting PDGF/PDGFR binding) as well as to promote an ongoing cycle of endothelial cell recruitment and proliferation. The end-results are blood vessels comprised of loosely connected endothelial cells with little-to-no pericyte coverage. Consequently, blood flow is severely restricted in areas of the tumor while fluid build-up (e.g., plasma protein extravasation) occurs in the tumor interstitium, all of which contributes to heightened hypoxia, acidosis, and interstitial pressure. These TME dynamics in late-stage disease may help account for melanoma's intrinsic resistance to chemo/radiotherapies [31]. First, the delivery of anti-tumor strategies is impaired due to deficiencies in the tumor-derived blood supply and increased interstitial pressure. The hypoxic environment also directly contributes to a reduced efficacy of drug function such as in the case of radiotherapies. Lastly, conventional strategies that incorporate cytotoxic drugs have a diminished effect on tumor cells selected for growth under hypoxic and acidic conditions.

3. Improving treatment strategies

3.1. Vascular reconditioning hypothesis

Correcting deficiencies in the tumor vasculature could potentially circumvent many of the problems that serve to limit the effective treatment of late-stage metastatic melanoma patients as outlined above. Historically, vasculature disruption was hypothesized to starve tumors, leading to apoptosis/necrosis and lesional regression. In reality, anti-vasculature measures appear to primarily modulate the overall tumor blood vessel architecture through actions on immature endothelial cells [32]. These effects lead to transient improvements in blood flow (thereby, diminishing hypoxia and acidosis) and reduced interstitial pressure in the tumor mass [31]. In phase II clinical trials, patients with either metastatic melanoma or colorectal cancer have experienced improved response rates when bevacizumab (an anti-VEGF monoclonal antibody therapy) was combined with a standard of care treatment such as chemotherapy [33-37]. Although bevacizumab monotherapy exhibits minimal clinical impact [38], the antibody appears to exert a helper action by improving the bioavailability/activity of co-delivered cytotoxic drugs via its disruption of the melanoma-associated vasculature. This overarching paradigm has been formally tested in a number of preclinical models showing the improved distribution and efficacy of anti-tumor agents subsequent to tumor blood vessel "normalization" [29]. One caveat to this strategy is the need to consider the optimal schedule for application of each modality to yield superior anti-tumor efficacy. Our laboratory has recently reported that delayed TKI administration in a therapeutic melanoma mouse model negated protection from a dendritic cell (DC) vaccine based on subcutaneous tumor growth kinetics [39]. These studies and others indicate a window of therapeutic opportunity where anti-vasculature measures are highly effective in enhancing co-administered anti-tumor therapies. Melanomas, however, would be expected to become refractory to the action of anti-vascular drugs based on the selection of mature blood vessels that are effectively stabilized by pericytes [32]. As noted with molecular targeting strategies, tumor cells are also likely selected based on their ability to induce angiogenesis via alternate signaling pathways that do not overlap those sensitive to the originally-administered agents. In the absence of an effective second line strategy, increased tumor growth following anti-vasculature monotherapy may instead occur [40].

3.2. Immunotherapy and melanoma

The immune system provides a promising platform for consideration of inclusion in combined anti-melanoma therapies as it holds many theoretical advantages over standard treatment options such as chemotherapy or bulk cytokine (biologic modifier) administration. Namely, immunotherapies can be tailored to specifically target and kill tumor cells while leaving the surrounding normal tissue intact. Immune memory (recall) can also aid in sustained therapeutic action as a result of active vaccination, allowing for the maintenance of sub-clinical residual disease (in the adjuvant setting) or the prevention of recurrent tumor variants (i.e., through mechanisms of immune cross-priming and epitope spreading in the protective T cell repertoire). Several clinical studies have highlighted the proof-of-principle for immunotherapy in mediating objective clinical responses in melanoma patients. Therapies incorporating ipilimumab and bevacizumab have been discussed in preceding sections. Impressive clinical results have also been obtained using *ex vivo* expanded tumor infiltrating lymphocytes (TIL; T cells) in combination with rhIL-2 and non-lethal irradiation therapy, although this is a highly specialized process limited to a few locations worldwide [41, 42]. Durable complete responses (CR) (RECIST) have been observed in 22% of patients undergoing this form of treatment and most responses have been durable for > 3 years irrespective of prior treatments. Not all patients are suited to this approach, however, due to the technical constraints of resecting and culturing TIL (approximately 45% of patients are eligible at this stage) and severe toxicities associated with IL-2 administration and lymphodepletion.

The general failure of immunotherapeutic strategies to date likely involves a number of issues. As noted, melanoma is a vascularized cancer that maintains an aberrant blood vessel system. Immunologic strategies that rely on the anti-tumor properties of effector cells such as CD8+ T cells or antibodies may be unable to penetrate areas of the tumor based on the abnormal dynamics of blood flow and high interstitial pressure. Other melanoma characteristics such as reduced oxygen content and low pH serve to further reduce the function of cytotoxic CD8+ T cells if they should even be recruited into the TME. First-line strategies that recondition the melanoma-associated vasculature would be expected to overcome such obstacles and allow for the improved delivery and cytotoxic action of immunotherapeutic moieties.

Melanoma is an inherently immunogenic tumor, given the anti-tumor properties of resected TIL *in vitro* [43] and clinical observations that patients with higher frequencies of TIL have improved overall survival [43, 44]. However, the late-stage TME is also quite immunosuppressive. Due in part to the hypoxic nature of the TME, immunosuppressive cells such as regulatory T cells (Tregs), TAMs, and MDSCs become enriched within the tumor and reinforce their own survival/function while coordinately opposing the survival/function of protective T effector cells and Type-1 polarized DCs via soluble mediators and direct cell-to-cell contact [45, 46]. Elaboration of cytokines such as IL-10 and TGF-β sustain Tregs and inhibit T cell Type-1 polarization and DC maturation [47-49]. T cells are further suppressed by MDSC secretion of reactive oxygen and nitrogen species, TGF-β, VEGF, and arginase (i.e., through L-arginine depletion) [50]. Additionally, melanoma cells can express inhibitory molecules such as PD-L1 on their cell surface that interacts with T cell-expressed PD1, leading to T cell dysfunction and death [51]. Melanoma cells might also prevent DC processing/ presentation or T cell targeting through defects in the antigen presenting machinery and/or antigen loss. Therefore, combined immunotherapies must counteract the suppressive TME at some level (e.g., ipilimumab's anti-CTLA-4 mode of action). By reversing the balance of immunosuppression toward inflammatory Type-1 immunity, one can envision improved clinical benefits for coordinately-applied cancer vaccines. Yet, the optimization of the vaccine sub-component of such regimens remains an area of intense study [52].

3.3. Focus on dendritic cell vaccination

DCs provide a theoretical advantage over other vaccine types since they potently stimulate antigen-specific *de novo* and memory recall T cell responses [47]. Under steady-state conditions, a mature DC first migrates out of the periphery and into the TME where antigen is sampled and processed/presented in the form of MHC class I/II-peptide complexes [53]. After upregulating CCR7 expression, antigen-loaded DC become competent to migrate to tissue-draining lymph nodes, where it may provide an antigenic target, costimulation (e.g., DC CD80/86 binding the T cell receptor CD28), and cytokines to allow for the activation of antigen-specific CD4+ and/or CD8+ T cells. These educated effector T cells then return to the blood circulation where a portion of these cells may enter the tumor and perform anti-tumor activities.

Effective vaccination against melanoma antigens (many of which are non-mutated and expressed by normal melanocytes) presents a formidable challenge. Indeed, most tumor-associated antigens are on the whole less immunogenic than tumor specific antigens that arise as a result of viral infection (e.g., HPV induced cervical cancer). Assuming that host central and peripheral tolerance mechanisms have not deleted the appropriate T cell repertoire, the maturation status of the DC may be key to whether specific anti-melanoma T cell responses can be invoked at all. For example, improperly matured DCs may engage responder T cells and induce either anergy or death rather than T cell activation, expansion, and differentiation into effector cells. In addition, the immunosuppressive TME can adversely condition both endogenous DC and T cell survival/function. Immuno-oncologists have attempted to tackle these confounding issues by adoptive transfer of *ex vivo* manipulated DCs (and T cells) that exhibit preferred (normal) bioactivity. In the case of DCs, these cells may be harvested as blood precursors from cancer patients and subsequently polarized to a Type-1 phenotype through genetic manipulation or exposure to a cocktail of inflammatory-prone soluble mediators in culture. After further loading with target antigens associated with tumor cell growth and progression, this cellular vaccine may be reinfused back into the patient. Fully-mature DCs generated in this fashion are able to efficiently home to draining lymph nodes and activate/instruct resident effector-prone T cells while remaining functionally-resistant to TME inhibitory factors such as IL-10, TGF-β, VEGF, IL-6, and PGE_2 [54]. The framework for the autologous DC delivery strategy in cancer patients has been validated to some degree with the FDA-approved cellular immunotherapy designated sipuleucel-T. In this protocol, peripheral blood mononuclear cells (PBMCs) are harvested from men with castration-resistant prostate cancer and incubated with a fusion protein containing prostatic acid phosphatase and GM-CSF, a cytokine important for DC maturation [55, 56]. The stimulated PBMCs are then delivered back into patients every two weeks for a total of three injections. In a phase III double-blind multicenter trial, sipuleucel-T resulted in a median survival advantage of 4.1 months in 22% of individuals versus the placebo group [55]. Sipuleucel-T promoted heightened Type-I T cell and antibody responses against the vaccine fusion protein in a majority of patients presumably due to the enhanced maturation state of infused activated DCs [56]. Overall survival correlated with improved specific immunity in responding patients suggesting that sipuleucel-T's mechanism of action includes immune targeting of prostate carcinoma cells by vaccine-induced T cells.

Many clinical studies have highlighted the ability of DC-based adoptive therapy to boost resident anti-tumor T cell responses and to mediate corollary clinical activity in patients with melanoma [57-65]. In one of the first reported DC-based therapy trials in the melanoma setting, DCs were harvested from patients (regardless of their HLA type), cultured in the presence of rhGM-CSF and rhIL-4 for one week, and pulsed with melanoma-associated peptides (e.g., HLA-A2 restricted gp100, tyrosinase, and Melan-A/MART1 peptides) or autologous tumor lysates [59]. The cellular vaccines were delivered into tumor uninvolved inguinal lymph nodes at least 4 times at weekly intervals. Eleven out of 16 (69%) enrolled patients developed DTH reactions to intradermal injections of DCs loaded with either vaccine-derived peptides or tumor lysates following DC vaccine therapy. Subsequent analysis of infiltrating T cells in representative biopsied DTH sites revealed peptide-specific reactivity to antigenic components of the vaccine. Overall, 2 CR and 3 PR were observed with these same patients also exhibiting vaccine-specific reactivity as evidenced in DTH testing. In a separate phase I clinical trial reported by Ribas and colleagues, GM-CSF/IL-4 *ex vivo* cultured DCs were loaded with a Melan-A/MART1 peptide and delivered intradermally into metastatic melanoma patients a total of 3 times every 2 weeks alongside tremelimumab (anti-CTLA-4) treatment [66]. Tetramer and ELISPOT analysis revealed increases in the frequency of peripheral Melan-A/MART1-reactive CD8+ T cells as a consequence of specific vaccination in 9 of 15 (60%) individuals, although tremelimumab therapy did not appear to enhance Melan-A/MART1 T cell frequency and function. Four vaccinated patients experienced objective clinical responses (2 CR, 2 PR) with 3 individuals also displaying an improved MART-1 T cell response post-DC vaccination. Although such studies provide proof-of principle, major improvements are still needed in order to achieve durable clinical responses and prolonged survival rates in a majority of patients undergoing autologous DC therapy. A potential improvement to DC activity *in vivo* may reside with how DCs are manipulated *ex vivo* following leukopheresis. In cases where DCs are stimulated to an underwhelmed (use of GM-CSF/IL-4) or exhausted (use of PGE_2) Type-1 state, effector T cells suffer from an inability to effectively mediate anti-tumor responses [49]. One promising DC polarizing method incorporates IL-1β, TNF-α, IFN-α, IFN-γ, and poly-I:C in the *ex vivo* culturing phase to effectively mature DCs (designated α-DC1). Twenty-two patients with recurrent malignant glioma were administered up to 4 vaccinations intranodally of α-DC1 loaded with glioma associated antigens at 2 week intervals [67]. At the conclusion of the immunization cycle, 58% of evaluable patients demonstrated a response to at least one antigenic component of the vaccine based on PBMC specific activity through IFN-γ ELISPOT or tetramer analysis. Upregulated gene expression profiles of Type-1 cytokines (e.g., IFN-α, IFN-γ) and chemokines (e.g., CXCL10) were also observed in PBMCs from α-DC1 treated patients, suggesting that the vaccine therapy enhanced the cytolytic activity and trafficking ability of immune cells. Progression free survival was extended to 12 months in 9 of 22 patients receiving the α-DC1 vaccine. The ability of α-DC1 to produce IL-12 (and, hence, stimulate CD4+ and CD8+ T cell function) correlated to prolonged progression free survival. Based on the safety profile and relative success of this trial, the α-DC1 generation protocol is currently being evaluated in a phase I trial in patients with metastatic melanoma (NCT00390338).

Another way to improve the immunogenicity of autologous DC-based therapy involves the choice of antigenic target for presentation to T cells (i.e., therapeutic selection of the responding anti-tumor T cell repertoire for expansion). Most DC-based vaccine trials have incorporated melanoma-associated antigens such as gp100, tyrosinase, Melan-A/MART1 and MAGE in the vaccine formulation. Despite the surprisingly high immunogenic nature of these "self" antigens in vaccinated patients, tumor cells can continue to grow progressively by evading the effector T cell system via various well-described mechanisms [46, 48, 53]. For instance, the tumor mass is composed of a heterogeneous mixture of cancer cells that exhibit a range of defects/deficiencies in the antigen presentation machinery that limits effective presentation of tumor antigen-derived peptides in MHC complexes and leads to poor recognition by the immune system. As such, a fraction of tumor cells may become "invisible" to the adaptive immune system, resulting in the negative selection of treatment-resistant tumor cells in progressor lesions [68]. This scenario can be avoided in part by the use of vaccines incorporating antigens that represent proteins required for maintenance of the transformed state, progressive growth, or metastasis. Alternatively, one may consider the inclusion of antigens expressed not by tumor cells themselves but by the supportive stromal cells (whose phenotype is uniquely modified by the TME) that enable the formation of large bulk tumors. We hypothesize that peptides associated with tumor angiogenesis (summarized in Table 1) may provide an ideal source of targets for DC/peptide vaccine design. In effect, targeting the underlying tumor stroma (e.g., vascular cells, pericytes) would disrupt melanoma growth and promote tumor-specific immunity and protection. Our laboratory has previously demonstrated the ability to successfully treat HLA-A2+ transgenic mice bearing established colon carcinoma or melanomas using DC-based vaccines containing antigens differentially associated with the tumor vasculature [69]. Animals administered peptide-loaded DC vaccines displayed enhanced protection from established tumor growth and ability, in instances of complete regression, to provide durable protection from dormant disease. Interestingly, active vaccination against tumor stromal antigens led to the corollary cross-priming of T cell responses directed against alternate vascular-associated antigens that were not originally comprised in the vaccine therapy as well as *bona fide* tumor cell-associated antigens. Normal donors and melanoma patients also exhibited immune reactivity to many of the stromal antigens upon *in vitro* sensitization, indicating that operational tolerance to such "self" antigens may be broken using a DC/peptide-based vaccination approach [70]. Importantly, this vaccine strategy appears safe in treated mice since we have not observed deleterious immunologic responses against the normal tissue vasculature, disruptions to the normal cutaneous wound healing process, or aberrations in the fertility/litter size of pre-vaccinated female animals [69, 70].

Stromal antigen	Cell expression	AA positions	Peptide sequence	CD8+ T cell response		
				HLA-A2+ transgenic mice	HLA-A2+ normal donors	HLA-A2+ melanoma patients
DLK1	P	269-277	RLTPGVHEL	++	+	++
		310-318	ILGVLTSLV	++	+	++
		328-336	FLNKCETWV	+++	+	++
EphA2	VEC	883-891	TLADFDPRV	+++	+	++
HBB	P	31-39	RLLVVYPWT	+	+	++
		105-114	RLLGNVLVCV	+	+	+
NG2	P	770-778	TLSNLSFPV	-	-	++
		2238-2246	LILPLLFYL	+	-	++
NP1	P	331-339	GLLRFVTAV	+	+	+++
		433-441	GMLGMVSGL	++	+	+++
		869-877	VLLGAVCGV	+++	+	+
NP2	P	214-222	DIWDGIPHV	-	-	++
		328-336	YLQVDLRFL	-	-	++
PDGFRβ	P	890-898	ILLWEIFTL	+++	+	+
PSMA	VEC	441-450	LLQERGVAYI	+	-	+
RGS5	P	5-13	LAALPHSCL	+	-	++
TEM1	VEC/P	691-700	LLVPTCVFLV	+	++	++
VEGFR1	VEC/P	770-778	TLFWLLLTL	++	+	+

Table 1. Candidate melanoma-associated vascular peptides for DC vaccine design. CD8+ T cell response summaries are provided from previous work by our laboratory [69, 70]. Naïve HLA-A2+ transgenic mice were vaccinated bi-weekly with DCs pre-pulsed with the appropriate antigen-derived peptide. One week following the second DC vaccine, splenic CD8+ T cells were harvested and co-cultured 48 hours with the HLA-A2+ T2 cell line pulsed with the relevant peptide. CD8+ T cell elaboration of IFN-γ (as a read-out for Type-1 activity) was then determined through ELISA. Human CD8+ T cell responses to stromal peptides were determined by first isolating PBMCs and stimulating cells in the presence of antigen-loaded autologous DCs for 1 week. Normal donor samples underwent 2 rounds of IVS while PBMCs obtained from melanoma patients were subjected to 1 round of IVS. CD8+ T cell IFN-γ expression was assessed as similarly described for HLA-A2+ transgenic mice. Abbreviations used: AA, amino acid; P, pericyte; VEC, vascular endothelial cell; -, No observed activity; +, low activity; ++, medium activity; +++, high activity; IVS, *in vitro* sensitization

3.4. Combining small molecule drugs with DC vaccination

In addition to empirically improving DC vaccine design (e.g., via the *ex vivo* conditioning of the APC and a rationale selection of the included antigenic targets), the effectiveness of such treatments would be expected to improve by mitigating the functional constraints on vaccine-induced T effector cells imposed by the generally suppressive TME. As previously mentioned, the aberrant dynamics of the tumor vascular architecture and enrichment of regulatory cell populations (e.g., MDSC, Treg) in the TME consort to diminish the recruitment, vitality, and tumoricidal activity of immune cells *in situ*. Therefore, the conditional abrogation of the negative attributes of the TME would be predicted to improve infiltration and function of vaccine-expanded T cell populations, leading to more durable objective clinical responses in melanoma patients as diagramed in Figure 1. What follows are examples of three FDA-approved TKI drugs that could be utilized in DC-based vaccine combination immunotherapies to achieve this goal.

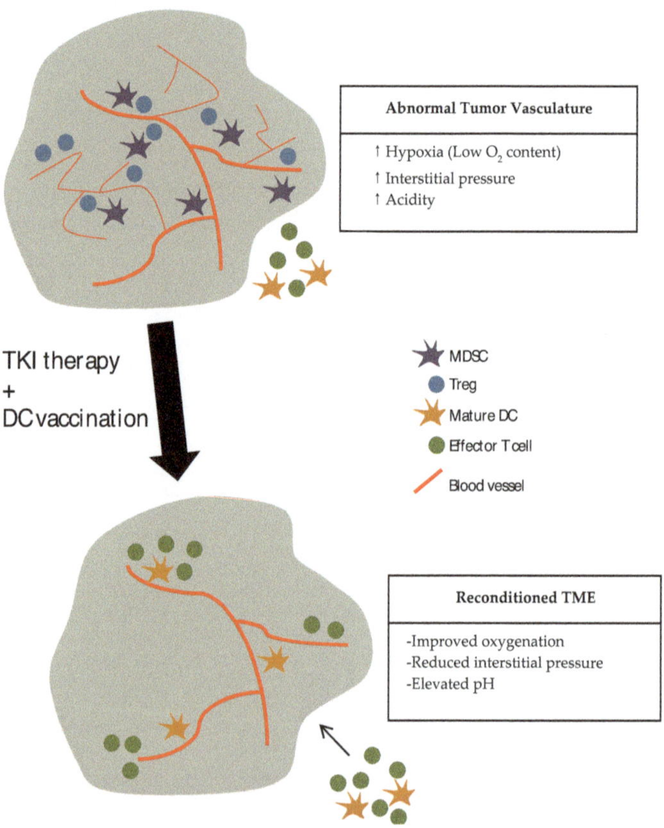

Figure 1. Paradigm for effective combination treatment of melanoma. Established vascularized cancers such as melanoma are entrenched with a chaotic blood vessel network and immunosuppressive cell populations. These TME properties serve to prevent the intratumoral delivery and function of single-agent cytotoxic therapies, including specific active vaccination. In cases of combined therapeutic strategies where the melanoma-associated vasculature is first modulated through TKI drug sensitization, for example, immature blood vessels (i.e., endothelial cells loosely decorated by or absent in pericyte coverage) may be disrupted, resulting in a normoxic TME with reduced interstitial pressure and acidity. Frequencies of MDSC and Treg cells are also minimized through mechanisms that are not entirely clear.

Consequently, vaccine-initiated effector T cells can better traffick into tumors and exert their anti-tumor functions. Mature DCs are also able to infiltrate the tumor lesion and sample material from dying cells or necrotic tissue for cross-presentation purposes to unknown/untargeted tumor associated antigens, leading to activation of a broad T cell repertoire that is competent to promote durable anti-tumor immunity. Abbreviations used: TKI, tyrosine kinase inhibitor; MDSC, myeloid-derived suppressor cell; Treg, regulatory T cell; DC, dendritic cell; TME, tumor microenvironment

Sunitinib binds to and inhibits a range of tyrosine kinases including the vascular associated molecules VEGFR and PDGFR. The drug is approved for use in patients with metastatic renal cell carcinoma (mRCC) or gastrointestinal stromal tumors, where most patients respond favorably to treatment in the short-term [71, 72]. In one recently reported phase I trial, metastatic melanoma patients harboring KIT mutations were administered sunitinib using the FDA-approved regimen of 50 mg/day for 4 weeks followed by 2 weeks off drug [73]. Out of 10 evaluable patients, 1 individual had a CR that lasted 15 months while 2 PR endured between 1-7 months. A separate clinical study, reported on the ability of sunitinib to work in concert with docetaxel therapy in patients with solid tumors including melanoma [74]. Two PR were confirmed in a total of 12 metastatic melanoma patients treated with the combination regimen, supporting a potential tumor vascular "reconditioning" role of sunitinib in improving the delivery and function of cytotoxic therapies within the TME. Our own animal studies support a similar paradigm for combination immunotherapies [39]. Protection from established melanoma progression (based on tumor growth kinetics and survival) were enhanced in mice receiving both sunitinib and DC/peptide-based vaccination versus either agent administered as a monotherapy. Sunitinib co-treatment facilitated the recruitment of DC-"primed" Type-1 CD8+ T cells into melanoma lesions based in part on the upregulated expression of VCAM-1 (on vascular endothelial cells) and CXCR3 ligand chemokines (e.g., CXCL9, CXCL10, CXCL11) within the TME. This TKI also reduced frequencies of immunosuppressive cell populations such as MDSC and Tregs in the tumor and tumor draining lymph node (TDLN), which was associated with increased cytotoxic potential mediated by vaccine-induced CD8+ T cells. Sunitinib therapy has similarly been reported to prevent the peripheral accumulations of MDSCs and Tregs in mRCC patients [75-77]. Although the molecular mechanism underlying these alterations remains an open question, sunitinib inhibits STAT3 activation (via inhibition of upstream tyrosine kinases) which may prove core to its perceived anti-tumor actions [39, 75].

Axitinib is a potent TKI targeting VEGFRs (VEGFR1, 2, and 3) that support tumor angiogenesis [30, 78]. Following the completion of a recent phase III trial [79], axitinib was granted approval by the FDA as a second-line therapy for mRCC patients refractory to first-line treatment options including sunitinib. Axitinib has also been used to treat patients with melanoma. Pre-clinical studies have supported a role for axitinib monotherapy to disrupt angiogenesis and tumor formation in xenograft melanoma models [80]. A multicenter phase II trial also justified the continued use of axitinib-based treatment in metastatic melanoma patients [81]. Individuals receiving this TKI experienced reductions of VEGFR2 and VEGFR3 and increased levels of soluble VEGF in their plasma. Treatment with axitinib was associated with an overall objective response rate of 18.8%, which is comparable to historical response rates for chemotherapy and IL-2-based therapies. Given the relative clinical success for axitinib monotherapy, we assessed the impact of axitinib on DC/peptide-based vaccination on established melanoma growth in murine models [82]. Melanoma-bearing mice administered axitinib and specific vaccines were protected from tumor growth and displayed enhanced survival for up to 80 days following melanoma implantation. Axitinib-sensitization improved the trafficking and retention of vaccine-induced CD8+ T cells in the TME, with the Type-1 functionality (as assessed by IFNγ expression) of CD8+ T cells elevated in both the tumor site and the TDLN. Similar to our observations with sunitinib [39], axitinib reduced systemic frequencies of MDSCs and Tregs and promoted a Type-1 TME, as evidenced by the upregulated expression of Tbet, IFN-γ, CXCR3, and CXCL10 gene transcripts.

Dasatinib has already been reported to selectively abrogate mutated KIT activity in human melanomas [19, 83]. This TKI also inhibits other tyrosine kinases such as the Src family of kinases (impacting PI3K-AKT signaling) involved in melanoma adhesion, motility, and invasion [84, 85]. As a monotherapy, dasatinib was well-tolerated in melanoma patients, yielding an objective response rate comparable to alternate current first-line treatment options [18]. Dasatinib diminishes tumor angiogenesis by inhibiting the tyrosine kinases EphA2 and PDGFR that play significant roles in endothelial and pericyte biology, respectively [84]. In unpublished results from our laboratory, dasatinib mediates anti-TME effects that are similar to sunitinib and axitinib in melanoma-bearing mice [39, 82]. Animals treated with dasatinib undergo a restructuring of the tumor vasculature in association with reduced hypoxia and MDSC/Treg frequencies and increased accumulation of T effector cells in the TME, particularly when combined with a DC/peptide-based vaccine. The combined therapy also yielded greatest objective clinical benefit when compared with either monotherapeutic approach. Overall, these studies have supported the design of a pilot phase II trial (dasatinib + DC/tumor stromal antigen-based vaccine) at the University of Pittsburgh planned to begin enrolling patients in Q4 2012. In this trial, HLA-A2+ patients with advanced-stage melanoma will be administered dasatinib and an autologous αDC1/peptide vaccine, with frequencies of antigen-specific T cells monitored in patient blood and tumor biopsies over time along with objective clinical responses.

4. Conclusions

The emergence of ipilimumab and vemurafenib as treatment alternatives to the long-standing DTIC-, IL-2-, and IFN-α-based therapies attests to progress made in treating patients with metastatic melanoma. Although the genetic heterogeneity of melanoma cells has confounded high-throughput sequencing technologies, patterns of molecular aberrations are becoming clearer and help support the clinical application of FDA-approved small molecule drugs (such as TKIs) as therapeutic options in eligible patients. Select TKIs (e.g., sunitinib, axitinib, dasatinib) not only directly inhibit melanoma growth and progression by specifically disrupting cell intrinsic signaling pathways, but these drugs indirectly perturb tumorigenesis based on their "normalizing" effects on the TME. Central to this therapeutic paradigm is the ability of the drugs to recondition the chaotic architecture and fluid dynamics of the blood vasculature in the TME. The short-term consequences of TKI sensitization are impressive and include a reversal of hypoxia, acidosis, and interstitial pressure in the TME, which allows for a corollary improvement in the accumulation and action of co-applied cytotoxic therapies (including immunotherapies).

Combinational immunotherapies hold great promise in minimizing/preventing the emergence and progression of (same) therapy-resistant melanoma populations, as has typically been observed in cases of single-agent treatment strategies. These approaches also have potential to result in a state of perpetual disease dormancy which may extend patient overall survival [69]. The current challenge to the field is to determine the best combination (dosing and scheduling) of agents to best affect a state of durable clinical benefit in the advance-stage disease setting. From our work, and that of many others, immunotherapy represents one promising component of such combined treatment strategies, particularly when integrated with agents that act as immune adjuvants, inhibitors of immune regulatory cells, and "normalizers" of the TME. Preclinical studies have clearly justified the combined strategy of TKI drug therapy alongside specific DC/peptide-based vaccination. In particular, TKI administration essentially serves as an "immune adjuvant" by reversing the inherent immunosuppression of the TME upon diminishing frequencies of suppressive cell populations and physically manipulating the tumor vasculature architecture. Vaccine-initiated effector T cells are then able to more effectively infiltrate a tumor lesion in order to perform their clinically-beneficial cytolytic functions. Prospective clinical trials will test the validity of this operational biologic paradigm on patient outcome and define a series of safe and effective combination treatment options for melanoma patients.

Acknowledgments

This work was supported by NIH grants P01 CA100327, R01 CA114071, R01 CA140375 and P50 CA121973 (to W.J.S.) and the University of Pittsburgh Cancer Center Support Grant (CCSG; P30 CA047904). D.B.L. was supported by a Postdoctoral Fellowship (PF-11-151-01-LIB) from the American Cancer Society.

Author details

Devin B. Lowe[1], Jennifer L. Taylor[1] and Walter J. Storkus[1,2*]

*Address all correspondence to: storkuswj@upmc.edu

1 Dermatology and Immunology, University of Pittsburgh School of Medicine, Pittsburgh, PA, USA

2 University of Pittsburgh Cancer Institute, Pittsburgh, PA, USA

References

[1] American Cancer Society. http://www.cancer.org/Research/CancerFactsFigures/CancerFactsFigures/cancer-facts-figures-2012 (accessed 14 August 2012).

[2] Tremante E, Ginebri A, Lo Monaco E, Frascione P, Di Filippo F, Terrenato I, et al. Melanoma molecular classes and prognosis in the postgenomic era. Lancet Oncol. 2012;13(5) e205-11.

[3] Lacy KE, Karagiannis SN, Nestle FO. Advances in the treatment of melanoma. Clin Med. 2012;12(2) 168-71.

[4] Hodi FS, O'Day SJ, McDermott DF, Weber RW, Sosman JA, Haanen JB, et al. Improved survival with ipilimumab in patients with metastatic melanoma. N Engl J Med. 2010;363(8) 711-23.

[5] Robert C, Thomas L, Bondarenko I, O'Day S, M DJ, Garbe C, et al. Ipilimumab plus dacarbazine for previously untreated metastatic melanoma. N Engl J Med. 2011;364(26) 2517-26.

[6] Flaherty KT, Hodi FS, Fisher DE. From genes to drugs: targeted strategies for melanoma. Nat Rev Cancer. 2012;12(5) 349-61.

[7] Chapman PB, Hauschild A, Robert C, Haanen JB, Ascierto P, Larkin J, et al. Improved survival with vemurafenib in melanoma with BRAF V600E mutation. N Engl J Med. 2011;364(26) 2507-16.

[8] Ernstoff MS. Been there, not done that--melanoma in the age of molecular therapy. N Engl J Med. 2011;364(26) 2547-8.

[9] Sosman JA, Kim KB, Schuchter L, Gonzalez R, Pavlick AC, Weber JS, et al. Survival in BRAF V600-mutant advanced melanoma treated with vemurafenib. N Engl J Med. 2012;366(8) 707-14.

[10] Hoek KS. Exploring melanoma's massively parallel universe. Pigment Cell Melanoma Res. 2010;23(3) 306-7.

[11] Bennett DC. How to make a melanoma: what do we know of the primary clonal events? Pigment Cell Melanoma Res. 2008;21(1) 27-38.

[12] Mehnert JM, Kluger HM. Driver Mutations in Melanoma: Lessons Learned From Bench-to-Bedside Studies. Curr Oncol Rep. 2012;14(5) 449-57.

[13] Colombino M, Capone M, Lissia A, Cossu A, Rubino C, De Giorgi V, et al. BRAF/NRAS Mutation Frequencies Among Primary Tumors and Metastases in Patients With Melanoma. J Clin Oncol. 2012;30(20) 2522-9.

[14] Furney SJ, Turajlic S, Fenwick K, Lambros MB, MacKay A, Ricken G, et al. Genomic characterisation of acral melanoma cell lines. Pigment Cell Melanoma Res. 2012;25(4) 488-92.

[15] Jazirehi AR, Wenn PB, Damavand M. Therapeutic implications of targeting the PI3Kinase/AKT/mTOR signaling module in melanoma therapy. Am J Cancer Res. 2012;2(2) 178-91.

[16] Mikhail M, Velazquez E, Shapiro R, Berman R, Pavlick A, Sorhaindo L, et al. PTEN expression in melanoma: relationship with patient survival, Bcl-2 expression, and proliferation. Clin Cancer Res. 2005;11(14) 5153-7.

[17] Meyer S, Fuchs TJ, Bosserhoff AK, Hofstadter F, Pauer A, Roth V, et al. A seven-marker signature and clinical outcome in malignant melanoma: a large-scale tissue-microarray study with two independent patient cohorts. PLoS One. 2012;7(6) e38222.

[18] Algazi AP, Weber JS, Andrews SC, Urbas P, Munster PN, DeConti RC, et al. Phase I clinical trial of the Src inhibitor dasatinib with dacarbazine in metastatic melanoma. Br J Cancer. 2012;106(1) 85-91.

[19] Woodman SE, Trent JC, Stemke-Hale K, Lazar AJ, Pricl S, Pavan GM, et al. Activity of dasatinib against L576P KIT mutant melanoma: molecular, cellular, and clinical correlates. Mol Cancer Ther. 2009;8(8) 2079-85.

[20] Kluger HM, Dudek AZ, McCann C, Ritacco J, Southard N, Jilaveanu LB, et al. A phase 2 trial of dasatinib in advanced melanoma. Cancer. 2011;117(10) 2202-8.

[21] Woodman SE, Lazar AJ, Aldape KD, Davies MA. New strategies in melanoma: molecular testing in advanced disease. Clin Cancer Res. 2012;18(5) 1195-200.

[22] Wilson TR, Fridlyand J, Yan Y, Penuel E, Burton L, Chan E, et al. Widespread potential for growth-factor-driven resistance to anticancer kinase inhibitors. Nature. 2012;487(7408) 505-9.

[23] Straussman R, Morikawa T, Shee K, Barzily-Rokni M, Qian ZR, Du J, et al. Tumour micro-environment elicits innate resistance to RAF inhibitors through HGF secretion. Nature. 2012;487(7408) 500-4.

[24] Flaherty KT, Puzanov I, Kim KB, Ribas A, McArthur GA, Sosman JA, et al. Inhibition of mutated, activated BRAF in metastatic melanoma. 2010;N Engl J Med. 363(9) 809-19.

[25] Rini BI, Atkins MB. Resistance to targeted therapy in renal-cell carcinoma. Lancet Oncol. 2009;10(10) 992-1000.

[26] Montemurro M, Bauer S. Treatment of gastrointestinal stromal tumor after imatinib and sunitinib. Curr Opin Oncol. 2011;23(4) 367-72.

[27] Puzanov I, Burnett P, Flaherty KT. Biological challenges of BRAF inhibitor therapy. Mol Oncol. 2011;5(2) 116-23.

[28] Leong SP, Mihm MC, Jr., Murphy GF, Hoon DS, Kashani-Sabet M, Agarwala SS, et al. Progression of cutaneous melanoma: implications for treatment. Clin Exp Metastasis. In press, 2012.

[29] Goel S, Duda DG, Xu L, Munn LL, Boucher Y, Fukumura D, et al. Normalization of the vasculature for treatment of cancer and other diseases. Physiol Rev. 2011;91(3) 1071-121.

[30] Carmeliet P, Jain RK. Molecular mechanisms and clinical applications of angiogenesis. Nature. 2011;473(7347) 298-307.

[31] Jain RK. Normalization of tumor vasculature: an emerging concept in antiangiogenic therapy. Science. 2005;307(5706) 58-62.

[32] Helfrich I, Scheffrahn I, Bartling S, Weis J, von Felbert V, Middleton M, et al. Resistance to antiangiogenic therapy is directed by vascular phenotype, vessel stabilization, and maturation in malignant melanoma. J Exp Med. 2010;207(3) 491-503.

[33] Hurwitz H, Fehrenbacher L, Novotny W, Cartwright T, Hainsworth J, Heim W, et al. Bevacizumab plus irinotecan, fluorouracil, and leucovorin for metastatic colorectal cancer. N Engl J Med. 2004;350(23) 2335-42.

[34] Del Vecchio M, Mortarini R, Canova S, Di Guardo L, Pimpinelli N, Sertoli MR, et al. Bevacizumab plus fotemustine as first-line treatment in metastatic melanoma patients: clinical activity and modulation of angiogenesis and lymphangiogenesis factors. Clin Cancer Res. 2010;16(23) 5862-72.

[35] Hainsworth JD, Infante JR, Spigel DR, Peyton JD, Thompson DS, Lane CM, et al. Bevacizumab and everolimus in the treatment of patients with metastatic melanoma: a phase 2 trial of the Sarah Cannon Oncology Research Consortium. Cancer. 2010;116(17) 4122-9.

[36] Perez DG, Suman VJ, Fitch TR, Amatruda T, 3rd, Morton RF, Jilani SZ, et al. Phase 2 trial of carboplatin, weekly paclitaxel, and biweekly bevacizumab in patients with unresectable stage IV melanoma: a North Central Cancer Treatment Group study, N047A. Cancer. 2009;115(1) 119-27.

[37] Vihinen PP, Hernberg M, Vuoristo MS, Tyynela K, Laukka M, Lundin J, et al. A phase II trial of bevacizumab with dacarbazine and daily low-dose interferon-alpha2a as first line treatment in metastatic melanoma. Melanoma Res. 2010;20(4) 318-25.

[38] Giantonio BJ, Catalano PJ, Meropol NJ, O'Dwyer PJ, Mitchell EP, Alberts SR, et al. Bevacizumab in combination with oxaliplatin, fluorouracil, and leucovorin (FOLFOX4) for previously treated metastatic colorectal cancer: results from the Eastern Cooperative Oncology Group Study E3200. J Clin Oncol. 2007;25(12) 1539-44.

[39] Bose A, Taylor JL, Alber S, Watkins SC, Garcia JA, Rini BI, et al. Sunitinib facilitates the activation and recruitment of therapeutic anti-tumor immunity in concert with specific vaccination. Int J Cancer. 2011;129(9) 2158-70.

[40] Ebos JM, Lee CR, Cruz-Munoz W, Bjarnason GA, Christensen JG, Kerbel RS. Accelerated metastasis after short-term treatment with a potent inhibitor of tumor angiogenesis. Cancer Cell. 2009;15(3) 232-9.

[41] Rosenberg SA, Yang JC, Sherry RM, Kammula US, Hughes MS, Phan GQ, et al. Durable complete responses in heavily pretreated patients with metastatic melanoma using T-cell transfer immunotherapy. Clin Cancer Res. 2011;17(13) 4550-7.

[42] Restifo NP, Dudley ME, Rosenberg SA. Adoptive immunotherapy for cancer: harnessing the T cell response. Nat Rev Immunol. 2012;12(4) 269-81.

[43] Yannelli JR, Wroblewski JM. On the road to a tumor cell vaccine: 20 years of cellular immunotherapy. Vaccine. 2004;23(1) 97-113.

[44] Clemente CG, Mihm MC, Jr., Bufalino R, Zurrida S, Collini P, Cascinelli N. Prognostic value of tumor infiltrating lymphocytes in the vertical growth phase of primary cutaneous melanoma. Cancer. 1996;77(7) 1303-10.

[45] Ostrand-Rosenberg S, Sinha P, Beury DW, Clements VK. Cross-talk between myeloid-derived suppressor cells (MDSC), macrophages, and dendritic cells enhances tumor-induced immune suppression. Semin Cancer Biol. 2012;22(4) 275-81.

[46] Lowe DB, Storkus WJ. Chronic inflammation and immunologic-based constraints in malignant disease. Immunotherapy. 2011;3(10) 1265-74.

[47] Karthaus N, Torensma R, Tel J. Deciphering the message broadcast by tumor-infiltrating dendritic cells. Am J Pathol. 2012;181(3) 733-42.

[48] Mayer CT, Berod L, Sparwasser T. Layers of dendritic cell-mediated T cell tolerance, their regulation and the prevention of autoimmunity. Front Immunol. 2012;3 183.

[49] Kalinski P, Edington H, Zeh HJ, Okada H, Butterfield LH, Kirkwood JM, et al. Dendritic cells in cancer immunotherapy: vaccines or autologous transplants? Immunol Res. 2011;50(2-3) 235-47.

[50] Lechner MG, Liebertz DJ, Epstein AL. Characterization of cytokine-induced myeloid-derived suppressor cells from normal human peripheral blood mononuclear cells. J Immunol. 2010;185(4) 2273-84.

[51] Topalian SL, Drake CG, Pardoll DM. Targeting the PD-1/B7-H1(PD-L1) pathway to activate anti-tumor immunity. Curr Opin Immunol. 2012;24(2) 207-12.

[52] Klebanoff CA, Acquavella N, Yu Z, Restifo NP. Therapeutic cancer vaccines: are we there yet? Immunol Rev. 2011;239(1) 27-44.

[53] Palucka K, Banchereau J. Cancer immunotherapy via dendritic cells. Nat Rev Cancer. 2012;12(4) 265-77.

[54] Kalinski P. Regulation of immune responses by prostaglandin E2. J Immunol. 2012;188(1) 21-8.

[55] Kantoff PW, Higano CS, Shore ND, Berger ER, Small EJ, Penson DF, et al. Sipuleucel-T immunotherapy for castration-resistant prostate cancer. N Engl J Med. 2010;363(5) 411-22.

[56] Sheikh NA, Petrylak D, Kantoff PW, Dela Rosa C, Stewart FP, Kuan LY, et al. Sipuleucel-T immune parameters correlate with survival: an analysis of the randomized phase 3 clinical trials in men with castration-resistant prostate cancer. Cancer Immunol Immunother. In press, 2012.

[57] Palucka AK, Ueno H, Connolly J, Kerneis-Norvell F, Blanck JP, Johnston DA, et al. Dendritic cells loaded with killed allogeneic melanoma cells can induce objective clinical responses and MART-1 specific CD8+ T-cell immunity. J Immunother. 2006;29(5) 545-57.

[58] O'Rourke MG, Johnson M, Lanagan C, See J, Yang J, Bell JR, et al. Durable complete clinical responses in a phase I/II trial using an autologous melanoma cell/dendritic cell vaccine. Cancer Immunol Immunother. 2003;52(6) 387-95.

[59] Nestle FO, Alijagic S, Gilliet M, Sun Y, Grabbe S, Dummer R, et al. Vaccination of melanoma patients with peptide- or tumor lysate-pulsed dendritic cells. Nat Med. 1998;4(3) 328-32.

[60] Thurner B, Haendle I, Roder C, Dieckmann D, Keikavoussi P, Jonuleit H, et al. Vaccination with mage-3A1 peptide-pulsed mature, monocyte-derived dendritic cells expands specific cytotoxic T cells and induces regression of some metastases in advanced stage IV melanoma. J Exp Med. 1999;190(11) 1669-78.

[61] Salcedo M, Bercovici N, Taylor R, Vereecken P, Massicard S, Duriau D, et al. Vaccination of melanoma patients using dendritic cells loaded with an allogeneic tumor cell lysate. Cancer Immunol Immunother. 2006;55(7) 819-29.

[62] Schuler-Thurner B, Schultz ES, Berger TG, Weinlich G, Ebner S, Woerl P, et al. Rapid induction of tumor-specific type 1 T helper cells in metastatic melanoma patients by vaccination with mature, cryopreserved, peptide-loaded monocyte-derived dendritic cells. J Exp Med. 2002;195(10) 1279-88.

[63] Ridolfi L, Petrini M, Fiammenghi L, Granato AM, Ancarani V, Pancisi E, et al. Dendritic cell-based vaccine in advanced melanoma: update of clinical outcome. Melanoma Res. 2011;21(6) 524-9.

[64] Steele JC, Rao A, Marsden JR, Armstrong CJ, Berhane S, Billingham LJ, et al. Phase I/II trial of a dendritic cell vaccine transfected with DNA encoding melan A and gp100 for patients with metastatic melanoma. Gene Ther. 2011;18(6) 584-93.

[65] Ribas A, Camacho LH, Lee SM, Hersh EM, Brown CK, Richards JM, et al. Multicenter phase II study of matured dendritic cells pulsed with melanoma cell line lysates in patients with advanced melanoma. J Transl Med. 2010;8 89.

[66] Ribas A, Comin-Anduix B, Chmielowski B, Jalil J, de la Rocha P, McCannel TA, et al. Dendritic cell vaccination combined with CTLA4 blockade in patients with metastatic melanoma. Clin Cancer Res. 2009;15(19) 6267-76.

[67] Okada H, Kalinski P, Ueda R, Hoji A, Kohanbash G, Donegan TE, et al. Induction of CD8+ T-cell responses against novel glioma-associated antigen peptides and clinical

activity by vaccinations with {alpha}-type 1 polarized dendritic cells and polyinosinic-polycytidylic acid stabilized by lysine and carboxymethylcellulose in patients with recurrent malignant glioma. J Clin Oncol. 2011;29(3) 330-6.

[68] Schreiber RD, Old LJ, Smyth MJ. Cancer immunoediting: integrating immunity's roles in cancer suppression and promotion. Science. 2011;331(6024) 1565-70.

[69] Zhao X, Bose A, Komita H, Taylor JL, Chi N, Lowe DB, et al. Vaccines targeting tumor blood vessel antigens promote CD8(+) T cell-dependent tumor eradication or dormancy in HLA-A2 transgenic mice. J Immunol. 2012;188(4) 1782-8.

[70] Zhao X, Bose A, Komita H, Taylor JL, Kawabe M, Chi N, et al. Intratumoral IL-12 gene therapy results in the crosspriming of Tc1 cells reactive against tumor-associated stromal antigens. Mol Ther. 2011;19(4) 805-14.

[71] Najjar YG, Rini BI. Novel agents in renal carcinoma: a reality check. Ther Adv Med Oncol. 2012;4(4) 183-94.

[72] Koshenkov VP, Rodgers SE. Adjuvant therapy of gastrointestinal stromal tumors. Curr Opin Oncol. 2012;24(4) 414-8.

[73] Minor DR, Kashani-Sabet M, Garrido M, O'Day SJ, Hamid O, Bastian BC. Sunitinib therapy for melanoma patients with KIT mutations. Clin Cancer Res. 2012;18(5) 1457-63.

[74] de Jonge MJ, Dumez H, Kitzen JJ, Beuselinck B, Verweij J, Courtney R, et al. Phase I safety and pharmacokinetic study of SU-014813 in combination with docetaxel in patients with advanced solid tumours. Eur J Cancer. 2011;47(9) 1328-35.

[75] Ko JS, Rayman P, Ireland J, Swaidani S, Li G, Bunting KD, et al. Direct and differential suppression of myeloid-derived suppressor cell subsets by sunitinib is compartmentally constrained. Cancer Res. 2010;70(9) 3526-36.

[76] Ko JS, Zea AH, Rini BI, Ireland JL, Elson P, Cohen P, et al. Sunitinib mediates reversal of myeloid-derived suppressor cell accumulation in renal cell carcinoma patients. Clin Cancer Res. 2009;15(6) 2148-57.

[77] Finke JH, Rini B, Ireland J, Rayman P, Richmond A, Golshayan A, et al. Sunitinib reverses type-1 immune suppression and decreases T-regulatory cells in renal cell carcinoma patients. Clin Cancer Res. 2008;14(20) 6674-82.

[78] Olsson AK, Dimberg A, Kreuger J, Claesson-Welsh L. VEGF receptor signalling - in control of vascular function. Nat Rev Mol Cell Biol. 2006;7(5) 359-71.

[79] Rini BI, Escudier B, Tomczak P, Kaprin A, Szczylik C, Hutson TE, et al. Comparative effectiveness of axitinib versus sorafenib in advanced renal cell carcinoma (AXIS): a randomised phase 3 trial. Lancet. 2011;378(9807) 1931-9.

[80] Hu-Lowe DD, Zou HY, Grazzini ML, Hallin ME, Wickman GR, Amundson K, et al. Nonclinical antiangiogenesis and antitumor activities of axitinib (AG-013736), an or-

al, potent, and selective inhibitor of vascular endothelial growth factor receptor tyrosine kinases 1, 2, 3. Clin Cancer Res. 2008;14(22) 7272-83.

[81] Fruehauf J, Lutzky J, McDermott D, Brown CK, Meric JB, Rosbrook B, et al. Multicenter, phase II study of axitinib, a selective second-generation inhibitor of vascular endothelial growth factor receptors 1, 2, and 3, in patients with metastatic melanoma. Clin Cancer Res. 2011;17(23) 7462-9.

[82] Bose A, Lowe DB, Rao A, Storkus WJ. Combined vaccine+axitinib therapy yields superior antitumor efficacy in a murine melanoma model. Melanoma Res. 2012;22(3) 236-43.

[83] Antonescu CR, Busam KJ, Francone TD, Wong GC, Guo T, Agaram NP, et al. L576P KIT mutation in anal melanomas correlates with KIT protein expression and is sensitive to specific kinase inhibition. Int J Cancer. 2007;121(2) 257-64.

[84] Buettner R, Mesa T, Vultur A, Lee F, Jove R. Inhibition of Src family kinases with dasatinib blocks migration and invasion of human melanoma cells. Mol Cancer Res. 2008;6(11) 1766-74.

[85] Jilaveanu LB, Zito CR, Aziz SA, Chakraborty A, Davies MA, Camp RL, et al. In vitro studies of dasatinib, its targets and predictors of sensitivity. Pigment Cell Melanoma Res. 2011;24(2) 386-9.

Section 2

Melanoma Related Features

Chapter 10

Immunomodulation

Konstantinos Arnaoutakis, Dorothy A. Graves,
Laura F. Hutchins and Thomas Kieber-Emmons

Additional information is available at the end of the chapter

1. Introduction

Immune treatment for melanoma has roots in clinical observations surrounding regression of normal nevi, the appearance of halo nevi, the correlation of vitiligo with outcome, the occurrence of spontaneous regression of primary melanomas, nodal metastases of unknown primary lesions and the occurrence of metastases many years after resection of a primary lesion. Coupling these observations with the observations on the power of the immune system to reject transplanted organs and control leukemia after allogeneic bone marrow transplant, the possibility of harnessing and directing this power has been a source of both excitement and disappointment.

In examining the natural history of normal nevi, it is noted that they undergo a life cycle in which growth occurs during childhood in the border of the epidermis and dermis (junctional nevi). With increasing age the melanocytes move deeper into the dermis. As adult life continues they regress in old age. It is not evident that this type of regression has an immune basis.

Another type of regression called halo nevi is more definitively tied to the immune system [1]. Akasu, et. al have described halo nevi regression in four stages characterized initially by pan-T lymphocytes in stage one and the addition of KP-1 positive cells as well as FX IIIa-positive cells in stage two. Stage three continues with increased numbers of FX IIIa-positive cells and the addition of Langerhans cells. Finally upon complete regression in stage four there is a moderate mononuclear infiltrate comprised predominantly of T cells [2]. The role of natural killer (NK) cells has been studied in normal and malignant melanocytic lesions. The highest concentration of NK cells was seen in regressing malignant lesions followed by regressing normal nevi [3]. This type of "spontaneous" regression is observed in other benign skin lesions such as keratoachanthomas, and the pathologic studies give insight into the possibility of stimulating similar immune action against malignancies [1, 2].

The autoimmune condition of vitiligo has been associated with regression of metastases as well as better outcomes associated with immunotherapy. Vitiligo is mediated through autoantibodies. Antibodies against tyrosinase have been observed in patients with melanoma as well as vitiligo not associated with melanoma. Other autoimmune effects are well documented with immunotherapeutic treatments, indicating the ability of the therapy to break tolerance to self-antigens [4-7].

Spontaneous regression is observed in primary melanoma [8, 9]. Statistics vary on the incidence but may be as high as 20%, especially if cases of unknown primary are included. When remnants of primary lesions are found, they frequently are partially regressed and show histologic evidence of infiltration by lymphocytes. Although some have observed a worse clinical outcome with partially regressed primary lesions, patients with nodal metastases and unknown primaries tend to have a better outcome. The latter observation is attributed to improved immune surveillance compared to patients with intact primaries [10-14]. Regression of metastases is less common and has anecdotally been tied to infections or surgeries. Regression of metastases seems to predict a better overall outcome [15, 16].

The issue of late metastases from primary melanoma is well documented but much harder to explain. Issues within the tumor microenvironment remain incompletely explored, but high on the list of explanations is the possibility that the immune system is able to control proliferation until some as yet undocumented effect allows escape [17, 18].

Early studies with nonspecific therapies described below produced enough positive results to keep interest in melanoma immunotherapy alive. However, progress in the clinic has been slow until very recently. Many issues have presented challenges to progress. Among them is an incomplete understanding of the normal immune system, including immune tolerance and the effects of the tumor microenvironment on the immune response. Drug development required technology to produce biologic agents, and that capability has only recently been perfected. Issues of study design also need to be kept in mind. Subject selection can be difficult since these studies require immune competence but disease advanced enough to answer the question in a reasonable time frame with a reasonable number of subjects.

2. Biomarkers and endpoints

Biomarkers and surrogate endpoints are tools to obtain information about disease status or response to interventions. The mainstay of efficacy determination in cancer therapeutic clinical trials has been the regression of known tumor masses listed as complete response (CR), partial response (PR), stable disease (SD) or progressive disease (PD) along with various survival endpoints: overall survival (OS), disease free survival (DFS) and progression free survival (PFS). Each of these endpoints is defined by the study. The response criteria have been standardized by various systems. The World Health Organization (WHO) developed the most commonly used system called response criteria for solid tumors (RECIST) [19]. Recent developments in assessing response during trials utilizing the drug, ipilimumab, have served to highlight differences in direct cytotoxic chemotherapy responses and those seen with immunotherapy. The responses in tumor measurement seen in the ipilimumab trials did not correspond to the survival endpoints. Subjects had prolonged survival with delayed or no tumor measurement changes. These observations have led to a new system for assessing immune based therapies called immune-related response criteria (irRC) [20].

Biomarkers can serve to assess efficacy, but it is difficult to find results that consistently correlate with clinical response. Some assays can serve as immunologic endpoints in addition to or instead of tumor regression, PFS and OS in clinical studies. The most frequent measurements include: antibody titers, delayed type hypersensitivity (DTH) skin tests, enzyme-linked immunosorbent assay (ELISA), enzyme-linked immunospot assay (ELISPOT), tetramer markers of antigen specific T cells and other assays indicating that the therapy induced a response toward its target [21-25].

All of these issues should be considered in assessing the past studies and in the planning of future studies. As we will discuss, progress has been made and enthusiasm is at an all-time high.

2.1. Patient selection

Predicting response to treatment is probably the best way to increase benefit from a variety of different immunotherapy agents that are currently approved or under investigation for the treatment of early stage (as adjuvant therapy) or advanced melanoma. Identifying patients that are likely to respond to these agents would spare patients unnecessary toxicities and encourage more research in the field.

Response to treatment may be determined by clinical characteristics or by the presence or level of biomarkers in the serum or tissue that predict a robust response to immunotherapy agents. Clinical characteristics such as ulcerated lesions appear to get more benefit from interferon (IFN) in the adjuvant setting [26]. In addition, Eastern Cooperative Oncology Group (ECOG) performance status, the number of involved organs and sites of metastases appear to be treatment factors predicting response to interleukin 2 (IL-2) in some studies [27].

The appearance of serum autoantibodies or clinical manifestations of autoimmunity during treatment with IFNα-2b was associated with improved outcomes in patients with melanoma [28]. In addition, multiplexed analysis of serum cytokines appeared to be potentially useful as a predictive marker of response to IFNα-2b in patients with high-risk operable melanoma [29]. A serum proteomic analysis has been found to possibly predict response to IL-2 treatment [30]. In this study, high pretreatment serum vascular endothelial growth factor (VEGF) and fibronectin levels were predictive of resistance to treatment. A marker of potential interest in ipilimumab therapy appears to be the absolute lymphocyte count [31]. Absolute lymphocyte counts that exceeded 1×10^9/L at the time of the third ipilimumab dose were associated with a survival benefit at one year. Immune responses to NY-ESO-1, a cancer-testis antigen, also appear to correlate with clinical benefit from ipilimumab [32].

Gene signatures within the tumor have also shown some correlation with clinical benefit both for IL-2 and vaccination [33, 34]. Little is known about some of the newer drugs such as the CTLA-4 antagonists (ipilimumab) or other checkpoint inhibitors. It has been suggested that the presence of PD-L1 expression detected by immunohistochemistry may predict response to PD-1 antibody therapy [35].

Undoubtedly, utilizing serum and tissue biomarkers for response to treatment is much more challenging for immunotherapy than in the field of molecular targeted therapies. For example V600E BRAF mutations predict treatment response in patients who receive vemurafenib, a BRAF inhibitor. In melanoma immunotherapy, however, no serum or tissue biomarkers have yet been prospectively studied in the context of a clinical trial.

3. Immunoregulatory barriers, immune tolerance and tumor microenvironment

The immune system is designed to protect our bodies from foreign agents. This protection is selective, such that host tissues are recognized as self and preserved (termed immunologic tolerance), while other agents are recognized as foreign and targeted for killing. Cancer cells, however, present the immune system with a unique challenge. While some, such as virally transformed cells, express foreign viral proteins on their surface, most tumors express normal proteins and carbohydrates. Efforts to understand how tumors survive immunosurveillance versus how and when they are targeted for killing have preoccupied scientists for well over half a century. This section explores what we currently know about the complex interplay between the immune system and cancer cells as it relates to immunotherapy.

We know now that tumor cells are immunogenic but efficacy is limited due to the lack of robustness of the response. There are two primary reasons for this: 1) due to the nature of the immunogens (self antigens) and 2) the active role-played by tumors to suppress the response. The mammalian anti-tumor response engages both the humoral and cell-mediated arms of the immune system through both specific (adaptive) and non-specific (innate) effectors. While cytotoxic T lymphocytes (CTLs), NK cells and T helper (TH) cells are viewed as the most significant players in the anti-tumor response, they are not alone [36]. Antigen presenting cells (APCs - macrophages and dendritic cells) are absolutely essential to stimulate a variety of anti-tumor responses across tumor types, and anti-tumor antibodies are often easily found in patients with melanoma and many other solid tumors, indicating a strong humoral response following stimulation by antigen specific TH cells [37]. There is accumulating evidence that the CD4+ T cell population is far more involved in the anti-tumor response than previously thought [38, 39]. When APCs present antigen to TH cells in the context of a major histocompatibility complex (MHC) molecule on their surface, TH cells become activated and can stimulate B cells to result in the proliferation of antibody-producing plasma cells and CTLs to result in direct killing of the tumor cells. NK cells and macrophages can also directly kill tumor cells alone or with the help of antibodies or complement.

3.1. Melanoma antigenicity

The goal of cancer immunotherapy is to provoke the immune system to generate a tumor cell rejection strength response and to prevent recurrence of cancer by establishing long-term effector cell memory. In order for the immune system to mount an attack against melanoma, it must first recognize the involved tumor cells as foreign or in need of clearing (a danger signal); it can then target them for killing. Tumor cells, like all cells, display a variety of proteins on their cell surface, and when antigen is presented in the context of MHC, the cell may be recognized by the T cell receptor (TCR) on an effector T lymphocyte. Tumor cells in general and melanoma tissues specifically, are antigenically diverse, and their ability to survive correlates with the ability of the tumor antigens to avoid detection by the immune system [40, 41]. Highly antigenic tumor cells are killed off rather quickly, due to the immune system's ability to recognize the tumor cells and mount an effective immune response, while poorly antigenic tumor cells thrive. Tumor specific transplantation antigens (TSTAs) generally convey strong immunogenicity. These are antigens expressed on the surface of tumor cells that are specific to that tumor or type of tumor. However, the majority of antigens associated with melanoma cells are tumor associated transplantation antigens, or TATAs. TATAs are antigens that are associated with tumor cells, but not unique to tumor cells. TATAs are far better at preserving a tumor cell under the radar of the immune system, because these antigens are not danger signals.

Within the tumor microenvironment, tolerance may be naturally overcome by antigen expression levels or the timing of antigen expression. Melanomas overexpress many antigens that are present in normal melanocytes but at lower levels, and expression of these antigens suggest a progression of differentiation from normal melanocytes to melanomas. For example, a melanoma expressing a mutant triosephosphate isomerase protein was discovered to bind MHC class II at five times greater affinity than the wild type oligopeptide, resulting in both a significant increase in surface expression and an increase in immunogenicity [42]. Some melanoma cells overexpress the transferrin receptor by a factor of 100 [43]. Some human melanomas overexpress the gangliosides relative to levels seen in normal melanocytes, illustrating that overexpression of carbohydrates can attract the attention of the immune system, similar to protein antigens [44].

Much of melanoma's antigenicity comes from the more than 100 identified melanoma TATAs. Melan-A/MART-1, gp100 and tyrosinase are well studied differentiation antigens expressed in both primary and metastatic melanoma [45-53].

Melanoma cells may also express oncofetal antigens which are normally displayed during embryogenesis but only expressed in select tissues, if at all, in adults. These include the cancer germ-line/cancer-testis (CT) antigens. MAGE-A family members and NY-ESO-1 are the most significant members of this group to date, and expression of MAGE-A1 and MAGE-A4 increases with tumor progression [47, 54, 55]. NY-ESO-1 is only expressed in adults in testis and placenta tissue, however, it is expressed in up to 40% of late stage melanomas and is highly immunogenic [56]. MAGE-6 is expressed in more than 70% of metastatic melanomas [57].

Identification of melanoma TATAs is crucial as a key strategy for immunotherapy. Administration of vaccines that deliver TATAs can push the immune system into overcoming tolerance. T cells specific for TATAs have been identified in melanoma patients, and spontaneously occurring circulating T cells reactive to Melan-A and NY-ESO-1 were recently found to be predictive of better survival [58]. A recent study reported an analysis of the human leukocyte antigen 1 (HLA-I) peptidomes from melanomas in four patients, and while finding that melanoma antigenicity was highly variable, the investigators also found that the peptidomes were highly immunogenic, identifying new potential peptides for melanoma vaccines [41].

3.2. Immunoevasion strategies

Tumor cells increase their odds of survival by lowering their immunological profiles. TH cells, CTLs and antibodies specific for TATAs are readily detectable in the blood, lymph nodes and tumors of cancer patients. Despite tolerance, the immune system can mount an immune response to these antigens, but tumors and/or tumor cells may persist, so all the efforts of the immune system are not enough to clear tumor cells. The immunoevasion strategies utilized by melanomas are impressive and generally include down-regulation of TATAs on the tumor cell surface, secretion of immunosuppressive cytokines that affect APCs and shedding of material that promotes the stimulation of the inhibitory regulatory T cells (Tregs). Together, these strategies create a toleragenic tumor microenvironment that is both adaptive to immune pressures and predictive of clinical outcomes.

Many tumor cells stop displaying TATAs or TSTAs on their surface to escape immune recognition [59]. Expression of MART-1, gp100 and tyrosinase generally decreases as melanoma progresses [60]. Following immunization with gp100 or MART-1 peptides, melanoma metastases lost expression of the corresponding TATA, suggesting that TATAs can be downregulated in direct response to a specific CTL anti-tumor response [45]. This strategy is specifically adaptive to removing known CTL targets from the tumor population and selects for proliferation of tumor cells that do not bear antigens yet targeted by the CTL response.

Tumor cells may additionally repress expression of MHC class I proteins by repressing MHC I gene expression or posttranslational modifications [59]. In fact, many human tumors demonstrate a decreased expression of MHC I, and the loss of MHC I expression is often associated with more invasive and metastatic tumors [61, 62]. In melanoma, MHC I expression correlates with disease progression, and the lack of HLA I expression and lack of response to T cell based immunotherapy may be linked to acquired β2-microglobulin gene defects [63-65]. C-myc oncogene overexpression in melanoma also correlates with HLA I downregulation [66]. The one caveat of this strategy, however, is that a total lack of MHC expression invites attack by NK cells [67]. To circumvent this, tumor cells often only lower MHC I expression, retaining some minimal expression to protect themselves while not alarming the immune system.

Tumors in general create microenvironments with depressed immune activity such that few functional cytotoxic cells are found near the developing tumor. One strategy for this involves the poorly understood regulation of lymphocyte types within the tumor microenvironment. Moderate to large numbers of tumor infiltrating lymphocytes (TILs) have been associated with improved survival in melanoma patients; however this has not been observed consistently [68, 69]. While most patients with melanoma have TILs, the mere presence of TILs is obviously not sufficient to mount an effective anti-tumor response [70]. Tumor cells are able to attract a particular type of T cell that is immunosuppressive. Tregs can directly inhibit and kill CTLs and TH cells, and they functionally drive the tumor's T helper Type 2 (Th-2) immune environment by producing the immunosuppressive cytokines IL-10 and tumor growth factor beta (TGF-β) while suppressing CTL production of immunostimulatory T helper Type 1 (Th-1) cytokines interferon gamma (IFN γ) and IL-2 [71]. Tregs also negatively regulate effector dendritic cells and NK cells. In melanoma, depletion of Tregs prior to infusion with activated T lymphocytes (adoptive cell therapy) measurably improves response rates [72].

Melanoma cells may also create an immunosuppressed microenvironment through galectin expression [73]. Deregulation of galectins is common in human tumors. Expression of galectin 3 correlates with melanoma metastasis and poorer disease outcomes, perhaps through induction of TIL apoptosis. Galectin 1 may also induce apoptosis of T cells and this may be an important mechanism of tumor evasion for melanoma. Additionally, galectins 1 and 3 convey resistance to apoptosis in tumor cells, though this is less studied in melanoma.

Immunosuppression similar to that found in the tumor microenvironment can also be found in the sentinel lymph node [71, 74]. Tregs are found in higher numbers in metastatic melanoma sentinel lymph nodes, and as in the tumor microenvironment, this appears to be mediated by Th-2 cytokines IL-6, IL-8, IL-10 and TGF-β, among others. This locoregional immunosupporession is thought to be necessary for metastasis and prepares the lymphatic environment for the arrival and survival of metastastic cells [75]. While dendritic cells are detectable in melanoma sentinel lymph nodes, they may be present in lower number and/or contain a higher percentage of immature dendritic cells that lack the costimulatory molecules necessary for effective T cell activation [74, 76].

IL-10 and TGF-β are immunosuppressive cytokines utilized by melanoma to create an immunosuppressive microenvironment and progress disease toward metastasis [77, 78]. Both cytokines can induce T cells to undergo apoptosis; TGF-β can additionally induce apoptosis in dendritic cells and macrophages. Normal melanocytes are subject to TGF-β anti-proliferative regulation, and loss of this phenotype is thought to be a crucial step toward melanoma development [77]. Neutrophils from patients with melanoma constitutively and spontaneously synthesize IL-10 through activation by serum amyloid A 1 (SAA-1) which is enriched in melanoma tissue [79].

There are a variety of other general tumor microenvironment conditions and immunoevasion strategies that melanomas employ to ensure their survival. Hypoxia occurs in solid tumor masses and is well known to create an immunosuppressive tumor microenvironment [80]. Tumor cells can also alter the expression of stress proteins that bind NK cells for targeted killing. Melanoma cells predominantly express the MICA and ULBP2 stress proteins, and a correlation has been found between poor prognosis and expression of soluble ULBP2 that is competitive for NK cell binding [81, 82]. Heat shock proteins are well known to promote tumor growth, invasion and metastasis through a variety of mechanisms [83]. Expression of heat shock proteins 90 and 40 (hsp90 and hsp40) in melanoma tissue correlates with advanced disease and patient survival, in the case of hsp40 [84].

It is important to remember that while immune evasion and creation of an immunsuppressive tumor microenvironment is highly variable among melanomas, the ability of the tumor to effectively create a strong toleragenic microenvironment correlates with clinical outcome. Toleragenic tumor microenvironments are associated with sentinel lymph node involvement and more advanced disease [74]. Efforts to overcome this tolerance and re-capitulate the balance of immune system regulators to a state of anti-tumor effectiveness comprise the field of immunotherapy, and success in this therapeutic approach holds tremendous promise for not only halting tumor progression but for turning back the clock to ultimately result in tumor clearance.

3.3. Immunotherapy strategies

Most immunotherapy efforts strive to activate T cells and specifically CTLs. Therapeutic melanoma vaccines may enhance antigen presentation directly through peptides or DNA. A synthetic peptide vaccine targeted to the melanoma gp100 TATA, for example, has resulted in good objective clinical responses [85]. Vaccines may also rely on the assistance of dendritic cells, a key stimulator of immune cells [86-88]. The goal is to utilize TSTA or TATA antigens to provoke the development and proliferation of cytotoxic cells directed against tumor cells, thereby overcoming tolerance.

Adoptive cell transfer or therapy (ACT) is a passive immunotherapeutic approach in which a patient's antigen-specific cells are expanded and activated *ex vivo* and then reintroduced following radiation or chemotherapy [89]. TILs, autologous T cell clones, donor anti-tumor lymphocytes and genetically engineered lymphocytes have all been used in this strategy. Some encouraging results have been seen in melanoma patients with advanced disease [90]. In three separate trials, autologous TILs provided through ACT and administered with IL-2 to metastatic melanoma patients resulted in up to a 72% objective response rate, and 22% of the 93 subjects had complete tumor regression [91]. ACT employing autologous T cells targeting NY-ESO-1 resulted in objective responses in five of 11 metastatic melanoma patients and two complete regressions at one-year post-procedure [92]. While it is argued that ACT is more effective in metastatic melanoma than ipilimumab (see below), it is practically more complex to administer and less accessible for a majority of patients [90].

Cytokines have shown efficacy in high risk local and metastatic melanoma patients as well. IL-2 and IFNα-2b have been investigated the most. IL-2 alone produces a durable remission in some patients, though it is often associated with significant side effects, and better outcomes may be obtained by combining it with other therapeutic approaches [93]. A pooled analysis of nearly 2,000 stage IIB and III melanoma patients indicated that adjuvant high dose IFNα-2b prolongs relapse free survival in patients [94].

At present, the greatest promise for metastatic melanoma patients lies in immunomodulatory antibody therapy against immunological checkpoints. Immunotherapies that employ this targeting strategy are recent and have yielded some of the most promising clinical responses in decades. Immunological checkpoints are negative regulators of the immune system. Cytotoxic T lymphocyte antigen 4 (CTLA4) is found on naïve T cells and Tregs; upon activation it turns off TCR signaling and serves to stop activation of targeted T cells. Antibodies to CTLA4 prevent this from happening and prolong and intensify T cell activation [36]. Ipilimumab was approved by the U.S. Food and Drug Administration (FDA) in 2012 for the treatment of metastatic melanoma owing to the overall survival benefit observed in a phase III study that has now resulted in durable responses lasting 8 years and beyond [95]. Although ipilimumab is the only FDA-approved checkpoint inhibitor indicated for treatment of melanoma, there are others in the pipeline [96]. Tremelimumab is another CTLA4 antibody, and there are several programmed death ligand 1 (PD-1) antibodies undergoing clinical development as well [97, 98]. Though both CTLA4 and PD-1 antibodies have demonstrated significant improvement in clinical outcome for metastatic melanoma patients, they are not effective in all patients and cause a new and unique spectrum of side effects termed "immune-related adverse events."

4. Nonspecific immune therapy and adjuvants

The success of anti-tumor and antiviral vaccines often requires the use of an adjuvant, a substance that significantly enhances the immune response to a coadministered antigen. Only a handful of adjuvants have both sufficient potency and acceptable toxicity for clinical investigation. The critical roles of vaccine adjuvants lie in their ability to: (1) enable the use of otherwise impotent antigens; (2) extend the benefits of vaccination to poor responders (e.g., older or immune-compromised patients); and (3) effect dose-sparing of rare and expensive antigens in short supply (e.g., during an epidemic) [99]. Vaccine adjuvants for the most part can be evaluated as such only when they are associated with a vaccine. Early therapies were nonspecific and were thought to produce a general immune response. Many current vaccine trials utilize nonspecific immune stimulants as adjuncts.

4.1. BCG

Adjuvant therapy of melanoma assumes that treatment will be more effective when the tumor burden is small. Mycobacterium bovis bacillus Calmette-Guérin (BCG) is an old vaccine/adjuvant used in countries where tuberculosis is widespread. First used in humans in 1921, BCG is made from a strain of weakened bovine tuberculosis bacterium. The local and systemic effect of BCG has been known for decades and is an immunomodulating agent for melanoma. BCG therapy induces a massive local immune response characterized by the expression of multiple cytokines. A significant correlation between a reduced risk of melanoma and BCG and vaccinia vaccination in early childhood or infectious diseases later in life has already been reported from the FEBrile Infections and Melanoma (FEBIM) multicenter case-control study [100]. Such observations suggest that BCG can augment immune responses and be used in adjuvant therapy strategies.

Phase II trials indicate that active specific immunotherapy can alter the natural course of American Joint Committee on Cancer [AJCC] Stage III and IV melanoma following surgical resection of nodal or distant metastases. Initial adjuvant immunotherapy trials demonstrated a greater disease-free interval in patients treated with BCG compared with historical controls [101]. In one study 149 patients at high risk of recurrence after surgical treatment of local or regional malignant melanoma were given BCG for 2 years and were followed up for a median of 28 months from the start of immunotherapy [101]. Studies such as these suggest that improved survival rates following recurrence might be explained by the pattern of recurrence; suggesting local or regional sites might be more responsive to treatment. Mechanistic studies suggest that tumor necrosis factor (TNF)-related apoptosis-inducing ligand (TRAIL) is induced by BCG treatment. Subsequently, BCG and components of the mycobacterial cell wall can directly stimulate the release of soluble TRAIL through toll-like receptor-2 (TLR2) recognition that is augmented by IFN. Based on the need for a Th-1 cytokine response to BCG therapy for therapeutic results, it might be proposed that cells migrating in response to BCG treatment release TRAIL. In addition, IFN acts to augment and prolong the amount of TRAIL released by effector cells, resulting in an effective therapeutic outcome.

Early trials of BCG-based immunotherapy for melanoma consistently showed a trend toward improved clinical outcomes in patients treated with BCG compared with observation alone (reviewed by [102]). However, mature results of a phase III randomized trial of BCG versus observation and BCG plus dacarbazine versus BCG in the adjuvant therapy of AJCC stage I-III melanoma (E1673: an ECOG trial) ascribes no benefit for BCG for this patient population [103]. As early as 1976 BCG was tested as an immunotherapy systemic adjunct to surgery in malignant melanoma [104]. In 1984 a polyvalent BCG formulation along with Canvaxin began testing in phase II trials as postsurgical adjuvant therapy for stage III melanoma [105], with results from such trials summarized as no apparent benefit from vaccination [106, 107].

Although experiments with animals have demonstrated that BCG mediates anti-tumor activity, most randomized adjuvant clinical trials have failed to show significant benefit to patients with malignant melanoma. This may be because there is no accepted clinical technique for monitoring *in vivo* BCG activity. As a result the optimal route of administration and dose of BCG have not been truly determined as well as the optimal BCG strain. Attempts to improve the efficacy of BCG therapy have been made. One approach introduced the gene encoding the 65 kDa hsp of Mycobacterium tuberculosis into a mouse malignant melanoma cell line (B16) as proof of principle [108].The 65 kDa hsp was expressed after gene transduction and significantly enhanced the anti-tumor effect of BCG immunotherapy, further indicating that CD4+ T cells play an important role in this anti-tumor effect.

4.2. DETOX

Many adjuvants currently under evaluation for use in cancer vaccines activate relevant APCs, such as dendritic cells and macrophages, via TLRs and promote effective uptake, processing and presentation of antigen to T-cells in draining lymph nodes. The Gram-negative bacterial cell constituent lipopolysaccharide (LPS) is known to possess strong immunostimulatory properties and has been evaluated as an adjuvant for promoting immune responses to minimally immunogenic antigens, including TATAs. The relatively recent discovery of TLRs and the identification of TLR4, in particular, as the signaling receptor for lipid A have allowed for a better understanding of how this immunostimulant functions with regard to induction of innate and adaptive immune responses. Local TLR stimulation is an attractive approach to induce anti-tumor immunity. Tumor cells respond to TLR ligands with an increase in MHC class I expression and induce IL-6 secretion *in vitro*. Melanoma cells are typically characterized as having low expression of MHC I. Consequently TLR ligands interacting with melanoma cells might enhance MHC class I expression, along with their targeting by melanoma specific CTLs. Although several lipid A species, including LPS and synthetic analogs, have been developed and tested as monotherapeutics for the treatment of cancer, monophosphoryl lipid A (MPL), a ligand for TLR4 has been evaluated as a cancer vaccine adjuvant in published human clinical trials. MPL comprises the lipid A portion of Salmonella minnesota LPS [109]. LPS and MPL induce similar cytokine profiles, but MPL is at least 100-fold less toxic.

DETOX, an adjuvant consisting of MPL and purified mycobacterial cell-wall skeleton (CWS) is another vaccine potentiating agent. MPL (Corixa Corp., Seattle, Washington, USA) adjuvant is a chemically modified LPS derivative that displays greatly reduced toxicity while maintaining most of the immunostimulatory activity of LPS [110] signaling through TLR4 to stimulate the innate immune system. MPL adjuvant has been used extensively in clinical trials as a component in prophylactic and therapeutic vaccines targeting infectious disease, cancer and allergies. MPL has been administered to more than 300,000 human subjects in studies of next-generation vaccines, emerging as a safe and effective vaccine adjuvant. In one study DETOX markedly potentiated antibody but had little effect on DTH responses to melanoma vaccine immunization. It did not appear to improve DFS in comparison to alum in this non-randomized study [111]. DETOX has been formulated into Melacine (Corixa Corp.), a vaccine prepared from the lysate of two melanoma cell lines adjuvanted with DETOX. In clinical trials with Melacine, tumor progression is delayed in the vaccine-treated patients, although this was only observed in patients with certain HLA phenotypes.

The potency of local TLR treatment in therapy demonstrates that local treatment with TLR adjuvants like MPL might effectively restore anti-tumor immunity. Melacine is available for sale in Canada.

4.3. QS-21

Saponins are natural glycosides of steroid or triterpene which exhibit many different biological and pharmacological activities [112]. Notably, saponins can activate the mammalian immune system, and this has led to significant interest in their potential as vaccine adjuvants. The most widely used saponin-based adjuvants are Quil A and its derivative QS-21, isolated from the bark of the Quillaja saponaria Molina (Chilean soap bark tree); these have been evaluated in numerous clinical trials [113]. Their unique capacity to stimulate both the Th-1 immune response and the production of CTLs against exogenous antigens makes them ideal for use in subunit vaccines and vaccines directed against intracellular pathogens as well as cancer.

QS-21 possesses an ability to clinically augment significant antibody and T cell responses to vaccine antigens against a variety of infectious diseases, degenerative disorders and cancers. Currently, there exists no rapid *in vitro* biological screen for assessing the potential efficacy of saponin vaccine adjuvants, given that the mechanism by which saponins augment the immune response is unknown. As a result, evaluation of novel saponins as immunostimulants typically proceed directly to preclinical studies involving mouse vaccination with antigens [99, 112-114].

QS-21 appears to augment both Th-1 and Th-2 type responses and to favor the *in vivo* priming of antigen-specific CD8+ cytotoxic cells. QS-21 has been used in a variety of melanoma targeting vaccines [115]. QS-21 has been shown to be superior to some vaccine formulations such as GM2-KLH plus QS-21 vaccine compared to GM2/BCG vaccine [115]. Efforts to further advance QS-21 in the clinic, as well as to illuminate its unknown mechanism of action, require access to adjuvant-active samples of known composition [114]. The recent synthesis of active molecules of QS-21 has provided a robust method to produce this leading vaccine adjuvant in high purity as well as to produce novel synthetic QS-21 congeners designed to induce increased immune responsiveness and decreased toxicity [99, 112-114].

4.4. Montanide

Mineral oils are known to be very efficient adjuvants but can sometimes induce local reactions with reactive antigens. In contrast, non-mineral oils are well tolerated but less effective with poor immunogens. Mineral oils stay at the injection site and are progressively eliminated by competent cells like the macrophages. They can also be partially metabolized into fatty acids, triglycerides, phospholipids or sterols. Water in oil emulsions represent one of the new promising generations of adjuvants for immunotherapy [116-118]. In this class both Montanide ISA 51 and 720 have been tested in animals and thousands of individuals and found to be safe. Nevertheless, the proper antigen concentration has yet to be established [116-118]. Adverse effects usually depend on the concentration and nature of the antigen.

The mechanistic premise of emulsions is the "depot" effect, in which the adjuvant protects the antigen from both dilution and rapid degradation and elimination by the host. By localizing and slowly releasing intact antigen, the adjuvant permits a slow, prolonged exposure of the immune system cells to a low level of antigen. This prolonged exposure results in continued stimulation of antibody producing cells, resulting in the production of high levels of antibody by the host.

MONTANIDE™ ISA 51 VG has been used in Phase I and II clinical trials for vaccines against malaria, HIV, and various cancers. MONTANIDE™ ISA 51 VG, has been tested in AIDS and cancer vaccine trials which together represent more than 10,000 patients and around 100,000 injections. A survey of ongoing clinical trials listed in ClinicalTrials.gov revealed 36 trials currently accruing patients that are using the olive-derived Montanide ISA

51 IFA. The formulation is generally well-tolerated and induces transient local reactions. Some transient general reactions such as flu-like symptoms are also observed. The results suggest that numerous repeated vaccine doses can be safely administered. Immunization with tumor associated antigen peptides in combination with montanide expands tumor antigen-specific CD8+ T cells in melanoma patients [119-122].

4.5. Cyclophosphamide

High-dose cyclophosphamide (CY) has long been used as an anti-cancer agent, a conditioning regimen for hematopoietic stem cell transplantation and a potent immunosuppressive agent in autoimmune diseases including aplastic anemia. High-dose CY is highly toxic to lymphocytes but spares hematopoietic stem cells because of their abundant levels of aldehyde dehydrogenase, the major mechanism of CY inactivation. CY has emerged as a clinically feasible agent that can suppress Tregs and allow more effective induction of anti-tumor immune responses [123]. Tregs have become an important player in regulating anti-cancer immune responses, with poor prognoses often ascribed to their action [124].

Studies using low dose CY in combination with vaccine components and IL-12 continue to suggest that CY is a viable addition to affect immune responses [125]. Low-dose CY is found to selectively deplete CD4+CD25+ T cells (Tregs) and impede tolerance allowing for a more active immune response. CY preconditioning can enhance the CD8+ T cell response to peptide vaccination, thus leading to enhanced anti-tumor effects against pre-existing tumors [126]. CY markedly enhanced the magnitude of secondary but not primary CTL response induced by vaccines and synergized with vaccine in therapy but not in prophylaxis tumor models [127].

4.6. Conclusions

The major issues that need to be addressed are designing more effective melanoma vaccines with a mix of melanoma-associated antigens that can stimulate clinically beneficial anti-tumor immune responses and finding an adjuvant that can safely, easily and powerfully boost the frequency and magnitude of these responses.

5. Cytokine therapy

Cytokine therapy has had an important position in the treatment of melanoma in the adjuvant and metastatic settings. Various cytokines have been studied with variable success. The most important cytokines in melanoma treatment thus far have been IFN, IL-2, IL-21 and GM-CSF.

5.1. IFN

Interferon IFN is a pleotropic cytokine that exerts anti-tumor activity through numerous mechanisms. High-dose IFNα-2b was approved by the FDA in 1995 for adjuvant therapy of resected stage IIB and III melanoma based on the results of ECOG E1684 [128]. This was a randomized controlled study of IFNα-2b administered at doses of 20 megaunits/m^2/d intravenously (IV) 5 days per week for 1 month and 10 megaunits/m^2 3 times per week subcutaneously (s.c.) for 48 weeks versus observation in 287 patients. Through this study IFNα-2b was the first agent to show a significant benefit in relapse-free survival (RFS) and OS of high-risk melanoma patients in a randomized controlled trial. A subsequent study [129] (E1690) with a total of 642 patients evaluated the efficacy of high-dose IFNα-2b for 1 year (20 megaunits/m^2/d IV 5 days/week for 4 weeks; 10 megaunits/m^2 s.c. TIW for 48 weeks) and low-dose IFNα-2b (3 megaunits/d TIW) for 2 years versus observation in high-risk (stage IIB and III) melanoma with RFS and OS as end points. The results of the intergroup E1690 trial demonstrated a RFS benefit of IFNα-2b that was dose-dependent and significant for the high-dose INFα-2b. Neither high-dose nor low dose IFNα-2b demonstrated an OS benefit compared with observation at the time.

Pooled data from E1684 and E1690 showed that RFS, but not OS, was significantly prolonged for patients treated with high dose IFN versus observation [94]. Long term OS data from E1684 also shows a diminishing level of statistical significance (P=.02 at 7 years, but P=. 09 at 12.6 years' median follow-up) [94]. Additional studies by the Eastern Organisation for Research and Treatment of Cancer (EORTC) [130] with adjuvant pegylated IFNα-2b (6 μg/kg per week for 8 weeks followed by 3 μg/kg per week for an intended duration of 5 years) showed a similarly significant and sustained effect on RFS.

The effect of IFNα on OS has been criticized strongly since only two studies (E1684 and E1694) have shown a survival benefit. In contrast, several other studies mentioned above have shown RFS as the only benefit. A recent meta-analysis [131] showed statistically significant improvement in both RFS and OS. The meta-analysis included 14 randomized controlled trials published between 1990 and 2008 and involved 8,122 patients, of which 4,362 were allocated to the IFNα arm. Subgroup analysis and meta-regression did not identify an optimal IFNα dose, the optimal treatment duration or a subset of patients more responsive than others to the adjuvant therapy. Therefore, the role of IFN in the adjuvant setting remains controversial by many. The National Comprehensive Cancer Network (NCCN) has a 2B recommendation for the use of IFN as an adjuvant treatment, and enrollment in clinical trials is encouraged.

Single-agent IFN has demonstrated modest activity in patients with metastatic malignant melanoma with response rates between 10%-20% [132]. Most of the responses were transient and usually restricted to cutaneous metastases [133]. Therefore, its use in the metastatic setting has been employed more frequently in combination with chemotherapy (biochemotherapy) with improved response rates but without a well documented survival benefit [134]. Other cytokines have been subsequently evaluated, and the interest in IFN has been shifted to the adjuvant setting as mentioned above.

5.2. IL-2

One of the most promising immune stimulating cytokines has been interleukin 2 (IL-2). High dose IL-2 produces not only PRs but also CRs. Overall objective response rates (ORR) are approximately 16% with IL-2 with a 6% CR rate [93]. Importantly, some patients achieved durable CRs which led to the approval of high-dose IL-2 for patients with metastatic melanoma. Responses occurred with all sites of disease and in patients with large tumor burdens (unlike previously with IFN). Disease progression was not observed in any patient responding for longer than 30 months, and in some cases where disease progression was observed, durable disease free status was achieved with metastasectomy.

The use of high-dose IL-2, however, is limited by its severe toxicity; 2.2% of the patients in the National Cancer Institute (NCI) trial series died from treatment-related toxicities with bacterial sepsis being the predominant cause of death. No deaths were observed in the NCI series when antibiotic prophylaxis was implemented. However, the incidence of grade 3-4 toxicities remains high, ranging between 1-64%. Alternate regimens have been employed including low dose IL-2 alone or in combination with IFN-α or chemotherapy. However, there is evidence that suggests that high dose IL-2 is a more efficacious regimen. A phase II study showed durable CRs with high-dose bolus IL-2 in patients with metastatic melanoma who have experienced progression after biochemotherapy [135]. In addition, IL-2 based biochemotherapy regimens have not shown significantly better results than chemotherapy alone, presumptively due to the fact that high dose IL-2 is not utilized [136].

5.3. IL-21

The role of other cytokines has also been explored. IL-21 has recently emerged as a promising cytokine [137]. In an open-label, multicenter phase II study, IL-21 was given as a bolus injection on days 1 through 5 on alternate weeks using three different dosing regimens in 40 patients with malignant melanoma. Cohort 1 received 50 μg/kg per day by outpatient IV bolus injection for 5 days of each week during weeks 1, 3, and 5 of an 8-week cycle. Cohort 2 received 30 μg/kg per day on the same schedule, and cohort 3 received 50 μg/kg per day for 5 days of each week during weeks 1 and 3 of a 6-week cycle. The primary objective of the study was to assess efficacy (ORR and PFS) of IL-21 in this population. The ORR to IL-21 was 22.5%. The median PFS was 4.3 months and the median OS was 12.4 months, suggesting that this is an active agent that warrants further investigation. The 30 μg/kg per day dose and schedule was generally well tolerated as an outpatient regimen, with the most common adverse events being flu-like symptoms and rash, most of which were grade 1 or 2.

5.4. GM-CSF

Granulocyte macrophage-colony stimulating factor (GM-CSF) has also been studied mostly in the adjuvant setting. Forty-eight patients with stage III or IV melanoma were treated in a phase II trial with long-term, chronic, intermittent GM-CSF after complete surgical resection of disease [138]. The median survival duration was 37.5 months in the study patients versus 12.2 months in the matched controls. OS and DFS were significantly prolonged in patients who received GM-CSF compared with matched historical controls, and treatment was well tolerated with acceptable toxicity. A phase III prospective, randomized, placebo-controlled study (E4697) failed to show an OS benefit but improved DFS in patients with completely resected high-risk melanoma with minimal toxicity [139].

5.5. Conclusions

Immune stimulating cytokines have historically been an important part of the therapeutic armamentarium for early stage and metastatic melanoma due to the importance of the immune system in this disease. The currently approved IFN and IL-2 treatments in the adjuvant and metastatic settings, respectively, provide modest but reproducible clinical benefits. Their use is limited by toxicity and the lack of clearly defined predictive-to-treatment tools. In the near future, the development of novel molecular and immune treatments might limit their role. However, the durable responses that we see in some patients should not be ignored, and the search for predictive biomarkers should continue.

6. Vaccine therapy

The purpose of cancer vaccines is to evoke an immune response against malignant cells. One of the earliest approaches was taken more than 100 years ago when Dr. William Coley treated patients with Coley's Toxin derived from bacteria [22]. Although clinical success in individual trials has been uncommon, a meta-analysis of 56 clinical trials showed that evidence of an immune response predicted a better outcome [140]. Vaccines are of various types, each with advantages and disadvantages. The following discussion will be divided by the vaccine type, and when available, clinical data in advanced and adjuvant settings.

6.1. Autologous whole cell vaccines

Vaccines derived from the patient's own cancer should have the advantage of presenting the complete array of tumor antigens, both internal and external. There should be less chance of the remaining tumor mutating sufficiently to avoid detection. These vaccines should be able to produce both humoral and cellular immunity [141]. Autologous vaccines are produced by irradiating resected tumors or by establishing cell lines from resected specimens [22]. This approach is difficult from a technical and regulatory standpoint. It is further hampered by limiting eligible patients to those with accessible cancer and those who can wait for the vaccine development [141]. These vaccines have used the cells themselves with adjuvants or cells modified to produce cytokines.

An autologous whole cell vaccine is exemplified in work done by Berd, et. al. Early reports demonstrated clinical response to an irradiated autologous tumor cell vaccine given with BCG as an adjuvant. Subsequently, low dose CY preceded vaccination. In that study there were 5 responses in the 40 subjects assessable for response. The responses were associated with DTH responses [142]. In the next series of studies the vaccine was modified by the hapten, dinitrophenyl (DNP), and BCG and CY were maintained. Sixty two subjects with resected nodal metastases were vaccinated and compared to historical controls. There was a perceived benefit in disease progression and survival, especially in subjects over the age of

50 years [143]. In an expansion of this initial trial to 214 subjects, there was an improvement in OS in patients who developed a positive DTH response (59.3% vs 29.3%; $p < 0.001$). Forty-seven percent of subjects had a DTH response [144].

Work done by the National Biotherapy Study Group utilizing patient specific autologous tumor cell lines in patients with melanoma has been summarized [145]. This series of studies utilized different adjuvants including BCG, IFNγ and GM-CSF. Once again, benefit was seen in groups developing a positive DTH response [145-147]. Additional non-randomized studies show positive outcomes as well, but without randomization, the results are difficult to weigh [148-151]. Some studies have genetically modified the tumor cells to secret cytokines. These trials have also been non-randomized but have shown positive results [152, 153]. A randomized trial using an autologous tumor vaccine processed to extract hsps compared to physician's choice was conducted in 322 patients with metastatic disease. There was no difference between the two groups overall, but subjects with M1a disease had longer survival when treated with vaccine [154].

6.2. Allogeneic whole cell vaccines

Allogeneic whole cell vaccines are produced by a cell line or cell lines. Other features are similar to the autologous cell vaccines. The advantage of this approach is that it is more readily available and would prevent delays in treatment that are necessitated by the autologous vaccines. However the antigens may not match those of the patient's melanoma [141].

A vaccine developed by Dr. Donald Morton beginning in 1984 from three irradiated melanoma cell lines has been studied the most extensively. It is named Canvaxin (CancerVax Corp., Carlsbad, California, USA). There were extensive phase II trials done in patients with stage IV disease demonstrating response to therapy. However, when tested in randomized multicenter trials in resected stage III and IV melanoma patients, there was no benefit noted. However, the trials were stopped prior to their planned accrual by the data safety monitoring board for futility [141, 155-157]. Other allogeneic vaccines including VACCIMEL (produced from three melanoma cell lines) have had less mature study and similar biomarker results [158].

6.3. Tumor lysate vaccines

Tumor lysate vaccines have similar advantages and disadvantages of allogeneic vaccines. The vaccinia melanoma oncolysate (VMO) vaccine is prepared from four allogeneic cell lines infected with the vaccinia virus to increase immunogenicity. The cells are then lysed by sonication prior to administration. VMO yielded encouraging phase II results, however, there was no statistically significant increase in DFS when studied in an adjuvant setting [157, 159].

A second tumor lysate vaccine, called Melacine (Corixa Corp., Seattle Washington, USA) is also a cell lysate vaccine which has been tested in two large randomized trials. One adjuvant trial conducted by the Southwest Oncology Group (SWOG) studied 600 eligible patients treated with Melacine along with the adjuvant DETOX versus observation. To be eligible the subjects had to have intermediate thickness lesions and negative nodes; however, sentinel lymph node biopsy was not required, and therefore, the staging in this trial would be considered inadequate by today's standards. Survival in the overall analysis showed no difference between treatment and observation, however, a subgroup of patients expressing certain MHC classes showed a five-year survival rate of 83% compared to 59% in the observation group. This subset analysis was statistically significant [160-163]. An Ad Hoc Melanoma Working Group reported a separate study in stage III resected patients comparing high dose IFN for one year versus low lose IFN plus Melacine with DETOX for 2 years. Six hundred subjects were registered. There was no difference in outcome [164]. As described above, high dose IFN had been shown previously to be superior to observation.

6.4. Protein vaccines

Protein vaccines using purified proteins have the potential for a broader spectrum of antigens, but they can be more complex to manufacture and monitor for response [157]. The use of hsps, which have a normal function in chaperoning proteins as they are processed into peptides, has also been explored with peptide vaccines [154] and may have a role in identifying new antigenic targets [165]. A trial using NY-ESO was found to produce a strong immunologic response after vaccination. There were better clinical outcomes compared to placebo in those given the protein vaccine compared to placebo. The adjuvant used in the trial was ISCOMATRIX [166].

6.5. Ganglioside antigen vaccines

Gangliosides are non-protein antigens (glycosphingolipids containing sialic acids) that have been shown to elicit antibodies. They are present on melanoma cells (GM2, GD2, GD3) [157, 167]. The GM2 antigen plus BCG versus BCG alone was studied in stage III resected patients. There was no difference in DFS, but subjects with IgM antibodies against the antigen had better outcome [167]. GM2 conjugated to a keyhole limpet hemocyanin (KLH) and administered with the adjuvant QS-21 had better immunogenicity [168]. This same vaccine was compared to high dose IFN in an Intergroup adjuvant trial in patients with resected stage IIB or III melanoma. The trial ended when an interim analysis showed therapeutic inferiority in the vaccine arm [169].

6.6. Peptide vaccines

Peptide vaccines have the advantage of being easy to manufacture and have an excellent safety record. However, there are challenges that impact their effectiveness. These include the identification of epitopes that stimulate a T cell response, selecting an appropriate adjuvant, breaking tolerance without causing limiting autoimmunity, handling MHC restriction and assessing the need for multi-epitope vaccines [170]. Peptide vaccines have been reported to increase survival following resection of metastatic lesions [171] and have been shown to have increased immune efficacy with various adjuvants [172, 173]. Use of multiple peptides has been another strategy [121, 174, 175]. An ECOG study testing a multi-epitope vaccine with GM-CSF and/or IFNα-2b showed that an immune response to the vaccine correlated with outcome but that the cytokines did not affect outcome [176].

One of the most studied peptide vaccines is a modified gp100 peptide antigen. This vaccine has been studied in locally advanced stage III or stage IV patients comparing IL-2 to IL-2 plus vaccine. The results showed a statistically significant improvement in response rate and PFS in the vaccine arm [177]. This is in contrast to a report from the Cytokine Working Group analysis of three phase II trials looking at a similar vaccine with IL-2 showing no benefit to the addition of the vaccine [178]. Another phase III study comparing ipilimumab plus gp100 vaccine versus gp100 plus placebo versus ipilimumab plus placebo failed to show a benefit to the addition of the vaccine, and the vaccine alone was inferior [95].

6.7. Monoclonal antibodies

Anti-idiotype vaccines consist of monoclonal antibodies that mimic an antigen. The theoretical hypothesis is sound [179-181], but trials have been limited [182-184]. These vaccines have not been tested prospectively.

6.8. Viral vaccines

Viral vectors can boost the immunogenicity of the vaccines they carry [141, 185]. However the presence of neutralizing antibodies in the host could play a role [186]. Novel methods of utilizing this mode of immune stimulation are still being explored [187, 188]. A randomized trial in stage III resected patients utilizing a vaccinia viral lysate vaccine failed to show benefit [189]. Transduction of cell lines to produce expression of B7-1and IL-2 have been accomplished and show promising immunostimulatory effects [190, 191]. These techniques are difficult to pursue from a technical and regulatory standpoint. Recombinant viral vaccines have also been used to prime dendritic cells [192].

6.9. DNA vaccines

DNA vaccines have the advantage of specificity for the target for which they encode, which can simplify monitoring, but in general they have not done well in breaking tolerance [141, 193-195]. Two groups have reported on vaccines that rely on production of GM-CSF. Dranoff has reported on a vaccine utilizing melanoma cell lines engineered to produce GM-CSF and has noted improved anti-tumor effects [196]. A different approach using an intralesional vaccination with an oncolytic herpesvirus encoding GM-CSF has been developed and has had initial positive results [197, 198]. Another agent called Allovectin-7 consists of a plasmid containing DNA encoding for the MHC class I gene, HLA-B7. It was administered by intralesional injection. Early studies showed evidence of biologic activity [199]. Subsequent phase II studies showed efficacy locally as well as systemically [200-203]. A phase III study has not yet been reported.

7. Cellular therapy

The transfer of immunologically competent white blood cells or their precursors into the host (cellular adoptive immunotherapy, adoptive cell treatment, adoptive cell therapy [ACT]) has been studied extensively in patients with melanoma over the last 30 years. Since it was thought that the effect of IL-2 is potentiated by this form of therapy, various studies examined the role of combination regimens with lymphokine-activated killer cells (LAK cells) or TILs with or without lymphodepletion with mixed results.

7.1. TILs

Earlier studies with LAK cells [204] showed promise, improving the responses with IL-2. A randomized study [205] with IL-2 and LAK cells compared to IL-2 alone failed to show significant improvement in survival which tempered the initial enthusiasm. Subsequent studies with Tumor Infiltrating Lymphocytes (TILs) [206] showed some response to treatment (overall ORR in these patients was 34%) when combined with IL-2. Interestingly, there was no significant difference in the ORR in patients whose therapy with high-dose IL-2 had failed (32%) compared with patients not previously treated with IL-2 (34%). However, the responses appeared to be short-lived, probably due to the transient persistence of the transferred TILs [207].

The addition of lymphodepletion has been thought to promote the persistence of the transferred TILs by eliminating the regulatory cells. Pooled data from three clinical trials employing three different lymphodepleting regimens [91] showed high responses between 49-72%. Ninety-five percent of these patients had progressive disease following a prior systemic treatment. Twenty of the 93 patients (22%) achieved complete tumor regression, and 19 have ongoing complete regressions beyond 3 years. The actuarial 3- and 5-year survival rates for the entire group were 36% and 29%, respectively, but for the 20 complete responders were 100% and 93%. Factors associated with objective response included longer telomeres of the infused cells, the number of CD8+ CD27+ cells infused and the persistence of the infused cells in the circulation at one month. This treatment appears to also be helpful in the treatment of intracranial disease [208].

At this point, there is reserved enthusiasm about the role of TILs with lymphodepletion regimens. There are several programs within the United States [209] outside of the NCI, where this work was pioneered, and internationally more groups are starting to employ similar strategies.

7.2. Dendritic cells

Another form of ACT is the infusion of dendritic cells. There is a lot of interest in developing dendritic cell based immunotherapy strategies since the approval of sipuleucel-T, an autologous dendritic cell based immunotherapy in hormone refractory prostate cancer. Dendritic cells are believed to induce a Th-1 response which activates CTLs through processing and presenting of peptides derived from the tumor protein antigens. In a study that evaluated the role of dendritic cells pulsed with Mage-3A1 tumor peptide and a recall antigen, tetanus toxoid or tuberculin, 6 of 11 patients with advanced stage IV melanoma experienced significant regression of their metastases [210]. Resolution of skin metastases in two of the patients was accompanied by $CD8^+$ T cell infiltration, whereas nonregressing lesions lacked $CD8^+$ T cells.

In another trial [211] 16 patients with metastatic stage IV melanoma were treated with dendritic cells derived from incubation of peripheral blood mononuclear cells with IL-4 and GM-CSF and overnight pulsing with several peptides (tyrosinase, gp100 and MART-1). One patient had a complete remission of lung and pleural disease after two cycles of therapy. Two additional patients had SD, and two patients had mixed responses. In general, reviewing over 30 studies that employed dendritic cell-based treatments [212], it appears that clinical response (defined as CR, PR or SD) was significantly correlated with the use of peptide antigens, use of helper antigen or adjuvant and induction of tumor antigen specific T cells.

Although there appears to be a real effect of these treatments on tumor response in a subset of the treated patients, undoubtedly the success has not been universal and convincing [213]. This could be due to Tregs that counteract the effect of dendritic cells. In addition, melanoma can also mediate dendritic cell suppression possibly through the activation of the MEK1/2-p44/42 axis [214]. Finally, little is known about optimal dendritic cell generation, administration and immune monitoring which could hamper progress in this field.

8. Enhancement of cellular immunity

8.1. Checkpoint inhibitors

Monoclonal antibodies targeted against a number of regulatory immune system checkpoints are being evaluated in patients with advanced melanoma. The recently approved ipilimumab remains the prototype, but others are currently being evaluated in several trials.

8.2. Ipilimumab

Ipilimumab is a monoclonal antibody against cytotoxic T-lymphocyte antigen 4 (CTLA-4). In two phase III trials ipilimumab showed improved OS in patients with advanced melanoma. In the first one [95], 676 HLA-A*0201–positive patients with unresectable stage III or IV melanoma, whose disease had progressed while they were receiving therapy for metastatic disease were studied. More than 70% of the patients had M1c disease (presence of visceral metastases), and more than 36% had elevated lactate dehydrogenase levels. The patients were randomly assigned, in a 3:1:1 ratio, to receive ipilimumab plus gp100, ipilimumab alone or gp100 alone. Ipilimumab, at a dose of 3 mg/kg of body weight, was administered with or without gp100 every three weeks for up to four treatments. HLA-A*0201–positivity was required because of the use of the gp100 vaccine. Certain patients were allowed to have another course of treatment upon progression. The primary end point was OS.

The median OS was 10.0 months among patients receiving ipilimumab plus gp100, as compared with 6.4 months among patients receiving gp100 alone (hazard ratio for death, 0.68; P<0.001). The median OS with ipilimumab alone was 10.1 months (hazard ratio for death in comparison with gp100 alone, 0.66; P=0.003). No difference in OS was detected between the ipilimumab groups (hazard ratio with ipilimumab plus gp100, 1.04; P=0.76). The best OR or SD was seen in the ipilimumab-alone group (10.9%) and a disease control rate (the proportion of patients with a PR, CR or SD) of 28.5%. In the ipilimumab-alone group, 60.0% maintained an OR for at least two years. Responses to ipilimumab continued to improve beyond week 24: in the ipilimumab-alone group, two patients with SD improved to a PR, and three with a PR improved to a CR. Interestingly, among 31 patients given reinduction therapy with ipilimumab, a PR, CR or SD was achieved by 21 weeks. Grade 3 or 4 immune-related adverse events occurred in 10 to 15% of patients treated with ipilimumab and in 3% treated with gp100 alone. There were 14 deaths related to the study drugs (2.1%), and seven were associated with immune-related adverse events.

In the second phase III study [215], 502 patients with previously untreated metastatic melanoma were assigned in a 1:1 ratio to receive 10 mg/kg ipilimumab plus 850 mg/m^2 dacarbazine or 850 mg/m^2 dacarbazine plus placebo, given at weeks 1, 4, 7 and 10, followed by 850 mg/m^2 dacarbazine alone every three weeks through week 22. Patients with SD or an OR and no dose-limiting toxic effects received ipilimumab or placebo every 12 weeks thereafter as maintenance therapy. Similarly with the previous study a significant number of patients had poor prognosis based on the presence of visceral metastases and increased lactate dehydrogenase. The primary end point was OS.

OS was significantly longer in the group receiving ipilimumab plus dacarbazine than in the group receiving dacarbazine plus placebo (11.2 months vs. 9.1 months), with higher survival rates in the ipilimumab–dacarbazine group at one year (47.3% vs. 36.3%), two years (28.5% vs. 17.9%), and three years (20.8% vs. 12.2%) (hazard ratio for death, 0.72; P<0.001). The rate of disease control (PR, CR or SD) did not differ significantly between the two groups: 33.2% in the ipilimumab–dacarbazine group and 30.2% in the dacarbazine group (P=0.41). The rate of best OR (PR or CR) was 15.2% in the ipilimumab–dacarbazine group and 10.3% in the dacarbazine group (P=0.09). However, the median duration of response among all patients with a PR or CR was 19.3 months (95% CI, 12.1 to 26.1) in the ipilimumab–dacarbazine group and 8.1 months (95% CI, 5.19 to 19.8) in the dacarbazine group (P=0.03). In addition, some patients in the study who were receiving ipilimumab had an improvement from PR to CR after six months. Grade 3 or 4 adverse events occurred in 56.3% of patients treated with ipilimumab plus dacarbazine, as compared with 27.5% treated with dacarbazine and placebo (P<0.001). No drug-related deaths or gastrointestinal perforations occurred in the ipilimumab–dacarbazine group.

Patients with untreated brain metastases were excluded from both phase III studies. However, phase II data indicate that ipilimumab has activity in patients with brain metastases [216]. The currently approved dose is 3 mg/kg based on the registration trial [95], however other doses and schedules [217] have been used that do not appear to produce significantly different results but appear to increase toxicity.

The experience with ipilimumab has shown that a subgroup of patients may experience a late response and more interestingly, some patients exhibit apparent disease progression after 12 weeks of ipilimumab followed by subsequent disease regression [218]. Therefore, traditional criteria (e.g. RECIST) may not apply in the evaluation of patients who receive ipilimumab or similar treatments, and different criteria may need to be established in the interpretation of efficacy data in clinical trials [20].

Based on the favorable results from the ipilimumab studies, other anti-CTLA4 antibodies are currently being evaluated such as tremelimumab. Tremelimumab has a longer half-life than ipilimumab and is dosed less frequently. Phase II data showed results similar to ipilimumab with durable responses suggesting a potential role for tremelimumab in melanoma [219]. However, a phase III trial comparing tremelimumab and chemotherapy failed to demonstrate an improvement in OS [220].

8.3. Toxicity with ipilimumab

The toxicity of ipilimumab appears to be related to the increased activation of the immune system. A variety of immune mediated adverse events have been observed. Some of them are life-threatening and the most common are enterocolitis, hepatitis, dermatitis and endocrinopathies, but others such as neurologic complications, ocular symptoms, hematologic manifestations, vasculitis, et al are also observed.The prompt administration of corticosteroids is paramount when these are observed, and in some cases treatment interruption or permanent discontinuation is required. A relationship between the development of side effects and anti-tumor activity has been proposed by several investigators [218].

8.4. PD-1

Another regulatory checkpoint is Programmed Death-1 receptor (PD-1). Its inhibition is currently being evaluated in clinical trials. The PD-1 and PD ligand-1 (PD-L1) interaction is believed to affect T cell anti-tumor immunity. Many tumors express high levels of PD-L1. When PD-L1 interacts with the PD-1 receptor on T cells, T cell function is impaired through a variety of mechanisms including induction of apoptosis, suppression of proliferation and inhibition of T cell cytokine production [96]. There are several ways to target PD-1; one way is targeting the PD-1 receptor and another is targeting the PD-1 ligand. There are several molecules currently under investigation that target the PD-1 receptor directly (BMS-936558, CT-011, MK-3475). In a recent study [98], BMS-936558 showed significant anti-tumor activity in a variety of solid tumors. In melanoma patients response rates were 28% and appeared to be durable. Interestingly, of 17 patients with PD-L1–negative tumors, none had an OR while 9 of 25 patients (36%) with PD-L1–positive tumors had an OR (P=0.006). CT-011 has demonstrated favorable results in hematologic malignancies but has not been well studied in melanoma patients yet [221], although there is an ongoing phase I study being conducted at present. The role of MK-3475 in melanoma is also currently being evaluated in a phase I trial. Another molecule which is not probably directly targeting the PD-1 is AMP-224; it is a fusion protein of B7-DC and an antibody Fc portion. It is not a monoclonal antibody like the three checkpoint agents mentioned previously, and no data has been reported yet regarding its efficacy in human trials. PD-L1 monoclonal antibodies have emerged as another strategy to affect the PD-1/PD L-1 pathway. A multi-center phase I study evaluating the role of BMS-936559 in patients with advanced cancers including melanoma showed a 17% response rate in melanoma patients with some of those being durable responses [97].

8.5. Co-stimulatory agonists

4-1BB or CD137 is a member of the TNF receptor (TNFR) family and provides a costimulatory signal important to the effective generation of many types of T cell responses. A completed phase I study in melanoma with BMS-663513, a fully human anti-CD137 agonist monoclonal antibody, showed that this agent was well tolerated and three PRs were seen [222].

OX-40 is another member of the TNFR family. An agonist molecule is also under investigation, but mature data are not yet available [223].

8.6. Conclusions

Checkpoint inhibitors and co-stimulatory agonists are improving anti-tumor cellular immunity. In a similar way to the more non-specific activation through cytokines, responses are durable but are not seen in all patients. This brings up issues such as appropriate patient selection, biomarker development and optimization of the dose, frequency and administration in order to optimize efficacy.

9. Combination approaches

Combination approaches have been traditionally used in the treatment of melanoma (for example different cytokines together or cytokines with chemotherapy). It is quite interesting that the results of this strategy have not been yet as successful as expected. While new agents are developed and we understand more about their function, these strategies may become more successful. At this point there is a lot of interest combining checkpoint inhibitors with other checkpoint blocking agents, co-stimulatory agonists, chemotherapy, targeted agents (such as B-type Raf kinas [BRAF] inhibitors) and radiotherapy. Interestingly, the BRAF inhibitors appear to improve T cell recognition of melanoma [224] which reinforces a rational combination of targeted therapy and immunotherapy. The results are not yet mature and studies are ongoing, but there is preclinical and retrospective data that support this model of treatment [224-227]. The following combination strategies have shown some recent benefit and promise.

9.1. Anti-CTLA4 and IFNa

A phase II study [227] combining tremelimumab and high dose IFN in patients with advanced melanoma showed an ORR of 24% with 4 patients obtaining a CR. Toxicity was acceptable and the median OS was 21 months. The University of Pittsburgh group is now contemplating a neoadjuvant and adjuvant therapy that employs an anti-CTLA4 and IFN-α combination strategy.

9.2. Anti-CTLA4 and GM-CSF

A phase II study through ECOG combining ipilimumab and GM-CSF is currently ongoing. Previous studies [228] with periodic infusions of anti-CTLA-4 antibodies after vaccination with irradiated, autologous tumor cells engineered to secrete GM-CSF have yielded favorable results with acceptable toxicity.

9.3. IL-2 and gp-100

A phase III trial evaluated the combination of IL-2 and the gp100 peptide vaccine in advanced melanoma. This combination therapy increased the response rate (16% vs. 6%) with more CRs in the combination arm and a trend toward increased OS [177]. Interestingly, the single arm responses were lower than expected. A similarly designed study employing ipilimumab did not show significant benefit in the combination arm [95].

10. Conclusion

Immunotherapy holds the promise of "the cure" for cancer. Glimpses of this outcome have been seen throughout the past century but may be best exemplified in melanoma therapy. Although attempts in the past have not had satisfactory results, the knowledge gained along with the ability to develop biologically active drugs is bearing fruit in the current generation of clinical trials. The few positive results have kept the interest for cancer immunotherapy alive which has also helped us to achieve a better understanding of the immune system in relationship to cancer treatment. The improvement in outcome seen with gp100 plus IL-2 is impressive, and the power of the anti-cancer and autoimmune toxicities seen with ipilimumab is dramatic. The excitement stems not only from the clinical results that were obtained but also by our ability to successfully manipulate the complex immune system in a different way than before. Undoubtedly, there are a lot of unanswered questions including why are there still a large number of patients who do not achieve responses with immunotherapy and eventually die from advanced disease? However, unlike immunotherapy applied to other advanced setting solid tumors, immunotherapy in advanced melanoma has resulted in some durable responses and possibly cures.

The future of immunotherapy in melanoma and other tumor types would ideally involve research in a broad range of directions. An optimization of the IL-2 based treatments is needed to improve the number of durable responses. Results from the current work at NCI augmenting IL-2 treatment with lymphodepletion are quite encouraging. Identification of serum or tissue biomarkers is also urgently needed. Biomarker research is often complex, but this work should reveal a better understanding of the tumor itself as well as the host. The checkpoint inhibitors such as ipilimumab and tremelimumab have opened the door for research into other immunologic checkpoints such as PD-1 and co-stimulatory signals. The need for a reliable melanoma biomarker is again paramount, and the significance of PD-L1 expression that is currently under investigation is anticipated with interest. Studying mechanisms of resistance in all cancer immunotherapeutics is equally important.

The combination of different immunotherapeutics with each other, with molecularly targeted agents or with conventional treatments such as chemotherapy or radiation therapy, may not be the simple process that combination strategies with vaccines were in the past, but this approach is quite attractive and rational and will help us further understand the role of the immune system in this disease. In a similar fashion, sequential therapy, using different agents at different times might improve clinical response and survival. Appropriate first line selection is also quite challenging since there are currently three approved agents in BRAF V600E mutated patients (high does IL-2, ipilimumab and vemurafenib) and two for BRAF wild type patients (high dose IL-2 and ipilimumab). A randomized clinical trial of ipilimumab followed by vemurafenib versus vemurafenib followed by ipilimumab is planned through the NCI Cooperative Group mechanisms [218]. Future clinical trials will hopefully provide some answers to these questions. In the design of clinical trials, the importance of refining the RECIST criteria for immunotherapy agents cannot be overemphasized. Overall, this is an exciting time for cancer immunologists and clinicians who treat patients with melanoma. The future for innovative trials of new agents and combinations is brighter than ever before.

Acknowledgements

The authors would like to thank Linda Ray for her invaluable administrative support.

Author details

Konstantinos Arnaoutakis, Dorothy A. Graves, Laura F. Hutchins and
Thomas Kieber-Emmons

Division of Hematology/Oncology and Department of Pathology University of Arkansas for Medical Sciences, Little Rock, AR, Winthrop P. Rockefeller Cancer Institute, USA

References

[1] I. B. Bayer-Garner, D. Ivan, M. R. Schwartz and J. A. Tschen, "The immunopathology of regression in benign lichenoid keratosis, keratoacanthoma and halo nevus," *Clin. Med. Res.*, vol. 2, pp. 89-97, May, 2004.

[2] R. Akasu, L. From and H. J. Kahn, "Characterization of the mononuclear infiltrate involved in regression of halo nevi," *J. Cutan. Pathol., vol. 21, pp. 302-311, Aug, 1994.*

[3] K. McKay, P. C. Moore, B. R. Smoller and K. M. Hiatt. Association between natural killer cells and regression in melanocytic lesions. Hum. *Pathol. [All @ UAMS; LRVA (latest 10 years)].* 42(12), pp. 1960-1964. 2011. Available: http://ovidsp.ovid.com/ovidweb.cgi?T=JS&CSC=Y&NEWS=N&PAGE=fulltext&D=medl&AN=21676435.

[4] N. Arpaia, N. Cassano and G. A. Vena. Regressing cutaneous malignant melanoma and vitiligo-like depigmentation. Int. J. Dermatol. [Part @ UAMS (Click Library Holdings)]. 45(8), pp. 952-956. 2006. Available: http://ovidsp.ovid.com/ovidweb.cgi?T=JS&CSC=Y&NEWS=N&PAGE=fulltext&D=med4&AN=16911383.

[5] M. G. Bouwhuis, A. Gast, A. Figl, A. M. Eggermont, K. Hemminki, D. Schadendorf and R. Kumar. Polymorphisms in the CD28/CTLA4/ICOS genes: Role in malignant melanoma susceptibility and prognosis?. Cancer Immunology, Immunotherapy [Not locally available; ask about Interlibrary Loan]. *59(2),* pp. 303-312. 2010. Available: http://ovidsp.ovid.com/ovidweb.cgi?T=JS&CSC=Y&NEWS=N&PAGE=fulltext&D=medl&AN=19672595.

[6] P. Fishman, O. Merimski, E. Baharav and Y. Shoenfeld. Autoantibodies to tyrosinase: The bridge between melanoma and vitiligo. *Cancer* [All @ UAMS; LRVA (latest 10 years)]. 79(8), pp. 1461-1464. 1997. Available: http://ovidsp.ovid.com/ovidweb.cgi?T=JS&CSC=Y&NEWS=N&PAGE=fulltext&D=med4&AN=9118024.

[7] K. A. Chianese-Bullock, E. M. Woodson, H. Tao, S. A. Boerner, M. Smolkin, W. W. Grosh, P. Y. Neese, P. Merrill, G. R. Petroni and C. L. Slingluff Jr. Autoimmune toxicities associated with the administration of antitumor vaccines and low-dose interleukin-2. *Journal of Immunotherapy* [All @ UAMS]. 28(4), pp. 412-419. 2005. Available: http://ovidsp.ovid.com/ovidweb.cgi?T=JS&CSC=Y&NEWS=N&PAGE=fulltext&D=medc&AN=16000961.

[8] C. Printz, "Spontaneous regression of melanoma may offer insight into cancer immunology," *J. Natl. Cancer Inst.,* vol. 93, pp. 1047-1048, Jul 18, 2001.

[9] W. A. High, D. Stewart, C. R. Wilbers, C. J. Cockerell, M. P. Hoang and J. E. Fitzpatrick, "Completely regressed primary cutaneous malignant melanoma with nodal and/or visceral metastases: a report of 5 cases and assessment of the literature and diagnostic criteria," *J. Am. Acad. Dermatol.,* vol. 53, pp. 89-100, Jul, 2005.

[10] K. K. Anbari, L. M. Schuchter, L. P. Bucky, R. Mick, M. Synnestvedt, D. Guerry 4th, R. Hamilton and A. C. Halpern, "Melanoma of unknown primary site: presentation, treatment, and prognosis--a single institution study. University of Pennsylvania Pigmented Lesion Study Group," *Cancer,* vol. 79, pp. 1816-1821, May 1, 1997.

[11] B. Schlagenhauff, W. Stroebel, U. Ellwanger, F. Meier, C. Zimmermann, H. Breuninger, G. Rassner and C. Garbe, "Metastatic melanoma of unknown primary origin shows prognostic similarities to regional metastatic melanoma: recommendations for initial staging examinations," *Cancer,* vol. 80, pp. 60-65, Jul 1, 1997.

[12] G. H. Baab and C. M. McBride. Malignant melanoma: The patient with an unknown site of primary origin. *Archives of Surgery* [All @ UAMS; LRVA (latest 10 years)].

110(8), pp. 896-900. 1975. Available: http://ovidsp.ovid.com/ovidweb.cgi?T=JS&CSC=Y&NEWS=N&PAGE=fulltext&D=med1&AN=1156155.

[13] M. F. Demierre. Thin melanomas and regression, thick melanomas and older men: Prognostic implications and perspectives on secondary prevention. *Arch. Dermatol.* [All @ UAMS; Part @ ACH(Click Lib.Holdings) & LRVA(10 yrs)]. *138(5),* pp. 678-682. 2002. Available: http://ovidsp.ovid.com/ovidweb.cgi?T=JS&CSC=Y&NEWS=N&PAGE=fulltext&D=med4&AN=12020232.

[14] J. K. O'Neill, R. Khundar, L. Knowles, N. Scott-Young and A. Orlando. Melanoma with an unknown primary--a case series. Journal of Plastic, Reconstructive & Aesthetic Surgery: JPRAS [Online Access Only (Click E Journal Holdings for Information)]. *63(12),* pp. 2071-2080. 2010. Available: http://ovidsp.ovid.com/ovidweb.cgi?T=JS&CSC=Y&NEWS=N&PAGE=fulltext&D=medl&AN=20335085.

[15] M. King, D. Spooner and D. C. Rowlands. Spontaneous regression of metastatic malignant melanoma of the parotid gland and neck lymph nodes: A case report and a review of the literature. *Clinical Oncology (Royal College of Radiologists)* [Online Access Only (Click E Journal Holdings for Information)]. 13(6), pp. 466-469. 2001. Available: http://ovidsp.ovid.com/ovidweb.cgi?T=JS&CSC=Y&NEWS=N&PAGE=fulltext&D=med4&AN=11824888.

[16] L. V. Kalialis, K. T. Drzewiecki and H. Klyver. Spontaneous regression of metastases from melanoma: Review of the literature. *Melanoma Res.* [Online Access Only (Click E Journal Holdings for Information)]. 19(5), pp. 275-282. 2009. Available: http://ovidsp.ovid.com/ovidweb.cgi?T=JS&CSC=Y&NEWS=N&PAGE=fulltext&D=medl&AN=19633580.

[17] N. J. Crowley and H. F. Seigler, "Late recurrence of malignant melanoma. Analysis of 168 patients," *Ann. Surg.,* vol. 212, pp. 173-177, Aug, 1990.

[18] M. H. Schmid-Wendtner, J. Baumert, M. Schmidt, B. Konz, D. Holzel, G. Plewig and M. Volkenandt, "Late metastases of cutaneous melanoma: an analysis of 31 patients," *J. Am. Acad. Dermatol.,* vol. 43, pp. 605-609, Oct, 2000.

[19] E. A. Eisenhauer, P. Therasse, J. Bogaerts, L. H. Schwartz, D. Sargent, R. Ford, J. Dancey, S. Arbuck, S. Gwyther, M. Mooney, L. Rubinstein, L. Shankar, L. Dodd, R. Kaplan, D. Lacombe and J. Verweij, "New response evaluation criteria in solid tumours: revised RECIST guideline (version 1.1)," *Eur. J. Cancer,* vol. 45, pp. 228-247, Jan, 2009.

[20] J. D. Wolchok, A. Hoos, S. O'Day, J. S. Weber, O. Hamid, C. Lebbe, M. Maio, M. Binder, O. Bohnsack, G. Nichol, R. Humphrey and F. S. Hodi, "Guidelines for the evaluation of immune therapy activity in solid tumors: immune-related response criteria," *Clin. Cancer Res.,* vol. 15, pp. 7412-7420, Dec 1, 2009.

[21] J. Weber and A. Aparicio. Novel immunologic approaches to the management of malignant melanoma. Curr. *Opin. Oncol. 13(2),* pp. 124-128. 2001.

[22] Faries and D. L. Morton. Therapeutic vaccines for melanoma - current status. Biodrugs [Not locally available; ask about Interlibrary Loan]. *19(4),* pp. 247-260. 2005. Available: http://ovidsp.ovid.com/ovidweb.cgi?T=JS&CSC=Y&NEWS=N&PAGE=fulltext&D=ipab&AN=42-19506.

[23] L. A. DiFronzo, R. K. Gupta, R. Essner, L. J. Foshag and D. L. Morton. Enhanced humoral immune response correlates with improved disease-free and overall survival in american joint committee on cancer stage II melanoma patients receiving adjuvant polyvalent vaccine. *Journal of Clinical Oncology* [All @ UAMS; LRVA (latest 10 years)]. *20(15),* pp. 3242-3248. 2002. Available: http://ovidsp.ovid.com/ovidweb.cgi?T=JS&CSC=Y&NEWS=N&PAGE=fulltext&D=ipab&AN=39-16839.

[24] E. Hsueh, R. Gupta, K. Qi and D. Morton. Correlation of specific immune responses with survival in melanoma patients with distant metastases receiving polyvalent melanoma cell vaccine. Journal of Clinical Oncology 16(9), pp. 2913-2920. 1998.

[25] K. Shafer-Weaver, S. Rosenberg, S. Strobl, W. Gregory Alvord, M. Baseler and A. Malyguine. Application of the granzyme B ELISPOT assay for monitoring cancer vaccine trials. Journal of Immunotherapy [All @ UAMS]. 29(3), pp. 328-335. 2006. Available: http://ovidsp.ovid.com/ovidweb.cgi?T=JS&CSC=Y&NEWS=N&PAGE=fulltext&D=medc&AN=16699376.

[26] A. Eggermont, S. Suciu, A. Testori, P. Patel and A. Spatz, "Ulceration of primary melanoma and responsiveness to adjuvant interferon therapy: analysis of the adjuvant trials EORTC 18952 and EORTC 18991 in 2,644 patients," *J. Clin. Oncol., vol. 27, pp. 9007, 2009.*

[27] D. Schadendorf, S. M. Algarra, L. Bastholt, G. Cinat, B. Dreno, A. M. Eggermont, E. Espinosa, J. Guo, A. Hauschild, T. Petrella, J. Schachter and P. Hersey. Immunotherapy of distant metastatic disease. Annals of Oncology [Online Access Only (Click E Journal Holdings for Information)]. 20(Suppl 6), pp. 41-50. 2009. Available: http://ovidsp.ovid.com/ovidweb.cgi?T=JS&CSC=Y&NEWS=N&PAGE=fulltext&D=medl&AN=19617297.

[28] H. Gogas, J. Ioannovich, U. Dafni, C. Stavropoulou-Giokas, K. Frangia, D. Tsoutsos, P. Panagiotou, A. Polyzos, O. Papadopoulos, A. Stratigos, C. Markopoulos, D. Bafaloukos, D. Pectasides, G. Fountzilas and J. M. Kirkwood, "Prognostic significance of autoimmunity during treatment of melanoma with interferon," *N. Engl. J. Med.,* vol. 354, pp. 709-718, Feb 16, 2006.

[29] Z. R. Yurkovetsky, J. M. Kirkwood, H. D. Edington, A. M. Marrangoni, L. Velikokhatnaya, M. T. Winans, E. Gorelik and A. E. Lokshin, "Multiplex analysis of serum cytokines in melanoma patients treated with interferon-alpha2b," *Clin. Cancer Res.,* vol. 13, pp. 2422-2428, Apr 15, 2007.

[30] M. Sabatino, S. Kim-Schulze, M. C. Panelli, D. Stroncek, E. Wang, B. Taback, D. W. Kim, G. Deraffele, Z. Pos, F. M. Marincola and H. L. Kaufman, "Serum vascular en-

dothelial growth factor and fibronectin predict clinical response to high-dose interleukin-2 therapy," *J. Clin. Oncol., vol. 27, pp. 2645-2652, Jun 1, 2009.*

[31] G. Y. Ku, J. Yuan, D. B. Page, S. E. Schroeder, K. S. Panageas, R. D. Carvajal, P. B. Chapman, G. K. Schwartz, J. P. Allison and J. D. Wolchok, "Single-institution experience with ipilimumab in advanced melanoma patients in the compassionate use setting: lymphocyte count after 2 doses correlates with survival," *Cancer,* vol. 116, pp. 1767-1775, Apr 1, 2010.

[32] J. Yuan, M. Adamow, B. A. Ginsberg, T. S. Rasalan, E. Ritter, H. F. Gallardo, Y. Xu, E. Pogoriler, S. L. Terzulli, D. Kuk, K. S. Panageas, G. Ritter, M. Sznol, R. Halaban, A. A. Jungbluth, J. P. Allison, L. J. Old, J. D. Wolchok and S. Gnjatic. Integrated NY-ESO-1 antibody and CD8+ T-cell responses correlate with clinical benefit in advanced melanoma patients treated with ipilimumab. *Proc. Natl. Acad. Sci. U. S. A.* [All @ UAMS; LRVA (latest 10 years)]. *108(40),* pp. 16723-16728. 2011. Available: http://ovidsp.ovid.com/ovidweb.cgi?T=JS&CSC=Y&NEWS=N&PAGE=fulltext&D=medl&AN=21933959.

[33] T. F. Gajewski, J. Louahed and V. G. Brichard. Gene signature in melanoma associated with clinical activity: A potential clue to unlock cancer immunotherapy. *Cancer Journal* [Online Access Only (Click E Journal Holdings for Information)]. 16(4), pp. 399-403. 2010. Available: http://ovidsp.ovid.com/ovidweb.cgi?T=JS&CSC=Y&NEWS=N&PAGE=fulltext&D=medl&AN=20693853.

[34] R. J. Sullivan, Y. Hoshida, J. Brunet, S. Tahan, J. Aldridge, C. Kwabi, E. Gardiner, D. McDermott, T. Golub and M. B. Atkins, "A single center experience with high-dose (HD) IL-2 treatment for patients with advanced melanoma and pilot investigation of a novel gene expression signature as a predictor of response," *J. Clin. Oncol., vol. 27, pp. 9003, 2009.*

[35] J. R. Brahmer, C. G. Drake, I. Wollner, J. D. Powderly, J. Picus, W. H. Sharfman, E. Stankevich, A. Pons, T. M. Salay, T. L. McMiller, M. M. Gilson, C. Wang, M. Selby, J. M. Taube, R. Anders, L. Chen, A. J. Korman, D. M. Pardoll, I. Lowy and S. L. Topalian. Phase I study of single-agent anti-programmed death-1 (MDX-1106) in refractory solid tumors: Safety, clinical activity, pharmacodynamics, and immunologic correlates. *Journal of Clinical Oncology* [All @ UAMS; LRVA (latest 10 years)]. *28(19),* pp. 3167-3175. 2010. Available: http://ovidsp.ovid.com/ovidweb.cgi?T=JS&CSC=Y&NEWS=N&PAGE=fulltext&D=medl&AN=20516446.

[36] I. Mellman, G. Coukos and G. Dranoff, "Cancer immunotherapy comes of age," *Nature,* vol. 480, pp. 480-489, Dec 21, 2011.

[37] M. G. Lewis, R. L. Ikonopisov, R. C. Nairn, T. M. Phillips, G. H. Fairley, D. C. Bodenham and P. Alexander, "Tumour-specific antibodies in human malignant melanoma and their relationship to the extent of the disease," *Br. Med. J.,* vol. 3, pp. 547-552, Sep 6, 1969.

[38] F. Avogadri and J. D. Wolchok, "Selecting antigens for cancer vaccines," *Nat. Biotechnol.*, vol. 30, pp. 328-329, Apr 10, 2012.

[39] P. Muranski, A. Boni, P. A. Antony, L. Cassard, K. R. Irvine, A. Kaiser, C. M. Paulos, D. C. Palmer, C. E. Touloukian, K. Ptak, L. Gattinoni, C. Wrzesinski, C. S. Hinrichs, K. W. Kerstann, L. Feigenbaum, C. C. Chan and N. P. Restifo, "Tumor-specific Th17-polarized cells eradicate large established melanoma," *Blood*, vol. 112, pp. 362-373, Jul 15, 2008.

[40] F. S. Hodi, "Well-defined melanoma antigens as progression markers for melanoma: insights into differential expression and host response based on stage," *Clin. Cancer Res.*, vol. 12, pp. 673-678, Feb 1, 2006.

[41] S. Jarmalavicius, Y. Welte and P. Walden, "High immunogenicity of the HLA peptidomes of melanoma tumor cells," *J. Biol. Chem.*, Aug 6, 2012.

[42] R. Pieper, R. E. Christian, M. I. Gonzales, M. I. Nishimura, G. Gupta, R. E. Settlage, J. Shabanowitz, S. A. Rosenberg, D. F. Hunt and S. L. Topalian, "Biochemical identification of a mutated human melanoma antigen recognized by CD4(+) T cells," *J. Exp. Med.*, vol. 189, pp. 757-766, Mar 1, 1999.

[43] J. P. Brown, R. G. Woodbury, C. E. Hart, I. Hellstrom and K. E. Hellstrom, "Quantitative analysis of melanoma-associated antigen p97 in normal and neoplastic tissues," *Proc. Natl. Acad. Sci. U. S. A.*, vol. 78, pp. 539-543, Jan, 1981.

[44] P. Fredman, K. Hedberg and T. Brezicka, "Gangliosides as therapeutic targets for cancer," *BioDrugs*, vol. 17, pp. 155-167, 2003.

[45] E. Jager, M. Ringhoffer, J. Karbach, M. Arand, F. Oesch and A. Knuth, "Inverse relationship of melanocyte differentiation antigen expression in melanoma tissues and CD8+ cytotoxic-T-cell responses: evidence for immunoselection of antigen-loss variants in vivo," *Int. J. Cancer*, vol. 66, pp. 470-476, May 16, 1996.

[46] E. Jager, M. Ringhoffer, H. P. Dienes, M. Arand, J. Karbach, D. Jager, C. Ilsemann, M. Hagedorn, F. Oesch and A. Knuth. Granulocyte-macrophage-colony-stimulating factor enhances immune responses to melanoma-associated peptides in vivo. *International Journal of Cancer* [All @ UAMS]. 67(1), pp. 54-62. 1996. Available: http://ovidsp.ovid.com/ovidweb.cgi?T=JS&CSC=Y&NEWS=N&PAGE=fulltext&D=med4&AN=8690525.

[47] C. Barrow, J. Browning, D. MacGregor, I. D. Davis, S. Sturrock, A. A. Jungbluth and J. Cebon, "Tumor antigen expression in melanoma varies according to antigen and stage," *Clin. Cancer Res.*, vol. 12, pp. 764-771, Feb 1, 2006.

[48] Y. Kawakami, S. Eliyahu, C. Jennings, K. Sakaguchi, X. Kang, S. Southwood, P. F. Robbins, A. Sette, E. Appella and S. A. Rosenberg, "Recognition of multiple epitopes in the human melanoma antigen gp100 by tumor-infiltrating T lymphocytes associated with in vivo tumor regression," *J. Immunol.*, vol. 154, pp. 3961-3968, Apr 15, 1995.

[49] T. Boon, P. G. Coulie, B. J. Van den Eynde and P. van der Bruggen, "Human T cell responses against melanoma," *Annu. Rev. Immunol.*, vol. 24, pp. 175-208, 2006.

[50] R. F. Wang and S. A. Rosenberg, "Human tumor antigens for cancer vaccine development," *Immunol. Rev.*, vol. 170, pp. 85-100, Aug, 1999.

[51] D. Valmori, M. J. Pittet, C. Vonarbourg, D. Rimoldi, D. Lienard, D. Speiser, R. Dunbar, V. Cerundolo, J. C. Cerottini and P. Romero, "Analysis of the cytolytic T lymphocyte response of melanoma patients to the naturally HLA-A*0201-associated tyrosinase peptide 368-376," *Cancer Res.*, vol. 59, pp. 4050-4055, Aug 15, 1999.

[52] K. S. Lang, C. C. Caroli, A. Muhm, D. Wernet, A. Moris, B. Schittek, E. Knauss-Scherwitz, S. Stevanovic, H. G. Rammensee and C. Garbe, "HLA-A2 restricted, melanocyte-specific CD8(+) T lymphocytes detected in vitiligo patients are related to disease activity and are predominantly directed against MelanA/MART1," *J. Invest. Dermatol., vol. 116, pp. 891-897, Jun, 2001.*

[53] P. P. Lee, C. Yee, P. A. Savage, L. Fong, D. Brockstedt, J. S. Weber, D. Johnson, S. Swetter, J. Thompson, P. D. Greenberg, M. Roederer and M. M. Davis, "Characterization of circulating T cells specific for tumor-associated antigens in melanoma patients," *Nat. Med.*, vol. 5, pp. 677-685, Jun, 1999.

[54] E. Zorn and T. Hercend, "A MAGE-6-encoded peptide is recognized by expanded lymphocytes infiltrating a spontaneously regressing human primary melanoma lesion," *Eur. J. Immunol.*, vol. 29, pp. 602-607, Feb, 1999.

[55] M. Monte, M. Simonatto, L. Y. Peche, D. R. Bublik, S. Gobessi, M. A. Pierotti, M. Rodolfo and C. Schneider, "MAGE-A tumor antigens target p53 transactivation function through histone deacetylase recruitment and confer resistance to chemotherapeutic agents," *Proc. Natl. Acad. Sci. U. S. A.*, vol. 103, pp. 11160-11165, Jul 25, 2006.

[56] S. Gnjatic, H. Nishikawa, A. A. Jungbluth, A. O. Gure, G. Ritter, E. Jager, A. Knuth, Y. T. Chen and L. J. Old, "NY-ESO-1: review of an immunogenic tumor antigen," *Adv. Cancer Res.*, vol. 95, pp. 1-30, 2006.

[57] V. Vantomme, P. Boel, E. De Plaen, T. Boon and P. van der Bruggen, "A new tumor-specific antigenic peptide encoded by MAGE-6 is presented to cytolytic T lymphocytes by HLA-Cw16," *Cancer. Immun.*, vol. 3, pp. 17, Dec 10, 2003.

[58] B. Weide, H. Zelba, E. Derhovanessian, A. Pflugfelder, T. K. Eigentler, A. M. Di Giacomo, M. Maio, E. H. Aarntzen, I. J. de Vries, A. Sucker, D. Schadendorf, P. Buttner, C. Garbe and G. Pawelec, "Functional T cells targeting NY-ESO-1 or Melan-A are predictive for survival of patients with distant melanoma metastasis," *J. Clin. Oncol., vol. 30, pp. 1835-1841, May 20, 2012.*

[59] H. T. Khong and N. P. Restifo, "Natural selection of tumor variants in the generation of "tumor escape" phenotypes," *Nat. Immunol.*, vol. 3, pp. 999-1005, Nov, 2002.

[60] T. J. de Vries, A. Fourkour, T. Wobbes, G. Verkroost, D. J. Ruiter and G. N. van Muijen, "Heterogeneous expression of immunotherapy candidate proteins gp100,

MART-1, and tyrosinase in human melanoma cell lines and in human melanocytic lesions," *Cancer Res.*, vol. 57, pp. 3223-3229, Aug 1, 1997.

[61] F. Garrido, F. Ruiz-Cabello, T. Cabrera, J. J. Perez-Villar, M. Lopez-Botet, M. Duggan-Keen and P. L. Stern, "Implications for immunosurveillance of altered HLA class I phenotypes in human tumours," *Immunol. Today*, vol. 18, pp. 89-95, Feb, 1997.

[62] I. Algarra, A. Collado and F. Garrido, "Altered MHC class I antigens in tumors," *Int. J. Clin. Lab. Res.*, vol. 27, pp. 95-102, 1997.

[63] M. Bernal, F. Ruiz-Cabello, A. Concha, A. Paschen and F. Garrido, "Implication of the beta2-microglobulin gene in the generation of tumor escape phenotypes," *Cancer Immunol. Immunother., vol. 61, pp. 1359-1371, Sep, 2012.*

[64] N. P. Restifo, F. M. Marincola, Y. Kawakami, J. Taubenberger, J. R. Yannelli and S. A. Rosenberg, "Loss of functional beta 2-microglobulin in metastatic melanomas from five patients receiving immunotherapy," *J. Natl. Cancer Inst.*, vol. 88, pp. 100-108, Jan 17, 1996.

[65] K. Taniguchi, M. Petersson, P. Hoglund, R. Kiessling, G. Klein and K. Karre, "Interferon gamma induces lung colonization by intravenously inoculated B16 melanoma cells in parallel with enhanced expression of class I major histocompatibility complex antigens," *Proc. Natl. Acad. Sci. U. S. A.*, vol. 84, pp. 3405-3409, May, 1987.

[66] R. Versteeg, K. M. Kruse-Wolters, A. C. Plomp, A. van Leeuwen, N. J. Stam, H. L. Ploegh, D. J. Ruiter and P. I. Schrier, "Suppression of class I human histocompatibility leukocyte antigen by c-myc is locus specific," *J. Exp. Med.*, vol. 170, pp. 621-635, Sep 1, 1989.

[67] K. Karre, "NK cells, MHC class I molecules and the missing self," *Scand. J. Immunol.*, vol. 55, pp. 221-228, Mar, 2002.

[68] R. J. Tuthill, J. M. Unger, P. Y. Liu, L. E. Flaherty, V. K. Sondak and Southwest Oncology Group, "Risk assessment in localized primary cutaneous melanoma: a Southwest Oncology Group study evaluating nine factors and a test of the Clark logistic regression prediction model," *Am. J. Clin. Pathol., vol. 118, pp. 504-511, Oct, 2002.*

[69] D. A. Oble, R. Loewe, P. Yu and M. C. Mihm Jr, "Focus on TILs: prognostic significance of tumor infiltrating lymphocytes in human melanoma," *Cancer. Immun.*, vol. 9, pp. 3, Apr 2, 2009.

[70] C. M. Balch, S. J. Soong, J. E. Gershenwald, J. F. Thompson, D. S. Reintgen, N. Cascinelli, M. Urist, K. M. McMasters, M. I. Ross, J. M. Kirkwood, M. B. Atkins, J. A. Thompson, D. G. Coit, D. Byrd, R. Desmond, Y. Zhang, P. Y. Liu, G. H. Lyman and A. Morabito, "Prognostic factors analysis of 17,600 melanoma patients: validation of the American Joint Committee on Cancer melanoma staging system," *J. Clin. Oncol., vol. 19, pp. 3622-3634, Aug 15, 2001.*

[71] T. E. Grotz, A. S. Mansfield, J. W. Jakub and S. N. Markovic, "Regional lymphatic immunity in melanoma," *Melanoma Res.*, vol. 22, pp. 9-18, Feb, 2012.

[72] M. E. Dudley, J. C. Yang, R. Sherry, M. S. Hughes, R. Royal, U. Kammula, P. F. Robbins, J. Huang, D. E. Citrin, S. F. Leitman, J. Wunderlich, N. P. Restifo, A. Thomasian, S. G. Downey, F. O. Smith, J. Klapper, K. Morton, C. Laurencot, D. E. White and S. A. Rosenberg, "Adoptive cell therapy for patients with metastatic melanoma: evaluation of intensive myeloablative chemoradiation preparative regimens," *J. Clin. Oncol., vol. 26, pp. 5233-5239, Nov 10, 2008.*

[73] R. R. Braeuer, E. Shoshan, T. Kamiya and M. Bar-Eli, "The sweet and bitter sides of galectins in melanoma progression," *Pigment Cell. Melanoma Res.*, vol. 25, pp. 592-601, Sep, 2012.

[74] M. W. Ma, R. C. Medicherla, M. Qian, E. Vega-Saenz de Miera, E. B. Friedman, R. S. Berman, R. L. Shapiro, A. C. Pavlick, P. A. Ott, N. Bhardwaj, Y. Shao, I. Osman and F. Darvishian, "Immune response in melanoma: an in-depth analysis of the primary tumor and corresponding sentinel lymph node," *Mod. Pathol., vol. 25, pp. 1000-1010, Jul, 2012.*

[75] A. S. Mansfield, S. G. Holtan, T. E. Grotz, J. B. Allred, J. W. Jakub, L. A. Erickson and S. N. Markovic, "Regional immunity in melanoma: immunosuppressive changes precede nodal metastasis," *Mod. Pathol., vol. 24, pp. 487-494, Apr, 2011.*

[76] M. E. Polak, P. Johnson, S. Di Palma, B. Higgins, J. Hurren, N. J. Borthwick, M. J. Jager, D. Mccormick and I. A. Cree, "Presence and maturity of dendritic cells in melanoma lymph node metastases," *J. Pathol.*, vol. 207, pp. 83-90, Sep, 2005.

[77] A. Busse and U. Keilholz, "Role of TGF-beta in melanoma," *Curr. Pharm. Biotechnol.*, vol. 12, pp. 2165-2175, Dec, 2011.

[78] K. Asadullah, W. Sterry and H. D. Volk, "Interleukin-10 therapy--review of a new approach," *Pharmacol. Rev.*, vol. 55, pp. 241-269, Jun, 2003.

[79] C. De Santo, R. Arscott, S. Booth, I. Karydis, M. Jones, R. Asher, M. Salio, M. Middleton and V. Cerundolo, "Invariant NKT cells modulate the suppressive activity of IL-10-secreting neutrophils differentiated with serum amyloid A," *Nat. Immunol.*, vol. 11, pp. 1039-1046, Nov, 2010.

[80] A. Facciabene, X. Peng, I. S. Hagemann, K. Balint, A. Barchetti, L. P. Wang, P. A. Gimotty, C. B. Gilks, P. Lal, L. Zhang and G. Coukos, "Tumour hypoxia promotes tolerance and angiogenesis via CCL28 and T(reg) cells," *Nature,* vol. 475, pp. 226-230, Jul 13, 2011.

[81] N. Schwinn, D. Vokhminova, A. Sucker, S. Textor, S. Striegel, I. Moll, N. Nausch, J. Tuettenberg, A. Steinle, A. Cerwenka, D. Schadendorf and A. Paschen, "Interferon-gamma down-regulates NKG2D ligand expression and impairs the NKG2D-mediated cytolysis of MHC class I-deficient melanoma by natural killer cells," *Int. J. Cancer,* vol. 124, pp. 1594-1604, Apr 1, 2009.

[82] A. Paschen, A. Sucker, B. Hill, I. Moll, M. Zapatka, X. D. Nguyen, G. C. Sim, I. Gutmann, J. Hassel, J. C. Becker, A. Steinle, D. Schadendorf and S. Ugurel, "Differential

clinical significance of individual NKG2D ligands in melanoma: soluble ULBP2 as an indicator of poor prognosis superior to S100B," *Clin. Cancer Res.*, vol. 15, pp. 5208-5215, Aug 15, 2009.

[83] S. K. Calderwood, M. A. Khaleque, D. B. Sawyer and D. R. Ciocca, "Heat shock proteins in cancer: chaperones of tumorigenesis," *Trends Biochem. Sci.*, vol. 31, pp. 164-172, Mar, 2006.

[84] C. Shipp, B. Weide, E. Derhovanessian and G. Pawelec, "Hsps are up-regulated in melanoma tissue and correlate with patient clinical parameters," *Cell Stress Chaperones*, Aug 8, 2012.

[85] S. A. Rosenberg, J. C. Yang, D. J. Schwartzentruber, P. Hwu, F. M. Marincola, S. L. Topalian, N. P. Restifo, M. E. Dudley, S. L. Schwarz, P. J. Spiess, J. R. Wunderlich, M. R. Parkhurst, Y. Kawakami, C. A. Seipp, J. H. Einhorn and D. E. White, "Immunologic and therapeutic evaluation of a synthetic peptide vaccine for the treatment of patients with metastatic melanoma," *Nat. Med.*, vol. 4, pp. 321-327, Mar, 1998.

[86] J. C. Yang, "Melanoma vaccines," *Cancer J.*, vol. 17, pp. 277-282, Sep-Oct, 2011.

[87] W. J. Lesterhuis, E. H. Aarntzen, I. J. De Vries, D. H. Schuurhuis, C. G. Figdor, G. J. Adema and C. J. Punt, "Dendritic cell vaccines in melanoma: from promise to proof?" *Crit. Rev. Oncol. Hematol., vol. 66, pp. 118-134, May, 2008.*

[88] J. Banchereau and R. M. Steinman, "Dendritic cells and the control of immunity," *Nature*, vol. 392, pp. 245-252, Mar 19, 1998.

[89] M. E. Dudley and S. A. Rosenberg, "Adoptive-cell-transfer therapy for the treatment of patients with cancer," *Nat. Rev. Cancer.*, vol. 3, pp. 666-675, Sep, 2003.

[90] S. Lee and K. Margolin, "Tumor-Infiltrating Lymphocytes in Melanoma," *Curr. Oncol. Rep.*, Aug 10, 2012.

[91] S. A. Rosenberg, J. C. Yang, R. M. Sherry, U. S. Kammula, M. S. Hughes, G. Q. Phan, D. E. Citrin, N. P. Restifo, P. F. Robbins, J. R. Wunderlich, K. E. Morton, C. M. Laurencot, S. M. Steinberg, D. E. White and M. E. Dudley, "Durable complete responses in heavily pretreated patients with metastatic melanoma using T-cell transfer immunotherapy," *Clin. Cancer Res.*, vol. 17, pp. 4550-4557, Jul 1, 2011.

[92] P. F. Robbins, R. A. Morgan, S. A. Feldman, J. C. Yang, R. M. Sherry, M. E. Dudley, J. R. Wunderlich, A. V. Nahvi, L. J. Helman, C. L. Mackall, U. S. Kammula, M. S. Hughes, N. P. Restifo, M. Raffeld, C. C. Lee, C. L. Levy, Y. F. Li, M. El-Gamil, S. L. Schwarz, C. Laurencot and S. A. Rosenberg, "Tumor regression in patients with metastatic synovial cell sarcoma and melanoma using genetically engineered lymphocytes reactive with NY-ESO-1," *J. Clin. Oncol., vol. 29, pp. 917-924, Mar 1, 2011.*

[93] M. B. Atkins, M. T. Lotze, J. P. Dutcher, R. I. Fisher, G. Weiss, K. Margolin, J. Abrams, M. Sznol, D. Parkinson, M. Hawkins, C. Paradise, L. Kunkel and S. A. Rosenberg, "High-dose recombinant interleukin 2 therapy for patients with metastatic melano-

ma: analysis of 270 patients treated between 1985 and 1993," *J. Clin. Oncol., vol. 17, pp. 2105-2116, Jul, 1999.*

[94] J. M. Kirkwood, J. Manola, J. Ibrahim, V. Sondak, M. S. Ernstoff, U. Rao and Eastern Cooperative Oncology Group, "A pooled analysis of eastern cooperative oncology group and intergroup trials of adjuvant high-dose interferon for melanoma," *Clin. Cancer Res.*, vol. 10, pp. 1670-1677, Mar 1, 2004.

[95] F. S. Hodi, S. J. O'Day, D. F. McDermott, R. W. Weber, J. A. Sosman, J. B. Haanen, R. Gonzalez, C. Robert, D. Schadendorf, J. C. Hassel, W. Akerley, A. J. van den Eertwegh, J. Lutzky, P. Lorigan, J. M. Vaubel, G. P. Linette, D. Hogg, C. H. Ottensmeier, C. Lebbe, C. Peschel, I. Quirt, J. I. Clark, J. D. Wolchok, J. S. Weber, J. Tian, M. J. Yellin, G. M. Nichol, A. Hoos and W. J. Urba, "Improved survival with ipilimumab in patients with metastatic melanoma," *N. Engl. J. Med.*, vol. 363, pp. 711-723, Aug 19, 2010.

[96] M. A. Postow, J. Harding and J. D. Wolchok, "Targeting immune checkpoints: releasing the restraints on anti-tumor immunity for patients with melanoma," *Cancer J.*, vol. 18, pp. 153-159, Mar-Apr, 2012.

[97] J. R. Brahmer, S. S. Tykodi, L. Q. Chow, W. J. Hwu, S. L. Topalian, P. Hwu, C. G. Drake, L. H. Camacho, J. Kauh, K. Odunsi, H. C. Pitot, O. Hamid, S. Bhatia, R. Martins, K. Eaton, S. Chen, T. M. Salay, S. Alaparthy, J. F. Grosso, A. J. Korman, S. M. Parker, S. Agrawal, S. M. Goldberg, D. M. Pardoll, A. Gupta and J. M. Wigginton, "Safety and activity of anti-PD-L1 antibody in patients with advanced cancer," *N. Engl. J. Med.*, vol. 366, pp. 2455-2465, Jun 28, 2012.

[98] S. L. Topalian, F. S. Hodi, J. R. Brahmer, S. N. Gettinger, D. C. Smith, D. F. McDermott, J. D. Powderly, R. D. Carvajal, J. A. Sosman, M. B. Atkins, P. D. Leming, D. R. Spigel, S. J. Antonia, L. Horn, C. G. Drake, D. M. Pardoll, L. Chen, W. H. Sharfman, R. A. Anders, J. M. Taube, T. L. McMiller, H. Xu, A. J. Korman, M. Jure-Kunkel, S. Agrawal, D. McDonald, G. D. Kollia, A. Gupta, J. M. Wigginton and M. Sznol, "Safety, activity, and immune correlates of anti-PD-1 antibody in cancer," *N. Engl. J. Med.*, vol. 366, pp. 2443-2454, Jun 28, 2012.

[99] M. M. Adams, P. Damani, N. R. Perl, A. Won, F. Hong, P. O. Livingston, G. Ragupathi and D. Y. Gin, "Design and synthesis of potent Quillaja saponin vaccine adjuvants," *J Am Chem Soc*, vol. 132, pp. 1939-45, Feb 17, 2010.

[100] B. Krone, K. F. Kolmel, J. M. Grange, G. Mastrangelo, B. M. Henz, I. N. Botev, M. Niin, C. Seebacher, D. Lambert, R. Shafir, E. M. Kokoschka, U. R. Kleeberg, O. Gefeller and A. Pfahlberg, "Impact of vaccinations and infectious diseases on the risk of melanoma--evaluation of an EORTC case-control study," *Eur J Cancer*, vol. 39, pp. 2372-8, Nov, 2003.

[101] H. K. Silver, E. M. Ibrahim, J. A. Evers, J. W. Thomas, R. N. Murray and J. J. Spinelli, "Adjuvant BCG immunotherapy for stage I and II malignant melanoma," *Can Med Assoc J*, vol. 128, pp. 1291-5, Jun 1, 1983.

[102] J. H. Stewart 4th and E. A. Levine. Role of bacillus calmette-guerin in the treatment of advanced melanoma. Expert Review of Anticancer Therapy [Not locally available; ask about Interlibrary Loan]. *11(11),* pp. 1671-1676. 2011. Available: http:// ovidsp.ovid.com/ovidweb.cgi?T=JS&CSC=Y&NEWS=N&PAGE=full-text&D=medl&AN=22050015.

[103] S. S. Agarwala, D. Neuberg, Y. Park and J. M. Kirkwood, "Mature results of a phase III randomized trial of bacillus Calmette-Guerin (BCG) versus observation and BCG plus dacarbazine versus BCG in the adjuvant therapy of American Joint Committee on Cancer Stage I-III melanoma (E1673): a trial of the Eastern Oncology Group," *Cancer,* vol. 100, pp. 1692-8, Apr 15, 2004.

[104] D. L. Morton, F. R. Eilber, E. C. Holmes, F. C. Sparks and K. Ramming, "BCG immunotherapy as a systemic adjunct to surgery in malignant melanoma," *Med Clin North Am,* vol. 60, pp. 431-9, May, 1976.

[105] D. L. Morton, L. J. Foshag, D. S. Hoon, J. A. Nizze, E. Famatiga, L. A. Wanek, C. Chang, D. G. Davtyan, R. K. Gupta and R. Elashoff, "Prolongation of survival in metastatic melanoma after active specific immunotherapy with a new polyvalent melanoma vaccine," *Ann Surg,* vol. 216, pp. 463-82, Oct, 1992.

[106] D. L. Morton, E. C. Hsueh, R. Essner, L. J. Foshag, S. J. O'Day, A. Bilchik, R. K. Gupta, D. S. Hoon, M. Ravindranath, J. A. Nizze, G. Gammon, L. A. Wanek, H. J. Wang and R. M. Elashoff, "Prolonged survival of patients receiving active immunotherapy with Canvaxin therapeutic polyvalent vaccine after complete resection of melanoma metastatic to regional lymph nodes," *Ann Surg,* vol. 236, pp. 438-48; discussion 448-9, Oct, 2002.

[107] S. Hoshimoto, M. B. Faries, D. L. Morton, T. Shingai, C. Kuo, H. J. Wang, R. Elashoff, N. Mozzillo, M. C. Kelley, J. F. Thompson, J. E. Lee and D. S. Hoon, "Assessment of prognostic circulating tumor cells in a phase III trial of adjuvant immunotherapy after complete resection of stage IV melanoma," *Ann Surg,* vol. 255, pp. 357-62, Feb, 2012.

[108] I. Hara, N. Sato, H. Miyake, M. Muramaki, S. Hikosaka and S. Kamidono, "Introduction of 65 kDa antigen of Mycobacterium tuberculosis to cancer cells enhances antitumor effect of BCG therapy," *Microbiol Immunol,* vol. 48, pp. 289-95, 2004.

[109] C. W. Cluff, "Monophosphoryl lipid A (MPL) as an adjuvant for anti-cancer vaccines: clinical results," *Adv Exp Med Biol,* vol. 667, pp. 111-23, 2010.

[110] J. T. Evans, C. W. Cluff, D. A. Johnson, M. J. Lacy, D. H. Persing and J. R. Baldridge, "Enhancement of antigen-specific immunity via the TLR4 ligands MPL adjuvant and Ribi.529," *Expert Rev Vaccines,* vol. 2, pp. 219-29, Apr, 2003.

[111] N. Schultz, R. Oratz, D. Chen, A. Zeleniuch-Jacquotte, G. Abeles and J. C. Bystryn, "Effect of DETOX as an adjuvant for melanoma vaccine," *Vaccine,* vol. 13, pp. 503-8, Apr, 1995.

[112] H. X. Sun, Y. Xie and Y. P. Ye, "Advances in saponin-based adjuvants," *Vaccine*, vol. 27, pp. 1787-96, Mar 13, 2009.

[113] G. Ragupathi, J. R. Gardner, P. O. Livingston and D. Y. Gin, "Natural and synthetic saponin adjuvant QS-21 for vaccines against cancer," *Expert Rev Vaccines*, vol. 10, pp. 463-70, Apr, 2011.

[114] K. Deng, M. M. Adams, P. Damani, P. O. Livingston, G. Ragupathi and D. Y. Gin, "Synthesis of QS-21-xylose: establishment of the immunopotentiating activity of synthetic QS-21 adjuvant with a melanoma vaccine," *Angew Chem Int Ed Engl*, vol. 47, pp. 6395-8, 2008.

[115] P. O. Livingston, "Approaches to augmenting the immunogenicity of melanoma gangliosides: from whole melanoma cells to ganglioside-KLH conjugate vaccines," *Immunol Rev*, vol. 145, pp. 147-66, Jun, 1995.

[116] J. Aucouturier, L. Dupuis, S. Deville, S. Ascarateil and V. Ganne, "Montanide ISA 720 and 51: a new generation of water in oil emulsions as adjuvants for human vaccines," *Expert Rev Vaccines*, vol. 1, pp. 111-8, Jun, 2002.

[117] J. Aucouturier, S. Ascarateil and L. Dupuis, "The use of oil adjuvants in therapeutic vaccines," *Vaccine*, vol. 24 Suppl 2, pp. S2-44-5, Apr 12, 2006.

[118] E. J. Huijbers, J. Femel, K. Andersson, H. Bjorkelund, L. Hellman and A. K. Olsson, "The non-toxic and biodegradable adjuvant Montanide ISA 720/CpG can replace Freund's in a cancer vaccine targeting ED-B--a prerequisite for clinical development," *Vaccine*, vol. 30, pp. 225-30, Jan 5, 2012.

[119] J. Fourcade, P. Kudela, P. A. Andrade Filho, B. Janjic, S. R. Land, C. Sander, A. Krieg, A. Donnenberg, H. Shen, J. M. Kirkwood and H. M. Zarour, "Immunization with analog peptide in combination with CpG and montanide expands tumor antigen-specific CD8+ T cells in melanoma patients," *J Immunother*, vol. 31, pp. 781-91, Oct, 2008.

[120] J. Karbach, S. Gnjatic, A. Bender, A. Neumann, E. Weidmann, J. Yuan, C. A. Ferrara, E. Hoffmann, L. J. Old, N. K. Altorki and E. Jager, "Tumor-reactive CD8+ T-cell responses after vaccination with NY-ESO-1 peptide, CpG 7909 and Montanide ISA-51: association with survival," *Int J Cancer*, vol. 126, pp. 909-18, Feb 15, 2010.

[121] K. A. Chianese-Bullock, J. Pressley, C. Garbee, S. Hibbitts, C. Murphy, G. Yamshchikov, G. R. Petroni, E. A. Bissonette, P. Y. Neese, W. W. Grosh, P. Merrill, R. Fink, E. M. Woodson, C. J. Wiernasz, J. W. Patterson and S. C. L. Jr, "MAGE-A1-, MAGE-A10-, and gp100-derived peptides are immunogenic when combined with granulocyte-macrophage colony-stimulating factor and montanide ISA-51 adjuvant and administered as part of a multipeptide vaccine for melanoma," *J Immunol*, vol. 174, pp. 3080-6, Mar 1, 2005.

[122] S. N. Markovic, V. J. Suman, J. N. Ingle, J. S. Kaur, H. C. Pitot, C. L. Loprinzi, R. D. Rao, E. T. Creagan, M. R. Pittelkow, J. B. Allred, W. K. Nevala and E. Celis, "Peptide vaccination of patients with metastatic melanoma: improved clinical outcome in pa-

tients demonstrating effective immunization," *Am J Clin Oncol*, vol. 29, pp. 352-60, Aug, 2006.

[123] D. T. Le and E. M. Jaffee, "Regulatory T-cell modulation using cyclophosphamide in vaccine approaches: a current perspective," *Cancer Res*, vol. 72, pp. 3439-44, Jul 15, 2012.

[124] E. Elkord, E. M. Alcantar-Orozco, S. J. Dovedi, D. Q. Tran, R. E. Hawkins and D. E. Gilham, "T regulatory cells in cancer: recent advances and therapeutic potential," *Expert Opin Biol Ther*, vol. 10, pp. 1573-86, Nov, 2010.

[125] Q. Y. Guo, M. Yuan, J. Peng, X. M. Cui, G. Song, X. Sui and S. B. Lu, "Antitumor activity of mixed heat shock protein/peptide vaccine and cyclophosphamide plus interleukin-12 in mice sarcoma," *J Exp Clin Cancer Res*, vol. 30, pp. 24, 2011.

[126] F. Ghiringhelli, N. Larmonier, E. Schmitt, A. Parcellier, D. Cathelin, C. Garrido, B. Chauffert, E. Solary, B. Bonnotte and F. Martin, "CD4+CD25+ regulatory T cells suppress tumor immunity but are sensitive to cyclophosphamide which allows immunotherapy of established tumors to be curative," *Eur J Immunol*, vol. 34, pp. 336-44, Feb, 2004.

[127] M. L. Salem, A. N. Kadima, S. A. El-Naggar, M. P. Rubinstein, Y. Chen, W. E. Gillanders and D. J. Cole, "Defining the ability of cyclophosphamide preconditioning to enhance the antigen-specific CD8+ T-cell response to peptide vaccination: creation of a beneficial host microenvironment involving type I IFNs and myeloid cells," *J Immunother*, vol. 30, pp. 40-53, Jan, 2007.

[128] J. M. Kirkwood, M. H. Strawderman, M. S. Ernstoff, T. J. Smith, E. C. Borden and R. H. Blum, "Interferon alfa-2b adjuvant therapy of high-risk resected cutaneous melanoma: the Eastern Cooperative Oncology Group Trial EST 1684," *J. Clin. Oncol., vol. 14, pp. 7-17, Jan, 1996.*

[129] J. M. Kirkwood, J. G. Ibrahim, V. K. Sondak, J. Richards, L. E. Flaherty, M. S. Ernstoff, T. J. Smith, U. Rao, M. Steele and R. H. Blum, "High- and low-dose interferon alfa-2b in high-risk melanoma: first analysis of intergroup trial E1690/S9111/C9190," *J. Clin. Oncol., vol. 18, pp. 2444-2458, Jun, 2000.*

[130] A. M. Eggermont, S. Suciu, M. Santinami, A. Testori, W. H. Kruit, J. Marsden, C. J. Punt, F. Sales, M. Gore, R. Mackie, Z. Kusic, R. Dummer, A. Hauschild, E. Musat, A. Spatz, U. Keilholz and EORTC Melanoma Group, "Adjuvant therapy with pegylated interferon alfa-2b versus observation alone in resected stage III melanoma: final results of EORTC 18991, a randomised phase III trial," *Lancet*, vol. 372, pp. 117-126, Jul 12, 2008.

[131] S. Mocellin, S. Pasquali, C. R. Rossi and D. Nitti, "Interferon alpha adjuvant therapy in patients with high-risk melanoma: a systematic review and meta-analysis," *J. Natl. Cancer Inst.*, vol. 102, pp. 493-501, Apr 7, 2010.

[132] C. I. Falkson, G. Falkson and H. C. Falkson, "Improved results with the addition of interferon alfa-2b to dacarbazine in the treatment of patients with metastatic malignant melanoma," *J. Clin. Oncol., vol. 9, pp. 1403-1408, Aug, 1991.*

[133] E. T. Creagan, D. L. Ahmann, S. J. Green, H. J. Long, S. Frytak, J. R. O'Fallon and L. M. Itri, "Phase II study of low-dose recombinant leukocyte A interferon in disseminated malignant melanoma," *J. Clin. Oncol., vol. 2, pp. 1002-1005, Sep, 1984.*

[134] N. J. Ives, R. L. Stowe, P. Lorigan and K. Wheatley, "Chemotherapy compared with biochemotherapy for the treatment of metastatic melanoma: a meta-analysis of 18 trials involving 2,621 patients," *J. Clin. Oncol., vol. 25, pp. 5426-5434, Dec 1, 2007.*

[135] A. A. Tarhini, J. M. Kirkwood, W. E. Gooding, C. Cai and S. S. Agarwala, "Durable complete responses with high-dose bolus interleukin-2 in patients with metastatic melanoma who have experienced progression after biochemotherapy," *J. Clin. Oncol., vol. 25, pp. 3802-3807, Sep 1, 2007.*

[136] D. F. McDermott and M. B. Atkins, "More support for the judicious use of high-dose interleukin-2 in patients with advanced melanoma," *J. Clin. Oncol., vol. 25, pp. 3791-3793, Sep 1, 2007.*

[137] T. M. Petrella, R. Tozer, K. Belanger, K. J. Savage, R. Wong, M. Smylie, S. Kamel-Reid, V. Tron, B. E. Chen, N. N. Hunder, L. Hagerman, W. Walsh and E. A. Eisenhauer, "Interleukin-21 Has Activity in Patients With Metastatic Melanoma: A Phase II Study," *J. Clin. Oncol., Aug 20, 2012.*

[138] L. E. Spitler, M. L. Grossbard, M. S. Ernstoff, G. Silver, M. Jacobs, F. A. Hayes and S. J. Soong, "Adjuvant therapy of stage III and IV malignant melanoma using granulocyte-macrophage colony-stimulating factor," *J. Clin. Oncol., vol. 18, pp. 1614-1621, Apr, 2000.*

[139] D. H. Lawson, S. J. Lee, A. A. Tarhini, K. A. Margolin, M. S. Ernstoff and J. M. Kirkwood, "Phase III cooperative group study of yeast-derived granulocyte macrophage colony-stimulating factor (GM-CSF) versus placebo as adjuvant treatment of patients with completely resected stage III-IV melanoma," *J Clin Oncol,* vol. 28, pp. 8504, 2010.

[140] M. Chi and A. Z. Dudek. Vaccine therapy for metastatic melanoma: Systematic review and meta-analysis of clinical trials. *Melanoma Res. 21(3),* pp. 165-174. 2011.

[141] A. M. Terando, M. B. Faries and D. L. Morton. Vaccine therapy for melanoma: Current status and future directions. *Vaccine* 25pp. B4-B16. 2007.

[142] D. BERD, H. MAGUIRE, P. MCCUE and M. MASTRANGELO. Treatment of metastatic melanoma with an autologous tumor-cell vaccine - clinical and immunological results in 64 patients. *Journal of Clinical Oncology 8(11),* pp. 1858-1867. 1990.

[143] D. Berd, H. Maguire, L. Schuchter, R. Hamilton, W. Hauck, T. Sato and M. Mastrangelo. Autologous hapten-modified melanoma vaccine as postsurgical adjuvant treatment after resection of nodal metastases. Journal of Clinical Oncology 15(6), pp. 2359-2370. 1997.

[144] D. Berd, T. Sato, H. C. Maguire, J. Kairys and M. J. Mastrangelo. Immunopharmacologic analysis of an autologous, hapten-modified human melanoma vaccine. Journal of Clinical Oncology [All @ UAMS; LRVA (latest 10 years)]. *22(3)*, pp. 403-415. 2004. Available: http://ovidsp.ovid.com/ovidweb.cgi?T=JS&CSC=Y&NEWS=N&PAGE=fulltext&D=ipab&AN=41-07931.

[145] R. O. Dillman, C. DePriest, C. DeLeon, N. M. Barth, L. S. Schwartzberg, L. D. Beutel, P. M. Schiltz and S. K. Nayak. Patient-specific vaccines derived from autologous tumor cell lines as active specific immunotherapy: Results of exploratory phase I/II trials in patients with metastatic melanoma. *Cancer Biotherapy and Radiopharmaceuticals 22(3)*, pp. 309-321. 2007.

[146] R. Dillman, S. Selvan, P. Schiltz, C. Peterson, K. Allen, C. DePriest, E. McClay, N. Barth, P. Sheehy, C. de Leon and L. Beutel. Phase I/II trial of melanoma patient-specific vaccine of proliferating autologous tumor cells, dendritic cells, and GM-CSF: Planned interim analysis. *Cancer Biotherapy and Radiopharmaceuticals 19(5)*, pp. 658-665. 2004.

[147] R. O. Dillman, L. D. Beutel, N. M. Barth, C. de Leon, A. A. O'Connor, C. DePriest and S. K. Nayak. Irradiated cells from autologous tumor cell lines as patient-specific vaccine therapy in 125 patients with metastatic cancer: Induction of delayed-type hypersensitivity to autologous tumor is associated with improved survival. *Cancer Biother. Radiopharm. [Not locally available; ask about Interlibrary Loan]. 17(1)*, pp. 51-66. 2002. Available: http://ovidsp.ovid.com/ovidweb.cgi?T=JS&CSC=Y&NEWS=N&PAGE=fulltext&D=med4&AN=11915174.

[148] A. Anichini, C. Vegetti and R. Mortarini. The paradox of T-cell-mediated antitumor immunity in spite of poor clinical outcome in human melanoma. Cancer Immunology, Immunotherapy [Not locally available; ask about Interlibrary Loan]. *53(10)*, pp. 855-864. 2004. Available: http://ovidsp.ovid.com/ovidweb.cgi?T=JS&CSC=Y&NEWS=N&PAGE=fulltext&D=med4&AN=15175905.

[149] E. G. Elias, C. M. Suter and D. S. Fabian. Adjuvant immunotherapy in melanoma with irradiated autologous tumor cells and low dose cyclophosphamide. J. Surg. Oncol. [Part @ UAMS (Click Library Holdings)]. 64(1), pp. 17-22. 1997. Available: http://ovidsp.ovid.com/ovidweb.cgi?T=JS&CSC=Y&NEWS=N&PAGE=fulltext&D=med4&AN=9040795.

[150] E. G. Elias, J. L. Zapas, E. C. McCarron, S. L. Beam, J. H. Hasskamp and W. J. Culpepper. Sequential administration of GM-CSF (sargramostim (R)) and IL-2 +/- autologous vaccine as adjuvant therapy in cutaneous melanoma: An interim report of a phase II clinical trial. *Cancer Biotherapy and Radiopharmaceuticals 23(3)*, pp. 285-291. 2008.

[151] O. Eton, D. Kharkevitch, M. Gianan, M. Ross, K. Itoh, M. Pride, C. Donawho, A. Buzaid, P. Mansfield, J. Lee, S. Legha, C. Plager, N. Papadopoulos, A. Bedikian, R. Benjamin and C. Balch. Active immunotherapy with ultraviolet B-irradiated autologous

whole melanoma cells plus DETOX in patients with metastatic melanoma. *Clinical Cancer Research 4(3),* pp. 619-627. 1998.

[152] R. Soiffer, T. Lynch, M. Mihm, K. Jung, C. Rhuda, J. C. Schmollinger, F. S. Hodi, L. Liebster, P. Lam, S. Mentzer, S. Singer, K. K. Tanabe, A. B. Cosimi, R. Duda, A. Sober, A. Bhan, J. Daley, D. Neuberg, G. Parry, J. Rokovich, L. Richards, J. Drayer, A. Berns, S. Clift, L. K. Cohen, R. C. Mulligan and G. Dranoff, "Vaccination with irradiated autologous melanoma cells engineered to secrete human granulocyte-macrophage colony-stimulating factor generates potent antitumor immunity in patients with metastatic melanoma," *Proc. Natl. Acad. Sci. U. S. A.,* vol. 95, pp. 13141-13146, Oct 27, 1998.

[153] S. Nawrocki, P. Murawa, J. Malicki, M. Kapcinska, K. Gryska, D. Izycki, A. Kaczmarek, M. Laciak, A. Czapczyk, A. Karczewska, S. Rose-John and A. Mackiewicz, "Genetically modified tumour vaccines (GMTV) in melanoma clinical trials," *Immunol. Lett., vol. 74, pp. 81-86, Sep 15, 2000.*

[154] A. Testori, J. Richards, E. Whitman, G. B. Mann, J. Lutzky, L. Camacho, G. Parmiani, G. Tosti, J. M. Kirkwood, A. Hoos, L. Yuh, R. Gupta and P. K. Srivastava. Phase III comparison of vitespen, an autologous tumor-derived heat shock protein gp96 peptide complex vaccine, with physician's choice of treatment for stage IV melanoma: The C-100-21 study group. *Journal of Clinical Oncology 26(6),* pp. 955-962. 2008.

[155] V. Sondak, M. Sabel and J. Mule. Allogeneic and autologous melanoma vaccines: Where have we been and where are we going? *Clinical Cancer Research 12(7),* pp. 2337S-2341S. 2006.

[156] E. Hsueh and D. Morton. Antigen-based immunotherapy of melanoma: Canvaxin therapeutic polyvalent cancer vaccine. *Semin. Cancer Biol. 13(6),* pp. 401-407. 2003.

[157] D. Berd and G. Parmiani. Human tumor vaccines go molecular. summary of american association for cancer research symposium, march 20,1995. *Cancer Immunology, Immunotherapy* [Not locally available; ask about Interlibrary Loan]. *41(3),* pp. 199-200. 1995. Available: http://ovidsp.ovid.com/ovidweb.cgi?T=JS&CSC=Y&NEWS=N&PAGE=fulltext&D=med3&AN=7553690.

[158] M. M. Barrio, P. T. de Motta, J. Kaplan, E. M. von Euw, A. I. Bravo, R. D. Chacon and J. Mordoh, "A phase I study of an allogeneic cell vaccine (VACCIMEL) with GM-CSF in melanoma patients," *J. Immunother.,* vol. 29, pp. 444-454, Jul-Aug, 2006.

[159] M. K. Wallack, S. D. Scoggin and M. Sivanandham, "Active specific immunotherapy with vaccinia melanoma oncolysate," *Mt. Sinai J. Med.,* vol. 59, pp. 227-233, May, 1992.

[160] M. S. Mitchell, W. Harel, J. Kan-Mitchell, L. G. LeMay, P. Goedegebuure, X. Q. Huang, F. Hofman and S. Groshen. Active specific immunotherapy of melanoma with allogeneic cell lysates. rationale, results, and possible mechanisms of action. *Ann. N. Y. Acad. Sci.* [Part @ UAMS (Click Library Holdings)]. *690*pp. 153-166. 1993.

Available: http://ovidsp.ovid.com/ovidweb.cgi?T=JS&CSC=Y&NEWS=N&PAGE=fulltext&D=med3&AN=8368734.

[161] V. K. Sondak, P. Y. Liu, R. J. Tuthill, R. A. Kempf and L. E. Flaherty. Adjuvant immunotherapy of resected, intermediate-thickness, node-negative melanoma with an allogeneic tumor vaccine: Overall results of a randomized trial of the southwest oncology group. *Journal of Clinical Oncology* [All @ UAMS; LRVA (latest 10 years)]. *20(8),* pp. 2058-2066. 2002. Available: http://ovidsp.ovid.com/ovidweb.cgi?T=JS&CSC=Y&NEWS=N&PAGE=fulltext&D=ipab&AN=39-11023.

[162] V. K. Sondak, J. Sosman, J. M. Unger, P. Y. Liu, J. Thompson, R. Tuthill, R. Kempf and L. Flaherty. Significant impact of HLA class I allele expression on outcome in melanoma patients treated with an allogeneic melanoma cell lysate vaccine. final analysis of SWOG-9035 [abstract]. *Annual Meeting Proceedings of the American Society of Clinical Oncology 707p*2004. Available: http://ovidsp.ovid.com/ovidweb.cgi?T=JS&CSC=Y&NEWS=N&PAGE=fulltext&D=cctr&AN=CN-00544014.

[163] J. A. Sosman, J. M. Unger, P. Y. Liu, L. E. Flaherty and SW Oncology Grp. Adjuvant immunotherapy of resected, intermediate-thickness, node-negative melanoma with an allogeneic tumor vaccine: Impact of HLA class I antigen expression on outcome. *Journal of Clinical Oncology* [All @ UAMS; LRVA (latest 10 years)]. *20(8),* pp. 2067-2075. 2002. Available: http://ovidsp.ovid.com/ovidweb.cgi?T=JS&CSC=Y&NEWS=N&PAGE=fulltext&D=ipab&AN=39-10980.

[164] M. S. Mitchell, J. Abrams, J. A. Thompson, M. Kashani-Sabet, R. C. DeConti, W. Hwu, M. B. Atkins, E. Whitman, M. S. Ernstoff, F. G. Haluska, J. G. Jakowatz, T. K. Das Gupta, J. M. Richards, W. E. Samlowski, J. J. Costanzi, F. R. Aronson, A. B. Deisseroth, A. Z. Dudek and V. E. Jones. Randomized trial of an allogeneic melanoma lysate vaccine with low-dose interferon alfa-2b compared with high-dose interferon alfa-2b for resected stage III cutaneous melanoma. *Journal of Clinical Oncology 25(15),* pp. 2078-2085. 2007.

[165] J. D. Wolchok and P. O. Livingston. Vaccines for melanoma: Translating basic immunology into new therapies. *Lancet Oncology* [Part @ UAMS (Click Library Holdings)]. 2(4), pp. 205-211. 2001. Available: http://ovidsp.ovid.com/ovidweb.cgi?T=JS&CSC=Y&NEWS=N&PAGE=fulltext&D=med4&AN=11905765.

[166] I. D. Davis, W. Chen, H. Jackson, P. Parente, M. Shackleton, W. Hopkins, Q. Chen, N. Dimopoulos, T. Luke, R. Murphy, A. M. Scott, E. Maraskovsky, G. McArthur, D. MacGregor, S. Sturrock, T. Y. Tai, S. Green, A. Cuthbertson, D. Maher, L. Miloradovic, S. V. Mitchell, G. Ritter, A. A. Jungbluth, Y. T. Chen, S. Gnjatic, E. W. Hoffman, L. J. Old and J. S. Cebon, "Recombinant NY-ESO-1 protein with ISCOMATRIX adjuvant induces broad integrated antibody and CD4(+) and CD8(+) T cell responses in humans," *Proc. Natl. Acad. Sci. U. S. A.,* vol. 101, pp. 10697-10702, Jul 20, 2004.

[167] P. O. Livingston, G. Y. Wong, S. Adluri, Y. Tao, M. Padavan, R. Parente, C. Hanlon, M. J. Calves, F. Helling and G. Ritter. Improved survival in stage III melanoma pa-

tients with GM2 antibodies: A randomized trial of adjuvant vaccination with GM2 ganglioside. *Journal of Clinical Oncology : Official Journal of the American Society of Clinical Oncology* [All @ UAMS; LRVA (latest 10 years)]. *12(5),* pp. 1036-1044. 1994. Available: http://ovidsp.ovid.com/ovidweb.cgi?T=JS&CSC=Y&NEWS=N&PAGE=fulltext&D=cctr&AN=CN-00100781.

[168] F. Helling, S. Zhang, A. Shang, S. Adluri and M. Calves. GM2-KLH conjugate vaccine: Increased immunogenicity in melanoma patients after administration with immunological adjuvant QS-21. *Cancer Res.* [All @ UAMS; LRVA (latest 10 years)]. *55(Jul 1),* pp. 2783-2788. 1995. Available: http://ovidsp.ovid.com/ovidweb.cgi?T=JS&CSC=Y&NEWS=N&PAGE=fulltext&D=ipab&AN=33-06593.

[169] J. M. Kirkwood, J. G. Ibrahim, J. A. Sosman, V. K. Sondak, S. S. Agarwala, M. S. Ernstoff and U. Rao. High-dose interferon alfa-2b significantly prolongs relapse-free and overall survival compared with the GM2-KLH/QS-21 vaccine in patients with resected stage IIB-III melanoma: Results of intergroup trial E1694/S9512/C509801. *Journal of Clinical Oncology* [All @ UAMS; LRVA (latest 10 years)]. *19(9),* pp. 2370-2380. 2001. Available: http://ovidsp.ovid.com/ovidweb.cgi?T=JS&CSC=Y&NEWS=N&PAGE=fulltext&D=med4&AN=11331315.

[170] C. Buteau, S. Markovic and E. Celis. Challenges in the development of effective peptide vaccines for cancer. Mayo Clin. *Proc. 77(4),* pp. 339-349. 2002.

[171] S. Tagawa, E. Cheung, W. Banta, C. Gee and J. Weber. Survival analysis after resection of metastatic disease followed by peptide vaccines in patients with stage IV melanoma. *Cancer 106(6),* pp. 1353-1357. 2006.

[172] P. Lee, F. Wang, J. Kuniyoshi, V. Rubio, T. Stuges, S. Groshen, C. Gee, R. Lau, G. Jeffery, K. Margolin, V. Marty and J. Weber. Effects of interleukin-12 on the immune response to a multipeptide vaccine for resected metastatic melanoma. *Journal of Clinical Oncology 19(18),* pp. 3836-3847. 2001.

[173] F. O. Smith, S. G. Downey, J. A. Klapper, J. C. Yang, R. M. Sherry, R. E. Royal, U. S. Kammula, M. S. Hughes, N. P. Restifo, C. L. Levy, D. E. White, S. M. Steinberg and S. A. Rosenberg. Treatment of metastatic melanoma using interleukin-2 alone or in conjunction with vaccines. Clinical Cancer Research 14(17), pp. 5610-5618. 2008.

[174] C. L. Slingluff, G. R. Petroni, K. A. ChianeseBullock, M. E. Smolkin, S. Hibbitts, C. Murphy, N. Johansen, W. W. Grosh, G. V. Yamshchikov, P. Y. Neese, J. W. Patterson, R. Fink and P. K. Rehm. Immunologic and clinical outcomes of a randomized phase II trial of two multipeptide vaccines for melanoma in the adjuvant setting. Clinical Cancer *Research : An Official Journal of the American Association for Cancer Research* [All @ UAMS]. *13(21),* pp. 6386-6395. 2007. Available: http://ovidsp.ovid.com/ovidweb.cgi?T=JS&CSC=Y&NEWS=N&PAGE=fulltext&D=cctr&AN=CN-00620609.

[175] V. Corbiere, J. Chapiro, V. Stroobant, W. Ma, C. Lurquin, B. Lethe, N. van Baren, B. J. Van den Eynde, T. Boon and P. G. Coulie. Antigen spreading contributes to MAGE

vaccination-induced regression of melanoma metastases. *Cancer Res. 71(4),* pp. 1253-1262. 2011.

[176] J. M. Kirkwood, S. Lee, S. J. Moschos, M. R. Albertini, J. C. Michalak, C. Sander, T. Whiteside, L. H. Butterfield and L. Weiner. Immunogenicity and antitumor effects of vaccination with peptide vaccine+/-granulocyte-monocyte colony-stimulating factor and/or IFN-alpha2b in advanced metastatic melanoma: Eastern cooperative oncology group phase II trial E1696. *Clinical Cancer Research : An Official Journal of the American Association for Cancer Research* [All @ UAMS]. *15(4),* pp. 1443-1451. 2009. Available: http://ovidsp.ovid.com/ovidweb.cgi?T=JS&CSC=Y&NEWS=N&PAGE=full-text&D=cctr&AN=CN-00688685.

[177] D. J. Schwartzentruber, D. H. Lawson, J. M. Richards, R. M. Conry, D. M. Miller, J. Treisman, F. Gailani, L. Riley, K. Conlon, B. Pockaj, K. L. Kendra, R. L. White, R. Gonzalez, T. M. Kuzel, B. Curti, P. D. Leming, E. D. Whitman, J. Balkissoon, D. S. Re-intgen, H. Kaufman, F. M. Marincola, M. J. Merino, S. A. Rosenberg, P. Choyke, D. Vena and P. Hwu, "Gp100 Peptide Vaccine and Interleukin-2 in Patients with Ad-vanced Melanoma," *N. Engl. J. Med.,* vol. 364, pp. 2119-2127, Jun 2, 2011.

[178] J. A. Sosman, C. Carrillo, W. J. Urba, L. Flaherty and Ernstoff. Three phase II cytokine working group trials of gp100 (210M) peptide plus high-dose interleukin-2 in pa-tients with HLA-A2-positive advanced melanoma. *Journal of Clinical Oncology* [All @ UAMS; LRVA (latest 10 years)]. *26(14),* pp. 2292-2298. 2008. Available: http://ovidsp.ovid.com/ovidweb.cgi?T=JS&CSC=Y&NEWS=N&PAGE=full-text&D=ipab&AN=45-13437.

[179] M. Bhattacharya-Chatterjee, S. K. Chatterjee and K. A. Foon. Anti-idiotype vaccine against cancer. Immunol. *Lett. [Part @ UAMS (Click Library Holdings)].* 74(1), pp. 51-58. 2000. Available: http://ovidsp.ovid.com/ovidweb.cgi?T=JS&CSC=Y&NEWS=N&PAGE=fulltext&D=med4&AN=10996628.

[180] S. Ferrone. Anti-idiotypes in melanoma. Hybridoma [Online Access Only (Click E Journal Holdings for Information)]. 12(5), pp. 509-514. 1993. Available: http://ovidsp.ovid.com/ovidweb.cgi?T=JS&CSC=Y&NEWS=N&PAGE=full-text&D=med3&AN=8300123.

[181] R. L. Metheringham, V. A. Pudney, B. Gunn, M. Towey, I. Spendlove and L. G. Dur-rant. Antibodies designed as effective cancer vaccines. *MAbs 1(1),* pp. 71-85. 2009. Available: http://ovidsp.ovid.com/ovidweb.cgi?T=JS&CSC=Y&NEWS=N&PAGE=fulltext&D=medl&AN=20046577.

[182] K. A. Foon, G. Sen, L. Hutchins, O. L. Kashala, R. Baral, M. Banerjee, M. Chakraborty, J. Garrison, R. A. Reisfeld and M. Bhattacharya-Chatterjee. Antibody responses in melanoma patients immunized with an anti-idiotype antibody mimicking disialo-ganglioside GD2. *Clinical Cancer Research* [All @ UAMS]. *4(5),* pp. 1117-1124. 1998. Available: http://ovidsp.ovid.com/ovidweb.cgi?T=JS&CSC=Y&NEWS=N&PAGE=fulltext&D=med4&AN=9607568.

[183] K. A. Foon, J. Lutzky, R. N. Baral, J. R. Yannelli, L. Hutchins, A. Teitelbaum, O. L. Kashala, R. Das, J. Garrison, R. A. Reisfeld and M. Bhattacharya-Chatterjee. Clinical and immune responses in advanced melanoma patients immunized with an anti-idiotype antibody mimicking disialoganglioside GD2. *Journal of Clinical Oncology* [All @ UAMS; LRVA (latest 10 years)]. *18(2),* pp. 376-384. 2000. Available: http://ovidsp.ovid.com/ovidweb.cgi?T=JS&CSC=Y&NEWS=N&PAGE=fulltext&D=med4&AN=10637253.

[184] P. B. Chapman, D. Wu, G. Ragupathi, S. Lu, L. Williams, W. J. Hwu, D. Johnson and P. O. Livingston. Sequential immunization of melanoma patients with GD3 ganglioside vaccine and anti-idiotypic monoclonal antibody that mimics GD3 ganglioside. Clinical Cancer *Research : An Official Journal of the American Association for Cancer Research* [All @ UAMS]. *10(14),* pp. 4717-4723. 2004. Available: http://ovidsp.ovid.com/ovidweb.cgi?T=JS&CSC=Y&NEWS=N&PAGE=fulltext&D=cctr&AN=CN-00502094.

[185] S. A. Rosenberg, J. C. Yang, D. J. Schwartzentruber, P. Hwu, S. L. Topalian, R. M. Sherry, N. P. Restifo, J. R. Wunderlich, C. A. Seipp, L. Rogers-Freezer, K. E. Morton, S. A. Mavroukakis, L. Gritz, D. L. Panicali and D. E. White. Recombinant fowlpox viruses encoding the anchor-modified gp100 melanoma antigen can generate antitumor immune responses in patients with metastatic melanoma. *Clinical Cancer Research* [All @ UAMS]. *9(8),* pp. 2973-2980. 2003. Available: http://ovidsp.ovid.com/ovidweb.cgi?T=JS&CSC=Y&NEWS=N&PAGE=fulltext&D=medc&AN=12912944.

[186] S. A. Rosenberg, Y. Zhai, J. C. Yang, D. J. Schwartzentruber and D. E. White. Immunizing patients with metastatic melanoma using recombinant adenoviruses encoding MART-1 or gp100 melanoma antigens. J. Natl. Cancer Inst. [All @ UAMS; LRVA (latest 10 years)]. *90(Dec 16),* pp. 1894-1900. 1998. Available: http://ovidsp.ovid.com/ovidweb.cgi?T=JS&CSC=Y&NEWS=N&PAGE=fulltext&D=ipab&AN=37-00699.

[187] M. Adamina, R. Rosenthal, W. P. Weber, D. M. Frey, C. T. Viehl, M. Bolli, R. W. Huegli, A. L. Jacob, M. Heberer, D. Oertli, W. Marti, G. C. Spagnoli and P. Zajac. Intranodal immunization with a vaccinia virus encoding multiple antigenic epitopes and costimulatory molecules in metastatic melanoma. Molecular Therapy 18(3), pp. 651-659. 2010.

[188] B. W. Bridle, J. E. Boudreau, B. D. Lichty, J. Brunelliere, K. Stephenson, S. Koshy, J. L. Bramson and Y. Wan. Vesicular stomatitis virus as a novel cancer vaccine vector to prime antitumor immunity amenable to rapid boosting with adenovirus. Molecular Therapy: The Journal of the American Society of Gene Therapy [Online Access Only (Click E Journal Holdings for Information)]. *17(10),* pp. 1814-1821. 2009. Available: http://ovidsp.ovid.com/ovidweb.cgi?T=JS&CSC=Y&NEWS=N&PAGE=fulltext&D=medl&AN=19603003.

[189] P. Hersey, A. S. Coates, W. H. McCarthy, J. F. Thompson and R. J. Simes. Adjuvant immunotherapy of patients with high-risk melanoma using vaccinia viral lysates of melanoma: Results of a randomized trial. *Journal of Clinical Oncology* [All @ UAMS; LRVA (latest 10 years)]. *20(20),* pp. 4181-4190. 2002. Available: http://

ovidsp.ovid.com/ovidweb.cgi?T=JS&CSC=Y&NEWS=N&PAGE=full-text&D=ipab&AN=40-02647.

[190] A. Mazzocchi, C. Melani, L. Rivoltini, C. Castelli, M. Del Vecchio, C. Lombardo, M. Colombo and G. Parmiani. Simultaneous transduction of B7-1 and IL-2 genes into human melanoma cells to be used as vaccine: Enhancement of stimulatory activity for autologous and allogeneic lymphocytes. *Cancer Immunology Immunotherapy 50(4),* pp. 199-211. 2001.

[191] H. Kaufman, G. DeRaffele, J. Mitcham, D. Moroziewicz, S. Cohen, K. Hurst-Wicker, K. Cheung, D. Lee, J. Divito, M. Voulo, J. Donovan, K. Dolan, K. Manson, D. Panicali, E. Wang, H. Horig and F. Marincola. Targeting the local tumor microenvironment with vaccinia virus expressing B7.1 for the treatment of melanoma. J. Clin. Invest. 115(7), pp. 1903-1912. 2005.

[192] C. J. Kim, J. Cormier, M. Roden, L. Gritz, G. P. Mazzara, P. Fetsch, Y. Hijazi, K. H. Lee, S. A. Rosenberg and F. M. Marincola. Use of recombinant poxviruses to stimulate anti-melanoma T cell reactivity. Annals of Surgical Oncology [Part @ UAMS (Click Library Holdings)]. *5(1),* pp. 64-76. 1998. Available: http://ovidsp.ovid.com/ovidweb.cgi?T=JS&CSC=Y&NEWS=N&PAGE=fulltext&D=med4&AN=9524710.

[193] Sabel and V. K. Sondak. Tumor vaccines - A role in preventing recurrence in melanoma? American Journal of Clinical Dermatology [Not locally available; ask about Interlibrary Loan]. *3(9),* pp. 609-616. 2002. Available: http://ovidsp.ovid.com/ovidweb.cgi?T=JS&CSC=Y&NEWS=N&PAGE=fulltext&D=ipab&AN=40-06431.

[194] G. J. Prud'homme. DNA vaccination against tumors. J. Gene Med. [Not locally available; ask about Interlibrary Loan]. *7(1),* pp. 3-17. 2005. Available: http://ovidsp.ovid.com/ovidweb.cgi?T=JS&CSC=Y&NEWS=N&PAGE=full-text&D=med4&AN=15538731.

[195] D. B. Lowe, M. H. Shearer, C. A. Jumper and R. C. Kennedy. Towards progress on DNA vaccines for cancer. Cellular and Molecular Life Sciences 64(18), pp. 2391-2403. 2007.

[196] G. Dranoff. GM-CSF-secreting melanoma vaccines. Oncogene [Part @ UAMS (Click Library Holdings)]. 22(20), pp. 3188-3192. 2003. Available: http://ovidsp.ovid.com/ovidweb.cgi?T=JS&CSC=Y&NEWS=N&PAGE=fulltext&D=med4&AN=12789295.

[197] H. L. Kaufman, D. W. Kim, G. DeRaffele, J. Mitcham, R. S. Coffin and S. Kim-Schulze. Local and distant immunity induced by intralesional vaccination with an oncolytic herpes virus encoding GM-CSF in patients with stage IIIc and IV melanoma. *Annals of Surgical Oncology 17(3),* pp. 718-730. 2010.

[198] H. L. Kaufman and S. D. Bines, "OPTIM trial: a Phase III trial of an oncolytic herpes virus encoding GM-CSF for unresectable stage III or IV melanoma," *Future Oncol.,* vol. 6, pp. 941-949, Jun, 2010.

[199] A. T. Stopeck, E. M. Hersh, E. T. Akporiaye, D. T. Harris, T. Grogan, E. Unger, J. Warneke, S. F. Schluter and S. Stahl, "Phase I study of direct gene transfer of an allogeneic histocompatibility antigen, HLA-B7, in patients with metastatic melanoma," *J. Clin. Oncol., vol. 15, pp. 341-349, Jan, 1997.*

[200] A. T. Stopeck, A. Jones, E. M. Hersh, J. A. Thompson, D. M. Finucane, J. C. Gutheil and R. Gonzalez. Phase II study of direct intralesional gene transfer of allovectin-7, an HLA-B7/beta2-microglobulin DNA-liposome complex, in patients with metastatic melanoma. *Clinical Cancer Research* [All @ UAMS]. *7(8),* pp. 2285-2291. 2001. Available: http://ovidsp.ovid.com/ovidweb.cgi?T=JS&CSC=Y&NEWS=N&PAGE=fulltext&D=med4&AN=11489803.

[201] R. Gonzalez, L. Hutchins, J. Nemunaitis, M. Atkins and P. O. Schwarzenberger, "Phase 2 trial of Allovectin-7 in advanced metastatic melanoma," *Melanoma Res.,* vol. 16, pp. 521-526, Dec, 2006.

[202] A. Y. Bedikian, J. Richards, D. Kharkevitch, M. B. Atkins, E. Whitman and R. Gonzalez, "A phase 2 study of high-dose Allovectin-7 in patients with advanced metastatic melanoma," *Melanoma Res.,* vol. 20, pp. 218-226, Jun, 2010.

[203] R. Chowdhery and R. Gonzalez, "Immunologic therapy targeting metastatic melanoma: allovectin-7," *Immunotherapy,* vol. 3, pp. 17-21, Jan, 2011.

[204] S. A. Rosenberg, M. T. Lotze, L. M. Muul, A. E. Chang, F. P. Avis, S. Leitman, W. M. Linehan, C. N. Robertson, R. E. Lee and J. T. Rubin, "A progress report on the treatment of 157 patients with advanced cancer using lymphokine-activated killer cells and interleukin-2 or high-dose interleukin-2 alone," *N. Engl. J. Med.,* vol. 316, pp. 889-897, Apr 9, 1987.

[205] S. A. Rosenberg, M. T. Lotze, J. C. Yang, S. L. Topalian, A. E. Chang, D. J. Schwartzentruber, P. Aebersold, S. Leitman, W. M. Linehan and C. A. Seipp, "Prospective randomized trial of high-dose interleukin-2 alone or in conjunction with lymphokine-activated killer cells for the treatment of patients with advanced cancer," *J. Natl. Cancer Inst.,* vol. 85, pp. 622-632, Apr 21, 1993.

[206] S. A. Rosenberg, J. R. Yannelli, J. C. Yang, S. L. Topalian, D. J. Schwartzentruber, J. S. Weber, D. R. Parkinson, C. A. Seipp, J. H. Einhorn and D. E. White, "Treatment of patients with metastatic melanoma with autologous tumor-infiltrating lymphocytes and interleukin 2," *J. Natl. Cancer Inst.,* vol. 86, pp. 1159-1166, Aug 3, 1994.

[207] A. I. Riker, S. Radfar, S. Liu, Y. Wang and H. T. Khong, "Immunotherapy of melanoma: a critical review of current concepts and future strategies," *Expert Opin. Biol. Ther.,* vol. 7, pp. 345-358, Mar, 2007.

[208] J. J. Hong, S. A. Rosenberg, M. E. Dudley, J. C. Yang, D. E. White, J. A. Butman and R. M. Sherry, "Successful treatment of melanoma brain metastases with adoptive cell therapy," *Clin. Cancer Res.,* vol. 16, pp. 4892-4898, Oct 1, 2010.

[209] Anonymous NCI. Available: http://www.cancer.gov/ncicancerbulletin/050112/page4.

[210] B. Thurner, I. Haendle, C. Roder, D. Dieckmann, P. Keikavoussi, H. Jonuleit, A. Bender, C. Maczek, D. Schreiner, P. von den Driesch, E. B. Brocker, R. M. Steinman, A. Enk, E. Kampgen and G. Schuler, "Vaccination with mage-3A1 peptide-pulsed mature, monocyte-derived dendritic cells expands specific cytotoxic T cells and induces regression of some metastases in advanced stage IV melanoma," *J. Exp. Med.*, vol. 190, pp. 1669-1678, Dec 6, 1999.

[211] R. Lau, F. Wang, G. Jeffery, V. Marty, J. Kuniyoshi, E. Bade, M. E. Ryback and J. Weber, "Phase I trial of intravenous peptide-pulsed dendritic cells in patients with metastatic melanoma," *J. Immunother.*, vol. 24, pp. 66-78, Jan-Feb, 2001.

[212] L. Engell-Noerregaard, T. H. Hansen, M. H. Andersen, P. Thor Straten and I. M. Svane, "Review of clinical studies on dendritic cell-based vaccination of patients with malignant melanoma: assessment of correlation between clinical response and vaccine parameters," *Cancer Immunol. Immunother., vol. 58, pp. 1-14, Jan, 2009.*

[213] D. Schadendorf, S. Ugurel, B. Schuler-Thurner, F. O. Nestle, A. Enk, E. B. Brocker, S. Grabbe, W. Rittgen, L. Edler, A. Sucker, C. Zimpfer-Rechner, T. Berger, J. Kamarashev, G. Burg, H. Jonuleit, A. Tuttenberg, J. C. Becker, P. Keikavoussi, E. Kampgen, G. Schuler and DC study group of the DeCOG, "Dacarbazine (DTIC) versus vaccination with autologous peptide-pulsed dendritic cells (DC) in first-line treatment of patients with metastatic melanoma: a randomized phase III trial of the DC study group of the DeCOG," *Ann. Oncol.*, vol. 17, pp. 563-570, Apr, 2006.

[214] D. T. Alexandrescu, T. E. Ichim, N. H. Riordan, F. M. Marincola, A. Di Nardo, F. D. Kabigting and C. A. Dasanu, "Immunotherapy for melanoma: current status and perspectives," *J. Immunother.*, vol. 33, pp. 570-590, Jul-Aug, 2010.

[215] R. Thomas, J. Padmanabha, M. Chambers, S. McFadyen, E. Walpole, G. Nielssen and M. Smithers. Metastatic lesions in the joint associated with acute inflammatory arthritis after dendritic cell immunotherapy for metastatic melanoma. *Melanoma Res.* [Online Access Only (Click E Journal Holdings for Information)]. 11(2), pp. 167-173. 2001. Available: http://ovidsp.ovid.com/ovidweb.cgi?T=JS&CSC=Y&NEWS=N&PAGE=fulltext&D=med4&AN=11333127.

[216] D. P. Lawrence, O. Hamid, D. F. McDermott, I. Puzanov, M. Sznol, J. Clark, T. Logan, F. S. Hodi, K. N. Heller and K. A. Margolin, "Phase II trial of ipilimubab monotherapy in melanoma patients with brain metastasis," *J. Clin. Oncol., vol. 28, pp. 8523, 2010.*

[217] J. D. Wolchok, B. Neyns, G. Linette, S. Negrier, J. Lutzky, L. Thomas, W. Waterfield, D. Schadendorf, M. Smylie, T. Guthrie Jr, J. J. Grob, J. Chesney, K. Chin, K. Chen, A. Hoos, S. J. O'Day and C. Lebbe, "Ipilimumab monotherapy in patients with pretreated advanced melanoma: a randomised, double-blind, multicentre, phase 2, dose-ranging study," *Lancet Oncol.*, vol. 11, pp. 155-164, Feb, 2010.

[218] K. T. Flaherty, J. A. Sosman and M. B. Atkins, "New options and new questions: How to select sequence therapies for patients with metastatic melanoma," *ASCO Educational Book*, pp. 524-530, 2012.

[219] J. M. Kirkwood, P. Lorigan, P. Hersey, A. Hauschild, C. Robert, D. McDermott, M. A. Marshall, J. Gomez-Navarro, J. Q. Liang and C. A. Bulanhagui, "Phase II trial of tremelimumab (CP-675,206) in patients with advanced refractory or relapsed melanoma," *Clin. Cancer Res.*, vol. 16, pp. 1042-1048, Feb 1, 2010.

[220] A. Ribas, A. Hauschild, R. Kefford, C. J. Punt, J. B. Haanen, M. Marmol, C. Garbe, J. Gomez-Navarro, D. Pavlov and M. Marshall, "Phase III, open-label, randomized, comparative study of tremelimumab (CP-675,206) and chemotherpay (temozolomide or dacarbazine) in patiens with advanced melanoma," *J. Clin. Oncol., vol. 26, pp. LBA9011, 2008.*

[221] D. M. Benson Jr, C. E. Bakan, A. Mishra, C. C. Hofmeister, Y. Efebera, B. Becknell, R. A. Baiocchi, J. Zhang, J. Yu, M. K. Smith, C. N. Greenfield, P. Porcu, S. M. Devine, R. Rotem-Yehudar, G. Lozanski, J. C. Byrd and M. A. Caligiuri, "The PD-1/PD-L1 axis modulates the natural killer cell versus multiple myeloma effect: a therapeutic target for CT-011, a novel monoclonal anti-PD-1 antibody," *Blood,* vol. 116, pp. 2286-2294, Sep 30, 2010.

[222] M. Sznol, F. S. Hodi, K. Margolin, D. F. McDermott, M. S. Ernstoff, J. M. Kirkwood, C. Wojtaszek, D. Feltquate and T. Logan, "Phase I study of BMS-663513, a fully human anti-CD137 agonist monoclonal antibody in patients with advanced cancer," *J. Clin. Oncol., vol. 26, pp. 3007, 2008.*

[223] B. Curti, A. Weinberg and N. Morris, "A phase I trial of monoclonal antibody to OX40 in patients with advanced cancer," *International Society for Biological Therapy of Cancer Annual Meeting,* 2007.

[224] A. Boni, A. P. Cogdill, P. Dang, D. Udayakumar, C. N. Njauw, C. M. Sloss, C. R. Ferrone, K. T. Flaherty, D. P. Lawrence, D. E. Fisher, H. Tsao and J. A. Wargo, "Selective BRAFV600E inhibition enhances T-cell recognition of melanoma without affecting lymphocyte function," *Cancer Res.*, vol. 70, pp. 5213-5219, Jul 1, 2010.

[225] M. A. Curran, W. Montalvo, H. Yagita and J. P. Allison, "PD-1 and CTLA-4 combination blockade expands infiltrating T cells and reduces regulatory T and myeloid cells within B16 melanoma tumors," *Proc. Natl. Acad. Sci. U. S. A.*, vol. 107, pp. 4275-4280, Mar 2, 2010.

[226] M. A. Curran, M. Kim, W. Montalvo, A. Al-Shamkhani and J. P. Allison, "Combination CTLA-4 blockade and 4-1BB activation enhances tumor rejection by increasing T-cell infiltration, proliferation, and cytokine production," *PLoS One,* vol. 6, pp. e19499, Apr 29, 2011.

[227] A. A. Tarhini, J. Cherian, S. J. Moschos, H. A. Tawbi, Y. Shuai, W. E. Gooding, C. Sander and J. M. Kirkwood, "Safety and efficacy of combination immunotherapy with interferon alfa-2b and tremelimumab in patients with stage IV melanoma," *J. Clin. Oncol., vol. 30, pp. 322-328, Jan 20, 2012.*

[228] F. S. Hodi, M. Butler, D. A. Oble, M. V. Seiden, F. G. Haluska, A. Kruse, S. Macrae, M. Nelson, C. Canning, I. Lowy, A. Korman, D. Lautz, S. Russell, M. T. Jaklitsch, N.

Ramaiya, T. C. Chen, D. Neuberg, J. P. Allison, M. C. Mihm and G. Dranoff, "Immunologic and clinical effects of antibody blockade of cytotoxic T lymphocyte-associated antigen 4 in previously vaccinated cancer patients," *Proc. Natl. Acad. Sci. U. S. A.*, vol. 105, pp. 3005-3010, Feb 26, 2008.

Chapter 11

The Menace of Melanoma: A Photodynamic Approach to Adjunctive Cancer Therapy

L.M. Davids and B. Kleemann

Additional information is available at the end of the chapter

1. Introduction

Metastatic malignant melanoma (MMM) remains one of the most dreaded skin cancers worldwide. Numerous factors contribute to its resistance to hosts of treatment regimes and despite significant scientific advances over the last decade in the field of chemotherapeutics and melanocytic targets, there still remains the need for improved therapeutic modalities. Photodynamic therapy (PDT), a minimally invasive therapeutic modality has been shown to be effective in a number of oncologic and non-oncologic conditions. Using second-generation stable, lipophillic photosensitizers with optimised activation wavelengths, PDT may be a promising tool for adjuvant therapy and even pre-treatment in combating melanoma. Potential targets for PDT in melanoma eradication include cell proliferation inhibition, activation of cell death and reduction in pro-survival autophagy, a decrease in the cellular melanocytic antioxidant system and a disruption in the endogenous multi-drug resistant (MDR) cellular machinery. This chapter highlights the current knowledge with respect to these characteristics and suggests that PDT be considered as a good candidate for adjuvant treatment in post-resected malignant metastatic melanoma. Furthermore, it suggests that primary consideration must be given to organelle-specific destruction in melanoma specifically targeting the melanosomes – the one organelle that is specific to cells of the melanocytic lineage that houses the toxic compound, melanin. We believe that using this combined knowledge may eventually lead to an effective therapeutic tool to combat this highly intractable disease.

1.1. Melanoma clinical statistics

Melanoma accounts for 4% of all dermatologic cancers but remains responsible for 80% of deaths from skin cancer with the average patient diagnosed with disseminated metastases surviving for an average of 5 years (Cancer facts and figures, 2003, Atlanta, American Cancer Society, 2003]. According to the World Health Organization (WHO) melanoma skin cancer has been increasing over the past decades with a global estimation of 132 000 melanoma-related skin cancers reported to occur each year. Over the past 50 years, melanoma incidence has risen by 3–8% per year in most people of European background, with the greatest increases in elderly men [1]. In Europe, the current estimates at 15-20 per 100 000 people predominating in the 20-35 year old age group in Caucasians [2]. South Africa, next to Australia, has one of the highest incidences of malignant melanoma in the world. Reliable statistics for South Africa are lacking, however currently an estimate figure for the South African Cape region is 69 new cases per year per population of 100 000 Caucasians (Australia is 65 per 100 000). This means that 1 in 1429 people will develop malignant melanoma. The age-standardised incidence of melanoma was 27.2 per 100 000 for males and 22.2 per 100 000 for females from 1990-1999 but this increased to 36.9 for males and 33.5 per 100 000 for females (2000-2003) (CANSA association of South Africa www.melanoma.co.za/D_doccnr_MFS.asp) (Table 1).

	Age-standardised incidence(10^5 /yr)	Lifetime risk (incidence)	Incidence trend over 10 years	Mortality trend over 10 years	Most common cancer (ranking)
Australia (2001)					
Men	41.4 (world)	1 in 25	22% increase	2% increase	4th
Women	31.1 (world)	1 in 35	12% increase	0% increase	3rd
South Africa (2000)					
Men	36.9 (world)	1 in 29	33% increase	1.5% increase	4th
Women	33.5 (world)	1 in 40	27% increase	1% increase	3rd
USA (2001)					
Men	21.4 (world)	1 in 53	31% increase	0% increase	5th
Women	13.8 (world)	1 in 78	25% increase	1% decrease	7th
UK (2000)					
Men	9.7 (world)	1 in 147	59% increase	20% increase	12th
Women	11.2 (world)	1 in 117	41% incraese	3% increase	7th

Table 1. Melanoma statistics in 2 southern and northern hemisphere countries

Despite extensive research and clinical trials, the prognosis and survival of metastatic melanoma remains dismal. Early detection of localized melanoma may be cured through surgery however there is no therapy for metastatic melanoma or melanoma with metastatic potential. In addition, recurrence rates of resected melanoma remain high. Because melanoma is inherently resistant to traditional forms of chemotherapy and radiotherapy [3], various strategies have been developed for treatments which include immunotherapy eg. interleukin-2 (IL-2) [4], radiotherapy [5] biochemotherapy [6-9] and gene therapy [4,10]. A limited number of these therapies have progressed to human clinical trials but their outcomes remain negligible. One promising therapy is high-dose interferon (IFN) alpha-2b therapy which has just recently been approved as the only adjuvant therapy for melanoma approved by the US Food and Drug Administration [11]. The other is the use of BRAF kinase inhibitors such as vemurafenib [12]. Despite convincing evidence of improved disease-free survival associated with this therapy, the overall survival remains negligible or very small [13-15]. In addition, a number of melanoma-specific and melanoma-associated tumor antigens such as gp100, MART-1 and MAGE3 have been cloned [16] and the hope is that these potential antigens may be developed to stimulate tumor-specific T cells to eliminate melanoma cells [17]. Despite these advances, there remains the need for the development of novel and effective approaches to treat melanoma and this review explores the possibility of using photodynamic therapy (PDT) as an adjuvant therapy alone or in combination with current therapeutics to combat melanoma.

1.2. Melanoma origins

Melanoma represents the malignant phenotype of a skin melanocyte. Melanoma occurs most frequently after intermittent exposure to UV radiation and in people with chronic sunburns. Epidemiologic data suggest that chronic or low-grade exposures to UV induce protection against DNA damage, whereas acute, intense UV exposure leads to DNA damage and concomitant genetic alterations in the melanocyte genome [18]. It develops as a result of accumulated abnormalities in genetic pathways within the melanocyte which give way to increased cell proliferation and prevent normal pathways of apoptosis in response to DNA damage. Furthermore, this damage results in the selection for genetic mutations that allow all aspects of the malignant phenotype, including stimulation of blood vessel growth, evasion of the immune response, tumour invasion, and metastasis [19]. Although the mechanisms of differential cancer cell killing are poorly understood [20], selection of cells that are resistant to apoptotic mechanisms might contribute to the resistance of melanoma cells to the cytotoxic effects of chemotherapy, radiotherapy, and immunotherapy, especially through the expression of apoptosis inhibitors such as B-cell lymphoma derived protein 2 (Bcl-2) and BclxL [21].

Melanocytes progress through a series of steps toward malignant transformation by the acquisition of various phenotypic features. The particular histological features characterising each step of progression are the visible manifestations of underlying genetic changes [22].

Originating from a benign nevus, melanocytes undergo aberrant growth within the lesion subsequently displaying irregular borders, a change in colour and often an associated allergic response. At this stage the lesion is considered dysplastic. At a molecular level, these changes are associated with abnormal activation of the mitogen-activated protein kinase (MAPK) signalling pathway resulting in somatic mutations in the N-RAS and BRAF genes which are associated with about 15 and 50% of melanomas, respectively [23,24]. There is complementarity between the presence of *NRAS* and *BRAF* mutations in any individual melanoma since each has the same effect of causing unrestrained cell proliferation.

In addition, mutations in both the cyclin-dependent kinase inhibitor 2A (CDKN2A) and the phosphatase and tensin homologue (PTEN) gene increases the probability of dysplastic naevi becoming malignant [25]. This genetic locus is frequently targeted for disruption in melanomas [26]. When defective, p16 is unable to inactivate CDK4 and CDK6, which phosphorylate Rb, releasing the transcription factor E2F and leading to cell cycle progression [27].The molecule that is usually central to protection against DNA damage, p53, is rarely mutated early in melanoma, which is possibly one of several adaptations to permit survival of cells responsible for generating sun-protective pigment, melanin [28]. Interestingly, by-products of melanin biosynthesis can themselves cause oxidative stress and contribute to malignant change.

Further progression of melanoma is associated with decreased differentiation and clonal proliferation leading to the radial growth phase (RGP). Clinically, RGP presents as patches or plaques which can measure up to 2.5cm. Superficial spreading melanoma lesions are slightly raised and show striking variations of red, blue, white, brown, and black coloration. In RGP, melanoma mitoses are frequently seen in the epidermis but rarely in the dermis. After complete surgical excision of the tumor, RGP melanomas are usually associated with longterm metastasis-free survival [29-33]. RGP cells can progress to vertical growth phase (VGP) cells which breach the basement membrane and invade the dermis as nodules or nests of cells. Vertical growth phase (VGP) melanomas usually present as gray-black, blue-black, or even amelanotic nodules. In late or developed VGP, melanomas form expansile nodules in the dermis with cytology different from melanoma cells in the overlying epidermis. Mitotic figures are variably present, and tumor aggregates may extend into the reticular dermis or even subcutaneous fat. Dermal tumoral nests are larger in VGP than in RGP. Moreover, these cells are considered to have metastatic potential. Interestingly, not all melanomas pass through each of these individual phases – RGP and VGP can both develop directly from melanocytes or naevi and both can progress directly to metastatic malignant melanoma [34]. Moreover, the transition from RGP to VGP in cutaneous melanoma isassociated with the loss of c-KIT expression and the gain of the melanoma cell adhesion molecule (MCAM/MUC18) [35].

Increased proliferation and survival, chemoresistance, the ability to resist apoptosis, the induction of autophagy and the presence of the pigment melanin have all been listed as reasons contributing to the high mortality rates associated with cutaneous melanoma. Each of these topics will be dealt with in the context of targeting them with PDT.

1.3. Photodynamic Therapy (PDT) as a cancer treatment

PDT is a minimally invasive therapeutic modality which has been shown to be effective in several types of cancer including non-melanoma skin cancer (NMSC) and other skin tumors such as lymphoma as well as non-oncological conditions such as psoriasis vulgaris, acne vulgaris and human papilloma virus-induced skin disease [36,37]. The basis of PDT is the systemic or topical application and preferential uptake of a photosensitizer (PS). The PS is then activated at a specific wavelength of light and in the presence of oxygen, produces reactive oxygen species (ROS). The accumulative presence of these cytotoxic photoproducts start a cascade of molecular and biochemical events resulting in cell death via apoptotic or necrotic mechanisms [38,39].

The main advantage of PDT over conventional cancer treatments are i) it has a very low systemic cumulative toxicity allowing repeated dosing, ii) its ability to destroy tumors selectively (this seems to be related to the lipophillic nature of photosensitizers). Due to this selectivity, damage to normal surrounding cells is minimal. Finally, iii) PDT can be applied alone or in combination as an adjuvant therapeutic modality with chemotherapy, surgery, radiotherapy and immunotherapy [40,41]. These properties have led to PDT receiving increased support from preclinical research [42,43]. PDT requires three elements to be efficacious - a good PS, a coherent light source and the presence of molecular oxygen. A large amount of data with regard to these three elements over the last few years have resulted in the development of more naturally-derived, efficacious, second-generation photosensitizers.

1.3.1. Photosensitizers and melanoma-PDT

Photosensitizers are critical to the successful eradication of malignant cells and numerous first and second-generation photosensitizers have been tested both clinically (in vivo) and in vitro over the past years (for a detailed summary of melanoma-PDT research see Table 2). The structure of many PS is based on the tetrapyrrol ring eg. protoporphyrin IX, Photofrin and chlorines related to it eg. phthalocyanines. Newer, more stable second-generation PS include natural hydroxyquinone chromophores such as hypericins and porphycenes [44-47]. It is now accepted that a good PS for PDT is – i) chemically pure with good stability, ii) preferentially accumulated and retained by target tissue, iii) minimal toxicity in the absence of light with maximal efficacy upon activation, iv) high quantum yield of $^1O_2$ with an associated high molecular extinction coefficient [40]. Due to these properties, a number of synthetic or natural compounds have thus far been studied for a variety of cancers however these have been limited to porphycenes (structural isomers of porphyrins) such as aminolevulinic acid (ALA, trade name, Levulan®) and methylaminolevulinic acid (MAL, trade name, Metvix®) for the treatment of squamous cell (SCC) and basal cell carcinomas (BCC) as well as actinic keratoses [48-50] (Table 2).

Type of study	Tumour/Cell line	Photosensitizer	Ref
in vitro	B16-F10 melanoma cells	magnetoliposomes (MLs) loaded with zinc phthalocyanine (ZnPc) complexed with cucurbituril (CB) (CB:ZnPc-MLs)	[51]
in vivo	mice carrying B16-F10 melanoma xenografts	butadiyne-linked conjugated porphyrin dimer (Oxdime)	[52]
in vivo	subcutaneous amelanotic melanoma transplanted in C57/BL6 mice	pheophorbide a (Pba) and monomethoxy-polyethylene glycol-Pba	[53]
in vitro	A375, UCT Mel-1 human melanoma cells	hypericin and kojic acid (depigmenting agent)	[54]
in vitro/ in vivo	B16F10 mouse melanoma cells and lung melanomas in C57BL/6 mice	aminolevulic acid, gaussia luciferase, and its' substrate coelenterazine; murine neural stem cells (NSCs) and rat umbilical cord matrix-derived stem cells (RUCMSCs) with a plasmid expressing gaussia luciferase	[55]
in vitro	C32 human melanoma cells	Ficus carica L. cultivar Dottato extracts	[56]
in vitro	Melanoma, keratinocyte and fibroblast cells	aluminum tetrasulfophthalocyanines	[57]
in vivo	B16-F1 and Cloudman S9 melanoma-bearing mice	chlorin e(6) and modular nanotransporters targeted to α-melanocyte-stimulating hormone (αMSH) and epidermal growth factor (EGF) receptor	[58]
in vivo	malignant melanoma mouse model	methylene blue	[59]
in vitro	A549 and S91 melanoma cells	halogenated sulfonamide bacteriochlorins	[60]
in vitro	A375 melanoma cells	carotenoids (neoxanthin, fucoxanthin and siphonaxanthin)	[61]
in vitro	melanoma cells	2 cationic octanuclear metalla-cubes dual photosensitizers and chemotherapeutics	[62]
in vitro	A375 melanoma cells	Cachrys pungens Jan extracts from Italy	[63]
in vitro	B16F10 murine melanoma	indocyanine green (ICG) and hyperthermia	[64]
in vitro	B78-H1 murine melanoma cells	pheophorbide a	[65]
in vitro	S91 Cloudman melanoma cells and DBA mice	synthetic chlorin derivative ($TCPCSO_3H$)	[66]
in vitro/ in vivo	Melanoma cells and xenograft melanoma model	cis-Dichlorobis [3,4,7,8-tetramethyl-1,10-phenanthroline) rhodium(III) chloride (OCTBP)	[67]
in vitro	M21 human melanoma cells	Hedyotis corymbosa extracts	[68]
in vitro	A375, UCT Mel-1 human melanoma cells	hypericin and phenylthiourea (depigmenting agent)	[69]
in vitro	melanoma, keratinocyte and fibroblast cells	zinc tetrasulfophthalocyanines (ZnTSPc)	[70]

Type of study	Tumour/Cell line	Photosensitizer	Ref
in vitro	melanoma cells	PDT and Lycopene, β-carotene, vitamin C, N-acetylcysteine, trolox, N-tert-butyl-α-phenylnitrone and HO-1 activity inhibitor zinc protoporphyrine IX (ZnPPIX)	[71]
in vivo	mice bearing mouse melanomas	verteporfin	[72]
in vitro/ in vivo	S91 mouse melanoma cells and DBA mice	5,10,15,20-tetrakis[2-chloro-5-sulfophenyl)bacteriochlorin (TCPBSO3H)	[66]
in vitro	WM451LU melanoma cells	photosensitizers and heme oxygenase I (HO-I) and poly(ADP-ribose) polymerase (PARP) inhibitors	[73]
in vitro	A375 melanoma cells	5-aminolevulinic acid [5-ALA) and novel metallophthalocyanine (MPc)	[74]
in vivo	transplanted B16 melanoma	novel derivatives of chlorin e[6]	[75]
in vitro/ in vivo	melanoma bearing mice	C(60)-(Glc)1 (D-glucose residue pendant fullerene) and C(60)-(6Glc)1 (a maltohexaose residue pendant fullerene)	[76]
in vitro	SK-MEL-188 (human melanoma) cells	chlorin and bacteriochlorin derivatives of 5,10,15,20-tetrakis[2-chloro-5-sulfophenyl)porphyrin	[77]
in vitro	B16 melanoma cells	IPL and IPL plus 5-ALA	[78]
in vitro	melanoma cells	bacteriochlorins and photofrin	[79]
in vitro	C57 mice bearing a sub-cutaneously transplanted melanoma	Zn(II)-phthalocyanine disulphide (C11Pc)	[80]
in vitro	WM 1552C human melanoma cells	liposomes (LP) and nanocapsules (NC) containing Chloroaluminum phthalocyanine (ClAlPc)	[81]
in vitro	A375 melanoma cells	5,15-Diarylporphyrins (1-5) and Photofrin	[82]
in vivo	B16 melanoma tumours on mice	2 doses of photosensitizer	[83]
in vitro	B16 mouse melanoma cells	chlordiazepoxide (CDZ)	[84]
in vitro/ in vivo	B78H1 amelanotic mouse melanoma cells and C57BL/6 mice bearing a subcutaneously transplanted B78H1 amelanotic melanoma.	octabutoxy-naphthalocyanines	[85]
in vitro	G361 human melanoma cells	zinc-5,10,15,20-tetrakis(4-sulphonatophenyl) porphyrine (ZnTPPS(4)), chloraluminium phtalocyanine disulfonate (ClAlPcS(2)) and 5-aminolevulinic acid (ALA)	[86]
in vitro	A375 human melanoma cells B16F10 mouse melanoma cells	Pc4 encapsulated in silica nanoparticles	[87]

Type of study	Tumour/Cell line	Photosensitizer	Ref
in vitro	Sk-Mel-28 human skin melanoma cells	indocyanine green	[88]
in vitro	UCT Mel-1 and A375 human melanoma cells	hypericin	[89]
in vitro	G361 human melanoma cells	chloroaluminum phthalocyanine (ClAlPc) and ultrasound	[90]
in vitro	A375 human melanoma cells	5-aminolevulinic acid (ALA)	[91]
in vitro/ in vivo	B16F1 mouse melanoma cells and C57BL6 mice bearing a subcutaneously injected B16F1 melanoma.	methylene blue	[92]
in vitro/ in vivo	B16F1 mouse melanoma cells and C57BL6 mice bearing a subcutaneously injected B16F1 melanoma.	carboranyl-containing chlorin (TPFC)	[93]
in vitro/ in vivo	human malignant melanoma cells (MMCs)	porfimer sodium	[94]
in vivo	B57BL/6 mice bearing a B16BL6 melanoma	porfimer sodium and antibodies neutralizing decay-accelerating factor (DAF), complement-receptor-1-related protein y (Crry), and protectin	[95]
in vitro	G361 human melanoma cells	porphyrines (TPPS4, ZnTPPS4 and PdTPPS4	[96]
in vitro/ in vivo	B-16 mouse melanoma cells and subcutaneous B-16 melanoma-bearing C57BL/6 mice	5,10,15,20-tetraphenylporphin-loaded PEG-PE micelles	[97]
in vitro	UCT Mel-1 and UCT Mel-3 human melanoma cells	hypericin	[98]
in vitro	Me300 human melanoma cells	Five 5,10,15,20-tetra[4-pyridyl)porphyrin (TPP) areneruthenium(II) derivatives and a p-cymeneosmium and two pentamethylcyclopentadienyliridium and -rhodium analogues	[99]
in vitro	B16F10 melanotic melanomas transplanted to nude mice	methyl 5-aminolevulinate (MAL) and depigmentation with violet light	[100]
in vitro	S-91 mouse melanoma cells	titanium dioxide modified with platinum(IV) chloride complexes ($TiO_2/PtCl_4$)	[101]
in vitro	G361 human melanoma cells	zinc-5,10,15,20-tetrakis(4-sulphonatophenyl) porphyrine (ZnTPPS4) and atomic force microscopy	[102]
in vitro	WM451Lu metastatic human melanoma cells	5-aminolevulinic acid (ALA)	[103]
in vitro	B16F1 mouse melanoma cells	meso-tetra[4-nido-carboranylphenyl)porphyrin (H2TCP)	[104]

Type of study	Tumour/Cell line	Photosensitizer	Ref
in vitro	B16F10 mouse melanoma cells	solketal-substituted phthalocyanine (Si(sol)2Pc in mPEG-b-p(HPMAm-Lac2) micelles	[105]
in vitro	B19 mouse and G361 human melanoma cells	phthalocyanine ClAlPcS(2)	[106]
in vitro	S91 mouse and SKMEL 188 human melanoma cells	5,10,15,20-tetrakis[2-chloro-3-sulfophenyl)porphyrin (TCPPSO(3)H),	[107]
in vivo	choroidal melanomas in 46 New Zealand albino rabbit eyes	hematoporphyrin monomethyl ether	[108]
in vitro	G361 human melanoma cells	3 porphyrin sensitizers (TPPS(4), ZnTPPS[4] and PdTPPS(4))	[109]
in vitro	YUSAC2/T34A-C4 human melanoma cell line	porfimer sodium	[110]
in vivo	subcutaneous B16BL6 melanoma-bearing C57BL/6 mice	BPD, ce6, Photofrin, and mTHPC and gamma-inulin	[111]
in vitro	A375 human melanoma cells	acridine orange	[112]
in vitro	Cloudman S91/I3 mouse melanoma cells	photofrin II (PfII- porfirmer sodium), verteporfin, and merocyanine 540 (MC540)	[113]
in vivo	A-Mel-3 melanomas implanted in the dorsal skin fold chamber of Syrian Golden hamsters	5-aminolaevulinic acid (ALA)	[114]
in vivo	B-16 melanoma-bearing C57BL/6 mice	ATX-S10 No (II) and intratumoral injection of naïve dendritic cells (IT-DC)	[115]
in vitro/ in vivo	B16F1 mouse melanoma cells and C57BL6 mice bearing a subcutaneously injected B16F1 melanoma.	Zn(ii)-phthalocyanine derivative bearing four 10B-enriched o-carboranyl units [10B-ZnB4Pc)	[116]
in vitro	human Beidegröm Melanoma (BM) cell line	porfirmer sodium (photofrin II)	[117]
in vitro	G361 human melanoma cells	ZnTPPS(4) sensitizer bound to cyclodextrin hpbetaCD	[118].
in vitro	B78H1 mouse melanoma cells	Ni(II)-octabutoxy-naphthalocyanine (NiNc)	[119]
in vitro	G361 human melanoma cells	ZnTPPS(4) sensitizer bound to cyclodextrin hpbetaCD	[120]
in vitro	M2R mouse melanoma cells	O-[Pd-bacteriochlorophyllide]-serine methyl ester (Pd-Bchl-Ser)	[121]
in vitro	B78H1 melanoma cells	liposome-delivered Ni(II)-octabutoxy-naphthalocyanine	[119]
in vitro	human choroidal melanoma (CM) cells	tetrahydroporphyrin tetratosylat (THPTS)	[122]

Type of study	Tumour/Cell line	Photosensitizer	Ref
in vivo	M2R mouse melanoma xenografts	WST11	[123]
in vitro	B16 mouse melanoma cells	5-aminolevulinic acid [5-ALA) ester derivatives	[124]
in vivo	B-16 melanoma-bearing C57BL/6 mice	metal-free sulfonated phthalocyanine (H(2)PcS(2.4))	[125]
in vitro	A375 human melanoma cells	alpha-methylene-gamma-butyrolactone-psoralen heterodimer 2	[126]
in vitro	B16 mouse melanoma cells	5-aminolevulinic acid (ALA)	[127]
in vivo	C57BL6 mice bearing a subcutaneously injected B16F10 melanoma	silkworm excreta (SPbalpha) porfirmer sodium	[128]
in vitro	M3Dau human melanoma cells	silicon-phthalocyanines (SiPc) and chloro-aluminium Pc (ClAlPc),	[129]
in vitro	Me45 human melanoma cells	meso-tetra-4-N-methylpyridyl-porphyrin iodide and 5,10-di-[4-acetamidophenyl)-15,20-di-[4-N-methylpyridyl) porphyrin	[130]
in vitro	G361 human melanoma cells	meso-tetrakis[4-sulphonatophenyl)porphine (TPPS4) and zinc metallocomplex (ZnTPPS4)	[131]
in vitro	G361 human melanoma cells	ATX-S10(Na)	[132]
in vivo	syrian Golden hamsters fitted with dorsal skinfold chambers containing A-Mel-3 melanoma cells	5-aminolaevulinic acid (ALA)	[133]
in vitro	B16 mouse melanoma cells	5-aminolaevulinic acid (ALA)	[134]
in vivo	UB900518 human melanoma cells transplanted on nude (*nu/nu*) CD-1 mice	Liposomal meso-tetrakis-phenylporphyrin (TPP)	[135]
in vivo	pigmented choroidal melanoma 44 New Zealand albino rabbit eyes	liposomal preparation of benzoporphyrin derivative (BPD), verteporfin	[136]
in vitro	S91 mouse and SKMEL 188 human melanoma cells	indocyanine green (ICG)	[137]
in vitro	B16A45 (B16) mouse melanoma cells	delta-aminolevulinic acid (ALA) and meta(tetrahydroxyphenyl)chlorin or m-THPC	[138]
in vitro	B16 mouse melanoma cells	m-THPC and four apoptosis inhibitors: BAPTA-AM, Forskolin, DSF, and Z.VAD.fmk	[47]
in vitro	Bro, SKMel-23, SKMel-28	5-aminolevulinic acid (ALA)	[139]
In vitro	SKMEL 188 human melanoma cells	tritolylporphyrin dimer (T-D).	[140]
in vivo	Syrian Golden hamsters fitted with dorsal skinfold chambers containing A-Mel-3 melanoma cells	5-aminolaevulinic acid (ALA)	[141]
in vivo	Nude CD1 mice bearing malignant M2R melanoma xenografts	bacteriochlorophyll-serine (Bchl-Ser),	[142]

Type of study	Tumour/Cell line	Photosensitizer	Ref
in vitro	SK-23 mouse melanoma and SK-Mel 28 human melanoma	methylene blue	[143]
in vitro	B78H1 melanoma cells	liposome-incorporated Ni(II)-octabutoxy-naphthalocyanine (NiNc),	[144]
in vitro	B78H1 melanoma cells	Cu(II)-hematoporphyrin (CuHp)	[145]
in vivo	Syrian Golden hamsters fitted with dorsal skinfold chambers containing A-Mel-3 melanoma cells	5-aminolaevulinic acid (ALA)	[146]
in vitro	M6 human melanoma cells	dichlorosilicon phthalocyanine (Cl2SiPc) and bis(tri-n-hexylsiloxy) silicon phthalocyanine (HexSiPc)	[147]
in vivo	C57/BL6 mice bearing a subcutaneously transplanted B1 melanoma	benzoporphyrin derivative monoacid ring A (verteporfin, BPD-MA)	[148]
in vitro	SkMel-23 melanoma cells	5-aminolaevulinic acid (ALA)	[149]
in vivo	C57/BL6 mice bearing a subcutaneously transplanted B16 melanoma	Si(i.v.)-naphthalocyanine (isoBO-SiNc)	[150]
in vivo	C57/BL6 mice bearing a subcutaneously transplanted B16 melanoma	aluminum phthalocyanine (AlpcS4	[151]
in vivo	C57/BL6 mice bearing a subcutaneously transplanted B16F10 melanoma	lutetium texaphyrin (PCI-0123),	[152]
in vivo	Syrian Golden hamsters fitted with dorsal skinfold chambers containing A-Mel-3 melanoma cells	9-acetoxy-2,7,12,17-tetrakis-(beta-methoxyethyl)-porphycene (ATMPn)	[153].
in vivo	C57/BL6 mice bearing a subcutaneously transplanted B16 melanoma	Si(IV)-methoxyethylene-glycol-naphthalocyanine	[154]
in vivo	Syrian Golden hamsters fitted with dorsal skinfold chambers containing A-Mel-3 melanoma cells	5-aminolaevulinic acid (ALA)	[155]
in vivo	10 choroidal melanomas in rabbits	liposomal preparation of benzoporphyrin derivative	[156]
in vivo	M2R mouse melanoma tumors implanted in CD1 nude mice	bacteriochlorophyll-serine (Bchl-Ser),	[157]
in vitro	uveal melanoma cells	hematoporphyrin esters (HPE)	[158]
in vivo	Syrian Golden hamsters fitted with dorsal skinfold chambers containing A-Mel-3 melanoma cells	5-aminolaevulinic acid (ALA)	[159]
in vivo	C57/BL6 mice bearing a subcutaneously transplanted B16 melanoma	Zn(II)-2,3 naphthalocyanine (ZnNc)	[160]

Type of study	Tumour/Cell line	Photosensitizer	Ref
in vivo	32 choroidal tumours in New Zealand albino rabbit eyes.	benzoporphyrin derivative	[161]
in vitro	G361,M18 and M6 human melanoma cells	hypericin	[162]
in vitro	melanoma cell lines	hypericin	[163]

Table 2. Comprehensive update of in vivo and in vitro photodynamic therapy studies from 1996-present.

For melanoma treatment, where PDT will be more effective as a post-operative adjunctive treatment, very few reports highlight its effectiveness even though laboratory studies using melanoma cells show promise. Clinically, PDT has shown promise in the treatment of both ocular amelanotic melanomas [164] and skin metastases [165] however, more extensive clinical studies need to be conducted before PDT is accepted as the adjunctive therapy of choice [166] (Table 3).

Type of study	Tumour	Pigmentary phenotype	Photosensitizer	Outcome of study	Ref
clinical	choroidal melanoma	unpigmented	verteporfin	Dramatic tumor regression over 2 months to a completely flat scar [1.3 mm thickness), and remained stable at 50 months of follow-up.	[167]
clinical	3 choroidal melanomas	pigmented	PDT and intravitreal bevacizumab	The tumors treated with PDT and bevacizumab showed a marked reduction in tumor vascularity. The tumors receiving PDT as a primary treatment were followed by progressive tumor growth that led to enucleation years after.	[168]
clinical	9 posteriorly located choroidal melanomas	unpigmented	verteporfin	Eight tumors demonstrated apparent complete regression over 1 month to 14 months with no recurrence during follow-up of between 34 months and 81 months. One case developed 2 separate local recurrences at 21 months and 34 months.	[169]
clinical	11 late stage melanomas (cutaneous metastases)	ND	indocyanine green and imiquimod (immune modifier)	Complete response was observed in 6 patients. All lesions in the treatment area of the patients responded to photo-immunotherapy, 8 of which achieved complete local response (CLR). CLR was observed in the non-treatment site (regional) lesions in four patients. Five patients were still alive at the time of last follow-up.	[170]

Type of study	Tumour	Pigmentary phenotype	Photosensitizer	Outcome of study	Ref
clinical	1 duodenal metastatic melanoma	ND	porfirmer sodium	Successful treatment.	[171]
clinical	6 brain metastasis of malignant melanoma	ND	porfirmer sodium	All 6 patients [100%) remained free of brain disease till death, 50% died of malignant melanoma elsewhere and 50% died of unrelated causes.	[172]
clinical	melanoma in situ	unigmented	methyl aminolevulinate (MAL)	Recurrence at the original tumour site 4 months after PDT.	[173]
clinical	choroidal melanoma	unpigmented	benzoporphyrin derivative (BPD)	The tumor fully disappeared 1 month after the treatment, the visual acuity improved from 4/16 to 4/4. The disease did not recur during 24-month follow-up.	[174]
clinical	2 late-stage melanoma. Patient 1 had the primary tumour and local metastases on the left arm and metastatic tumours in the lungs. Patient 2 had a head and neck melanoma with multiple local metastases, which had failed repeated attempts at surgical resection and high-dose radiation therapy.	pigmented	indocyanine green (ICG) + imiquimod (toll-like receptor agonist)	Patient 1 free of all clinically detectable tumours (including the lung metastases) "/>20 months after the first treatment cycle. Patient 2 has been free of any clinical evidence of the tumour for over 6 months.	[175]
clinical	4 uveal melanoma, PDT on actual tumour site	mildly to heavily pigmented	benzoporphyrin derivative (BPD)	Vascular occlusion and thrombosis in mildly pigmented melanoma but no response in pigmented ones.	[176]
clinical	25 small and medium choroidal melanomas	ND	indocyanine green and transpupillary thermotherapy	After a mean of 2.4 treatments (range, 1 to 5 treatments), all of the tumors but one showed a significant volume reduction without clinical evidence of recurrences. Complications included retinal vascular occlusions, edema and superficial scarring of the macula, and rhegmatogenous retinal detachment.	[177]

Type of study	Tumour	Pigmentary phenotype	Photosensitizer	Outcome of study	Ref
clinical	14 skin metastasis from malignant melanoma, despite multiple courses of chemotherapy	pigmented	chlorin e_6	Complete regression after the first PDT treatment in eight cases and complete regression after multiple treatments in six cases. 11 of 14 patients died due to the progression of the melanoma, the median survival time after surgery was 883 days.	[165]
clinical	38 choroidal melanomas	ND	indocyanine green (ICG)	Changes in microcirculation 6 months after PDT, as well as significant decrease of tumors thickness in ultrasonography (mean 38%), were detected in all cases. Complete regression of intrinsic vessels was demonstrated by ICGA in 26 cases, and partial regression of pathological vascularization was found in 12 patients.	[178]
clinical	4 choroidal melanomas	ND	benzoporphyrin derivative (BPD)	One tumor decreased in size and remained stable for 18 months. One tumor had no growth for 11 months. Two melanomas continued to grow, necessitating enucleation.	[179]
clinical	3 uveal melanoma, PDT on unaffected areas before enucleation	ND	benzoporphyrin derivative (BPD)	Vascular thrombosis. No damage to the photoreceptors.	[180]
clinical	36 uveal melanomas	various	hematoporphyrin derivative	76 % of tumours were not growing at the end of the first year, 62 % after the second year and 38% after the fifth year. No eyes were lost as a result of PDT. The degree of tumour pigmentation and patient age at therapy significantly influence the tumour response to PDT.	[181]

Table 3. Clinical reports and outcomes of photodynamic effectiveness of photodynamic therapy protocols including the melanoma pigmentary phenotype.

1.3.2. Hypericin, a second generation photosensitizer for PDT

Hypericin, a second generation PS isolated from the plant *Hypericum perforatum,* is a phenanthroperylenequinone with two broad peaks of absorption – 300-400nm (ultraviolet) and 500-600nm (white light) (Figure 1). This may be considered as a disadvantage as a number of current second-generation photosensitizers have absorption peaks beyond 630nm allowing for increased penetration into tissues [182]. However, white light, used to activate hypericin, does penetrate deep into the dermis of the skin. Moreover, activation with ultraviolet light could be a distinct advantage for the use of hypericin in daylight-mediated PDT. This type of PDT is more convenient for patients and clinicians and causes less pain. It poses a particularly interesting avenue to explore for hospitals in developing countries where space is limited and budgets are inadequate. Daylight-mediated PDT is an effective treatment for thin actinic keratosis, as shown in three randomized controlled clinical studies (reviewed in Wiegell et al., 2011) [183]. The potential of hypericin in clinical practice has been highlighted by reports on its use to treat squamous and basal cell carcinomas [184-187], pancreatic tumors [188], bladder carcinomas [189-193], nasophyrangeal tumors [194,195] and recently melanomas [196].

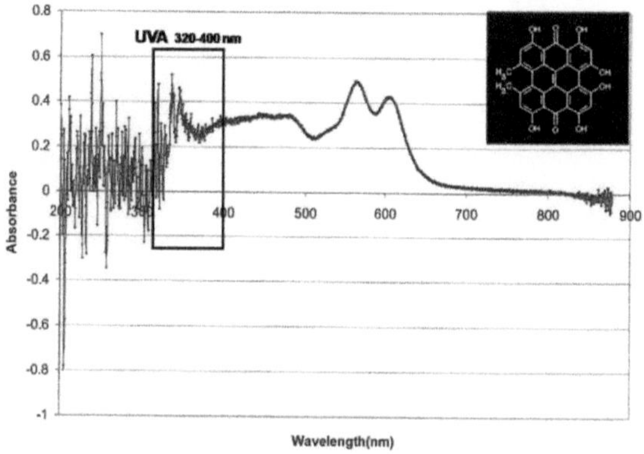

Figure 1. Absorbance spectrum of hypericin. Box, the wavelength of light used in our studies [98,197] representing one of the two activation peaks. Inset, chemical structure of hypericin.

1.3.3. Melanoma cell death and biological mechanisms induced by hypericin-PDT

Despite these promising studies, very few reports have highlighted hypericin's role in targeting melanoma. For the most part, cytotoxicity testing of new photosensitizers are tested on cell lines in vitro using assays such as the 3-[4,5-Dimethylthiazol-2-yl)-2,5-diphenyltetrazolium bromide (MTT), which is a colorimetric assays for measuring the activity of enzymes that reduce MTT to formazan dyes, giving a purple color [198,199]. Other tests for cytotoxicity include dead cell protease tests. Despite being used as the "gold standard" for cytotoxicity testing, it must be borne in mind that these assays are based on cellular metabolic activity and could result in a false positive result were the treatment to produce a cytostatic effect in cells. Moreover, as these are colorimetric-based tests, the photosensitizer used itself may interfere with the wavelength at which these tests are read.

One of the first few reports testing 1 to 20mg/ml hypericin efficacy on squamous carcinoma, sarcoma and melanoma cell lines found that a combination of activating laser light sources resulted in a reduction in cell viability of 90% [163]. Following this, Hadjur et al. (1996) exposed human pigmented and unpigmented melanoma cell lines to hypericin and showed minimal cytotoxicity on uptake but upon activation with white light, increased cell death in all three cell lines. Their findings thus suggest that amelanotic melanomas may be more susceptible to hypericin-PDT than pigmented melanomas. Their possible reasons for this related to the presence of melanin and antioxidant status of melanomas [162].

Work from our laboratory has shown a pigmentation dependant susceptibility of melanoma cells to hypericin-PDT, with pigmented cells being less susceptible than unpigmented cells [54,98,200,201]. Upon depigmentation with tyrosinase inhibitors, kojic acid and phenylthiourea, pigmented melanoma cells become more susceptible to hypericin-PDT [54,69]. Moreover, 72 hours after hypericin-PDT the cell viability of the depigmented melanoma cells remained significantly less than the control cells. Over the same time period the cells not treated with kojic acid approached a cell viability similar to the control.

Melanin is a potent antioxidant which could be a reason for the increased resistance of pigmented melanoma cells to PDT due to the scavenging of ROS produced by this therapy. Indeed we have shown that after depigmenting melanoma cells with kojic acid more ROS is produced upon treatment with hypericin-PDT compared to pigmented melanoma cells which were not depigmented [54]. We did not find a difference between the caspase 3, 7 activity after hypericin-PDT for both the depigmented and pigmented melanoma cells, which was lower than control. This suggests that pigmented melanoma cells might induce a caspase-independent mode of cell death such as the activation of apoptosis-inducing factor (AIF). Moreover, these cells might also undergo necrosis, necroptosis or autophagy in response to hypericin-PDT. We have further shown induction of autophagy at 4hours after hypericin-PDT in both pigmented and unpigmented melanoma cells [197]. Interestingly, pigmented melanoma cells (UCT Mel-1) show higher levels of externalisation of Annexin V, an early apoptotic event, compared to mildy and unpigmented melanoma cells [501mel and A375, respectively) after hypericin-PDT (Figure 2). However, the cell death response of pigmented and unpigmented melanoma cells is very complex and does seem to be cell type dependant. A possible explanation for this may be that the cell lines used in our studies are from different genetic origins and they thus might differ in various biochemical characteristics, including their antioxidant systems. The subcellular localisation of the photosensitizer is another factor determining the cell death mode initiated by PDT. Upon activation by light, photosensitizers produce ROS which are short-lived species acting directly in their vicinity of production. Localisation to different cellular compartments thus induces different modes of cell death.

Note: Since the discovery of programmed cell death in the 1960's the cell death field has evolved immensely. Researchers have shifted from morphological classifications to using more biochemical criteria. The increase in cell death studies necessitated a systemic classification of cell death modalities, which led to the formation of the Nomenclature Committee on Cell Death (NCCD). The main mission of this committee is 'to provide a forum in which names describing distinct modalities of cell death are critically evaluated and recommendations on their definition and use are formulated, hoping that a non-rigid, yet uniform nomenclature will facilitate the communication among scientists and ultimately accelerate the pace of discovery' [202-204].

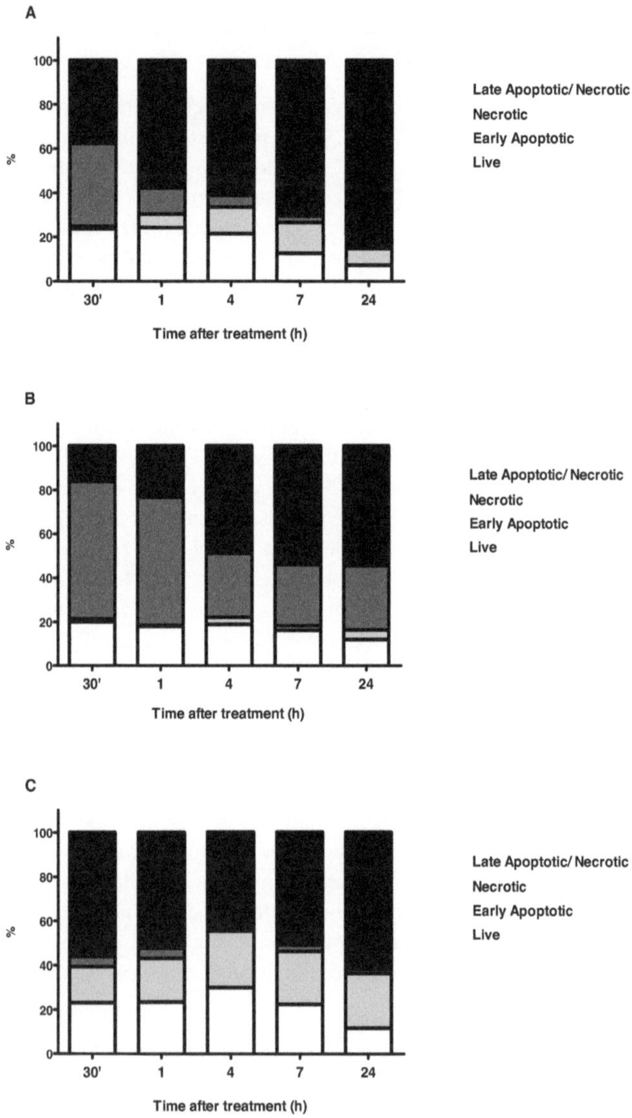

Figure 2. Graphs representing fluorescent activated cell sorting (FACS) analyses of melanoma cells at 30min, 1, 4, 7 and 24h after hypericin-PDT treatment (3μM hypericin with 1 J/cm^2 UVA). A: unpigmented A375, B: mildly pigmented 501mel and C: pigmented UCT Mel-1. Cells were stained for early apoptosis (FITC Annexin V, BD Biosciences) and necrosis (LIVE/DEAD Fixable Violet stain, Invitrogen). Different modes of cell death are represented as proportional percentages normalised to the control, black: late apoptotic/ necrotic, dark grey: necrotic, light grey: apoptotic, white: live; n=3.

1.4. PDT targets to treat melanoma

1.4.1. Cell proliferation and survival

It is now well established that one of the chief characteristics of cancer cells is their ability to overcome cellular control of proliferation [205]. In melanocytes, proliferation is caused by a combination of several mitogenic growth factors such as stem cell factor (SCF), epidermal growth factor (EGF), fibroblast growth factor (FGF) and hepatocyte growth factor (HGF) which cause a sustained extracellular receptor kinase (ERK) activity [206]. In melanoma, the RAS/Raf/MEK/ERK pathway is a key regulating pathway in proliferation with ERK being hyperactivated in up to 90% of human melanomas [207]. BRAF and PTEN mutations (see above) are co-incident in about 20% of cases [208]. The most common mutation in BRAF is a glutamic acid for valine substitution at position 600 (^{V600E}BRAF) [209]. This mutation leads to constitutive ERK signalling resulting in hyperproliferation and cell survival [210]. This pathway, through the EGF receptor as an extracellular ligand, has been a worthwhile target for PDT in that sustained activation of the ERK pathway protected cells from photofrin-based PDT as well as a reduction in the Raf protein levels in treated cells [211].

Nuclear factor kappa beta (NF-κβ) signalling leads to transcriptional regulation of a number of genes involved in responses ranging from proliferation, metastasis, and survival to inflammation. It therefore is an important target in PDT to stop aberrant cell proliferation. PDT-induced oxidative stress through increased ROS production has been shown to activate (NF-κβ) [212] and inactivate its inhibitor (Iκβ). Moreover, Ryter and Gomer showed increased NF-κβ binding in response to PDT stress in mouse cancer cells leading to a reduction in proliferation [213].

1.4.2. Inhibition of apoptosis

Apoptosis, a controlled mode of cell death, is characterised by cell shrinkage, chromatin condensation, DNA fragmentation, membrane blebbing and activation of caspases [214]. It is now well established that activation of the caspase cascade occurs through death receptor activation (extrinsic pathway) or through mitochondrial outer membrane permeabilization (intrinsic pathway). Both of these pathways have been shown to be activated through PDT. Several biochemical studies have established that PDT with different photosensitizers, including hypericin, utilise the mitochondrial-mediated pathway of caspase activation [215,216] although PDT has recently been shown to also engage caspase-independent pathways [217]. It is further known that several anti-cancer agents induce apoptosis and may share common pathways leading to cell killing with Fas/APO-1/CD95 [218,219]. Ali et al. (2002) elegantly showed that hypericin-PDT induces human nasopharyngeal cancer cells to undergo apoptosis through the Fas/FasL system. Moreover, they showed that the upregulation of Fas/FasL results in the release of cytochrome c into the cytoplasm with subsequent caspase induction – results that suggest that although apoptosis is considered a product of either an extrinsic or intrinsic mechanism; the overall response to PDT may be a combination of mechanisms [220].

Cancer cells are known to resist cell death by upregulation of anti-apoptotic proteins, mutations in pro-apoptotic proteins, inhibition of cell senescence or through protective mechanisms such as autophagy. PDT that is targeted for cancer therapy aims to invoke cell cytoxicity through attacking these characteristics – topics of a number of recent reviews [36,221-223].

Intriguingly, the emergence of a defined 'immunogenic apoptosis' seems to be a new 'subset' of apoptosis and autophagic cell death which has been shown to have the ability to release/expose damage-associated membrane proteins (DAMPs) [224-227]. Therapeutically, the immunogenicity of apoptosis is preferable for application rather than necrosis (or for that matter autophagic cell death) since necrosis can lead to harmful immunological reactions [228] (on the other hand, the extent of immunological impact of autophagic cell death is as yet uncharacterized, thereby making it an uncertain modality to use in the context of 'immunochemotherapy') [229]. The cell killing effectiveness is however dependent on parameters such as the PS used, the light dose and most importantly, the subcellular localization of the PS. It is crucial for photosensitizers to effectively enter the cell and accumulate in specific intracellular organelles in order to be efficient in their killing ability. Clearly, the final destination of the PS and its immediate vicinity will lead to different modes of cell death and consequently different efficiencies. Recent reports have highlighted that hypericin not only localises to different subcellular organelles but that this localization is exposure and dose-dependent in addition to being tumour cell-specific [230-234]. As a start however, the lipophillic nature of hypericin dictates its association with cellular membranes [235]. The fact that hypericin has been shown to associate with serum proteins (LDL and HDL lipoproteins [236] ensues that it enters cells quickly and is preferentially taken up by cancer cells in the 3-dimensional milieu as recent reports showed that these cells have high levels of LDL surface receptors [237]. This is further supported by a recent report showing that cholesterol serves as a key determinant for the uptake of hypericin into cellular membranes [238].

Noteworthy however is that even though high levels of hydrophobicity ensues, high levels of intracellular accumulation of the photosensitizer, changes in the physical structure of the PS due to aggregation and other modifications, may lead to reduced PDT efficiency [239]. Overall, the consensus emerging is that hypericin localises to three intracellular organelles namely, the endoplasmic reticulum (ER)-Golgi network [230,231,240,241], mitochondria (Mt) [242-245] and lysosomes [237,246] where through synergistic action, apoptosis is induced. More recent work by the Agostinis group show that hypericin-based PDT would produce photo-oxidative ER (p-ox ER stress) stress while 5-ALA (localizes in the mitochondria)-based PDT would produce photo-oxidative mitochondrial stress [36,247]. They also observed that Hyp-PDT induces 'pre-apoptotic' active exo-ATP secretion and late stage passive release of DAMPs like HSP70, HSP90 and CRT [223]. Overall they suggest that the potential of Hyp-PDT in causing exposure/secretion of 'critical' DAMPs add to the apoptotic cell death modality in a rather 'small club' of anti-cancerous therapeutic agents/modalities capable of exposing immunogenic signals like ecto-CRT [227,248].

1.4.3. Induction of autophagy

A recent finding is the induction of the cytoprotective programme of autophagy in melanomas in response to PDT-induced oxidative stress [89]. In addition, recent reports showed that cancer cells may respond to chemotherapeutics or other forms of oxidative stress such as PDT, through the induction of autophagy initially but continued stress leads to an overwhelming of the endogenous antioxidant enzymes along with a shift from autophagy to a possible senescent phenotype in an attempt to prolong cellular survival. Consequently however, the cell enters an apoptotic or necrotic mode of cell death [249-251]. Autophagy, defined as a cellular response to nutrient deprivation with consequent organelle breakdown, could converge with PDT at a number of cellular locations. Although more work relating to this aspect in melanomas is needed, reports on other cancer cells have shown that autophagy can be induced if the lysosomal system, needed for the clearance of ROS-damaged organelles, is affected by PDT [252]. Another cellular location is the mitochondria, where the PDT-induced loss of anti-apoptotic protein Bcl-2, may lead to an initation of autophagy [253].

1.4.4. Chemoresistance due to increased antioxidants

Cancer cells are considered to be under continuous oxidative stress which has been suggested to aid in tumor progression [254]. In support, several studies have shown tumor cell lines producing higher levels of ROS compared to their normal counterparts [255,256]. Due to this increased level of ROS and hence constitutive increased level of oxidative stress, it is not surprising that cancer cells have an extensive and advanced intracellular antioxidant network – a characteristic which further increases their chemoresistant property. Interestingly, the antioxidant status of melanomas differs from that of other skin cancers such as basal and squamous cell carcinomas in that their antioxidant activity levels (i.e. catalase, glutathione peroxidise, superoxide dismutase) are much higher [257]. In contrast, melanocytes, their normal untransformed phenotype, have lower levels of antioxidant activities and associated lower levels of resistance to oxidative stress [258]. It is therefore reasonable to postulate whether breaking this tolerance to oxidative stress may increase therapeutic efficacy in targeting melanoma. A number of studies have therefore suggested that treating melanoma by inhibiting cellular antioxidants may be efficacious [259-261]. One example of this was the addition of the superoxide dismutase (SOD) activity inhibitor, 2-methoxyestradiol (2-ME_2), to a mouse transplant model which induced growth arrest of melanoma cells after injection [262]. Paradoxically, several studies have suggested that antioxidants can enhance the action of cancer chemotherapeutics drugs in their in vitro models through inhibition of a variety of factors which contribute to the malignant phenotype [263,264]. A recent study however, using six different combinations of antioxidants and chemotherapeutic drugs in combination, failed to identify a single combination in which an antioxidant reduced the survival of malignant breast carcinoma cells [265]. To our knowledge the use of PDT as an inhibitor of antioxidants has not been tested in cancer cells.

1.4.5. Melanin and melanosomes as pro-survival agents

All the potential intracellular organelle targets for PDT mentioned above are consistent with most cancer cells. However, the one aspect that sets melanoma apart from other cancers is the presence of its cell-specific organelle called the melanosome and its associated product, melanin pigment. It is thus not inconceivable to believe that the intractability of this skin disease may in some way be related to this organelle and its function [266,267]. It follows logically then, that treatment regimes need to consider the melanosome as another potential target organelle in the fight against melanoma [268].

Melanosomes are membrane-bound organelles in melanocytic cells which house the pathway that results in the formation of the polymeric pigment, melanin [269,270]. The enzymes which participate in this pathway are translated in the cytoplasm and chaperoned to the melanosomes. Tyrosinase (TYR), the rate-limiting enzyme of the pathway, and its related proteins tyrosinase-related proteins 1 and 2 (TYRP-1 and TYRP-2) act in concert to first convert tyrosine to 3,4-dihydroxy-phenylalanine (DOPA) via tyrosine hydroxylase activity and then convert DOPA to DOPAquinone via dopa oxidase activity. Both of these activities occur via separate tyrosinase catalytic sites. During melanin synthesis toxic intermediates such as 5, 6-dihydroxyindole and 5,6-dihydroxyindole-2-carboxylic acid are produced. Structurally, the melanosomes are designed to compartmentalise these cytotoxic melanin intermediates from spilling into the cytoplasm [271]. Melanosomal biogenesis progresses through four distinct stages of maturation where the first two stages contain no melanin and the later stages constitute intermediates required to generate a matrix favourable for the formation of melanin [269,272]. The Pmel17/gp100/Silv/ME20 protein, a product of the Silver locus in melanocytic cells [273], is capable of polymerizing into fibrillar arrays that form the backbone of melanosomes. As a major component of the fibrillar matrix of early stage melanosomes, Pmel-17 serves as the best marker to follow intracellular trafficking steps that regulate melanosomal formation [274].

Moreover, as Pmel-17 facilitates melanin deposition and plays a pivotal role in melanosome biogenesis, it remains a strategic target when trying to combat melanoma through the fact that melanosomes are involved in scavenging endogenous cytotoxic metabolites and storing their waste products - a function that has been suggested to be a key in creating multi-drug resistance [267]. With the premise that melanosomes may be acting as cytotoxic drug "sinks" through the sequestration of chemotherapeutic drugs [267], it would be considered an effective therapy for a PS to enter the melanosomal membrane and damage the wall of the melanosome thus allowing the leakage of toxic melanin intermediates resulting in cell death. The drawback is that melanosomes, which are classified into stages along their biogenesis [269,270] only produce the toxic intermediates during their final maturing stages III and IV [268-270,275-277]. Most pigmented melanomas do however present with a majority of these end-stage melanosomes in their cytoplasm making the melanosomal membrane an attractive target for PDT. On the basis of this information, one may imagine that pigmented melanomas are therefore more susceptible to PDT-induced cell death. In contrast, our work has shown that pigmented melanomas are much less susceptible to hypericin-PDT than unpigmented/amelanotic melanomas despite hypericin readily entering the melanosomes [89].

We hypothesize that the reason for this is due to the presence of the pigment melanin. In support of this, pigmented human xenograft melanotic melanoma in mice, was shown to be far less responsive to PDT than amelanotic melanoma [278].

Melanin has been shown to act as both an oxidant and antioxidant [266,279] and in parallel studies, its presence in melanomas have been linked to chemoresistance. In support, further studies have shown that a lack of pigment in melanomas decreases their resistance to cell death. Our ongoing investigation into susceptibility to PDT-induced cell death in depigmented melanomas supports this hypothesis [54,69].

1.4.6. Cancer stem cells as future PDT targets

The cancer stem cell hypothesis purports the idea that a subset of cancer cells is capable of maintaining and driving disease progression [280,281]. With the identification of cancer stem cell populations in colon, breast and brain tumors [282-285], it is believed that these cells are integrally related to tumor formation, resistance to chemotherapy and escape from remission [286]. While the qualifications for melanoma stem cells have generally been defined as tumorigenicity in xenograft spheroid formation and self-renewal in non-adherent cultures, the markers used to identify these cells from the general tumor population remain debatable. A brief summary of these markers and their potential as targets for novel PDT-based therapy, follow.

ATP-binding cassette (ABC) transporters are a vast family of transmembrane proteins that have been studied for their ability to actively transport cytotoxic substances out of cells [287]. Intriguingly, some of these transporters have been demonstrated to be highly expressed in highly tumorigenic subpopulations of melanoma suggesting that they may be markers of melanoma stem cells [286]. One of these includes the ABCB5 transporter. Known for increased expression during melanoma progression in human tumor samples, ABCB5+ cells were able to resist treatment with doxorubicin [288]. While ABCB5+ cells were not able to renew in culture (a "stemness trait"), a subpopulation of cells that were indeed able to renew expressed the ABC transporter, Multi-drug Resistant-1 (MDR1) [289]. In vitro, MDR1+ cells exhibited less pigmentation than MDR1- cells, possessed the ability to continuously self-renew in soft agar and expressed the pluripotency and self-renewal regulators, human telomerase reverse transcriptase (hTERT) – all characteristics pointing towards "stemness". Interestingly, while MDR+ cells did exhibit cancer stem-cell like properties in vitro, they also co-expressed ABCB5 and ABCC2 mRNAs suggesting that a number of ABC transporters may be expressed in sub-populations [289]. To further add to the complication of delineating melanoma stem cell markers as potential targets for PDT is the fact that a number of recent markers are co-expressed with ABC transporters. These include CD133/prominin-1/AC133, which is co-expressed with ABCB5 and ABCG2 [288,290] and Nestin ([286].

Accumulating evidence suggests that another transporter, ABCG2, has physiological relevance in terms of photosensitivity and hence, PDT [291,292]. It has been shown that clinical photosensitizers and chemotherapeutic drugs have been transported out of cells by ABCG2 whereas this effect was abrogated by co-administration of its inhibitor, imatinib mesylate [293]. It is fascinating to speculate that a PDT protocol using a new, more stable photosensitizer such as hypericin may, through optimized concentrations, inhibit the action of the

ABCG2 transporter and thus create an intracellular pool of ROS resulting in efficacious cell death. This is definitely an avenue for exploration.

Overall, the ability to halt melanoma cancer progression through targeting melanoma stem cells could be extremely advantageous. However, with such a large number of potential markers and their interaction with PDT unknown, it may be a better option to focus on ABC transporters and investigate their susceptibility to second generation PS-based PDT as a means to an end for melanoma progression.

2. Conclusion and future directions

There is no doubt that our understanding of the molecular and cellular basis of melanoma has grown substantially over the past decade. However, due to its multifunctional nature, the nee d for better, improved therapies to combat or target melanoma remain essential. In addition, better understanding of the heterogenous nature of this diverse disease will likely lead to re-evaluation of the basic concepts underlying melanoma therapeutics development and clinical trial design. Till then however, novel adjuvant treatment modalities such as PDT using photostable, second-generation photosensitizers such as hypericin remain an option and need to be investigated further. Moreover, optimization of this type of therapy with regard to subcellular localization and its effect on cell death mechanisms within melanoma cells is needed. Targeting the integrity of melanocytes-specific organelles such as the melanosomes and producing an over-riding increase in ROS with consequent cytotoxicity remains a good therapeutic option but needs a systematic, scientific approach. Intriguingly, as more avenues of therapeutic targets such as melanoma stem cells and ABC transporters become illuminated, the ability to invoke cell death modalities in combination with PDT become more evident. Finally, it is clear that all these factors need to be considered in synergy if progress is to be made toward combating the menace that is metastatic melanoma.

Acknowledgements

This work was supported by the University of Cape Town Research Committee, the National Research Foundation of South Africa (LMD) and Postgraduate funding (BK) from the NRF and DAAD.

Author details

L.M. Davids and B. Kleemann

Redox Laboratory, Department of Human Biology; Faculty of Health Sciences; University of Cape Town Medical School; Cape Town, South Africa

References

[1] Armstrong B. Epidemiology of cutaneous melanoma and current trends. In: Thompson J, Morton D, Kroon B, editors. Textbook of Melanoma London, UK: Martin Dunitz; 2004. p. 65-80.

[2] Bataille V. Early detection of melanoma improves survival. Practitioner 2009 Oct; 253(1722):29-32, 3.

[3] Zbytek B, Carlson JA, Granese J, Ross J, Mihm MC, Slominski A. Current concepts of metastasis in melanoma. Expert Rev Dermatol 2008 Oct;3(5):569-585.

[4] Carlson JA, Ross JS, Slominski A, Linette G, Mysliborski J, Hill J, et al. Molecular diagnostics in melanoma. J Am Acad Dermatol 2005 May;52(5):743-75; quiz 775-8.

[5] Moncrieff MD, Martin R, O'Brien CJ, Shannon KF, Clark JR, Gao K, et al. Adjuvant postoperative radiotherapy to the cervical lymph nodes in cutaneous melanoma: is there any benefit for high-risk patients? Ann Surg Oncol 2008 Nov;15(11):3022-3027.

[6] Yamamura H, Ugawa S, Ueda T, Morita A, Shimada S. TRPM8 activation suppresses cellular viability in human melanoma. Am J Physiol Cell Physiol 2008 Aug; 295(2):C296-301.

[7] Chudnovsky Y, Khavari PA, Adams AE. Melanoma genetics and the development of rational therapeutics. J Clin Invest 2005 Apr;115(4):813-824.

[8] Slominski A, Tobin DJ, Shibahara S, Wortsman J. Melanin pigmentation in mammalian skin and its hormonal regulation. Physiol Rev 2004 Oct;84(4):1155-1228.

[9] Slominski A, Wortsman J, Carlson AJ, Matsuoka LY, Balch CM, Mihm MC. Malignant melanoma. Arch Pathol Lab Med 2001 Oct;125(10):1295-1306.

[10] Thompson JF, Scolyer RA, Kefford RF. Cutaneous melanoma. Lancet 2005 Feb 19-25;365(9460):687-701.

[11] McMasters KM, Edwards MJ, Ross MI, Reintgen DS, Martin RC,2nd, Urist MM, et al. Ulceration as a predictive marker for response to adjuvant interferon therapy in melanoma. Ann Surg 2010 Sep;252(3):460-5; discussion 465-6.

[12] Chapman PB, Hauschild A, Robert C, Haanen JB, Ascierto P, Larkin J, et al. Improved survival with vemurafenib in melanoma with BRAF V600E mutation. N Engl J Med 2011 Jun 30;364(26):2507-2516.

[13] Wheatley K, Ives N, Hancock B, Gore M, Eggermont A, Suciu S. Does adjuvant interferon-alpha for high-risk melanoma provide a worthwhile benefit? A meta-analysis of the randomised trials. Cancer Treat Rev 2003 Aug;29(4):241-252.

[14] Mocellin S, Pasquali S, Rossi CR, Nitti D. Interferon alpha adjuvant therapy in patients with high-risk melanoma: a systematic review and meta-analysis. J Natl Cancer Inst 2010 Apr 7;102(7):493-501.

[15] Janku F, Kurzrock R. Adjuvant interferon in high-risk melanoma: end of the era? J Clin Oncol 2010 Jan 10;28(2):e15-6; author reply e17-8.

[16] Boon T. Tumor antigens recognized by cytolytic T lymphocytes: present perspectives for specific immunotherapy. Int J Cancer 1993 May 8;54(2):177-180.

[17] Vogel TU, Visan L, Ljutic B, Gajewska B, Caterini J, Salha D, et al. Preclinical qualification of a new multi-antigen candidate vaccine for metastatic melanoma. J Immunother 2010 Oct;33(8):743-758.

[18] Gilchrest BA, Eller MS, Geller AC, Yaar M. The pathogenesis of melanoma induced by ultraviolet radiation. N Engl J Med 1999 Apr 29;340(17):1341-1348.

[19] Satyamoorthy K, Herlyn M. Cellular and molecular biology of human melanoma. Cancer Biol Ther 2002 Jan-Feb;1(1):14-17.

[20] Vogelstein B, Kinzler KW. Cancer genes and the pathways they control. Nat Med 2004 Aug;10(8):789-799.

[21] Soengas MS, Lowe SW. Apoptosis and melanoma chemoresistance. Oncogene 2003 May 19;22(20):3138-3151.

[22] Clark WH,Jr, Elder DE, Guerry D,4th, Epstein MN, Greene MH, Van Horn M. A study of tumor progression: the precursor lesions of superficial spreading and nodular melanoma. Hum Pathol 1984 Dec;15(12):1147-1165.

[23] Brunet A, Roux D, Lenormand P, Dowd S, Keyse S, Pouyssegur J. Nuclear translocation of p42/p44 mitogen-activated protein kinase is required for growth factor-induced gene expression and cell cycle entry. EMBO J 1999 Feb 1;18(3):664-674.

[24] Lin AW, Barradas M, Stone JC, van Aelst L, Serrano M, Lowe SW. Premature senescence involving p53 and p16 is activated in response to constitutive MEK/MAPK mitogenic signaling. Genes Dev 1998 Oct 1;12(19):3008-3019.

[25] Miller AJ, Mihm MC,Jr. Melanoma. N Engl J Med 2006 Jul 6;355(1):51-65.

[26] Kefford R, Bishop JN, Tucker M, Bressac-de Paillerets B, Bianchi-Scarra G, Bergman W, et al. Genetic testing for melanoma. Lancet Oncol 2002 Nov;3(11):653-654.

[27] Serrano M. The tumor suppressor protein p16INK4a. Exp Cell Res 1997 Nov 25;237(1):7-13.

[28] Gilchrest BA, Eller MS. DNA photodamage stimulates melanogenesis and other photoprotective responses. J Investig Dermatol Symp Proc 1999 Sep;4(1):35-40.

[29] Johnson TM, Dolan OM, Hamilton TA, Lu MC, Swanson NA, Lowe L. Clinical and histologic trends of melanoma. J Am Acad Dermatol 1998 May;38(5 Pt 1):681-686.

[30] Rossi CR, Foletto M, Vecchiato A, Alessio S, Menin N, Lise M. Management of cutaneous melanoma M0: state of the art and trends. Eur J Cancer 1997 Dec;33(14): 2302-2312.

[31] Slominski A, Ross J, Mihm MC. Cutaneous melanoma: pathology, relevant prognostic indicators and progression. Br Med Bull 1995 Jul;51(3):548-569.

[32] Clark WH,Jr, Elder DE, Guerry D,4th, Braitman LE, Trock BJ, Schultz D, et al. Model predicting survival in stage I melanoma based on tumor progression. J Natl Cancer Inst 1989 Dec 20;81(24):1893-1904.

[33] Guerry D,4th, Synnestvedt M, Elder DE, Schultz D. Lessons from tumor progression: the invasive radial growth phase of melanoma is common, incapable of metastasis, and indolent. J Invest Dermatol 1993 Mar;100(3):342S-345S.

[34] Gray-Schopfer V, Wellbrock C, Marais R. Melanoma biology and new targeted therapy. Nature 2007 Feb 22;445(7130):851-857.

[35] Jean D, Gershenwald JE, Huang S, Luca M, Hudson MJ, Tainsky MA, et al. Loss of AP-2 results in up-regulation of MCAM/MUC18 and an increase in tumor growth and metastasis of human melanoma cells. J Biol Chem 1998 Jun 26;273(26): 16501-16508.

[36] Buytaert E, Dewaele M, Agostinis P. Molecular effectors of multiple cell death pathways initiated by photodynamic therapy. Biochim Biophys Acta 2007 Sep;1776(1): 86-107.

[37] Babilas P, Schreml S, Landthaler M, Szeimies RM. Photodynamic therapy in dermatology: state-of-the-art. Photodermatol Photoimmunol Photomed 2010 Jun;26(3): 118-132.

[38] Dougherty TJ, Gomer CJ, Henderson BW, Jori G, Kessel D, Korbelik M, et al. Photodynamic therapy. J Natl Cancer Inst 1998 Jun 17;90(12):889-905.

[39] Henderson BW, Dougherty TJ. How does photodynamic therapy work? Photochem Photobiol 1992 Jan;55(1):145-157.

[40] Juarranz A, Jaen P, Sanz-Rodriguez F, Cuevas J, Gonzalez S. Photodynamic therapy of cancer. Basic principles and applications. Clin Transl Oncol 2008 Mar;10(3): 148-154.

[41] Ortel B, Shea CR, Calzavara-Pinton P. Molecular mechanisms of photodynamic therapy. Front Biosci 2009 Jan 1;14:4157-4172.

[42] Gomer CJ, Ferrario A, Luna M, Rucker N, Wong S. Photodynamic therapy: combined modality approaches targeting the tumor microenvironment. Lasers Surg Med 2006 Jun;38(5):516-521.

[43] Verma S, Watt GM, Mai Z, Hasan T. Strategies for enhanced photodynamic therapy effects. Photochem Photobiol 2007 Sep-Oct;83(5):996-1005.

[44] Detty MR, Gibson SL, Wagner SJ. Current clinical and preclinical photosensitizers for use in photodynamic therapy. J Med Chem 2004 Jul 29;47(16):3897-3915.

[45] Stockert JC, Canete M, Juarranz A, Villanueva A, Horobin RW, Borrell JI, et al. Porphycenes: facts and prospects in photodynamic therapy of cancer. Curr Med Chem 2007;14(9):997-1026.

[46] Bourre L, Rousset N, Thibaut S, Eleouet S, Lajat Y, Patrice T. PDT effects of m-THPC and ALA, phototoxicity and apoptosis. Apoptosis 2002 Jun;7(3):221-230.

[47] Thibaut S, Bourre L, Hernot D, Rousset N, Lajat Y, Patrice T. Effects of BAPTA-AM, Forskolin, DSF and Z.VAD.fmk on PDT-induced apoptosis and m-THPC phototoxicity on B16 cells. Apoptosis 2002 Apr;7(2):99-106.

[48] Szeimies RM, Karrer S, Radakovic-Fijan S, Tanew A, Calzavara-Pinton PG, Zane C, et al. Photodynamic therapy using topical methyl 5-aminolevulinate compared with cryotherapy for actinic keratosis: A prospective, randomized study. J Am Acad Dermatol 2002 Aug;47(2):258-262.

[49] Szeimies RM. Methyl aminolevulinate-photodynamic therapy for basal cell carcinoma. Dermatol Clin 2007 Jan;25(1):89-94.

[50] Szeimies RM, Morton CA, Sidoroff A, Braathen LR. Photodynamic therapy for nonmelanoma skin cancer. Acta Derm Venereol 2005;85(6):483-490.

[51] Bolfarini GC, Siqueira-Moura MP, Demets GJ. In vitro evaluation of combined hyperthermia and photodynamic effects using magnetoliposomes loaded with cucurbituril zinc phthalocyanine complex on melanoma. 2012 Jun 5.

[52] Khurana M, Ulrich S, Kim A, Moriyama Y, Netchev G, Akens MK, et al. Biodistribution and Pharmacokinetic Studies of a Porphyrin Dimer Photosensitizer (Oxdime) by Fluorescence Imaging and Spectroscopy in Mice Bearing Xenograft Tumors. Photochem Photo 2012 Jun 23.

[53] Rapozzi V, Zorzet S, Zacchigna M, Drioli S, Xodo LE. The PDT activity of free and pegylated pheophorbide a against an amelanotic melanoma transplanted in C57/BL6 mice. Invest New Drugs 2012 Jun 12.

[54] Sharma KV, Davids LM. Depigmentation in melanomas increases the efficacy of hypericin-mediated photodynamic-induced cell death. Photodiagnosis Photodyn Ther 2012 Jun;9(2):156-163.

[55] Shrestha TB, Seo GM, Basel MT, Kalita M, Wang H, Villanueva D, et al. Stem cell-based photodynamic therapy. Photochem Photobiol Sci 2012 Jul;11(7):1251-1258.

[56] Conforti F, Menichini G, Zanfini L, Tundis R, Statti GA, Provenzano E, et al. Evaluation of phototoxic potential of aerial components of the fig tree against human melanoma. Cell Prolif 2012 Jun;45(3):279-285.

[57] Maduray K, Odhav B, Nyokong T. In vitro photodynamic effect of aluminum tetrasulfophthalocyanines on melanoma skin cancer and healthy normal skin cells. Photodiagnosis Photodyn Ther 2012 Mar;9(1):32-39.

[58] Slastnikova TA, Rosenkranz AA, Gulak PV, Schiffelers RM, Lupanova TN, Khramtsov YV, et al. Modular nanotransporters: a multipurpose in vivo working platform for targeted drug delivery. Int J Nanomedicine 2012;7:467-482.

[59] Wagner M, Suarez ER, Theodoro TR, Machado Filho CD, Gama MF, Tardivo JP, et al. Methylene blue photodynamic therapy in malignant melanoma decreases expression of proliferating cell nuclear antigen and heparanases. Clin Exp Dermatol 2012 Jul; 37(5):527-533.

[60] Dabrowski JM, Arnaut LG, Pereira MM, Urbanska K, Simoes S, Stochel G, et al. Combined effects of singlet oxygen and hydroxyl radical in photodynamic therapy with photostable bacteriochlorins: evidence from intracellular fluorescence and increased photodynamic efficacy in vitro. Free Radic Biol Med 2012 Apr 1;52(7):1188-1200.

[61] Yoshii H, Yoshii Y, Asai T, Furukawa T, Takaichi S, Fujibayashi Y. Photo-excitation of carotenoids causes cytotoxicity via singlet oxygen production. Biochem Biophys Res Commun 2012 Jan 6;417(1):640-645.

[62] Schmitt F, Barry NP, Juillerat-Jeanneret L, Therrien B. Efficient photodynamic therapy of cancer using chemotherapeutic porphyrin-ruthenium metalla-cubes. Bioorg Med Chem Lett 2012 Jan 1;22(1):178-180.

[63] Menichini G, Alfano C, Provenzano E, Marrelli M, Statti GA, Menichini F, et al. Cachrys pungens Jan inhibits human melanoma cell proliferation through photo-induced cytotoxic activity. Cell Prolif 2012 Feb;45(1):39-47.

[64] Radzi R, Osaki T, Tsuka T, Imagawa T, Minami S, Okamoto Y. Morphological study in B16F10 murine melanoma cells after photodynamic hyperthermal therapy with indocyanine green (ICG). J Vet Med Sci 2012 Apr;74(4):465-472.

[65] Rapozzi V, Umezawa K, Xodo LE. Role of NF-kappaB/Snail/RKIP loop in the response of tumor cells to photodynamic therapy. Lasers Surg Med 2011 Sep;43(7): 575-585.

[66] Dabrowski JM, Krzykawska M, Arnaut LG, Pereira MM, Monteiro CJ, Simoes S, et al. Tissue uptake study and photodynamic therapy of melanoma-bearing mice with a nontoxic, effective chlorin. ChemMedChem 2011 Sep 5;6(9):1715-1726.

[67] Kim MR, Morrison H, Mohammed SI. Effect of a photoactivated rhodium complex in melanoma. Anticancer Drugs 2011 Oct;22(9):896-904.

[68] You BJ, Wu YC, Wu CY, Bao BY, Chen MY, Chang YH, et al. Proteomics displays cytoskeletal proteins and chaperones involvement in Hedyotis corymbosa-induced photokilling in skin cancer cells. Exp Dermatol 2011 Aug;20(8):653-658.

[69] Sharma KV, Bowers N, Davids LM. Photodynamic therapy-induced killing is enhanced in depigmented metastatic melanoma cells. Cell Biol Int 2011 Sep;35(9): 939-944.

[70] Maduray K, Karsten A, Odhav B, Nyokong T. In vitro toxicity testing of zinc tetrasulfophthalocyanines in fibroblast and keratinocyte cells for the treatment of melanoma cancer by photodynamic therapy. J Photochem Photobiol B 2011 May 3;103(2):98-104.

[71] Grimm S, Mvondo D, Grune T, Breusing N. The outcome of 5-ALA-mediated photodynamic treatment in melanoma cells is influenced by vitamin C and heme oxygenase-1. Biofactors 2011 Jan;37(1):17-24.

[72] Tammela T, Saaristo A, Holopainen T, Yla-Herttuala S, Andersson LC, Virolainen S, et al. Photodynamic ablation of lymphatic vessels and intralymphatic cancer cells prevents metastasis. Sci Transl Med 2011 Feb 9;3(69):69ra11.

[73] Kastle M, Grimm S, Nagel R, Breusing N, Grune T. Combination of PDT and inhibitor treatment affects melanoma cells and spares keratinocytes. Free Radic Biol Med 2011 Jan 15;50(2):305-312.

[74] Robertson CA, Abrahamse H, Evans D. The in vitro PDT efficacy of a novel metallophthalocyanine (MPc) derivative and established 5-ALA photosensitizing dyes against human metastatic melanoma cells. Lasers Surg Med 2010 Dec;42(10):766-776.

[75] Moisenovich MM, Ol'shevskaya VA, Rokitskaya TI, Ramonova AA, Nikitina RG, Savchenko AN, et al. Novel photosensitizers trigger rapid death of malignant human cells and rodent tumor transplants via lipid photodamage and membrane permeabilization. PLoS One 2010 Sep 15;5(9):e12717.

[76] Otake E, Sakuma S, Torii K, Maeda A, Ohi H, Yano S, et al. Effect and mechanism of a new photodynamic therapy with glycoconjugated fullerene. Photochem Photobiol 2010 Nov-Dec;86(6):1356-1363.

[77] Dabrowski JM, Arnaut LG, Pereira MM, Monteiro CJ, Urbanska K, Simoes S, et al. New halogenated water-soluble chlorin and bacteriochlorin as photostable PDT sensitizers: synthesis, spectroscopy, photophysics, and in vitro photosensitizing efficacy. ChemMedChem 2010 Oct 4;5(10):1770-1780.

[78] Chen P, Jiang X, Wei DP, Li L. The effects of intense pulsed light and 5-aminolevulinic acid on the cultured B16 marine melanoma cells. Sichuan Da Xue Xue Bao Yi Xue Ban 2010 Mar;41(2):280-283.

[79] Mroz P, Huang YY, Szokalska A, Zhiyentayev T, Janjua S, Nifli AP, et al. Stable synthetic bacteriochlorins overcome the resistance of melanoma to photodynamic therapy. FASEB J 2010 Sep;24(9):3160-3170.

[80] Camerin M, Magaraggia M, Soncin M, Jori G, Moreno M, Chambrier I, et al. The in vivo efficacy of phthalocyanine-nanoparticle conjugates for the photodynamic therapy of amelanotic melanoma. Eur J Cancer 2010 Jul;46(10):1910-1918.

[81] Barbugli PA, Siqueira-Moura MP, Espreafico EM, Tedesco AC. In vitro phototoxicity of liposomes and nanocapsules containing chloroaluminum phthalocyanine on human melanoma cell line. J Nanosci Nanotechnol 2010 Jan;10(1):569-573.

[82] Serra A, Pineiro M, Santos CI, Gonsalves AM, Abrantes M, Laranjo M, et al. In vitro photodynamic activity of 5,15-bis(3-hydroxyphenyl)porphyrin and its halogenated derivatives against cancer cells. Photochem Photobiol 2010 Jan-Feb;86(1):206-212.

[83] Nikitina RG, Mardynskaja VP, Morozova TG, Drozhzhina VV. A method for improving the efficiency of therapy for melanoma. Bull Exp Biol Med 2009 Aug;148(2): 238-240.

[84] Ouedraogo M, De Maesschalck E, Soentjens-Werts V, Dubois J. In vitro cytotoxicity study of oxaziridines generated after chlordiazepoxide, demoxepam, and desmethylchlordiazepoxide UV irradiation. Drug Chem Toxicol 2009;32(4):417-423.

[85] Camerin M, Rello-Varona S, Villanueva A, Rodgers MA, Jori G. Metallo-naphthalocyanines as photothermal sensitisers for experimental tumours: in vitro and in vivo studies. Lasers Surg Med 2009 Nov;41(9):665-673.

[86] Krestyn E, Kolarova H, Bajgar R, Tomankova K. Photodynamic properties of ZnTPPS(4), ClAlPcS(2) and ALA in human melanoma G361 cells. Toxicol In Vitro 2009 Aug 29.

[87] Zhao B, Yin JJ, Bilski PJ, Chignell CF, Roberts JE, He YY. Enhanced photodynamic efficacy towards melanoma cells by encapsulation of Pc4 in silica nanoparticles. Toxicol Appl Pharmacol 2009 Dec 1;241(2):163-172.

[88] Mamoon AM, Gamal-Eldeen AM, Ruppel ME, Smith RJ, Tsang T, Miller LM. In vitro efficiency and mechanistic role of indocyanine green as photodynamic therapy agent for human melanoma. Photodiagnosis Photodyn Ther 2009 Jun;6(2):105-116.

[89] Davids LM, Kleemann B, Cooper S, Kidson SH. Melanomas display increased cytoprotection to hypericin-mediated cytotoxicity through the induction of autophagy. Cell Biol Int 2009 Oct;33(10):1065-1072.

[90] Kolarova H, Tomankova K, Bajgar R, Kolar P, Kubinek R. Photodynamic and sonodynamic treatment by phthalocyanine on cancer cell lines. Ultrasound Med Biol 2009 Aug;35(8):1397-1404.

[91] Tsai T, Ji HT, Chiang PC, Chou RH, Chang WS, Chen CT. ALA-PDT results in phenotypic changes and decreased cellular invasion in surviving cancer cells. Lasers Surg Med 2009 Apr;41(4):305-315.

[92] Chen Y, Zheng W, Li Y, Zhong J, Ji J, Shen P. Apoptosis induced by methylene-blue-mediated photodynamic therapy in melanomas and the involvement of mitochondrial dysfunction revealed by proteomics. Cancer Sci 2008 Oct;99(10):2019-2027.

[93] Hao E, Friso E, Miotto G, Jori G, Soncin M, Fabris C, et al. Synthesis and biological investigations of tetrakis(p-carboranylthio-tetrafluorophenyl)chlorin (TPFC). Org Biomol Chem 2008 Oct 21;6(20):3732-3740.

[94] Chang CJ, Yu JS, Wei FC. In vitro and in vivo photosensitizing applications of Photofrin in malignant melanoma cells. Chang Gung Med J 2008 May-Jun;31(3):260-267.

[95] Korbelik M, Cecic I. Complement activation cascade and its regulation: relevance for the response of solid tumors to photodynamic therapy. J Photochem Photobiol B 2008 Oct 16;93(1):53-59.

[96] Kolarova H, Nevrelova P, Tomankova K, Kolar P, Bajgar R, Mosinger J. Production of reactive oxygen species after photodynamic therapy by porphyrin sensitizers. Gen Physiol Biophys 2008 Jun;27(2):101-105.

[97] Skidan I, Dholakia P, Torchilin V. Photodynamic therapy of experimental B-16 melanoma in mice with tumor-targeted 5,10,15,20-tetraphenylporphin-loaded PEG-PE micelles. J Drug Target 2008 Jul;16(6):486-493.

[98] Davids LM, Kleemann B, Kacerovska D, Pizinger K, Kidson SH. Hypericin phototoxicity induces different modes of cell death in melanoma and human skin cells. J Photochem Photobiol B 2008 May 29;91(2-3):67-76.

[99] Schmitt F, Govindaswamy P, Suss-Fink G, Ang WH, Dyson PJ, Juillerat-Jeanneret L, et al. Ruthenium porphyrin compounds for photodynamic therapy of cancer. J Med Chem 2008 Mar 27;51(6):1811-1816.

[100] Ma LW, Nielsen KP, Iani V, Moan J. A new method for photodynamic therapy of melanotic melanoma -- effects of depigmentation with violet light photodynamic therapy. J Environ Pathol Toxicol Oncol 2007;26(3):165-172.

[101] Janczyk A, Wolnicka-Glubisz A, Urbanska K, Kisch H, Stochel G, Macyk W. Photodynamic activity of platinum(IV) chloride surface-modified TiO2 irradiated with visible light. Free Radic Biol Med 2008 Mar 15;44(6):1120-1130.

[102] Tomankova K, Kolarova H, Vujtek M, Bajgar R. Photodynamic effect on melanoma cells investigated by atomic force microscopy. Gen Physiol Biophys 2007 Sep;26(3): 200-206.

[103] Frank J, Lornejad-Schafer MR, Schoffl H, Flaccus A, Lambert C, Biesalski HK. Inhibition of heme oxygenase-1 increases responsiveness of melanoma cells to ALA-based photodynamic therapy. Int J Oncol 2007 Dec;31(6):1539-1545.

[104] Fabris C, Vicente MG, Hao E, Friso E, Borsetto L, Jori G, et al. Tumour-localizing and -photosensitising properties of meso-tetra(4-nido-carboranylphenyl)porphyrin (H2TCP). J Photochem Photobiol B 2007 Dec 14;89(2-3):131-138.

[105] Rijcken CJ, Hofman JW, van Zeeland F, Hennink WE, van Nostrum CF. Photosensitiser-loaded biodegradable polymeric micelles: preparation, characterisation and in vitro PDT efficacy. J Control Release 2007 Dec 20;124(3):144-153.

[106] Kolarova H, Nevrelova P, Bajgar R, Jirova D, Kejlova K, Strnad M. In vitro photodynamic therapy on melanoma cell lines with phthalocyanine. Toxicol In Vitro 2007 Mar;21(2):249-253.

[107] Dabrowski JM, Pereira MM, Arnaut LG, Monteiro CJ, Peixoto AF, Karocki A, et al. Synthesis, photophysical studies and anticancer activity of a new halogenated water-soluble porphyrin. Photochem Photobiol 2007 Jul-Aug;83(4):897-903.

[108] Ji HX, Zhang F, Gao LQ, Jia LY, Xiong Y, Liang C, et al. Photodynamic therapy of pigmented choroidal melanomas in rabbits using hematoporphyrin monomethyl ether. Zhonghua Yan Ke Za Zhi 2007 Mar;43(3):212-216.

[109] Kolarova H, Lenobel R, Kolar P, Strnad M. Sensitivity of different cell lines to phototoxic effect of disulfonated chloroaluminium phthalocyanine. Toxicol In Vitro 2007 Oct;21(7):1304-1306.

[110] Ferrario A, Rucker N, Wong S, Luna M, Gomer CJ. Survivin, a member of the inhibitor of apoptosis family, is induced by photodynamic therapy and is a target for improving treatment response. Cancer Res 2007 May 15;67(10):4989-4995.

[111] Korbelik M, Cooper PD. Potentiation of photodynamic therapy of cancer by complement: the effect of gamma-inulin. Br J Cancer 2007 Jan 15;96(1):67-72.

[112] Hiruma H, Katakura T, Takenami T, Igawa S, Kanoh M, Fujimura T, et al. Vesicle disruption, plasma membrane bleb formation, and acute cell death caused by illumination with blue light in acridine orange-loaded malignant melanoma cells. J Photochem Photobiol B 2007 Jan 3;86(1):1-8.

[113] Nowak-Sliwinska P, Karocki A, Elas M, Pawlak A, Stochel G, Urbanska K. Verteporfin, photofrin II, and merocyanine 540 as PDT photosensitizers against melanoma cells. Biochem Biophys Res Commun 2006 Oct 20;349(2):549-555.

[114] Schacht V, Szeimies RM, Abels C. Photodynamic therapy with 5-aminolevulinic acid induces distinct microcirculatory effects following systemic or topical application. Photochem Photobiol Sci 2006 May;5(5):452-458.

[115] Saji H, Song W, Furumoto K, Kato H, Engleman EG. Systemic antitumor effect of intratumoral injection of dendritic cells in combination with local photodynamic therapy. Clin Cancer Res 2006 Apr 15;12(8):2568-2574.

[116] Friso E, Roncucci G, Dei D, Soncin M, Fabris C, Chiti G, et al. A novel 10B-enriched carboranyl-containing phthalocyanine as a radio- and photo-sensitising agent for boron neutron capture therapy and photodynamic therapy of tumours: in vitro and in vivo studies. Photochem Photobiol Sci 2006 Jan;5(1):39-50.

[117] Saczko J, Kulbacka J, Chwilkowska A, Drag-Zalesiniska M, Wysocka T, Lugowski M, et al. The influence of photodynamic therapy on apoptosis in human melanoma cell line. Folia Histochem Cytobiol 2005;43(3):129-132.

[118] Kolarova H, Macecek J, Nevrelova P, Huf M, Tomecka M, Bajgar R, et al. Photodynamic therapy with zinc-tetra(p-sulfophenyl)porphyrin bound to cyclodextrin induces single strand breaks of cellular DNA in G361 melanoma cells. Toxicol In Vitro 2005 Oct;19(7):971-974.

[119] Camerin M, Rello S, Villanueva A, Ping X, Kenney ME, Rodgers MA, et al. Photothermal sensitisation as a novel therapeutic approach for tumours: studies at the cellular and animal level. Eur J Cancer 2005 May;41(8):1203-1212.

[120] Macecek J, Kolarova H, Psotova J, Bajgar R, Huf M, Nevrelova P, et al. Assessment of cellular damage by comet assay after photodynamic therapy in vitro. Acta Medica (Hradec Kralove) 2004;47(4):327-329.

[121] Posen Y, Kalchenko V, Seger R, Brandis A, Scherz A, Salomon Y. Manipulation of redox signaling in mammalian cells enabled by controlled photogeneration of reactive oxygen species. J Cell Sci 2005 May 1;118(Pt 9):1957-1969.

[122] Schastak S, Jean B, Handzel R, Kostenich G, Hermann R, Sack U, et al. Improved pharmacokinetics, biodistribution and necrosis in vivo using a new near infra-red photosensitizer: tetrahydroporphyrin tetratosylat. J Photochem Photobiol B 2005 Mar 1;78(3):203-213.

[123] Mazor O, Brandis A, Plaks V, Neumark E, Rosenbach-Belkin V, Salomon Y, et al. WST11, a novel water-soluble bacteriochlorophyll derivative; cellular uptake, pharmacokinetics, biodistribution and vascular-targeted photodynamic activity using melanoma tumors as a model. Photochem Photobiol 2005 Mar-Apr;81(2):342-351.

[124] Vena FC, Turchiello RF, Laville I, Pigaglio S, Blais J, Tedesco AC. 5-aminolevulinic acid ester-induced protoporphyrin IX in a murine melanoma cell line. Lasers Med Sci 2004;19(2):119-126.

[125] Karmakova T, Feofanov A, Nazarova A, Grichine A, Yakubovskaya R, Luk'yanets E, et al. Distribution of metal-free sulfonated phthalocyanine in subcutaneously transplanted murine tumors. J Photochem Photobiol B 2004 Jul 19;75(1-2):81-87.

[126] Ropp S, Guy J, Berl V, Bischoff P, Lepoittevin JP. Synthesis and photocytotoxic activity of new alpha-methylene-gamma-butyrolactone-psoralen heterodimers. Bioorg Med Chem 2004 Jul 1;12(13):3619-3625.

[127] Ickowicz Schwartz D, Gozlan Y, Greenbaum L, Babushkina T, Katcoff DJ, Malik Z. Differentiation-dependent photodynamic therapy regulated by porphobilinogen deaminase in B16 melanoma. Br J Cancer 2004 May 4;90(9):1833-1841.

[128] Lim DS, Ko SH, Lee WY. Silkworm-pheophorbide alpha mediated photodynamic therapy against B16F10 pigmented melanoma. J Photochem Photobiol B 2004 Mar 19;74(1):1-6.

[129] Barge J, Decreau R, Julliard M, Hubaud JC, Sabatier AS, Grob JJ, et al. Killing efficacy of a new silicon phthalocyanine in human melanoma cells treated with photodynamic therapy by early activation of mitochondrion-mediated apoptosis. Exp Dermatol 2004 Jan;13(1):33-44.

[130] Szurko A, Kramer-Marek G, Widel M, Ratuszna A, Habdas J, Kus P. Photodynamic effects of two water soluble porphyrins evaluated on human malignant melanoma cells in vitro. Acta Biochim Pol 2003;50(4):1165-1174.

[131] Kolarova H, Mosinger J, Lenobel R, Kejlova K, Jirova D, Strnad M. In vitro toxicity testing of supramolecular sensitizers for photodynamic therapy. Toxicol In Vitro 2003 Oct-Dec;17(5-6):775-778.

[132] Nagata S, Obana A, Gohto Y, Nakajima S. Necrotic and apoptotic cell death of human malignant melanoma cells following photodynamic therapy using an amphiphilic photosensitizer, ATX-S10(Na). Lasers Surg Med 2003;33(1):64-70.

[133] Babilas P, Schacht V, Liebsch G, Wolfbeis OS, Landthaler M, Szeimies RM, et al. Effects of light fractionation and different fluence rates on photodynamic therapy with 5-aminolaevulinic acid in vivo. Br J Cancer 2003 May 6;88(9):1462-1469.

[134] Haddad R, Kaplan O, Greenberg R, Siegal A, Skornick Y, Kashtan H. Photodynamic therapy of murine colon cancer and melanoma using systemic aminolevulinic acid as a photosensitizer. Int J Surg Investig 2000;2(3):171-178.

[135] Jezek P, Nekvasil M, Skobisova E, Urbankova E, Jirsa M, Zadinova M, et al. Experimental photodynamic therapy with MESO-tetrakisphenylporphyrin (TPP) in liposomes leads to disintegration of human amelanotic melanoma implanted to nude mice. Int J Cancer 2003 Feb 20;103(5):693-702.

[136] Hu L, Wu X, Song Y, Young LH, Gragoudas ES. Photodynamic therapy of pigmented choroidal melanomas in rabbits. Zhonghua Yan Ke Za Zhi 2002 Aug;38(8):491-494.

[137] Urbanska K, Romanowska-Dixon B, Matuszak Z, Oszajca J, Nowak-Sliwinsk P, Stochel G. Indocyanine green as a prospective sensitizer for photodynamic therapy of melanomas. Acta Biochim Pol 2002;49(2):387-391.

[138] Bourre L, Rousset N, Thibaut S, Eleouet S, Lajat Y, Patrice T. PDT effects of m-THPC and ALA, phototoxicity and apoptosis. Apoptosis 2002 Jun;7(3):221-230.

[139] Lang K, Bolsen K, Stahl W, Ruzicka T, Sies H, Lehmann P, et al. The 5-aminolevulinic acid-induced porphyrin biosynthesis in benign and malignant cells of the skin. J Photochem Photobiol B 2001 Dec 1;65(1):29-34.

[140] Drzewiecka A, Urbanska K, Matuszak Z, Pineiro M, Arnaut LG, Habdas J, et al. Tritolylporphyrin dimer as a new potent hydrophobic sensitizer for photodynamic therapy of melanoma. Acta Biochim Pol 2001;48(1):277-282.

[141] Pahernik S, Langer S, Botzlar A, Dellian M, Goetz AE. Tissue distribution and penetration of 5-ALA induced fluorescence in an amelanotic melanoma after topical application. Anticancer Res 2001 Jan-Feb;21(1A):59-63.

[142] Zilberstein J, Schreiber S, Bloemers MC, Bendel P, Neeman M, Schechtman E, et al. Antivascular treatment of solid melanoma tumors with bacteriochlorophyll-serine-based photodynamic therapy. Photochem Photobiol 2001 Mar;73(3):257-266.

[143] Rice L, Wainwright M, Phoemix DA. Phenothiazine photosensitizers. III. Activity of methylene blue derivatives against pigmented melanoma cell lines. J Chemother 2000 Feb;12(1):94-104.

[144] Busetti A, Soncin M, Reddi E, Rodgers MA, Kenney ME, Jori G. Photothermal sensitization of amelanotic melanoma cells by Ni(II)-octabutoxy-naphthalocyanine. J Photochem Photobiol B 1999 Nov-Dec;53(1-3):103-109.

[145] Soncin M, Busetti A, Fusi F, Jori G, Rodgers MA. Irradiation of amelanotic melanoma cells with 532 nm high peak power pulsed laser radiation in the presence of the photothermal sensitizer Cu(II)-hematoporphyrin: a new approach to cell photoinactivation. Photochem Photobiol 1999 Jun;69(6):708-712.

[146] Langer S, Abels C, Botzlar A, Pahernik S, Rick K, Szeimies RM, et al. Active and higher intracellular uptake of 5-aminolevulinic acid in tumors may be inhibited by glycine. J Invest Dermatol 1999 May;112(5):723-728.

[147] Decreau R, Richard MJ, Verrando P, Chanon M, Julliard M. Photodynamic activities of silicon phthalocyanines against achromic M6 melanoma cells and healthy human melanocytes and keratinocytes. J Photochem Photobiol B 1999 Jan;48(1):48-56.

[148] Busetti A, Soncin M, Jori G, Rodgers MA. High efficiency of benzoporphyrin derivative in the photodynamic therapy of pigmented malignant melanoma. Br J Cancer 1999 Feb;79(5-6):821-824.

[149] Klotz LO, Fritsch C, Briviba K, Tsacmacidis N, Schliess F, Sies H. Activation of JNK and p38 but not ERK MAP kinases in human skin cells by 5-aminolevulinate-photodynamic therapy. Cancer Res 1998 Oct 1;58(19):4297-4300.

[150] Busetti A, Soncin M, Jori G, Kenney ME, Rodgers MA. Treatment of malignant melanoma by high-peak-power 1064 nm irradiation followed by photodynamic therapy. Photochem Photobiol 1998 Sep;68(3):377-381.

[151] Haddad R, Blumenfeld A, Siegal A, Kaplan O, Cohen M, Skornick Y, et al. In vitro and in vivo effects of photodynamic therapy on murine malignant melanoma. Ann Surg Oncol 1998 Apr-May;5(3):241-247.

[152] Woodburn KW, Fan Q, Kessel D, Luo Y, Young SW. Photodynamic therapy of B16F10 murine melanoma with lutetium texaphyrin. J Invest Dermatol 1998 May;110(5):746-751.

[153] Abels C, Szeimies RM, Steinbach P, Richert C, Goetz AE. Targeting of the tumor microcirculation by photodynamic therapy with a synthetic porphycene. J Photochem Photobiol B 1997 Oct;40(3):305-312.

[154] Mantareva V, Shopova M, Spassova G, Wohrle D, Muller S, Jori G, et al. Si(IV)-methoxyethylene-glycol-naphthalocyanine: synthesis and pharmacokinetic and photosensitizing properties in different tumour models. J Photochem Photobiol B 1997 Oct;40(3):258-262.

[155] Abels C, Fritsch C, Bolsen K, Szeimies RM, Ruzicka T, Goerz G, et al. Photodynamic therapy with 5-aminolaevulinic acid-induced porphyrins of an amelanotic melanoma in vivo. J Photochem Photobiol B 1997 Aug;40(1):76-83.

[156] Kim RY, Hu LK, Flotte TJ, Gragoudas ES, Young LH. Digital angiography of experimental choroidal melanomas using benzoporphyrin derivative. Am J Ophthalmol 1997 Jun;123(6):810-816.

[157] Zilberstein J, Bromberg A, Frantz A, Rosenbach-Belkin V, Kritzmann A, Pfefermann R, et al. Light-dependent oxygen consumption in bacteriochlorophyll-serine-treated melanoma tumors: on-line determination using a tissue-inserted oxygen microsensor. Photochem Photobiol 1997 Jun;65(6):1012-1019.

[158] Blom DJ, Schuitmaker HJ, de Waard-Siebinga I, Dubbelman TM, Jager MJ. Decreased expression of HLA class I on ocular melanoma cells following in vitro photodynamic therapy. Cancer Lett 1997 Jan 30;112(2):239-243.

[159] Fritsch C, Abels C, Goetz AE, Stahl W, Bolsen K, Ruzicka T, et al. Porphyrins preferentially accumulate in a melanoma following intravenous injection of 5-aminolevulinic acid. Biol Chem 1997 Jan;378(1):51-57.

[160] Michailov N, Peeva M, Angelov I, Wohrle D, Muller S, Jori G, et al. Fluence rate effects on photodynamic therapy of B16 pigmented melanoma. J Photochem Photobiol B 1997 Jan;37(1-2):154-157.

[161] Kim RY, Hu LK, Foster BS, Gragoudas ES, Young LH. Photodynamic therapy of pigmented choroidal melanomas of greater than 3-mm thickness. Ophthalmology 1996 Dec;103(12):2029-2036.

[162] Hadjur C, Richard MJ, Parat MO, Jardon P, Favier A. Photodynamic effects of hypericin on lipid peroxidation and antioxidant status in melanoma cells. Photochem Photobiol 1996 Aug;64(2):375-381.

[163] VanderWerf QM, Saxton RE, Chang A, Horton D, Paiva MB, Anderson J, et al. Hypericin: a new laser phototargeting agent for human cancer cells. Laryngoscope 1996 Apr;106(4):479-483.

[164] Donaldson MJ, Lim L, Harper CA, Mackenzie J, G Campbell W. Primary treatment of choroidal amelanotic melanoma with photodynamic therapy. Clin Experiment Ophthalmol 2005 Oct;33(5):548-549.

[165] Sheleg SV, Zhavrid EA, Khodina TV, Kochubeev GA, Istomin YP, Chalov VN, et al. Photodynamic therapy with chlorin e(6) for skin metastases of melanoma. Photodermatol Photoimmunol Photomed 2004 Feb;20(1):21-26.

[166] Baldea I, Filip AG. Photodynamic therapy in melanoma--an update. J Physiol Pharmacol 2012 Apr;63(2):109-118.

[167] Tuncer S, Kir N, Shields CL. Dramatic regression of amelanotic choroidal melanoma with PDT following poor response to brachytherapy. Ophthalmic Surg Lasers Imaging 2012 May 3;43(3):e38-40.

[168] Canal-Fontcuberta I, Salomao DR, Robertson D, Cantrill HL, Koozekanani D, Rath PP, et al. Clinical and histopathologic findings after photodynamic therapy of choroidal melanoma. Retina 2012 May;32(5):942-948.

[169] Campbell WG, Pejnovic TM. Treatment of amelanotic choroidal melanoma with photodynamic therapy. Retina 2012 Jul;32(7):1356-1362.

[170] Li X, Naylor MF, Le H, Nordquist RE, Teague TK, Howard CA, et al. Clinical effects of in situ photoimmunotherapy on late-stage melanoma patients: a preliminary study. Cancer Biol Ther 2010 Dec 1;10(11):1081-1087.

[171] Fasanella KE, McGrath K. Successful palliative treatment of duodenal metastatic melanoma with photodynamic therapy. Gastrointest Endosc 2009 Jan;69(1):182-184.

[172] Zilidis G, Aziz F, Telara S, Eljamel MS. Fluorescence image-guided surgery and repetitive Photodynamic Therapy in brain metastatic malignant melanoma. Photodiagnosis Photodyn Ther 2008 Dec;5(4):264-266.

[173] Chetty NC, Osborne V, Harland C. Amelanotic melanoma in situ: lack of sustained response to photodynamic therapy. Clin Exp Dermatol 2008 Mar;33(2):204-206.

[174] Soucek P, Cihelkova I. Primary treatment of choroidal amelanotic melanoma with photodynamic therapy--comment. Clin Experiment Ophthalmol 2006 Sep-Oct;34(7):721; author reply 721-2.

[175] Naylor MF, Chen WR, Teague TK, Perry LA, Nordquist RE. In situ photoimmunotherapy: a tumour-directed treatment for melanoma. Br J Dermatol 2006 Dec;155(6):1287-1292.

[176] Wachtlin J, Bechrakis NE, Foerster MH. Photodynamic therapy with verteporfin for uveal melanoma. Ophthalmologe 2005 Mar;102(3):241-246.

[177] Liggett PE, Lavaque AJ, Chaudhry NA, Jablon EP, Quiroz-Mercado H. Preliminary results of combined simultaneous transpupillary thermotherapy and ICG-based photodynamic therapy for choroidal melanoma. Ophthalmic Surg Lasers Imaging 2005 Nov-Dec;36(6):463-470.

[178] Kubicka-Trzaska A, Starzycka M, Romanowska-Dixon B, Morawski K. Use of indocyanine green for photodynamic therapy of choroidal melanoma--preliminary report. Klin Oczna 2003;105(3-4):132-135.

[179] Barbazetto IA, Lee TC, Rollins IS, Chang S, Abramson DH. Treatment of choroidal melanoma using photodynamic therapy. Am J Ophthalmol 2003 Jun;135(6):898-899.

[180] Schlotzer-Schrehardt U, Viestenz A, Naumann GO, Laqua H, Michels S, Schmidt-Erfurth U. Dose-related structural effects of photodynamic therapy on choroidal and retinal structures of human eyes. Graefes Arch Clin Exp Ophthalmol 2002 Sep;240(9):748-757.

[181] Favilla I, Favilla ML, Gosbell AD, Barry WR, Ellims P, Hill JS, et al. Photodynamic therapy: a 5-year study of its effectiveness in the treatment of posterior uveal mela-

noma, and evaluation of haematoporphyrin uptake and photocytotoxicity of melanoma cells in tissue culture. Melanoma Res 1995 Oct;5(5):355-364.

[182] Chen B, Xu Y, Agostinis P, De Witte PA. Synergistic effect of photodynamic therapy with hypericin in combination with hyperthermia on loss of clonogenicity of RIF-1 cells. Int J Oncol 2001 Jun;18(6):1279-1285.

[183] Wiegell SR, Fabricius S, Stender IM, Berne B, Kroon S, Andersen BL, et al. A randomized, multicentre study of directed daylight exposure times of 1(1/2) vs. 2(1/2) h in daylight-mediated photodynamic therapy with methyl aminolaevulinate in patients with multiple thin actinic keratoses of the face and scalp. Br J Dermatol 2011 May; 164(5):1083-1090.

[184] Alecu M, Ursaciuc C, Halalau F, Coman G, Merlevede W, Waelkens E, et al. Photodynamic treatment of basal cell carcinoma and squamous cell carcinoma with hypericin. Anticancer Res 1998 Nov-Dec;18(6B):4651-4654.

[185] Bublik M, Head C, Benharash P, Paiva M, Eshraghi A, Kim T, et al. Hypericin and pulsed laser therapy of squamous cell cancer in vitro. Photomed Laser Surg 2006 Jun; 24(3):341-347.

[186] Chung PS, Rhee CK, Kim KH, Paek W, Chung J, Paiva MB, et al. Intratumoral hypericin and KTP laser therapy for transplanted squamous cell carcinoma. Laryngoscope 2000 Aug;110(8):1312-1316.

[187] Chung PS, Saxton RE, Paiva MB, Rhee CK, Soudant J, Mathey A, et al. Hypericin uptake in rabbits and nude mice transplanted with human squamous cell carcinomas: study of a new sensitizer for laser phototherapy. Laryngoscope 1994 Dec;104(12): 1471-1476.

[188] Liu CD, Kwan D, Saxton RE, McFadden DW. Hypericin and photodynamic therapy decreases human pancreatic cancer in vitro and in vivo. J Surg Res 2000 Sep;93(1): 137-143.

[189] D'Hallewin MA, Kamuhabwa AR, Roskams T, De Witte PA, Baert L. Hypericin-based fluorescence diagnosis of bladder carcinoma. BJU Int 2002 May;89(7):760-763.

[190] D'Hallewin MA, De Witte PA, Waelkens E, Merlevede W, Baert L. Fluorescence detection of flat bladder carcinoma in situ after intravesical instillation of hypericin. J Urol 2000 Aug;164(2):349-351.

[191] Kubin A, Loew HG, Burner U, Jessner G, Kolbabek H, Wierrani F. How to make hypericin water-soluble. Pharmazie 2008 Apr;63(4):263-269.

[192] Sim HG, Lau WK, Olivo M, Tan PH, Cheng CW. Is photodynamic diagnosis using hypericin better than white-light cystoscopy for detecting superficial bladder carcinoma? BJU Int 2005 Jun;95(9):1215-1218.

[193] Kubin A, Meissner P, Wierrani F, Burner U, Bodenteich A, Pytel A, et al. Fluorescence diagnosis of bladder cancer with new water soluble hypericin bound to polyvinylpyrrolidone: PVP-hypericin. Photochem Photobiol 2008 Nov-Dec;84(6):1560-1563.

[194] Bhuvaneswari R, Gan YY, Yee KK, Soo KC, Olivo M. Effect of hypericin-mediated photodynamic therapy on the expression of vascular endothelial growth factor in human nasopharyngeal carcinoma. Int J Mol Med 2007 Oct;20(4):421-428.

[195] Olivo M, Du HY, Bay BH. Hypericin lights up the way for the potential treatment of nasopharyngeal cancer by photodynamic therapy. Curr Clin Pharmacol 2006 Sep; 1(3):217-222.

[196] Kacerovska D, Pizinger K, Majer F, Smid F. Photodynamic therapy of nonmelanoma skin cancer with topical hypericum perforatum extract--a pilot study. Photochem Photobiol 2008 May-Jun;84(3):779-785.

[197] Davids LM, Kleemann B, Cooper S, Kidson SH. Melanomas display increased cytoprotection to hypericin-mediated cytotoxicity through the induction of autophagy. Cell Biol Int 2009 Oct;33(10):1065-1072.

[198] Mosmann T. Rapid colorimetric assay for cellular growth and survival: application to proliferation and cytotoxicity assays. J Immunol Methods 1983 Dec 16;65(1-2):55-63.

[199] Cory AH, Owen TC, Barltrop JA, Cory JG. Use of an aqueous soluble tetrazolium/ formazan assay for cell growth assays in culture. Cancer Commun 1991 Jul;3(7): 207-212.

[200] Davids LM, Kleemann B. Combating melanoma: The use of photodynamic therapy as a novel, adjuvant therapeutic tool. Cancer Treat Rev 2010 Dec 16.

[201] Davids LM, du Toit E, Kidson SH, Todd G. A rare repigmentation pattern in a vitiligo patient: a clue to an epidermal stem-cell reservoir of melanocytes? Clin Exp Dermatol 2009 Mar;34(2):246-248.

[202] Kroemer G, El-Deiry WS, Golstein P, Peter ME, Vaux D, Vandenabeele P, et al. Classification of cell death: recommendations of the Nomenclature Committee on Cell Death. Cell Death Differ 2005 Nov;12 Suppl 2:1463-1467.

[203] Golstein P, Kroemer G. Cell death by necrosis: towards a molecular definition. Trends Biochem Sci 2007 Jan;32(1):37-43.

[204] Galluzzi L, Vitale I, Abrams JM, Alnemri ES, Baehrecke EH, Blagosklonny MV, et al. Molecular definitions of cell death subroutines: recommendations of the Nomenclature Committee on Cell Death 2012. Cell Death Differ 2012 Jan;19(1):107-120.

[205] Hanahan D, Weinberg RA. Hallmarks of cancer: the next generation. Cell 2011 Mar 4;144(5):646-674.

[206] Wellbrock C, Weisser C, Geissinger E, Troppmair J, Schartl M. Activation of p59(Fyn) leads to melanocyte dedifferentiation by influencing MKP-1-regulated mitogen-activated protein kinase signaling. J Biol Chem 2002 Feb 22;277(8):6443-6454.

[207] Cohen C, Zavala-Pompa A, Sequeira JH, Shoji M, Sexton DG, Cotsonis G, et al. Mitogen-actived protein kinase activation is an early event in melanoma progression. Clin Cancer Res 2002 Dec;8(12):3728-3733.

[208] Tsao H, Goel V, Wu H, Yang G, Haluska FG. Genetic interaction between NRAS and BRAF mutations and PTEN/MMAC1 inactivation in melanoma. J Invest Dermatol 2004 Feb;122(2):337-341.

[209] Davies H, Bignell GR, Cox C, Stephens P, Edkins S, Clegg S, et al. Mutations of the BRAF gene in human cancer. Nature 2002 Jun 27;417(6892):949-954.

[210] Gray-Schopfer VC, da Rocha Dias S, Marais R. The role of B-RAF in melanoma. Cancer Metastasis Rev 2005 Jan;24(1):165-183.

[211] Tong Z, Singh G, Rainbow AJ. Sustained activation of the extracellular signal-regulated kinase pathway protects cells from photofrin-mediated photodynamic therapy. Cancer Res 2002 Oct 1;62(19):5528-5535.

[212] Mercurio F, Manning AM. NF-kappaB as a primary regulator of the stress response. Oncogene 1999 Nov 1;18(45):6163-6171.

[213] Ryter SW, Gomer CJ. Nuclear factor kappa B binding activity in mouse L1210 cells following photofrin II-mediated photosensitization. Photochem Photobiol 1993 Nov; 58(5):753-756.

[214] Danial NN, Korsmeyer SJ. Cell death: critical control points. Cell 2004 Jan 23;116(2): 205-219.

[215] Oleinick NL, Morris RL, Belichenko I. The role of apoptosis in response to photodynamic therapy: what, where, why, and how. Photochem Photobiol Sci 2002 Jan;1(1): 1-21.

[216] Agostinis P, Buytaert E, Breyssens H, Hendrickx N. Regulatory pathways in photodynamic therapy induced apoptosis. Photochem Photobiol Sci 2004 Aug;3(8):721-729.

[217] Buytaert E, Callewaert G, Vandenheede JR, Agostinis P. Deficiency in apoptotic effectors Bax and Bak reveals an autophagic cell death pathway initiated by photodamage to the endoplasmic reticulum. Autophagy 2006 Jul-Sep;2(3):238-240.

[218] Fisher DE. Apoptosis in cancer therapy: crossing the threshold. Cell 1994 Aug 26;78(4):539-542.

[219] Micheau O, Solary E, Hammann A, Martin F, Dimanche-Boitrel MT. Sensitization of cancer cells treated with cytotoxic drugs to fas-mediated cytotoxicity. J Natl Cancer Inst 1997 Jun 4;89(11):783-789.

[220] Ali SM, Chee SK, Yuen GY, Olivo M. Hypericin induced death receptor-mediated apoptosis in photoactivated tumor cells. Int J Mol Med 2002 Jun;9(6):601-616.

[221] Reiners JJ,Jr, Agostinis P, Berg K, Oleinick NL, Kessel D. Assessing autophagy in the context of photodynamic therapy. Autophagy 2010 Jan;6(1):7-18.

[222] Dewaele M, Maes H, Agostinis P. ROS-mediated mechanisms of autophagy stimulation and their relevance in cancer therapy. Autophagy 2010 Oct 19;6(7).

[223] Garg AD, Krysko DV, Vandenabeele P, Agostinis P. DAMPs and PDT-mediated photo-oxidative stress: exploring the unknown. Photochem Photobiol Sci 2011 May;10(5): 670-680.

[224] Garg AD, Nowis D, Golab J, Vandenabeele P, Krysko DV, Agostinis P. Immunogenic cell death, DAMPs and anticancer therapeutics: an emerging amalgamation. Biochim Biophys Acta 2010 Jan;1805(1):53-71.

[225] Green DR, Ferguson T, Zitvogel L, Kroemer G. Immunogenic and tolerogenic cell death. Nat Rev Immunol 2009 May;9(5):353-363.

[226] Zitvogel L, Kepp O, Kroemer G. Decoding cell death signals in inflammation and immunity. Cell 2010 Mar 19;140(6):798-804.

[227] Zitvogel L, Kepp O, Senovilla L, Menger L, Chaput N, Kroemer G. Immunogenic tumor cell death for optimal anticancer therapy: the calreticulin exposure pathway. Clin Cancer Res 2010 Jun 15;16(12):3100-3104.

[228] Demaria S, Pikarsky E, Karin M, Coussens LM, Chen YC, El-Omar EM, et al. Cancer and inflammation: promise for biologic therapy. J Immunother 2010 May;33(4): 335-351.

[229] Garg AD, Nowis D, Golab J, Agostinis P. Photodynamic therapy: illuminating the road from cell death towards anti-tumour immunity. Apoptosis 2010 Mar 10.

[230] Buytaert E, Callewaert G, Hendrickx N, Scorrano L, Hartmann D, Missiaen L, et al. Role of endoplasmic reticulum depletion and multidomain proapoptotic BAX and BAK proteins in shaping cell death after hypericin-mediated photodynamic therapy. FASEB J 2006 Apr;20(6):756-758.

[231] Ritz R, Roser F, Radomski N, Strauss WS, Tatagiba M, Gharabaghi A. Subcellular colocalization of hypericin with respect to endoplasmic reticulum and Golgi apparatus in glioblastoma cells. Anticancer Res 2008 Jul-Aug;28(4B):2033-2038.

[232] Galanou MC, Theodossiou TA, Tsiourvas D, Sideratou Z, Paleos CM. Interactive transport, subcellular relocation and enhanced phototoxicity of hypericin encapsulated in guanidinylated liposomes via molecular recognition. Photochem Photobiol 2008 Sep-Oct;84(5):1073-1083.

[233] Ali SM, Olivo M. Bio-distribution and subcellular localization of Hypericin and its role in PDT induced apoptosis in cancer cells. Int J Oncol 2002 Sep;21(3):531-540.

[234] Ali SM, Chee SK, Yuen GY, Olivo M. Hypericin induced death receptor-mediated apoptosis in photoactivated tumor cells. Int J Mol Med 2002 Jun;9(6):601-616.

[235] English DS, Doyle RT, Petrich JW, Haydon PG. Subcellular distributions and excited-state processes of hypericin in neurons. Photochem Photobiol 1999 Mar;69(3):301-305.

[236] Crnolatac I, Huygens A, Agostinis P, Kamuhabwa AR, Maes J, van Aerschot A, et al. In vitro accumulation and permeation of hypericin and lipophilic analogues in 2-D and 3-D cellular systems. Int J Oncol 2007 Feb;30(2):319-324.

[237] Theodossiou TA, Hothersall JS, De Witte PA, Pantos A, Agostinis P. The Multifaceted Photocytotoxic Profile of Hypericin. Mol Pharm 2009 Sep 24.

[238] Ho YF, Wu MH, Cheng BH, Chen YW, Shih MC. Lipid-mediated preferential localization of hypericin in lipid membranes. Biochim Biophys Acta 2009 Jun;1788(6): 1287-1295.

[239] Mojzisova H, Bonneau S, Brault D. Structural and physico-chemical determinants of the interactions of macrocyclic photosensitizers with cells. Eur Biophys J 2007 Nov; 36(8):943-953.

[240] Buytaert E, Matroule JY, Durinck S, Close P, Kocanova S, Vandenheede JR, et al. Molecular effectors and modulators of hypericin-mediated cell death in bladder cancer cells. Oncogene 2008 Mar 20;27(13):1916-1929.

[241] Verfaillie T, Salazar M, Velasco G, Agostinis P. Linking ER Stress to Autophagy: Potential Implications for Cancer Therapy. Int J Cell Biol 2010;2010:930509.

[242] Thomas C, MacGill RS, Miller GC, Pardini RS. Photoactivation of hypericin generates singlet oxygen in mitochondria and inhibits succinoxidase. Photochem Photobiol 1992 Jan;55(1):47-53.

[243] Miccoli L, Beurdeley-Thomas A, De Pinieux G, Sureau F, Oudard S, Dutrillaux B, et al. Light-induced photoactivation of hypericin affects the energy metabolism of human glioma cells by inhibiting hexokinase bound to mitochondria. Cancer Res 1998 Dec 15;58(24):5777-5786.

[244] Theodossiou TA, Papakyriakou A, Hothersall JS. Molecular modeling and experimental evidence for hypericin as a substrate for mitochondrial complex III; mitochondrial photodamage as demonstrated using specific inhibitors. Free Radic Biol Med 2008 Dec 1;45(11):1581-1590.

[245] Utsumi T, Okuma M, Kanno T, Takehara Y, Yoshioka T, Fujita Y, et al. Effect of the antiretroviral agent hypericin on rat liver mitochondria. Biochem Pharmacol 1995 Aug 25;50(5):655-662.

[246] Buytaert E, Callewaert G, Vandenheede JR, Agostinis P. Deficiency in apoptotic effectors Bax and Bak reveals an autophagic cell death pathway initiated by photodamage to the endoplasmic reticulum. Autophagy 2006 Jul-Sep;2(3):238-240.

[247] Castano AP, Mroz P, Hamblin MR. Photodynamic therapy and anti-tumour immunity. Nat Rev Cancer 2006 Jul;6(7):535-545.

[248] Panaretakis T, Kepp O, Brockmeier U, Tesniere A, Bjorklund AC, Chapman DC, et al. Mechanisms of pre-apoptotic calreticulin exposure in immunogenic cell death. EMBO J 2009 Mar 4;28(5):578-590.

[249] Young AR, Narita M, Ferreira M, Kirschner K, Sadaie M, Darot JF, et al. Autophagy mediates the mitotic senescence transition. Genes Dev 2009 Apr 1;23(7):798-803.

[250] Lu Z, Luo RZ, Lu Y, Zhang X, Yu Q, Khare S, et al. The tumor suppressor gene ARHI regulates autophagy and tumor dormancy in human ovarian cancer cells. J Clin Invest 2008 Dec;118(12):3917-3929.

[251] Gewirtz DA. Autophagy, senescence and tumor dormancy in cancer therapy. Autophagy 2009 Nov;5(8):1232-1234.

[252] Nystrom T. Role of oxidative carbonylation in protein quality control and senescence. EMBO J 2005 Apr 6;24(7):1311-1317.

[253] Pattingre S, Tassa A, Qu X, Garuti R, Liang XH, Mizushima N, et al. Bcl-2 antiapoptotic proteins inhibit Beclin 1-dependent autophagy. Cell 2005 Sep 23;122(6):927-939.

[254] Coussens LM, Werb Z. Inflammation and cancer. Nature 2002 Dec 19-26;420(6917): 860-867.

[255] Szatrowski TP, Nathan CF. Production of large amounts of hydrogen peroxide by human tumor cells. Cancer Res 1991 Feb 1;51(3):794-798.

[256] Toyokuni S, Okamoto K, Yodoi J, Hiai H. Persistent oxidative stress in cancer. FEBS Lett 1995 Jan 16;358(1):1-3.

[257] Sander CS, Chang H, Hamm F, Elsner P, Thiele JJ. Role of oxidative stress and the antioxidant network in cutaneous carcinogenesis. Int J Dermatol 2004 May;43(5): 326-335.

[258] Lincoln DT, Ali Emadi EM, Tonissen KF, Clarke FM. The thioredoxin-thioredoxin reductase system: over-expression in human cancer. Anticancer Res 2003 May-Jun; 23(3B):2425-2433.

[259] Cen D, Gonzalez RI, Buckmeier JA, Kahlon RS, Tohidian NB, Meyskens FL,Jr. Disulfiram induces apoptosis in human melanoma cells: a redox-related process. Mol Cancer Ther 2002 Jan;1(3):197-204.

[260] Cen D, Brayton D, Shahandeh B, Meyskens FL,Jr, Farmer PJ. Disulfiram facilitates intracellular Cu uptake and induces apoptosis in human melanoma cells. J Med Chem 2004 Dec 30;47(27):6914-6920.

[261] Huang P, Feng L, Oldham EA, Keating MJ, Plunkett W. Superoxide dismutase as a target for the selective killing of cancer cells. Nature 2000 Sep 21;407(6802):390-395.

[262] Dobos J, Timar J, Bocsi J, Burian Z, Nagy K, Barna G, et al. In vitro and in vivo antitumor effect of 2-methoxyestradiol on human melanoma. Int J Cancer 2004 Dec 10;112(5):771-776.

[263] Russo GL. Ins and outs of dietary phytochemicals in cancer chemoprevention. Biochem Pharmacol 2007 Aug 15;74(4):533-544.

[264] Tyagi AK, Singh RP, Agarwal C, Chan DC, Agarwal R. Silibinin strongly synergizes human prostate carcinoma DU145 cells to doxorubicin-induced growth Inhibition, G2-M arrest, and apoptosis. Clin Cancer Res 2002 Nov;8(11):3512-3519.

[265] De Larco JE, Park CA, Dronava H, Furcht LT. Paradoxical roles for antioxidants in tumor prevention and eradication. Cancer Biol Ther 2010 Mar 8;9(5).

[266] Farmer PJ, Gidanian S, Shahandeh B, Di Bilio AJ, Tohidian N, Meyskens FL,Jr. Melanin as a target for melanoma chemotherapy: pro-oxidant effect of oxygen and metals on melanoma viability. Pigment Cell Res 2003 Jun;16(3):273-279.

[267] Chen KG, Valencia JC, Lai B, Zhang G, Paterson JK, Rouzaud F, et al. Melanosomal sequestration of cytotoxic drugs contributes to the intractability of malignant melanomas. Proc Natl Acad Sci U S A 2006 Jun 27;103(26):9903-9907.

[268] Chen KG, Leapman RD, Zhang G, Lai B, Valencia JC, Cardarelli CO, et al. Influence of melanosome dynamics on melanoma drug sensitivity. J Natl Cancer Inst 2009 Sep 16;101(18):1259-1271.

[269] Raposo G, Marks MS. The dark side of lysosome-related organelles: specialization of the endocytic pathway for melanosome biogenesis. Traffic 2002 Apr;3(4):237-248.

[270] Hearing VJ. Biogenesis of pigment granules: a sensitive way to regulate melanocyte function. J Dermatol Sci 2005 Jan;37(1):3-14.

[271] Baldea I. Melanocyte pigmentation – friend or foe on the route to melanoma. In: Tanaka Y, editor. Breakthroughs in Melanoma Research Rijeka, Croatia: InTech; 2011. p. 183-217.

[272] Solano F, Martinez-Esparza M, Jimenez-Cervantes C, Hill SP, Lozano JA, Garcia-Borron JC. New insights on the structure of the mouse silver locus and on the function of the silver protein. Pigment Cell Res 2000;13 Suppl 8:118-124.

[273] Kwon BS, Chintamaneni C, Kozak CA, Copeland NG, Gilbert DJ, Jenkins N, et al. A melanocyte-specific gene, Pmel 17, maps near the silver coat color locus on mouse chromosome 10 and is in a syntenic region on human chromosome 12. Proc Natl Acad Sci U S A 1991 Oct 15;88(20):9228-9232.

[274] Theos AC, Truschel ST, Raposo G, Marks MS. The Silver locus product Pmel17/gp100/Silv/ME20: controversial in name and in function. Pigment Cell Res 2005 Oct;18(5):322-336.

[275] Orlow SJ. Melanosomes are specialized members of the lysosomal lineage of organelles. J Invest Dermatol 1995 Jul;105(1):3-7.

[276] Raposo G, Tenza D, Murphy DM, Berson JF, Marks MS. Distinct protein sorting and localization to premelanosomes, melanosomes, and lysosomes in pigmented melanocytic cells. J Cell Biol 2001 Feb 19;152(4):809-824.

[277] Valencia JC, Hoashi T, Pawelek JM, Solano F, Hearing VJ. Pmel17: controversial indeed but critical to melanocyte function. Pigment Cell Res 2006 Jun;19(3):250-2; author reply 253-7.

[278] Nelson JS, McCullough JL, Berns MW. Photodynamic therapy of human malignant melanoma xenografts in athymic nude mice. J Natl Cancer Inst 1988 Mar 2;80(1): 56-60.

[279] Meyskens FL,Jr, Farmer P, Fruehauf JP. Redox regulation in human melanocytes and melanoma. Pigment Cell Res 2001 Jun;14(3):148-154.

[280] Shackleton M, Quintana E, Fearon ER, Morrison SJ. Heterogeneity in cancer: cancer stem cells versus clonal evolution. Cell 2009 Sep 4;138(5):822-829.

[281] Marotta LL, Polyak K. Cancer stem cells: a model in the making. Curr Opin Genet Dev 2009 Feb;19(1):44-50.

[282] Al-Hajj M, Wicha MS, Benito-Hernandez A, Morrison SJ, Clarke MF. Prospective identification of tumorigenic breast cancer cells. Proc Natl Acad Sci U S A 2003 Apr 1;100(7):3983-3988.

[283] Bonnet D, Dick JE. Human acute myeloid leukemia is organized as a hierarchy that originates from a primitive hematopoietic cell. Nat Med 1997 Jul;3(7):730-737.

[284] O'Brien CA, Pollett A, Gallinger S, Dick JE. A human colon cancer cell capable of initiating tumour growth in immunodeficient mice. Nature 2007 Jan 4;445(7123): 106-110.

[285] Singh SK, Hawkins C, Clarke ID, Squire JA, Bayani J, Hide T, et al. Identification of human brain tumour initiating cells. Nature 2004 Nov 18;432(7015):396-401.

[286] Abel EV, Aplin AE. Finding the root of the problem: the quest to identify melanoma stem cells. Front Biosci (Schol Ed) 2011 Jun 1;3:937-945.

[287] Jones PM, George AM. The ABC transporter structure and mechanism: perspectives on recent research. Cell Mol Life Sci 2004 Mar;61(6):682-699.

[288] Frank NY, Margaryan A, Huang Y, Schatton T, Waaga-Gasser AM, Gasser M, et al. ABCB5-mediated doxorubicin transport and chemoresistance in human malignant melanoma. Cancer Res 2005 May 15;65(10):4320-4333.

[289] Keshet GI, Goldstein I, Itzhaki O, Cesarkas K, Shenhav L, Yakirevitch A, et al. MDR1 expression identifies human melanoma stem cells. Biochem Biophys Res Commun 2008 Apr 18;368(4):930-936.

[290] Monzani E, Facchetti F, Galmozzi E, Corsini E, Benetti A, Cavazzin C, et al. Melanoma contains CD133 and ABCG2 positive cells with enhanced tumourigenic potential. Eur J Cancer 2007 Mar;43(5):935-946.

[291] Robey RW, Steadman K, Polgar O, Bates SE. ABCG2-mediated transport of photosensitizers: potential impact on photodynamic therapy. Cancer Biol Ther 2005 Feb; 4(2):187-194.

[292] Tamura A, An R, Hagiya Y, Hoshijima K, Yoshida T, Mikuriya K, et al. Drug-induced phototoxicity evoked by inhibition of human ABC transporter ABCG2: development of in vitro high-speed screening systems. Expert Opin Drug Metab Toxicol 2008 Mar; 4(3):255-272.

[293] Liu W, Baer MR, Bowman MJ, Pera P, Zheng X, Morgan J, et al. The tyrosine kinase inhibitor imatinib mesylate enhances the efficacy of photodynamic therapy by inhibiting ABCG2. Clin Cancer Res 2007 Apr 15;13(8):2463-2470.

Chapter 12

Study of the Anti-Photoaging Effect of Noni (*Morinda citrifolia*)

Hideaki Matsuda, Megumi Masuda, Kazuya Murata,
Yumi Abe and Akemi Uwaya

Additional information is available at the end of the chapter

1. Introduction

During the aging process, morphological changes in the human skin appear most noticeably in areas of frequent exposure to ultraviolet (UV) light from the sun, such as the face and hands. Chronic UV exposure induces photoaging, characterized by pigmented spots and wrinkles in the skin. Gradual destruction of the ozonosphere has raised photoaging risk. This has led to rapid growth of the anti-photoaging cosmetic market, especially among women with young and fair skin. Sunscreen agents are a first choice for protection against photoaging. However, a certain amount of UV irradiation penetrates skin dermis, and adverse effect may occur with use of these agents. Because of this, a current trend is the development of safer cosmetic ingredients that effectively inhibit the UV signaling pathways leading to photoaging [1].

Therefore, in this chapter we discuss searching for novel cosmetic ingredients from natural resources which prevent the generation of pigmented spots and wrinkles *via* antagonistic activities against UV signaling pathways. We focused this search on plants growing along the coasts of South Pacific islands, as they may have developed specific self-defense systems against harmful UV radiation. Following this strategy, we selected "noni" (*Morinda citrifolia* L., Rubiaceae).

2. Subtropical plant noni

Selected *M. citrifolia* as a subject is commonly called "noni", which is a subtropical plant distributed widely in the tropical/ subtropical zone, including Tahiti and Hawaii. The tree is a rapidly growing evergreen that is resistant to drought and poor soil conditions.

Noni has been utilized for various reasons in many areas. The root was used as dye in Japan, and the leaves and the seeds, as well as the fruit, were eaten frequently in Southeast Asia and the Pacific islands. Currently, the fruit juice and leaf tea are sold in the functional foods market. Noni is also used as an herbal medicine to promote health and beauty. The whole plant, from the root to fruit, has been used without waste for more than 2000 years as a panacea [2]. Therefore, noni was considered a "gift from God" by generations of Pacific Islanders.

In the last decade, many papers have reported the chemical constituents and biological activities of noni including hypotensive [3], hypoglycemic [4], and anticancer activities [5], which scientifically support traditional claims of noni. Noni has been used traditionally for the treatment of dermatoses such as ringworm, dry skin, acne, pustule, and other skin troubles. Moreover, ripe noni fruit juice has been drunk for cosmetic reasons. In some areas, the dried immature noni fruit, the leaves, or the seeds mixed with coconut oil have been used as an external treatment [6]. But studies reporting potential cosmetic uses of noni, such as inhibition of melanogenesis and reduction of wrinkles, have only recently been completed. Noni fruit contains a large number of seeds throughout its flesh. But during the production of noni fruit juice, the seeds are removed and discarded. Considering the potential utility of all parts of the plant, we investigated extracts from the fruit flesh, leaves, and seeds for active anti-photoaging agents.

3. Skin whitening effect of noni

3.1. Screening tests for melanogenesis inhibitory effect of noni

During photoaging, UV rays trigger melanogenesis and chromatosis. These processes generate pigmented spots by UV activation of melanocyte tyrosinase (a melanin synthesis enzyme) which then converts L-tyrosine to L-DOPA, followed by conversion to dopaquinone. Dopaquinone subsequently forms melanin through several steps, including auto-oxidation. As such, tyrosinase inhibitors may be useful for prevention of pigmented spots.

Initial evaluation of the anti-melanogenesis activity of noni was carried out using an *in vitro* tyrosinase inhibition assay with 50% ethanol extracts of fruit flesh (Fruit-ext), leaves (Leaf-ext), and seeds (Seed-ext). As oxidative reactions also contribute to melanogenesis [7], the 1-diphenyl-2-picrylhydrazyl (DPPH) assay was also performed to find whether noni has antioxidant activity.

3.1.1. *Tyrosinase inhibitory activities*

The results of the *in vitro* tyrosinase inhibition assay are shown in Table 1. At 20 to 500 μg/ml, Seed-ext inhibited tyrosinase activity, in a concentration-dependent manner. Fruit-ext exhibited weak activity only at 500 μg/ml, and Leaf-ext did not inhibit enzyme activity at any concentration [8].

3.1.2. DPPH radical scavenging activities

As oxidative reactions contribute to melanogenesis, the DPPH assay was performed to measure the antioxidant activity of noni. As shown in Table 2, Seed-ext exhibited potent DPPH radical scavenging activity, with an IC_{50} value of 12 μg/ml. Leaf-ext and Fruit-ext exhibited weaker antioxidant activities, with IC_{50} values of 113 and 240 μg/ml, respectively [8].

The results of the two assays reveal that Seed-ext has stronger tyrosinase inhibitory and antioxidant activity than Fruit-ext and Leaf-ext.

Samples	**Concentration**	**OD (×1000) [a)] at 475 nm**	**Inhibition (%)**
Control		472±4	
Fruit-ext	20 (μg/ml)	471±3	0
	100 (μg/ml)	451±2	5
	500 (μg/ml)	419±9[i]	11
Leaf-ext	20 (μg/ml)	471±2	0
	100 (μg/ml)	460±2	3
	500 (μg/ml)	442±1[i]	6
Seed-ext	20 (μg/ml)	449±5[i]	5
	100 (μg/ml)	394±4[i]	17
	500 (μg/ml)	365±4[i]	23
Kojic acid	10 (μM)	207±3[i]	56
	50 (μM)	77±3[i]	84

Table 1. Tyrosinase Inhibitory Activities of Fruit-ext, Leaf-ext, Seed-ext and Kojic Acid ([a)] OD: optical density. Each value represents the mean±S.E. of 3 experiments. Significantly different from control group, [i]: *p*<0.01.)

Samples	**Concentration**	**OD (×1000) [a)] at 520 nm**	**Inhibition (%)**	**IC_{50} value [b)]**
Control		974±21		
Fruit-ext	100 (μg/ml)	759±3[i]	22	240 (μg/ml)
	200 (μg/ml)	536±5[i]	45	
	400 (μg/ml)	188±3[i]	81	
Leaf-ext	50 (μg/ml)	765±4[i]	22	113 (μg/ml)
	100 (μg/ml)	570±3[i]	42	
	200 (μg/ml)	301±6[i]	69	
Seed-ext	5 (μg/ml)	771±2[i]	21	12 (μg/ml)
	10 (μg/ml)	537±7[i]	45	
	20 (μg/ml)	121±5[i]	88	
L-Ascorbic acid	20 (μM)	570±4[i]	41	23 (μM)
	50 (μM)	79±2[i]	92	

Table 2. DPPH Radical Scavenging Activities of Fruit-ext, Leaf-ext, Seed-ext and L-Ascorbic Acid ([a)] OD: optical density. Each value represents the mean±S.E. of 3 experiments. Significantly different from control group, [i]: *p*<0.01. [b)] IC_{50} value represents the concentration of sample required to scavenge 50% of DPPH free radical.)

3.2. Inhibitory effect of noni seeds on melanogenesis and its active compounds

According to the *in vitro* the screenings, Seed-ext may have melanogenesis inhibitory properties. Further examination of Seed-ext involved the use of B16 murine melanoma cells as an *in vitro* melanogenesis test model. In this assay, cells were stimulated by α-melanocyte stimulating hormone (α-MSH) and incubated for 72 hrs with the vehicle or test material [9]. As shown in Table 3, vehicle control treated cells, stimulated with α–MSH, significantly promoted melanogenesis compared to control that was not stimulated with α-MSH. At concentrations ranging from 12.5 to 200 μg/ml, Seed-ext inhibited α-MSH-stimulated melanogenesis in a concentration dependent manner without any significant effects on cell proliferation [10].

The tyrosinase inhibitory activity of Seed-ext was not as potent as that of other well known skin whitening agents. But in the B16 melanoma cells culture system, it inhibited melanin production. Thus, noni seed may be useful as an anti-photoaging cosmetic ingredient which prevents pigmented spots by interacting with a different active site than existing general skin whitening agents.

Samples	Concentration	α-MSH (μM)	Melanin content (μg/well)	Cell proliferation (%)
Control			1.6±0.4	61.9±1.2
Vehicle control		1	42.8±1.6[ii]	100.0±1.2[ii]
Seed-ext	12.5 (μg/ml)	1	29.0±0.6[i]	100.6±1.1
	50 (μg/ml)	1	21.1±0.6[i]	105.9±1.2
	200 (μg/ml)	1	11.9±0.6[i]	103.5±2.5
Kojic acid	100 (μM)	1	13.5±0.4[i]	107.4±1.9
	200 (μM)	1	6.9±0.4[i]	103.2±2.4

Table 3. Effects of Seed-ext and Kojic Acid on α-MSH-Stimulated Melanogenesis in B16 Melanoma Cells (Each value in melanin content represents the mean±S.E. of 3 experiments. Significantly different from the control group, [ii]: $p<0.01$. Significantly different from the vehicle control group, [i]: $p<0.01$. Each value in cell proliferation represents the mean ±S.E. of 3 experiments.)

As Seed-ext was confirmed to potently inhibit melanogenesis, activity guided isolation of the active compounds was carried out. Two lignans, 3,3'-bisdemethylpinoresinol (**1**) and americanin A (**2**), were isolated from noni seeds and found to be active constituents. As shown in Table 4, 10 and 20 μM of **1** displayed weak inhibition of cell proliferation. But 1.25 to 5 μM of **1** inhibited melanogenesis in a concentration dependent without any significant effects on cell proliferation. Also, 100 and 200 μM of **2** inhibited melanogenesis [10]. **1** (IC_{50} value: 0.3 mM) and **2** (IC_{50} value: 2.7 mM) exhibited tyrosinase inhibition, and **1** (IC_{50} value: 4 μM) and **2** (IC_{50} value: 11 μM) exhibited potent DPPH radical scavenging properties [8].

Samples	Concentration (μM)	α-MSH (μM)	Melanin content (μg/well)	Cell proliferation (%)
Run 1				
Control			4.5±0.8	55.2±1.3
Vehicle control		1	37.5±1.5[ii]	100.0±1.1[ii]
1	1.25	1	29.9±0.6[i]	97.8±0.4
	2.5	1	21.6±0.8[i]	101.0±1.7
	5	1	18.5±1.2[i]	99.1±0.7
	10	1	15.2±0.2[i]	88.8±1.2[i]
	20	1	13.2±0.8[i]	88.5±0.3[i]
Kojic acid	100	1	17.2±1.1[i]	97.1±1.3
	200	1	6.4±0.4[i]	98.2±1.4
Run 2				
Control			7.3±2.5	58.8±2.4
Vehicle control		1	39.0±0.9[ii]	100.0±5.1[ii]
2	12.5	1	39.3±0.7	101.6±1.0
	25	1	36.7±0.7	107.1±0.4
	50	1	33.9±0.8	103.3±0.9
	100	1	25.5±1.5[i]	99.4±4.5
	200	1	13.9±1.0[i]	102.8±1.4
Kojic acid	100	1	15.7±1.0[i]	101.9±3.8
	200	1	8.6±0.6[i]	98.4±2.7

Table 4. Effects of 3,3′-Bisdemethylpinoresinol (1), Americanin A (2) and Kojic Acid on α-MSH-Stimulated Melanogenesis in B16 Melanoma Cells (Each value in melanin content represents the mean±S.E. of 3 experiments. Significantly different from the control group, [ii]: $p<0.01$. Significantly different from the vehicle control group, [i]: $p<0.01$. Each value in cell proliferation represents the mean±S.E. of 3 experiments.)

Compared to kojic acid, which is a common skin whitening ingredient, **1** exhibited more potent inhibition of melanogenesis. This suggested that the anti-melanogenesis effect of **1** may be due to the suppression of tyrosinase protein expression in the cells, rather than inhibiting tyrosinase itself.

3.3. Effects of noni compounds; 3,3'-bisdemethylpinoresinol and americanin A on inhibitory melanogenesis activity

As the anti-melanogenesis of Seed-ext may be due to **1** and **2**, the inhibitory mechanism of these two lignans was studied with α-MSH stimulated B16 melanoma cells.

3.3.1. *Effects of 3,3′-bisdemethylpinoresinol and americanin A on tyrosinase expression in B16 melanoma cells*

First, the effect of **1** and **2** on tyrosinase expression in α-MSH stimulated B16 melanoma cells was investigated by using Western blot analysis. As shown in Fig. 1, the tyrosinase expression of the control at 72 hrs was enhanced remarkably. But after 72 hrs of treatment with **1** (5 μM) or **2** (200 μM), the enhancement of expression was notably suppressed without any significant effect on cell proliferation [10].

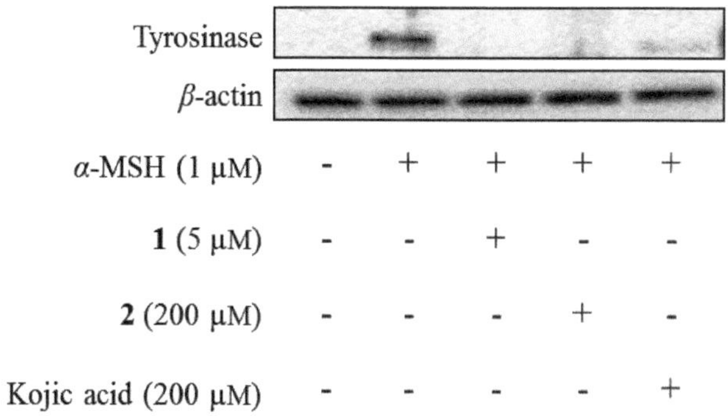

Figure 1. Effects of 3,3′-Bisdemethylpinoresinol (1), Americanin A (2) and Kojic Acid on Tyrosinase Expression in α-MSH-Stimulated B16 Melanoma Cells (The cells were treated with α-MSH (1 μM) in the presence of **1** (5 μM), **2** (200 μM) or kojic acid (200 μM) for 72 hrs. The level of tyrosinase expression was examined by Western blot analysis using specific antibody. Equal protein loading was confirmed by β-actin expression.)

3.3.2. *Inhibition of tyrosinase in B16 melanoma cells by 3,3′-bisdemethyl-pinoresinol and americanin A*

With suppressed expression of the enzyme, the activity of tyrosinase in the cell may decrease. Secondly, α-MSH stimulated B16 melanoma cells were cultivated during treatment with **1** or **2**. Next, the amount of melanin and tyrosinase activity in the cells were measured.

As shown in Fig. 2A, the intracellular melanin content of control group increased remarkably after cultivation for 24 to 72 hrs, whereas the content in cells treated with **1** (5 μM) or **2** (200 μM) decreased after 72 hrs. As shown in Fig. 2B, the tyrosinase activity in the α-MSH stimulated cells was also significantly inhibited by addition of **1** (5 μM) or **2** (200 μM) after 24 to 72 hrs incubation [10].

As just described, lignans **1** (5 μM) and **2** (200 μM) inhibited intracellular melanin contents induced by α-MSH. The results of Western blot analysis demonstrated that **1** and **2** remarkably inhibit tyrosinase stimulated by α-MSH. Moreover, as **1** and **2** reduced intracellular tyrosinase activity, it became clear that their melanogenesis inhibitory activity involved suppression of tyrosinase expression.

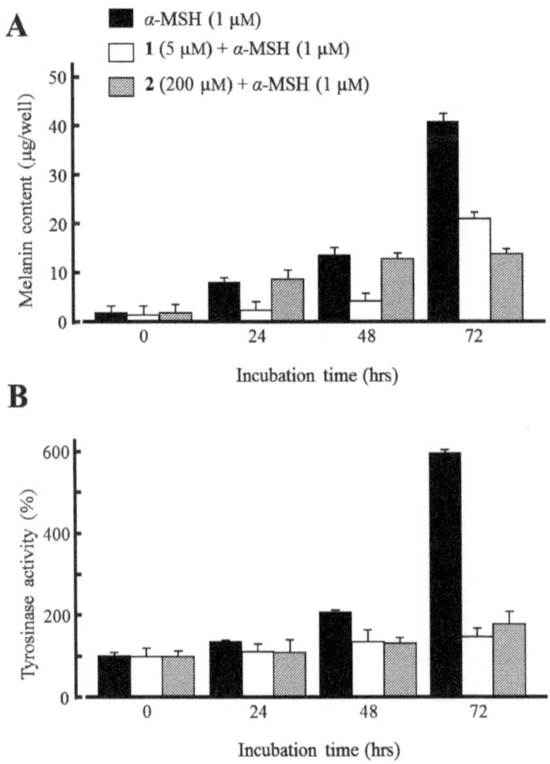

Figure 2. Effects of 3,3'-Bisdemethylpinoresinol (1) and Americanin A (2) on Melanogenesis and Tyrosinase Activity in α-MSH-Stimulated B16 Melanoma Cells (The cells were treated with α-MSH (1 μM, black column), **1** (5 μM, white column) and **2** (200 μM, slashed column) for the indicated times. (A) The melanin content was determined. (B) Tyrosinase activity was determined by measuring the formation of dopachrome. Data represent mean±S.E. of two different experiments each carried out in triplicate.)

3.3.3. Effect of 3,3'-bisdemethylpinoresinol and americanin A on phosphorylation of p38 MAPK

During melanogenesis in melanocytes, it is known that microphthalmia-associated transcription (MITF) is a transcription factor that regulates expression of the tyrosinase gene, and that melanins are produced by the activation of MITF [11]. Since mitogen-activated protein kinases (MAPKs) pathway is one of the intracellular signals that activates MITF, further research on this pathway was performed. It has been reported that phosphorylation of p38 MAPK activates MITF, whereas that of ERK1/2 and p70 S6K suppress MITF [12, 13]. The effects of **1** and **2** on the MAPK signaling activities of α-MSH-stimulated B16 melanoma cells were examined.

The levels of phosphorylation of p38 MAPK were compared, at 6 and 12 hrs after stimulation of B16 melanoma cells by α-MSH (1 μM). As shown in Fig. 3A, the analysis at 6 and 12 hrs reveals that the levels of phosphorylation of p38 MAPK in B16 cells were enhanced by α-MSH treatment in comparison to those without α-MSH. The treatment with lignan **1** (5 μM) or lignan **2** (200 μM) suppressed phosphorylation of p38 MAPK and enhanced that of ERK1/2 at 6 and 12 hrs after stimulated by α-MSH (Fig. 3B). However, both lignans had no effect on p70 S6K phosophorylation (Fig. 3B) [10].

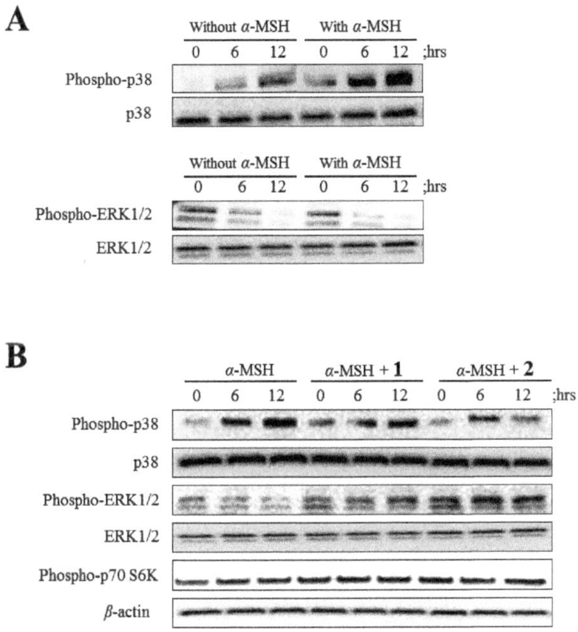

Figure 3. (A) Effect of α-MSH on Phosphorylation of p38 MAPK and ERK1/2 in B16 Melanoma Cells. (B) Effects of 3,3′-Bisdemethylpinoresinol (1) and Americanin A (2) on Phosphorylation of p38 MAPK, ERK1/2 and p70 S6K in α-MSH-Stimulated B16 Melanoma Cells ((A) The cells were treated with or without α-MSH (1 μM) for the indicated times. (B) The cells were treated with α-MSH (1 μM) in the presence of **1** (5 μM) or **2** (200 μM) for the indicated times. Phosphorylation of p38 MAPK, ERK1/2, and p70 S6K was assessed by Western blot analysis with using specific antibody for phosphorylated forms of p38 MAPK, ERK1/2, and p70 S6K. Equal protein loading was confirmed by β-actin expression.)

As the inhibitory mechanism of melanogenesis in α-MSH-stimulated B16 melanoma cells, These results strongly suggest that the lignans inhibit tyrosinase expression by suppressing p38 MAPK phosphorylation and enhancing ERK1/2, which then prevents activation of MITF.

4. Inhibitory effect of noni on wrinkle formation

It is thought that wrinkles form mainly by aging, but they are also caused by photoaging. The causes are degradation of moisture-retaining property of epidermis and transformation of dermal configuration due to altered elastic or collagen fibers in the cutis. Anti-wrinkle cosmetics are useful for comparatively slight wrinkles and fine lines. The main functions of anti-wrinkle cosmetics included normalization of moisture retention by the cornified layer, acceleration of keratinocyte turnover, and acceleration of collagen and elastin synthesis through proliferation and stimulation of fibroblasts. Recently, retinol and its analogs, so-called retinoids, have received increased attention and utilization as a cosmetic ingredient because they promote fibroblastic collagen production in the cutis and improve skin tension. Also, vitamin A reportedly accelerates turnover, which reduces hyperpigmented skin spots caused by melanin excreted by the epidermis, even though it has no inhibitory effects on activation of tyrosinase and melanogenesis. But retinoids irritate the skin and have adverse effects such as dermatitis. Therefore, safer reducing wrinkle ingredients are needed [1].

4.1. Wrinkle inhibition screening test of noni

One cause of photoaging wrinkle formation is the degradation of collagen, a main component of corium connective tissue [14]. The degradation of collagen is promoted by release of human leukocyte elastase (HLE) from infiltrated neutrophils into the skin by UV irradiation [15]. HLE cleaves the triple helix structure of type I collagen and degrades elastic fiber in human skin [16]. Thus, HLE inhibitors may be useful for the prevention of wrinkle formation.

4.1.1. Inhibitory effect of noni on HLE and its active compounds

The inhibitory effect of noni on wrinkle formation was investigated by measuring HLE inhibiting activity *in vitro*. As shown in Table 5, concentrations raging from 0.5 to 1.0 mg/ml of Seed-ext displayed HLE inhibitory activity in a concentration-dependent manner. Fruit-ext and Leaf-ext had no inhibitory activity at 1.0 mg/ml [8].

As Seed-ext exhibited potent HLE inhibitory activity compared with Fruit-ext and Leaf-ext, noni seeds appear to be the most source of cosmetic ingredients capable of preventing wrinkle formation during photoaging.

The active compounds in Seed-ext were isolated using the HLE inhibition bioassay as a fractionation guide. Ursolic acid (**3**) was isolated from Seed-ext and found to the active constituent. The IC_{50} value of **3** in the HLE inhibition assay was 0.07 mM. The IC_{50} value of phenylmethanesulfonyl fluoride (PMSF), the positive control, was 0.14 mM. Thus, **3** was more potent than the positive control (data not shown) [8].

Samples	Concentration	OD (×1000) [a] at 405 nm	Inhibition (%)	IC $_{50}$ value [b]
Control A [c]		946±23		
Fruit-ext	0.1 (mg/ml)	994±38 [i]	-8	
	0.5 (mg/ml)	1014±9 [i]	-10	
	1.0 (mg/ml)	1039±9 [i]	-12	
Leaf-ext	0.1 (mg/ml)	1014±16 [i]	-10	
	0.5 (mg/ml)	1023±18 [i]	-11	
	1.0 (mg/ml)	1042±36 [i]	-13	
Seed-ext	0.1 (mg/ml)	1052±20 [i]	-14	1.0 (mg/ml)
	0.5 (mg/ml)	722±21 [i]	22	
	1.0 (mg/ml)	467±30 [i]	50	
Control B [d]		925±9		
PMSF	0.08 (mM)	676±7 [ii]	29	0.14 (mM)
	0.15 (mM)	383±14 [ii]	60	
	0.50 (mM)	100±1 [ii]	90	

Table 5. HLE Inhibitory Activities of Fruit-ext, Leaf-ext, Seed-ext and PMSF ([a] OD: optical density. [b] IC_{50} value represents the concentration of sample required to inhibit 50% of HLE activity. [c] Control A is a control for extracts. [d] Control B is a control for PMSF. Each value represents the mean±S.E. of 3 experiments. Significantly different from control A group, [i]: $p<0.01$. Significantly different from control B group, [ii]: $p<0.01$.)

4.2. Inhibitory effect of noni seeds on matrix metalloproteinase-1 (MMP-1) secretion and its active compounds

Matrix metalloproteinases (MMPs) are matrix degrading enzymes associated with destructive processes including inflammation, tumor invasion and skin aging [1]. More than 20 subtypes of MMPs have been reported [17]. Among these, MMP-1, secreted from human skin fibroblasts, is mainly responsible for the degradation of dermal type I collagen in the photoaging process [18]. Also, HLE activates MMP-1 [19]. Thus, it is expected that MMP-1 and HLE inhibitors may be useful for the prevention of photoaging and subsequent wrinkle formation.

Since Seed-ext displayed strong HLE inhibitory activity, its ability to inhibit MMP-1 secretion was investigated in UV-irradiated normal human dermal fibroblasts (NHDFs). The amount of MMP-1 protein secreted from NHDFs into culture media was analyzed by Western blotting. UVA irradiation (5 J/cm^2) enhanced the secretion of MMP-1 from NHDFs in the vehicle control group at 9 to 48 hrs incubation, as compared to the control group without UVA-irradiation (Fig. 4). The group which was treated with Seed-ext (10 μg/ml) after UVA-irradiated NHDFs inhibited the secretion MMP-1 at 24 to 48 hrs, when compared to the vehicle control (Fig. 4) [20]. Seed-ext was not cytotoxic at 3 to 30 μg/ml.

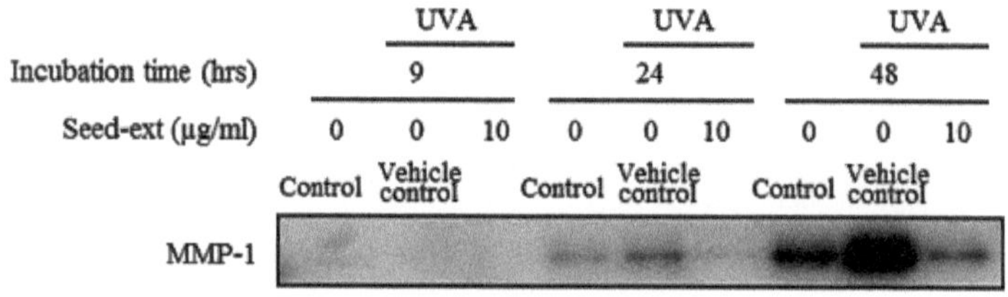

Figure 4. Effect of Seed-ext on MMP-1 Secretion from UVA-Irradiated NHDFs (Fibroblasts were exposed to UVA (5 J/cm^2) and then cultured in the serum free medium containing test samples for 9, 24, and 48 hrs. MMP-1 protein levels in the cultured medium at the indicated times were assessed by Western blot analysis using the antibody against human MMP-1. The blot is representative of three separate experiments and represents a single immunoblot.)

The active compounds responsible for the inhibitory effect of Seed-ext on MMP-1 secretion were searched for by following bioassay guided fractionation. As shown in Fig. 5A and 5B, 3,3'-bisdemethylpinoresinol (**1**), which is an active anti-melanogenesis compound, significantly inhibited the secretion MMP-1 at 3 μM. On the other hand, ursolic acid (**3**), which is an active anti-HLE compound, had no effect on MMP-1 secretion (data not shown). There was no cytotoxicity from **1** and **3** at 0.03, 0.1 and 0.3 μM [20].

It is clear that ursolic acid (**3**) inhibits HLE, whereas 3,3'-bisdemethylpinoresinol (**1**) inhibits MMP-1 secretion. Further, Seed-ext inhibits both MMP-1 secretion and HLE activity. There are very few plant extracts or compounds that have both inhibitory effects. Thus, noni seeds may be an ideal cosmetic ingredient to prevent wrinkle formation.

4.3. Inhibitory effect of 3,3′-bisdemethylpinoresinol on MMP-1 secretion

In UV irradiated skin, MMP-1 is a major collagenolytic enzyme responsible for collagen damage [21]. It has been reported that UV irradiation promotes expression of MMP-1 in NHDFs [22] and secretion into culture media [23]. It is also known that UV irradiation activates intracellular fibroblast signals, c-Jun-N-terminal kinase (JNK) and p38 mitogen-activated protein kinase (p38 MAPK) cascades, promotes phosphorylation of JNK and p38, enhances expression of c-Jun and c-Fos, followed by activation of activation protein-1 (AP-1), and, in the end, enhances expression of MMP-1 [14, 24]. In order to find the mechanism of inhibition of MMP-1, compound **1** was investigated for effects on intracellular MMP-1 expression and activation of MAPKs in UVA-irradiated NHDFs.

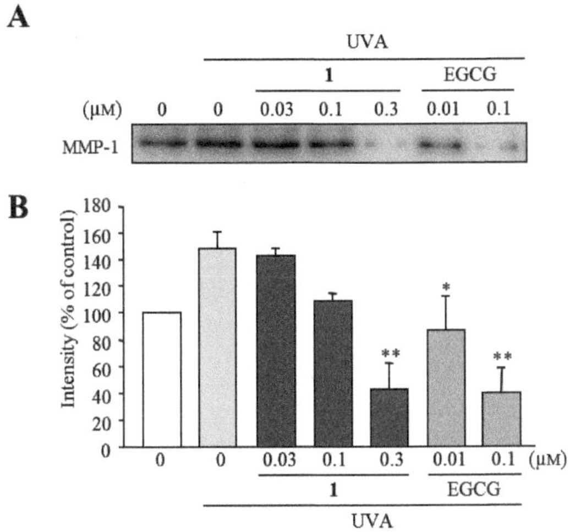

Figure 5. Effects of 3,3'-Bisdemethylpinoresinol (1) and and epigallocatechin-3-*O*-gallate (EGCG) on MMP-1 Secretion from UVA-Irradiated NHDFs (Fibroblasts were exposed to UVA (5 J/cm^2) and then cultured in the serum free medium containing test samples for 48 hrs. MMP-1 protein levels in the cultured medium were assessed by Western blot analysis using human MMP-1 specific antibody. (A) The blot is representative of three separate experiments and represents a single immunoblot. (B) All data is reported as mean±S.E. of three separate experiments. Significantly different from the vehicle control group, *: $p<0.05$, **: $p<0.01$.)

4.3.1. Effect of 3,3'-bisdemethylpinoresinol (1) on intracellular MMP-1 expression in UVA irradiation NHDFs

First, the effect of **1** on intracellular MMP-1 expression in UVA-irradiation was examined. In the vehicle control group, UVA irradiation enhanced the levels of intracellular MMP-1 expression at 24 and 48 hrs, with most of the MMP-1 expression being detected at 48 hrs (Fig. 6). But in the treatment group (addition of **1**, 0.3 μM), the expression was down-regulated at 48 hrs (Fig. 6A). The levels of MMP-1 secretion from UVA-irradiated NHDF into the culture medium increased at 48 hrs in the vehicle control group, whereas the treatment group (addition of **1**, 0.3 μM) obviously inhibited MMP-1 secretion (Fig. 6B) [20].

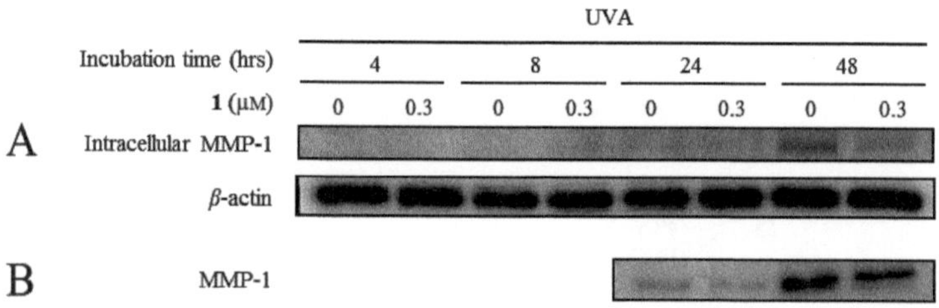

Figure 6. (A) Effect of 3,3′-Bisdemethylpinoresinol (1) on the Intracellular MMP-1 Expression in UVA-Irradiated NHDFs (B) Effect of 3,3′-Bisdemethylpinoresinol (1) on MMP-1 Secretion from UVA-Irradiated NHDFs ((A) Fibroblasts were exposed to UVA (5 J/cm^2) and then cultured in the serum free medium containing test samples for 4, 8, 24, and 48 hrs. Intracellular MMP-1 protein levels, at the indicated times, were assessed by Western blot analysis using human MMP-1 specific antibody. The blot is representative of two separate experiments and represents a single immunoblot. (B) Fibroblasts were exposed to UVA (5 J/cm^2) and then cultured in serum free medium containing test samples for 24 to 48 hrs. MMP-1 protein levels in cultured medium were assessed by Western blot analysis using human MMP-1 specific antibody. The blot is representative of two separate experiments and represents a single immunoblot.)

4.3.2. *Effect of 3,3′-bisdemethylpinoresinol on MAPKs phosphorylation in UVA-irradiated NHDFs*

The effect of **1** on activation of MAPKs was investigated by Western blot analysis. JNK and p38 MAPK phosophorylation in UVA irradiated NHDFs versus incubation time is shown in Fig. 7A. JNK phosophorylation was enhanced in a more rapid and transient manner at 0.5 to 1 hr after UVA irradiation, whereas that of p38 MAPK was enhanced at 0 to 1 hr. Therefore, the effect of **1** (0.1 and 0.3 μM) on JNK and p38 MAPK phosophorylation in UVA-irradiated NHDFs was examined at 0.5 hr after irradiation. As shown in Fig. 7B, **1** (0.1 μM) had no inhibitory effect of JNK and p38 MAPK, whereas **1** (0.3 μM) inhibited phosphorylation of both [20].

The results suggest that 1 inhibits MMP-1 secretion in UVA-irradiated NHDFs by decreasing JNK and p38 phosphorylation and suppressing c-Jun and c-Fos expression. This, subsequently, inhibits AP-1 and MMP-1 expression, resulting in a reduction in MMP- secretion.

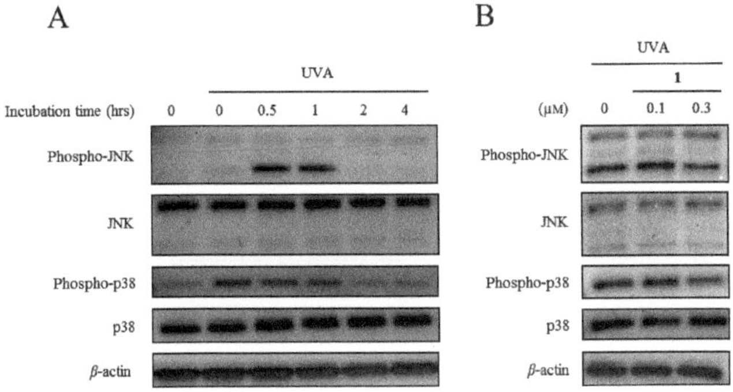

Figure 7. Time Course of MAPKs Phosphorylation in UVA-Irradiated NHDFs (B) Effect of 3,3′-Bisdemethylpinoresinol (1) on MAPKs Phosphorylation in UVA-Irradiated NHDFs ((A) Fibroblasts were exposed to UVA (5 J/cm^2) and then cultured in the serum free medium for the indicated time. Total cellular proteins were prepared for Western blot analysis of MAPKs and phospho-MAPKs proteins using the antibodies against phospho-form and total-form of JNK and p38. β-actin was used as an internal control. The blot is representative of three separate experiments and represents a single immunoblot. (B) Fibroblasts were exposed to UVA (5 J/cm^2) and then cultured in the serum free medium for 0.5 hr. Total cellular proteins were prepared for Western blot analysis of MAPKs and phospho-MAPKs proteins using the antibodies against phospho-form and total-form of JNK and p38. β-actin was used for internal control. The blot is representative of three separate experiments and represents a single immunoblot.)

5. Inhibitory effect of noni seeds on poor blood fluidity

In addition to melanogenesis and degradation of collagen by HLE and MMP-1, blood stagnation may also contribute to hyperpigmented spots on the skin. In oriental medicine, the clinical state of blood stasis in the venous system is called "Oketsu" in Japanese. Accumulation of wastes caused by blood stagnation in the skin leads to pigmentation. Degradation of blood flow, leading to dry skin and atrophy, also leads to wrinkle formation. Therefore, improved blood fluidity is likely to prevent formation of pigmented spots and wrinkles. As cosmetic ingredients that improve blood fluidity are desired for use in anti-photoaging products, the effect of noni seeds on poor blood fluidity was investigated.

5.1. Antithrombotic effect of noni seeds in a disseminated intravascular coagulation (DIC) rat model

The effect of noni seeds on excessive increased blood coagulation, accompanying poor blood fluidity, was examined by using a DIC rat model, induced by lipopolysaccharide (LPS) [25, 26].

Each Seed-ext (200 and 500 mg/kg) was administrated orally once a day to the rats for 7 successive days. LPS was injected on Day 7. Four hrs after injection, blood samples were collected from the abdominal great vein (vena cava). Whole blood passage time was measured by a micro channel array flow analyzer (MC-FAN). As shown in Table 6, the vehicle control group (LPS-induced) significantly prolonged blood passage time, in comparison with the control group. However, Seed-ext dose-dependently reduced passage time [27].

Platelet count, fibrinogen and fibrin degradation products (FDP) were also measured. Seed-ext had no effect on any of these hematological parameters (Table 6) [27].

Samples	Dose [a)]	Route [b)]	Blood passage time (s) [c)]	Platelets ($\times 10^4$/μl)	Fibrinogen (mg/dl)	FDP (μg/ml)
Control		*p.o.*	17±1	81.1±2.5	198.0±5.2	0.43±0.06
Vehicle control		*p.o.*	1813±34[ii]	18.4±1.1[ii]	96.6±3.9[ii]	2.06±0.17[ii]
Seed-ext	200 (mg/kg)	*p.o.*	1722±16[iii]	26.7±0.5[i]	96.7±2.9	1.86±0.11
	500 (mg/kg)	*p.o.*	1413±19[i]	22.5±0.8	105.2±2.7	1.75±0.07
Heparin	500 (U/kg)	i.v.	26±1[i]	46.1±2.8[i]	194.1±7.2[i]	0.52±0.15[iii]

Table 6. Effects of Seed-ext and Heparin on Blood Passage Time, Platelet Count, Fibrinogen, and FDP in Rats, after LPS Injection (Each value represents the mean±S.E. (*n*=7). Significantly different from the control group, [ii]: $p<0.01$. Significantly different from the vehicle control group, [iii]: $p<0.05$, [i]: $p<0.01$. [a)] For 7 successive days, 0.2% CMC-Na was administered orally to control and vehicle control groups. Each extract (200 and 500 mg/kg) was suspended with CMC-Na and administrated orally to each test group once daily for 7 successive days (Day 1-7). 1 hr after the final daily dose on Day 7, LPS (1 mg/kg, dissolved in saline, i.v.) was injected into the tail vein. Heparin (500 U/kg, dissolved in saline, i.v.) was administered intravenously to the rats 1 hr before LPS injection on Day 7 to the heparin group. [b)] *p.o.*: oral administration, i.v.: intravenous administration [c)] Blood passage time measured by MC-FAN as the time taken for the flow of 50 μl of sample mixture (1.8 ml of blood and 0.2 ml of 3.8% sodium citrate solution).

The results from the DIC rat model experiments suggest that Seed-ext improves poor blood fluidity. Therefore, noni seeds may help reduce pigmentation associated with blood stagnation.

5.2. Inhibitory effect of noni seeds, and active consituents, on platelet aggregation

Blood fluidity, as measured by using MC-FAN, is influenced by erythroid deformability, leukocytic adherence ability and thrombocytic agglutinability [28, 29]. Blood flow regulating factors in microcirculation have vascular systemic and blood component functions. Circulatory system function deteriorates with platelet aggregation induced coagulation, degradation of erythrocyte deformability, hemagglutination, elevation of plasma viscosity, and by degradation of fibrinolytic system activation [28, 29].

In order to examine the inhibitory effect of Seed-ext on blood coagulation, collagen-induced platelet aggregation [30] and polybrene-induced erythrocyte aggregation [31], *in vitro* tests were carried out. Seed-ext did not inhibit platelet aggregation (data not shown). But it did inhibit hemagglutination at concentrations ranging from 50 to 500 μg/ml (Table 7). As shown in Table 7, **3** inhibited platelet aggregation at 10 to 50 μM. Lingnans **1** and **2** had weak effects of platelet aggregation, when comparison to **3** [27].

The results suggest that one inhibitory mechanisms behind the effect of Seed-ext on poor blood fluidity in the DIC rat model may be anti-hemaggulatination by 1, 2, and 3.

Samples	**Concentration**	**Aggregation (%)**	**Inhibition (%)**
Control		45±1	
Seed-ext	50 (μg/ml)	27±1[i]	40
	200 (μg/ml)	8±1[i]	82
	500 (μg/ml)	9±1[i]	81
1	10 (μM)	42±1	7
	20 (μM)	39±1	13
	50 (μM)	34±1[i]	24
	100 (μM)	27±1[i]	41
2	10 (μM)	42±2	7
	20 (μM)	41±1	9
	50 (μM)	38±1	16
	100 (μM)	32±1[i]	29
3	5 (μM)	40±0	11
	10 (μM)	31±2[i]	31
	20 (μM)	10±5[i]	78
	50 (μM)	7±2[i]	84
Neuraminidase	7.8 (mU/ml)	36±2	19
	15.6 (mU/ml)	33±3[i]	27
	31.3 (mU/ml)	23±1[i]	48
	62.5 (mU/ml)	17±1[i]	63
	125 (mU/ml)	8±0[i]	82

Table 7. Effects of Seed-ext, **1**, **2**, **3** and Neuraminidase on Polybrene-Induced Erythrocyte Aggregation (Each value represents the mean±S.E. of 3 experiments. Significantly different from control group, [iii]: $p<0.05$, [i]: $p<0.01$.)

5.3. Fibrinolytic activity of noni seeds in rats

Activation of the fibrinolytic system improves blood flow by promoting the lysis of thrombi in blood vessel walls. To better understand the fibrinolytic potential of Seed-ext, as it relates to degradation of blood fluidity, the euglobulin lysis time (ELT) assay in normal rats was conducted. ELT is the time required for the disappearance of a fibrin clot produced by the addition of thrombin to the eugloblin fraction obtained from blood samples [32]. A reduction in ELT reveals activation of fibrinolysis activity, whereas an extension in ELT implies reduced activity [32].

Seed-ext was administrated orally, and 1 hr later, blood samples were collected. Then ELT was measured using eugloblin fractions from the sample. As shown in Table 8, Seed-ext significantly reduced ELT at dosages from 50 and 200 mg/kg in dose-dependent manner. This reveals that Seed-ext may have an enhancing effect on fibrinolysis activity [27].

Samples	Dose	Route	ELT (min)
Control A [a)]		*p.o.*	98±2
Seed-ext	50 (mg/kg)	*p.o.*	55±5[i]
	200 (mg/kg)	*p.o.*	42±7[i]
Control B [b)]		i.v.	97±2
Dextran sulphate sodium salt	5 (mg/kg)	i.v.	32±3[ii]

Table 8. Effects of Seed-ext and Dextran Sulphate Sodium Salt on ELT in Rats ([a)] Control A is a control for extracts. [b)] Control B is a control for dextran sulphate sodium salt. Each value represents the mean±S.E. of 7 rats. Significantly different from control A group, [i]: $p<0.01$. Significantly different from control B group, [ii]: $p<0.01$.)

Seed-ext has an inhibitory effect on hemagglutination. But it also activates fibrinolysis, suggesting that it may improve blood flow through anti-coagulation and fibrinolysis systems. As such, noni seeds may be a useful supplementary ingredient for the prevention of both pigmented spots and wrinkles caused by venous blood stagnation.

6. Conclusion

We are the first to investigate and find 4 inhibitory effects—namely tyrosinase, melanogenesis, HLE, and MMP-1—for noni seeds related to prevention of pigmented spots and wrinkles by photoaging. As a desirable anti-photoaging agent that is antagonistic to the UV signaling pathways of photoaging, Seed-ext may be a useful novel cosmetic ingredient for the prevention or treatment for pigmented spots and wrinkles. Since we found Seed-ext may improve blood fluidity, it may also be a useful supplemental ingredient aimed for beauty. However, further research, including clinical trials, is needed.

Noni fruit flesh and leaves have been used as functional foods, but the seeds have been discarded without utilization in most cases. Production of a cosmetic ingredient from noni seeds adds significant value to this largely unused natural resource.

Author details

Hideaki Matsuda[1], Megumi Masuda[1], Kazuya Murata[1], Yumi Abe[2] and Akemi Uwaya[2]

1 Faculty of Pharmacy, Kinki University, Japan

2 Research & Development, Morinda Worldwide, Inc., Japan

References

[1] Yaar M., Gilchrest B. A., Photoageing: mechanism, prevention and therapy., British Journal of Dermatology, 2007; 157, 874-887.

[2] Ross I. A., Medicinal Plants of the World Vol. II., Totowa: Humana press; 2001, p309-317.

[3] Youngken H. W., Jenkins H. J., Butler C. L., Studies on *Morinda citrifolia* L. II., Journal of the American Pharmaceutical Association, 1960; 49, 271-273.

[4] Kamiya K., Hamabe W., Harada S., Murakami R., Tokuyama S., Satake T., Chemical constituents of *Morinda citrifolia* roots exhibit hypoglycemic effects in streptozotocin-induced diabetic mice., Biological and Pharmaceutical Bulletin, 2008; 31(5), 935-938.

[5] Wang M. Y., Su C., Cancer preventive effect of *Morinda citrifolia* (Noni)., Annals of the New York Academy of Sciences, 2001; 952, 161-168.

[6] Pande M., Naiker M., Mills G., Singh N., Voro T., The Kura files: qualitative social survey., Pacific Health Dialog, 2005; 12(2), 85-93.

[7] Tobin D., Thody A. J., The superoxide anion may mediate short- but not long-term effects of ultraviolet radiation on melanogenesis., Experimental Dermatology, 1994; 3(3), 99-105.

[8] Masuda M., Murata K., Fukuhama A., Naruto S., Fujita T., Uwaya A., Isami F., Matsuda H., Inhibitory effects of constituents of *Morinda citrifolia* seeds on elastase and tyrosinase., Journal of Natural Medicines, 2009; 63(3), 267-273.

[9] Ohguchi K., Akao Y., Nozawa Y., Involvement of calpain in melanogenesis of mouse B16 melanoma cells., Molecular and Cellular Biochemistry, 2005; 275(1-2), 103-107.

[10] Masuda M., Itoh K., Murata K., Naruto S., Uwaya A., Isami F., Matsuda H., Inhibitory effects of *Morinda citrifolia* extract and its constituents on melanogenesis in murine B16 melanoma cells., Biological and Pharmaceutical Bulletin, 2012; 35(1), 78-83.

[11] Widlund H. R., Fisher D. E., Microphthalamia-associated transcription factor: a critical regulator of pigment cell development and survival., Oncogene, 2003; 22(20), 3035-3041.

[12] Kim D.-S., Hwang E.-S., Lee J.-E., Kim S.-Y., Kwon S.-B., Park K.-C., Sphingosine-1-phosphate decreases melanin synthesis via sustained ERK activation and subsequent MITF degradation., Journal of Cell Science, 2003; 116, 1699-1706.

[13] Smalley K., Eisen T., The involvement of p38 mitogen-activated protein kinase in the alpha-melanocyte stimulating hormone (alpha-MSH)-induced melanogenic and anti-proliferative effects in B16 murine melanoma cells., FEBS Letters, 2000; 476(3), 198-202.

[14] Rittié L., Fisher G. J., UV-light-induced signal cascades and skin aging., Ageing Research Reviews, 2002; 1(5), 705-720.

[15] Rijken F., Kiekens R. C. M., Bruijnzeel P. L. B., Skin-infiltrating neutrophils following exposure to solar-simulated radiation could play an important role in photoageing of human skin., British Journal of Dermatology, 2005; 152(2), 321-328.

[16] Kafienah W., Buttle D. J., Burnett D., Hollander A. P., Cleavage of native type I collagen by human neutrophil elastase., The Biochemical Journal, 1998; 330, 897-902.

[17] Grant G. M., Giambernardi T. A., Grant A. M., Klebe R. J., Overview of expression of matrix metalloproteinases (MMP-17, MMP-18, and MMP-20) in cultured human cells., Matrix Biology, 1999; 18(2), 145-148.

[18] Wang X.-Y., Bi Z.-G., UVB-irradiated human keratinocytes and interleukin-1alpha indirectly increase MAP kinase/AP-1 activation and MMP-1 production in UVA-irradiated dermal fibroblasts., Chinese Medical Journal, 2006; 119(10), 827-831.

[19] Takeuchi H., Gomi T., Shishido M., Watanabe H., Suenobu N., Neutrophil elastase contributes to extracellular matrix damage induced by chronic low-dose UV irradiation in a hairless mouse photoaging model., Journal of Dermatological Science, 2010; 60(3), 151-158.

[20] Masuda M., Murata K., Naruto S., Uwaya A., Isami F., Matsuda H., Matrix metalloproteinase-1 inhibitory activities of *Morinda citrifolia* seed extract and its constituents in UVA-irradiated human dermal fibroblasts., Biological and Pharmaceutical Bulletin, 2012; 35(2), 210-215.

[21] Brennan M., Bhatti H., Nerusu K. C., Bhagavathula N., Kang S., Fisher G. J., Varani J., Voorhees J. J., Matrix metalloproteinase-1 is the major collagenolytic enzyme responsible for collagen damage in UV-irradiated human skin., Photochemistry and Photobiology, 2003; 78(1), 43-48.

[22] Suganuma K., Nakajima H., Ohtsuki M., Imokawa G., Astaxanthin attenuates the UVA-induced up-regulation of matrix metalloproteinase-1 and skin fibroblast elastase in human dermal fibroblasts., Journal of Dermatological Science, 2010; 58(2), 136-142.

[23] Oh H.-I., Shim J.-S., Gwon S.-H., Kwon H.-J., Hwang J.-K., The effect of xanthorrhizol on the expression of matrix metalloproteinase-1 and type-I procollagen in ultraviolet-irradiated human skin fibroblasts., Phytotherapy Research, 2009; 23(9), 1299-1302.

[24] Fisher G. J., Talwar H. S., Lin J., Lin P., McPhillips F., Wang Z., Li X., Wan Y., Kang S., Voorhees J. J., Retinoic acid inhibits induction of c-Jun protein by ultraviolet radiation that occurs subsequent to activation of mitogen-activated protein kinase pathways in human skin *in vivo*., The Journal of Clinical Investigation, 1998; 101(6), 1432-1440.

[25] Schoendorf T. H., Rosenberg M., Beller F. K., Endotoxin-induced disseminated intravascular coagulation in nonpregnant rats. A new experimental model., The American Journal of Pathology, 1971; 65(1), 51-58.

[26] Chang G.-T., Min S.-Y., Kim J.-H., Kim S.-H., Kim J.-K., Kim C.-H., Anti-thrombic activity of Korean herbal medicine, Dae-Jo-Whan and its herbs., Vascular Pharmacology, 2005; 43(4), 283-288.

[27] Masuda M., Murata K., Itoh K., Naruto S., Uwaya A., Isami F., Matsuda H., Effects of *Morinda citrifolia* extract and its constituents on blood fluidity., Journal of Traditional Medicines, 2011, 28(2), 47-54.

[28] Seki K., Sumino H., Murakami M., Study on blood rheology measured by MC-FAN., Rinsho Byori, 2003; 51(8), 770-775.

[29] Itoh K., Masuda M., Naruto S., Murata K., Matsuda H., Effects of unripe *Citrus hassaku* fruits extract and its flavanone glycosides on blood fluidity., Biological and Pharmaceutical Bulletin, 2010; 33(4), 659-664.

[30] Born G. V. R., Cross M. J., The Aggregation of Blood Platelets., The Journal of Physiology, 1963; 168, 178-195.

[31] Sabio H., Levien M., Atkinson S., Continuous recording of red cell interactions., Thrombosis Research, 1983; 29(5), 537-540.

[32] Sakuragawa N., Euglobulin lysis time., Nihon Rinsho, 1997; 55, 139-144.

Chapter 13

Inhibiting S100B in Malignant Melanoma

Kira G. Hartman, Paul T. Wilder, Kristen Varney,
Alexander D. Jr. MacKerell, Andrew Coop,
Danna Zimmer, Rena Lapidus and David J. Weber

Additional information is available at the end of the chapter

1. Introduction

The development of new therapies for patients diagnosed with malignant melanoma is in high need. In this chapter, the design and testing of inhibitors are discussed for S100B, a calcium-binding protein that down-regulates the tumor suppressor p53. Because p53 is wild type in many malignant melanoma patients, the restoration of p53 with S100B inhibitors (SBiXs) represents a new and potentially effective strategy for sensitizing melanoma cells to p53-dependent apoptosis pathways and for targeting this deadly cancer. Such a strategy requires blocking of the S100B-p53 protein-protein interaction (PPI) and involves methods including computer aided drug design (CADD), screening technologies, nuclear magnetic resonance (NMR), X-ray crystallography, and medicinal chemistry approaches. The ultimate goal is to design a highly specific and potent inhibitor of S100B that has clinical value.

2. The S100 protein family

The S100 family of EF-hand calcium-binding proteins has more than 20 members, with the genes encoding these proteins present only in vertebrates [7]. S100 proteins (S100s) are expressed in both a cell type and tissue-specific manner to provide diverse functional roles including calcium homeostasis, cell-cell communication, cell proliferation, differentiation, cytoskeletal dynamics, and cell morphology [7-10]. On the other hand, dysregulation of S100 expression is observed in several types of cancers, including malignant melanoma [7-9]. They are also problematic when elevated in several cognitive disorders including those arising from traumatic brain injuries [12-16]. While S100 proteins themselves have no inherent enzymatic activity, they regulate important biological processes via specific Ca^{2+}-dependent protein-protein interactions [17,18].

The first members of the S100 family were discovered in 1965 in a subcellular fraction from bovine brain tissue and were named based on their solubility in 100% saturated ammonium sulfate. When this protein fraction was examined in detail, two similar, but distinct proteins were discovered and designated S100α and S100β that are now referred to as S100A1 and S100B, respectively [17,19]. As with S100A1 and S100B, other S100s have a similar molecular weight (9-12 kDa), have homologous amino acid sequences (>40%), and typically exist as symmetric homodimers, or as heterodimers, held together by noncovalent interactions as pairs of four-helix bundles [20,21]. Two EF-hand helix-loop-helix calcium-binding structural motifs, first defined using the "E" and "F" helices from the X-ray crystal structure of parvalbumin, are present in each S100 subunit [22]. The N-terminal *"S100"* or *"pseudo"* EF-hand (EF1) is comprised of 14 rather than the original 12 residues and this 14 amino acid sequence readily distinguishes S100s from other EF-hand calcium signaling proteins. The canonical EF-hand (EF2) is found at the C-terminus of each subunit and typically binds Ca^{2+} with a higher affinity than EF1. The two EF-hand domains are connected by a stretch of amino acid residues (<25 residues) termed the "hinge region". This "hinge" together with the C-terminal loop of the S100 protein contains the least amount of sequence homology and, therefore, represents the two regions that give each family member their individual target-binding specificity [7,8,23]. In addition to binding Ca^{2+}, several S100s bind Zn^{2+} at a separate site from the EF-hand calcium-binding domains. The Zn^{2+} site can also bind other metals (i.e. Mn^{2+}, Cu^{2+}, and others) and has two ligating residues contributed from each subunit at the dimer interface to provide tetrahedral coordination that is typical for Zn^{2+} [24]. However, for S100B, Zn^{2+}-binding is not sufficient to induce target binding on its own, but rather functions by increasing the affinity S100B has for Ca^{2+} and its target proteins [25,26].

Figure 1. Structures of apo- versus holo-S100B. Ribbon diagrams comparing the NMR solution structures of calcium-free (left) and calcium-bound S100B (right), illustrating the 90° reorientation of helices 3 and 3' in each subunit of S100B. Shown in yellow on one subunit is the S100B target binding site that is exposed after the Ca^{2+}-dependent conformational change.

3. S100B structure & interactions with ions

As with most S100 proteins, each 91 amino acid subunit of S100B has four alpha helices arranged into two helix-loop-helix (HLH) calcium-binding motifs connected by the flexible "hinge" region. Helix 1 and 2 make up the S100 EF-hand, while helix 3 and 4 form the canonical EF-hand (Figure 1). Each S100B subunit, therefore, binds two molecules of calcium, though with significantly different affinities [27]. While the canonical EF-hand binds Ca^{2+} with moderate affinity (K_D = 20 – 50 μM), the weaker S100 EF-hand binds Ca^{2+} with a much lower affinity (K_D = 200 – 500 μM) [27-30]. Calcium binding induces a dramatic conformational change in S100B where helix 3 rotates by 90º to become perpendicular to helix 4 (Figure 1). This change in conformation exposes a unique binding pocket, which in turn, binds to targets specific for each S100 protein generating a biological response [23]. However, it is clear that the dissociation constants of calcium from most S100s *in vitro*, including S100B, are too weak to compete on their own for free Ca^{2+} typically present in the cytosol (100 to 500 nM). Interestingly, it is now understood that the affinity of S100s for Ca^{2+} is increased by as much as 300-fold when bound to biologically relevant target proteins (i.e. at 100 nM free Ca^{2+}) suggesting that S100s typically only sequester free Ca^{2+} when their biologically relevant targets are present at optimal levels within the cell [31-34]. While the mechanism for this allosteric tightening of Ca^{2+} is not completely understood, it is known that when a target peptide derived from CapZ (termed TRTK-12) is bound to S100B, a loss in μs-ms motions occurs throughout the protein including in the side chain of a Ca^{2+}-coordinating residues. These results were consistent with the hypotheses that stabilizing motions, particularly for Ca^{2+}-coordinating residue(s) in EF2, could be responsible for the significant increase in Ca^{2+}-ion binding affinity observed when a target is bound to Ca^{2+}-S100B [35]. Likewise, the binding of S100B to Zn^{2+} (K_D = 90 ± 20 nM) stabilizes residues in the C-terminus of the protein, resulting in an increase in both Ca^{2+}- and target-binding affinities [28,36].

Thus, as with many EF-hand proteins, S100 signaling proteins do not bind Ca^{2+} with high affinity unless they are bound to their biologically relevant protein target(s) [32-34,37,38]. In other words, in the absence of a bound target, the Ca^{2+}-binding affinity for most S100 proteins is relatively low (i.e. in the μM range [1,17,27,39], but when bound to peptides (i.e. TRTK-12) or full-length targets, the Ca^{2+}-binding affinity can be increased by 5- to 300-fold, respectively [32-34,37,38,40]. This property is physiologically necessary because while there are over 600 EF-hand Ca^{2+}-binding domains within any given cell, Ca^{2+} homeostasis must be maintained with sufficient free Ca^{2+} ion concentrations for proper signaling (i.e. 100 to 500 nM). Thus, as a physiological control mechanism, S100s and many other EF-hand proteins do not sequester significant amounts of free Ca^{2+} unless their functionally relevant molecular target is available [29,34,38]. It is especially important for drug design that we continue to investigate and understand this phenomenon at the molecular level because S100 inhibitor binding must mimic the EF-hand-target complex and allosterically tighten Ca^{2+} ion binding affinity upon complex formation to be effective inside the cell [35,37]. For S100B, this includes targets such as p53, hdm2, hdm4, Rsk1 and RAGE, among others, which subsequently contributes to a Ca^{2+}-mediated growth response in a cell-specific manner, including those in skin and brain (Table 1).

4. S100B pathology

The protein S100B is found in melanocytes, glial cells, chondrocytes, and adipocytes, exhibiting both intra- and extracellular functionality. The cellular responses elicited by S100B can vary depending on several factors, including concentration (nM or μM), cell type, and cellular location [8,9]. Of particular concern is the role of elevated S100B in melanoma (Figure 2), the most deadly of all skin cancers, notorious for its resistence to chemotherapy and radiation. Clinical studies have established S100B as an effective biomarker for melanoma; however, this is only the case when highly specific S100B antibodies are used [12]. For example, in one study, samples from 412 melanoma patients at varying stages were compared to those diagnosed with non-melanoma skin cancers and inflammatory cutaneous diseases. Using a cutoff value of 0.2 μg/l serum S100B, a positive correlation was observed for patients having S100B levels above the cutoff level and advancement of tumor stage, indicative of a contribution by S100B to micro- and/or macro-metastases [41-43]. Though elevated S100B cannot be used to identify tumor thickness or lympth node status, it is predictive of poor patient prognosis, increased tumor recurrence, and low overall survival [9,41-44]. Subsequent studies reinforce these findings and consistently show elevated levels of S100B to be a sensitive and specific marker of melanoma progression with the ability to detect metastases or relapse at much earlier timepoints. S100B levels can also be used to monitor treatment strategies for rapid identification of whether a particular therapy is promising or for deciding to take an alternative approach [9]. While S100B is a useful prognostic indicator for melanoma, its use as a biomarker for several other cancers with elevated S100B is still under investigation; including colorectal cancer [45-47], several gliomas [48,49], mengiomas [50], non-small cell lung cancer (NSCLC) [51], renal cell carcinoma (RCC) [52], and thyroid carcinoma [53]. In addition, these clinical observations underscore the need to fully understand the role of elevated S100B in cancer, which is ongoing [2-4,54].

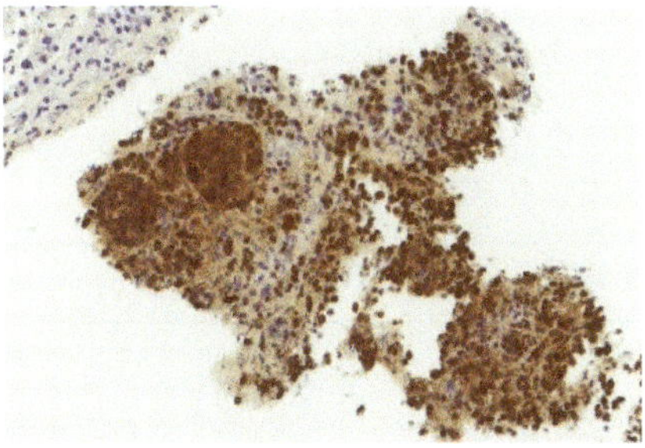

Figure 2. Staining for elevated S100B in a human malignant melanoma biopsy. Elevated S100B is stained brown in this human biopsy recorded for a patient before entering a S100B inhibitor clinical trial (SBi1). Patients are also tested for their p53 status and S100B:p53 ratio as recommended by Lin et al [2-4].

Although not considered in detail here, S100B also plays an important role in the brain, and as with cancer, several cognitive disorders show over-expression of S100B in brain tissue and are associated with pathological states including Alzheimer's disease (AD), Down's syndrome (DS), and schizophrenia [55-59]. One mechanism for this pathology is that elevated intracellular levels of S100B present in glial cells are excreted and regulate neighboring neuronal cell activity. At low levels, the presence of this extracellular S100B is sufficient to promote neurite extension and growth, while elevated S100B levels are toxic and lead to neuronal cell apoptosis [9,60]. As with skin cancer, the clinical utility of S100B as a marker to identify and characterize neurological diseases and traumas is complicated by overlapping expression of S100B and other S100s in several cell types, its multiple mechanisms of secretion, and its association with more than one neurodegenerative disorder [14]. However, as found for melanoma, lowering S100B levels upon drug delivery is one means used to evaluate drug efficacy for treating schizophrenia [16,61]. Furthermore, the development of S100B inhibitors themselves may be useful for the treatment of these neuropathies, making the identification of such compounds important for advancing efforts towards understanding and treating cancers and cognitive disorders in which S100B levels are at pathologically high levels [62].

Cellular Activity	Protein	References
Ca^{2+} Homeostasis	AHNAK*	[26]
Cell Cycle Regulation	Hdm2, Hdm4	[63]
	NDR	[64,65]
Cytoskeletal Regulation	Caldesmon*	[66]
	Calponin	[67]
	CapZα	[68]
	GFAP	[69]
	IQGAP1	[70]
	MARCKS*	[71]
	Src kinase	[26]
	τ-protein*	[72]
	Tubulin	[73]
Energy Metabolism	Fructose 1,6 bisphosphate aldolase	[74]
	Phosphoglucomutase	[75]
Growth & Survival	p53*	[1,28,76,77]

*PKC-mediated phosphorylation target proteins

Table 1. Targets of S100B

5. S100B targets

The ability of S100B to bind a diverse array of protein and enzyme targets is attributable to its broad consensus target-binding sequence [63]. S100B targets include proteins involved in calcium homeostasis, cell-cycle regulation, cytoskeletal regulation, energy metabolism, and growth/survival (Table 1). One common theme among several S100B-target interactions is that they regulate protein phosphorylation [78]. For example, S100B associates with nuclear Dbf2-related (NDR) protein by binding a region distinct from the active site and inducing a conformational change, which stimulates autophosphorylation, and ultimately activates the protein [64]. S100B also regulates phosphorylation by binding to kinase substrates such as those of protein kinase C (PKC) and sterically blocking phosphorylation [76,77,79] (Table 1). This includes the myristoylated alanine-rich C-kinase substrate (MARCKS), τ-protein, and caldesmon to name a few [66,80,81]. One noteable S100B target is the PKC substrate, p53, which is activated by phosphorylation in the C-terminal negative regulatory domain (NRD). In addition to blocking PKC-dependent phosphorylation, the S100B-p53 complex formation shifts the p53 tetramer to dimer to monomer equilibrium towards oligomer dissociation [76,78]. Thus, for p53, when S100B levels are too high, PKC-mediated activation of p53 is inhibited and p53 tetramers are dissociated. Consequently, p53 cannot bind DNA, which affects its transcriptional activity [2,28,76,77,82,83] and inhibits its ability to control cell cycle progression and apoptosis [2-4]. Other S100B targets include the E3 that designates p53 for ubiquitination, Hdm2, and the Hdm2 regulator, Hdm4 [63]. Thus, studies are underway to understand how S100B complexes involving Hdm2/Hdm4 contribute to lowering p53 levels in melanoma. Complicating this is the fact that both of these negative regulators of p53, Hdm2 and S100B, are themselves transcriptionally regulated by p53 [4,63]. This feedback regulatory mechanism results in time-dependent regulation of p53 that depends on having correct levels of all four proteins for proper regulation of cell cycle growth arrest and apoptosis [63]. Since elevated S100B disrupts the maintenance of p53 levels and promotes a cancerous phenotype, the development of small molecule inhibitors designed to target Ca^{2+}-bound S100B has become a high priority. Specifically, investigations are focused on the identification of compounds capable of blocking the Ca^{2+}-dependent S100B-p53 interaction in malignant melanoma (Figure 3). Ideally, administration of such compounds would reactivate p53 in malignant melanoma, as found for siRNA^{S100B}, to induce normal apoptosis pathways and reduce proliferation/survival of the cancer cells [2-4].

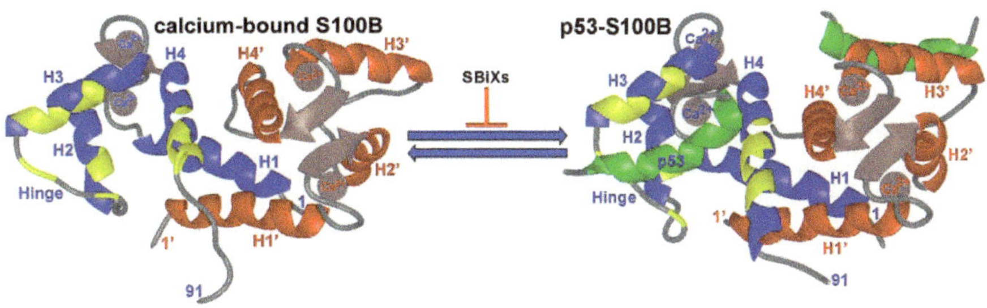

Figure 3. Illustration of the p53-binding site on S100B. Shown are ribbon diagrams Ca^{2+}-bound S100B (NMR), p53$^{367-388}$-bound Ca^{2+}-bound S100B (NMR, PDB entry 1DT7). The helices of S100B are colored in blue, while the p53$^{367-388}$ peptide is shown in red. Gray spheres represent the two calcium molecules per subunit. S100B inhibitors (SBiXs) are being developed to inhibit the Ca^{2+}-dependent formation of the S100B-p53 complex.

6. Targeting the S100B-p53 interaction

Binding of S100B to p53 blocks PKC-dependent phosphorylation, p53 tetramerization, and p53-dependent transcription activation [28,63,76,82,83]. Therefore, efforts to restore wild-type p53 activities in malignant melanoma are underway as part of a drug design strategy [28]. A combination of approaches is being used, including those involving target validation and screening, computer aided drug design, structural biology, medicinal chemistry, and *in vivo* biology and drug testing methods (Figure 4). In one case, a previously FDA approved drug was discovered to block the S100B-p53 interaction. The wealth of available data associated with this compound, including its use in animals and human clinical trials made repurposing it for use in malignant melanoma a fairly quick transition.

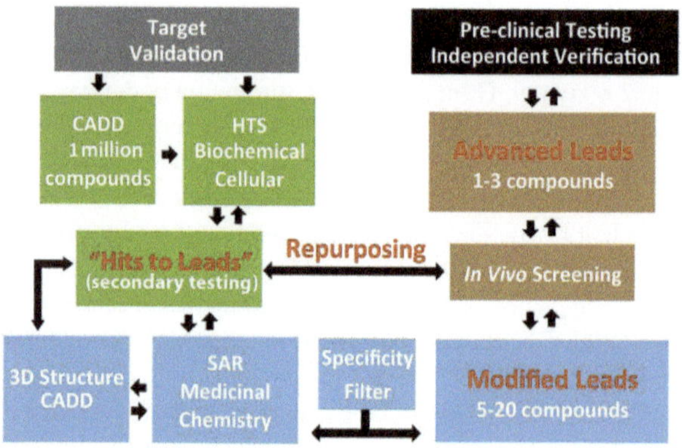

Figure 4. Summary of strategies for advancing hits from screening studies to leads, modified leads, and then advanced lead compounds. This schematic is a general guideline for the early stages of drug development. The data from these approaches is compiled and used to choose "candidate" compounds that are studied more extensively in humans for their toxicology and effectiveness in treating cancer. It is oftern advantageous to consider repurposing compounds that are already known to be safe in humans as a means to advance this process more quickly.

Screening for S100B inhibitors was initiated using computer-aided drug design methods (CADD) [28,84], and in all steps of identifying and prioritizing "hits" during these and other screens, the pharmacological activity of compounds was evaluated semi-quantitatively, providing an unbiased means of eliminating compounds that do not fulfill specific "drug-like" criteria [84,85]. Compounds identified in screens are also evaluated regarding their potential for absorption, distribution, and metabolism/excretion (ADME) properties [86]. Among many CADD approaches, a recent structure-based technique termed Site Identification by Ligand Competitive Saturation (SILCS) is now used extensively [87-89]. The simultaneous presence of benzene, propane and water in MD simulations of the target protein (ie. S100B) in this fragment-based computational approach identifies potential binding regions for aliphatic moieties, aromatic moieties and hydrogen bond donors and acceptors, while simultaneously allowing for increased flexibility and conformational changes to occur within the drug-binding site [87-89]. In addition, SILCS is very useful for strategically modifying "hits" or "lead compounds" to span a larger area of the protein surface [87,88]. CADD methods such as these are particularly important for blocking protein-protein interactions (PPIs) such as that for the S100B-p53 complex since at least three distinct target binding pockets have been identified on S100B (Figure 5) [27,29,30,37,63,68,90,91]. As a result, the drug pentamidine diisethionate (Pnt), which is referred to as SBi1 (designated SBiX, where 'X' is an arbitrary compound number), was identified at a very early stage of the screening process as an effective inhibitor of the S100B-p53 complex [84]. Pnt was approved by the FDA as an antimicrobial agent for the treatment of Pneumocystis carinii pneumonia (PCP), which allowed for repurposing of this drug for *in vivo* testing for efficacy in treating malignant melanoma (Figure 4). To this end, a clinical trial is ongoing at the University of Maryland Medical Center (UMMC) to determine the efficacy of Pnt in melanoma patients *(0794GCC: "Treatment of melanoma with wild-type p53 and detectable S100B using pentamidine (SBi1): a Phase II trial with correlative biomarker end-points"*; CA135624; PI: Dr. Ed Sausville, M.D.; Co-PI: Dr. David J. Weber). Although, there are promising results for the use of Pnt for the treatment of malignant melanoma, efforts have continued with the goal of engineering a compound with higher efficacy and more specificity for targeting S100B (versus other S100 proteins).

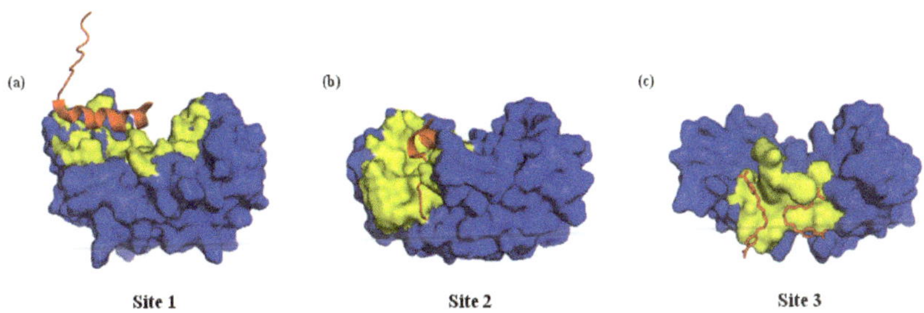

Figure 5. Three binding pockets are targeted on S100B. Surface representation of the structures of Ca^{2+}-S100B bound to (a) the C-terminal negative regulatory domain of p53 (PDB ID: 1DT7)(1), (b) TRTK-12 (PDB ID: 1MWN) [5], and (c) pentamidine, also referred to as SBi1 (PDB ID: 3CR4) [6]. Sites 1, 2, and 3 are labeled. The protein is depicted as a blue surface and the regions within 3 Å of the bound peptide or small molecule are colored yellow. TRTK-12, p53 peptide, and pentamidine are shown in red.

In addition to CADD, biochemical and cellular screening methods are continuously ongoing to identify "hits" that can be considered further as scaffolds for drug development (Figure 4). One sensitive method done *in vitro* is a fluorescence polarization competition assay (FPCA), which can identify PPI inhibitors in a high-throughput manner. This competition assay takes advantage of a small molecule inhibitor causing the dissociation of a small peptide-bound fluorophore from a larger protein-peptide complex. Specifically, SBiX inhibitors can readily be identified since the smaller, faster rotating free fluorophore-bound peptide will exhibit lower polarization when competed away by the SBiX and compared to the larger S100B-peptide complex. Importantly, the labeled-peptide must differ in molecular weight from the S100B-peptide complex to provide a reasonable dynamic range for the assay [92].

While it is important to show that an S100B-compound complex forms *in vitro*, it is also important to demonstrate that the SBiX has anti-cancer activity in cellular assays (i.e. growth inhibition, reduction in survival, increase apoptosis activity etc). In addition to showing compound efficacy in cells, these assays are important for providing information about other properties of the compound(s) including its membrane permeability and overall toxicity. One reliable method for identifying inhibitors of S100B-dependent pathways is via the creation of matched cell lines that only differ in S100B expression level. For example, MALME-3M melanoma cells were selected because they express elevated S100B protein levels and retain wild-type p53. Small interfering RNA (siRNA) was then stably transfected into the MALME-3M cells to give a scrambled siRNA control with high S100B levels and an isogenetically matched $siRNA^{S100B}$ construct resulting in low S100B (unpublished data). These matched cell lines provided a means for a large-scale screen of compound libraries to identify SBiXs with potency and specificity towards pathways involving S100B. The "hits" in this cellular assay were then routinely tested for direct binding and secondary cellular assays were completed by comparing the effect of these hits on primary malignant melanoma cells side-by-side with normal melanocytes [84]. Compounds that result in indiscriminate cell death were considered toxic rather than from specific inhibition of S100B or an S100B-dependent pathway and highlighted the importance of including normal melanocytes in every screen. Preferential growth inhibition of melanoma with high S100B as compared to little or no effect on the melanocytes or cells containing $siRNA^{S100B}$ was considered to be an early indication that the compound may have promising therapeutic value. This is exemplified with pentamidine, since treatment of C8146A primary melanoma cells resulted in significant cell growth inhibition, but little or no effect was noticed from this drug on normal melanocytes [84].

One of the most important requirements of any drug development program is to obtain physiological data at an early stage in the process to help determine whether a lead compound is effective and/or shows unanticipated toxicities *in vivo [93]*. This is particularly important for S100 inhibitors since there are over 20 structurally similar proteins in the S100 protein family, and they each regulate specific cellular pathway(s) [94,95]. To address these issues as quickly as possible, an *in vivo* screening assay was developed to test potential lead compounds for melanoma at an early stage in the drug development process. Once promising hits are designated as lead compounds via *in vitro* and cellular testing and secondary validation protocols, they need to be tested *in vivo*. Leads to be tested *in vivo* are chosen based on binding affinities (K_Ds) and/or specificity both in biochemical assays and in cellular assays. For the cellular assays, specificity and potential off-target effects are evaluated by comparing IC_{50} values of isogenic cell lines with or without S100B over-expression [96,97]. The vast majority of lead SBiXs are new chemical entities that require extensive optimization prior to entering *in vivo* testing, with the exception of those compounds that have been repurposed from other studies and trials. Animal models play a fundamental role in such *in vivo* testing. For example, a compound may need to be more lipophilic to pass through the cell membrane and reach its target or side groups may need to be added to allow for oral delivery or brain penetration. In the case of accessible tumors such as melanoma, drugs can be delivered directly to the tumor (intratumoral) without optimization for systemic delivery [93]. In addition, intratumoral delivery can achieve significantly higher drug concentrations at the site of action than can be obtained via systemic delivery. For this purpose a multi-allelic genetically engineered mouse model was chosen to test SBiX compounds since this model mimics spontaneous tumoriogenesis and heterogeneity as well as provide additional information necessary for additional target validation [98]. One such melanoma model is the RAS-induced INK4a/ARF$^{-/-}$ mouse [99], which was chosen for *in vivo* SBiX screening because it has: (i) an intact S100B-p53 signaling pathway (elevated S100B and wild type p53), (ii) an intact immune system, (iii) tumors which are amenable to intratumoral delivery, and (iv) a proven record in developing new melanoma therapies [99,100]. This screen utilizes 2-3 month old experimental Tyr::RAS^{G12V}/INK4a/ARF$^{-/-}$ male mice that develop spontaneous cutaneous melanomas in the pinna of the ears (30%), torso (23%), and tail (20%) without distant metastasis [99] and uses tumor proliferation rate as the primary outcome. Although the screen is not optimized for obtaining tolerability, PK or PD information, the gross/histological pathology, SBiX levels and p53 pathway reactivation in the tumors are monitored as is necessary to select more advanced leads that have potential for proceeding to pre-clinical testing (Table 2).

In the case of modified leads that have ADME properties favorable for systemic administration, concurrent tolerability (MTD) and pharmacokinetic (PK) assays are also conducted. MTD and PK trials are also performed to determine if a lead is suitable for pre-clinical testing or if it requires additional medicinal chemistry optimization and/or further evaluation prior to pre-clinical testing. If the compound is found to be toxic, then it is eliminated from further consideration. Should successful tumor shrinkage be observed in mice treated with the well-tolerated S100B inhibitors, an effort is then put in place to consider phase 1 or 2b human clinical trials.

Parameter	Leads	Modified Leads	Advanced Leads
K_D	<10 μM	<50 nM	<50 nM
IC_{50} in cells	<10 μM	<50 nM	<50 nM
Off target effects	$K_D \approx IC_{50}$	$K_D \approx IC_{50}$	$K_D \approx IC_{50}$
Activity in target (-/-) cells	<50%	<20%	<10%
CYP2D6 Metabolism	Not determined	No	No
P450 CYP induction	Not determined	<50% at 30 mM	<50% at 30 mM
Bioavailability	Not determined	Preferred oral	Preferred oral
Metabolic stability	Not determined	>80% after 1 hour	>80% after 1 hour
BSA Ligand K_D	Not determined	K_D> 10 mM	K_D> 10 mM
Specificity	>5:1	>50:1	>500:1

Table 2. Some criteria for leads, modified leads, and advanced leads

7. SBiX lead optimization

SBiX leads are typically optimized using structure-based drug design and by examining structure/activity relationships (SAR) using traditional medicinal chemistry approaches. Modified leads are also tested using cellular and *in vivo* assays described above to determine whether the modification improved efficacy, specificity, and other criteria listed in Table 2. Although several leads were identified for S100B and are undergoing optimization via a structure-based drug design approach, diverse scaffolds remain essential at this stage of development in case the existing lead compounds become intractable.

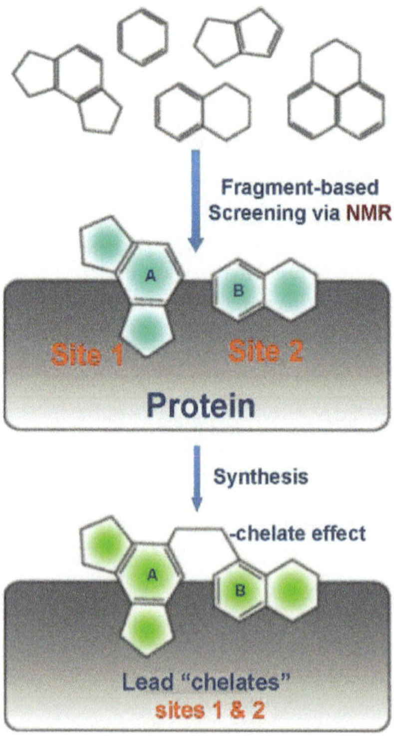

Figure 6. SAR by NMR [11]. NMR screens identify compounds that bind pockets "all over" the protein, which can be linked synthetically to obtain high affinity and specific SBiX inhibitors.

The availability of 3D structures of S100B-SBiX complexes allow for CADD to be used to select compounds from 3D chemical databases with an enhanced potential for binding to S100B [101-105] and/or to engineer compounds de novo via *in silico* methods [106,107]. In an iterative process, new S100B-drug complexes are solved, lead modifications to improve affinity predicted via CADD, predicted compounds synthesized and the resulting compounds experimentally evaluated. Work is also underway to develop novel inhibitors of S100B via a fragment-based approach that targets multiple binding sites on the protein identified by NMR, X-ray crystallography, and CADD techniques, including the new SILCS technique [87]. The SAR by NMR approach is now a standard method for quickly identifying ^{1}H-^{15}N and/or ^{1}H-^{13}C chemical shift perturbations in HSQC and/or TROSY spectra as a result of an S100B-small molecule interaction; this enables rapid, qualitative identification of binding site(s) on S100B for fragment-based design of new compounds that take advantage of the well-established "chelate effect" involved in linking fragments that bind neighboring sites [108,109] (Figure 6). For fast exchanging inhibitors, saturation transfer differences are collected to identify protons of the lead at the S100B-lead interface [84,110,111]. Thus, progress using a combination of functional-group optimization and the fragment-based approaches offers the potential for improvement in affinities/specificity, and for identifying novel leads. As new lead compounds are identified and structurally characterized (NMR, X-ray crystallography), SBiX affinity is considered as is scaffold diversity due to potential unforeseen problems with compounds that can occur during later-stage preclinical development (e.g. pharmacokinetic limitations, toxicity in humans). Therefore, as many as 3-6 chemical scaffolds are under consideration for development, and this number will be reduced as the project proceeds based on ADME properties, synthetic feasibility, and other pre-clinical/clinical information (Table 2). Such criteria include physiochemical properties related to bioavailability (molecular weight, clogP, TPSA, pKa, nitrogen atoms, carboxylates, H-bond donors, H-bond acceptors, rotatable bonds, H-bonds), and dose-limiting toxicities that may be predictive of the therapeutic index. Importantly, promising leads are routinely tested *in vivo* as early as possible to avoid wasted effort on toxic/ineffective compounds.

8. Summary

Ongoing collaborative efforts involving biology, structure determination, CADD and synthetic chemistry have lead to the development of a collection of inhibitors of S100B. These efforts include identification of the FDA approved compound pentamidine, which is currently being evaluated in human clinical trials. In addition, the work has identified several novel chemical scaffolds that are undergoing optimization and have laid the foundation for the application of fragment-based approaches to design additional novel scaffolds. Notably, while the goal of this research is to develop a potent inhibitor of S100B for the treatment of malignant melanoma, we anticipate that the knowledge gained to date will be of utility in designing specific inhibitors of other members of the S100 protein family for the treatment of a range of S100 associated disease states.

Acknowledgements

Support from the NIH (CA107331; to DJW), The Center for Biomolecular Therapeutics (CBT), and the University of Maryland Computer-Aided Drug Design Center is appreciated.

Author details

Kira G. Hartman[1], Paul T. Wilder[1,3,4], Kristen Varney[1,2,3], Alexander D. Jr. MacKerell[2,3,4], Andrew Coop[2,4], Danna Zimmer[1,3], Rena Lapidus[3,4] and David J. Weber[1,3,4*]

*Address all correspondence to: dweber@som.umaryland.edu

1 Department of Biochemistry and Molecular Biology, University of Maryland School of Medicine, Baltimore, MD, USA

2 Department of Pharmaceutical Sciences, University of Maryland School of Pharmacy, Baltimore, MD, USA

3 Center for Biomolecular Therapeutics, University of Maryland School of Medicine, Baltimore, MD, USA

4 University of Maryland Marlene and Stewart Greenebaum NCI Cancer Center, Baltimore, MD, USA

References

[1] Rustandi, R. R., Baldisseri, D. M., and Weber, D. J. (2000) *Nat Struct Biol* 7, 570-574

[2] Lin, J., Blake, M., Tang, C., Zimmer, D., Rustandi, R. R., Weber, D. J., and Carrier, F. (2001) *J Biol Chem* 276, 35037-35041

[3] Lin, J., Yang, Q., Wilder, P. T., Carrier, F., and Weber, D. J. (2010) *J Biol Chem* 285, 27487-27498

[4] Lin, J., Yang, Q., Yan, Z., Markowitz, J., Wilder, P. T., Carrier, F., and Weber, D. J. (2004) *J Biol Chem* 279, 34071-34077

[5] Rustandi, R. R., Baldisseri, D. M., Inman, K. G., Nizner, P., Hamilton, S. M., Landar, A., Zimmer, D. B., and Weber, D. J. (2002) *Biochemistry* 41, 788-796

[6] Charpentier, T. H., Wilder, P. T., Liriano, M. A., Varney, K. M., Pozharski, E., MacKerell, A. D., Jr., Coop, A., Toth, E. A., and Weber, D. J. (2008) *J Mol Biol* 382, 56-73

[7] Marenholz, I., Heizmann, C. W., and Fritz, G. (2004) *Biochem Biophys Res Commun* 322, 1111-1122

[8] Donato, R. (2001) *Int J Biochem Cell Biol* 33, 637-668

[9] Harpio, R., and Einarsson, R. (2004) *Clin Biochem* 37, 512-518

[10] Zimmer, D. B., Cornwall, E. H., Landar, A., and Song, W. (1995) *Brain Res Bull* 37, 417-429

[11] Fesik, S. W. (1993) *J Biomol NMR* 3, 261-269

[12] Gaynor, R., Herschman, H. R., Irie, R., Jones, P., Morton, D., and Cochran, A. (1981) *Lancet* 1, 869-871

[13] Van Eldik, L. J., and Griffen, W. S. T. (1994) *Biochimica et Biophysica Acta* 1223, 398-403

[14] Steiner, J., Bogerts, B., Schroeter, M. L., and Bernstein, H. G. (2011) *Clinical chemistry and laboratory medicine : CCLM / FESCC* 49, 409-424

[15] Steiner, J., Marquardt, N., Pauls, I., Schiltz, K., Rahmoune, H., Bahn, S., Bogerts, B., Schmidt, R. E., and Jacobs, R. (2011) *Brain Behav Immun* 25, 1233-1241

[16] Rothermundt, M., Ahn, J. N., and Jorgens, S. (2009) *Gen Physiol Biophys* 28 Spec No Focus, F76-81

[17] Kligman, D., and Hilt, D. C. (1988) *Trends in biochemical sciences* 13, 437-443

[18] Donato, R. (1991) *Cell Calcium* 12, 713-726

[19] Moore, B. W. (1965) *Biochemical and biophysical research communications* 19, 739-744

[20] Isobe, T., Ishioka, N., and Okuyama, T. (1981) *European Journal of Biochemistry* 115, 469-474

[21] Hunter, M. J., and Chazin, W. J. (1998) *J Biol Chem* 273, 12427-12435

[22] Kretsinger, R. H. (1979) *Adv Cyclic Nucleotide Res* 11, 1-26

[23] Drohat, A. C., Baldisseri, D. M., Rustandi, R. R., and Weber, D. J. (1998) *Biochemistry* 37, 2729-2740

[24] Baudier, J., Galsser, N., Haglid, K., and Gerard, D. (1984) *Biochimica et Biophysica Acta* 790, 164-173

[25] Barber, K. R., McClintock, K. A., Jamieson, G. A., Jr., Dimlich, R. V., and Shaw, G. S. (1999) *J Biol Chem* 274, 1502-1508

[26] Gentil, B. J., Delphin, C., Mbele, G. O., Deloulme, J. C., Ferro, M., Garin, J., and Baudier, J. (2001) *J Biol Chem* 276, 23253-23261

[27] Markowitz, J., Carrier, F., Varney, K. M., Mackerell, A. D., Jr., and Weber, D. J. (2005) *AACR Meeting Abstracts* 2005, 1140-a-

[28] Rustandi, R. R., Drohat, A. C., Baldisseri, D. M., Wilder, P. T., and Weber, D. J. (1998) *Biochemistry* 37, 1951-1960

[29] Markowitz, J., Rustandi, R. R., Varney, K. M., Wilder, P. T., Udan, R., Wu, S. L., Horrocks, W. D., and Weber, D. J. (2005) *Biochemistry* 44, 7305-7314

[30] Markowitz, J., Mackerell, A. D., Jr., Carrier, F., Charpentier, T. H., and Weber, D. J. (2005) *Curr Top Med Chem* 5, 1093-1108

[31] Ferreon, J. C., Lee, C. W., Arai, M., Martinez-Yamout, M. A., Dyson, H. J., and Wright, P. E. (2009) *Proc Natl Acad Sci U S A* 106, 6591-6596

[32] Wright, N. T., Cannon, B. R., Wilder, P. T., Morgan, M. T., Varney, K. M., Zimmer, D. B., and Weber, D. J. (2009) *Journal of molecular biology* 386, 1265-1277

[33] Wright, N. T., Inman, K. G., Levine, J. A., Cannon, B. R., Varney, K. M., and Weber, D. J. (2008) *J Biomol NMR* 42, 279-286

[34] Wright, N. T., Prosser, B. L., Varney, K. M., Zimmer, D. B., Schneider, M. F., and Weber, D. J. (2008) *J Biol Chem* 283, 26676-26683

[35] Liriano, M. A., Varney, K. M., Wright, N. T., Hoffman, C. L., Toth, E. A., Ishima, R., and Weber, D. J. (2012) *Journal of molecular biology*

[36] Wilder, P. T., Baldisseri, D. M., Udan, R., Vallely, K. M., and Weber, D. J. (2003) *Biochemistry* 42, 13410-13421

[37] Charpentier, T. H., Thompson, L. E., Liriano, M. A., Varney, K. M., Wilder, P. T., Pozharski, E., Toth, E. A., and Weber, D. J. (2010) *J Mol Biol* 396, 1227-1243

[38] Malashkevich, V. N., Varney, K. M., Garrett, S. C., Wilder, P. T., Knight, D., Charpentier, T. H., Ramagopal, U. A., Almo, S. C., Weber, D. J., and Bresnick, A. R. (2008) *Biochemistry* 47, 5111-5126

[39] Baudier, J., and Gerard, D. (1986) *J Biol Chem* 261, 8204-8212

[40] Wright, N. T., Cannon, B. R., Zimmer, D. B., and Weber, D. J. (2009) *Current chemical biology* 3, 138-145

[41] Hauschild, A., Engel, G., Brenner, W., Glaser, R., Monig, H., Henze, E., and Christophers, E. (1999) *The British journal of dermatology* 140, 1065-1071

[42] Hauschild, A., Engel, G., Brenner, W., Glaser, R., Monig, H., Henze, E., and Christophers, E. (1999) *Oncology* 56, 338-344

[43] Hauschild, A., Michaelsen, J., Brenner, W., Rudolph, P., Glaser, R., Henze, E., and Christophers, E. (1999) *Melanoma research* 9, 155-161

[44] Karnell, R., von Schoultz, E., Hansson, L. O., Nilsson, B., Arstrand, K., and Kagedal, B. (1997) *Melanoma Res* 7, 393-399

[45] Huang, M. Y., Wang, H. M., Chang, H. J., Hsiao, C. P., Wang, J. Y., and Lin, S. R. (2012) *DNA Cell Biol* 31, 43-49

[46] Huang, M. Y., Wang, H. M., Tok, T. S., Chang, H. J., Chang, M. S., Cheng, T. L., Wang, J. Y., and Lin, S. R. (2012) *DNA Cell Biol* 31, 625-635

[47] Hwang, C. C., Chai, H. T., Chen, H. W., Tsai, H. L., Lu, C. Y., Yu, F. J., Huang, M. Y., and Wang, J. Y. (2011) *Ann Surg Oncol* 18, 139-145

[48] Preusser, M., Hoischen, A., Novak, K., Czech, T., Prayer, D., Hainfellner, J. A., Baumgartner, C., Woermann, F. G., Tuxhorn, I. E., Pannek, H. W., Bergmann, M., Radl-

wimmer, B., Villagran, R., Weber, R. G., and Hans, V. H. (2007) *Am J Surg Pathol* 31, 1709-1718

[49] Gartner, W., Ilhan, A., Neziri, D., Base, W., Weissel, M., Wohrer, A., Heinzl, H., Waldhor, T., Wagner, L., and Preusser, M. (2010) *Neuro Oncol* 12, 1004-1008

[50] Hancq, S., Salmon, I., Brotchi, J., Gabius, H. J., Heizmann, C. W., Kiss, R., and Decaestecker, C. (2004) *Int J Oncol* 25, 1233-1240

[51] Pang, X., Min, J., Liu, L., Liu, Y., Ma, N., and Zhang, H. (2012) *Med Oncol*

[52] Yang, J. F., Zhang, X. Y., and Qi, F. (2004) *Zhong Nan Da Xue Xue Bao Yi Xue Ban* 29, 301-304

[53] Nagasaka, A., Umekawa, H., Hidaka, H., Iwase, K., Nakai, A., Ariyoshi, Y., Ohyama, T., Aono, T., Nakagawa, H., Ohtani, S., and et al. (1987) *Metabolism* 36, 388-391

[54] American Cancer Society. (2011)

[55] Van Eldik, L. J., and Wainwright, M. S. (2003) *Restor Neurol Neurosci* 21, 97-108

[56] Sorci, G., Bianchi, R., Riuzzi, F., Tubaro, C., Arcuri, C., Giambanco, I., and Donato, R. (2010) *Cardiovascular psychiatry and neurology* 2010

[57] Zimmer, D. B., Chaplin, J., Baldwin, A., and Rast, M. (2005) *Cell Mol Biol (Noisy-le-grand)* 51, 201-214

[58] Mori, T., Asano, T., and Town, T. (2010) *Cardiovascular psychiatry and neurology* 2010

[59] Mrak, R. E., and Griffin, W. S. (2004) *J Neuropathol Exp Neurol* 63, 679-685

[60] Castets, F., Griffin, W. S., Marks, A., and Van Eldik, L. J. (1997) *Brain Res Mol Brain Res* 46, 208-216

[61] Rothermundt, M., Ponath, G., and Arolt, V. (2004) *Int Rev Neurobiol* 59, 445-470

[62] Roltsch, E., Holcomb, L., Young, K. A., Marks, A., and Zimmer, D. B. (2010) *J Neuroinflammation* 7, 78

[63] Wilder, P. T., Lin, J., Bair, C. L., Charpentier, T. H., Yang, D., Liriano, M., Varney, K. M., Lee, A., Oppenheim, A. B., Adhya, S., Carrier, F., and Weber, D. J. (2006) *Biochim Biophys Acta* 1763, 1284-1297

[64] Millward, T. A., Heizmann, C. W., Schafer, B. W., and Hemmings, B. A. (1998) *Embo J* 17, 5913-5922

[65] Bhattacharya, S., Large, E., Heizmann, C. W., Hemmings, B., and Chazin, W. J. (2003) *Biochemistry* 42, 14416-14426

[66] Skripnikova, E. V., and Gusev, N. B. (1989) *FEBS Lett* 257, 380-382

[67] Wills, F. L., McCubbin, W. D., and Kay, C. M. (1993) *Biochemistry* 32, 2321-2328

[68] Inman, K. G., Yang, R., Rustandi, R. R., Miller, K. E., Baldisseri, D. M., and Weber, D. J. (2002) *J Mol Biol* 324, 1003-1014

[69] Bianchi, R., Garbuglia, M., Verzini, M., Giambanco, I., Ivanenkov, V. V., Dimlich, R. V., Jamieson, G. A., Jr., and Donato, R. (1996) *Biochimica et Biophysica Acta* 1313, 258-267

[70] Mbele, G. O., Deloulme, J. C., Gentil, B. J., Delphin, C., Ferro, M., Garin, J., Takahashi, M., and Baudier, J. (2002) *J Biol Chem* 277, 49998-50007

[71] Sheu, F. S., Huang, F. L., and Huang, K. P. (1995) *Arch Biochem Biophys* 316, 335-342

[72] Baudier, J., and Cole, R. D. (1988) *J. Biol. Chem.* 263, 5876-5883

[73] Donato, R. (1987) *Cell Calcium* 8, 283-297

[74] Zimmer, D. B., and Van Eldik, L. J. (1986) *J Biol Chem* 261, 11424-11428

[75] Landar, A., Caddell, G., Chessher, J., and Zimmer, D. B. (1996) *Cell Calcium* 20, 279-285

[76] Baudier, J., Delphin, C., Grunwald, D., Khochbin, S., and Lawrence, J. J. (1992) *Proc Natl Acad Sci U S A* 89, 11627-11631

[77] Wilder, P. T., Rustandi, R. R., Drohat, A. C., and Weber, D. J. (1998) *Protein Sci* 7, 794-798

[78] Donato, R., Cannon, B. R., Sorci, G., Riuzzi, F., Hsu, K., Weber, D. J., and Geczy, C. L. (2012) *Curr Mol Med*

[79] Brozzi, F., Arcuri, C., Giambanco, I., and Donato, R. (2009) *J Biol Chem* 284, 8797-8811

[80] Albert, K. A., Wu, W. C., Nairn, A. C., and Greengard, P. (1984) *Proc Natl Acad Sci U S A* 81, 3622-3625

[81] Baudier, J., Mochly-Rosen, D., Newton, A., Lee, S. H., Koshland, D. E., Jr., and Cole, R. D. (1987) *Biochemistry* 26, 2886-2893

[82] Sakaguchi, K., Sakamoto, H., Lewis, M. S., Anderson, C. W., Erickson, J. W., Appela, E., and Xie, D. (1997) *Biochemistry* 36, 10117-10124

[83] Sakaguchi, K., Sakamoto, H., Xie, D., Erickson, J. W., Lewis, M. S., Anderson, C. W., and Appella, E. (1997) *J Protein Chem* 16, 553-556

[84] Markowitz, J., Chen, I., Gitti, R., Baldisseri, D. M., Pan, Y., Udan, R., Carrier, F., MacKerell, A. D., Jr., and Weber, D. J. (2004) *J Med Chem* 47, 5085-5093

[85] Whitlow, J. L., Varughese, J. F., Zhou, Z., Bartolotti, L. J., and Li, Y. (2009) *Journal of molecular graphics & modelling* 27, 969-977

[86] Lipinski, C. A., Lombardo, F., Dominy, B. W., and Feeney, P. J. (2001) *Adv Drug Deliv Rev* 46, 3-26

[87] Guvench, O., and MacKerell Jr, A. D. (2009) *PLoS Comp. Biol.* 5, e1000435

[88] Raman, E. P., Yu, W., Guvench, O., and Mackerell, A. D. (2011) *J Chem Inf Model* 51, 877-896

[89] Foster, T. J., Mackerell, A. D., Jr., and Guvench, O. (2012) *J Comput Chem* 33, 1880-1891

[90] Charpentier, T. H., Wilder, P. T., Liriano, M. A., Varney, K. M., Zhong, S., Coop, A., Pozharski, E., MacKerell, A. D., Jr., Toth, E. A., and Weber, D. J. (2009) *Biochemistry* 48, 6202-6212

[91] Markowitz, J., MacKerell, A. D., Jr., and Weber, D. J. (2007) *Mini Rev Med Chem* 7, 609-616

[92] Wilder, P. T., Charpentier, T. H., Liriano, M. A., Gianni, K., Varney, K. M., Pozharski, E., Coop, A., Toth, E. A., Mackerell, A. D., and Weber, D. J. (2010) *International journal of high throughput screening* 2010, 109-126

[93] Zimmer, D. B., Lapidus, R.G., Weber, D.J. (2012) *Methods Mol Biol* in press

[94] Leclerc, E., and Heizmann, C. W. (2011) *Front Biosci (Schol Ed)* 3, 1232-1262

[95] Zimmer, D. B., and Weber, D. J. (2010) *Cardiovascular psychiatry and neurology* 2010

[96] Vitolo, M. I., Weiss, M. B., Szmacinski, M., Tahir, K., Waldman, T., Park, B. H., Martin, S. S., Weber, D. J., and Bachman, K. E. (2009) *Cancer Research* 69, 8275-8283

[97] Weiss, M. B., Vitolo, M. I., Mohseni, M., Rosen, D. M., Denmeade, S. R., Park, B. H., Weber, D. J., and Bachman, K. E. (2010) *Oncogene* 29, 4715-4724

[98] Singh, M., Lima, A., Molina, R., Hamilton, P., Clermont, A. C., Devasthali, V., Thompson, J. D., Cheng, J. H., Bou Reslan, H., Ho, C. C., Cao, T. C., Lee, C. V., Nannini, M. A., Fuh, G., Carano, R. A., Koeppen, H., Yu, R. X., Forrest, W. F., Plowman, G. D., and Johnson, L. (2010) *Nat Biotechnol* 28, 585-593

[99] Chin, L., Pomerantz, J., Polsky, D., Jacobson, M., Cohen, C., Cordon-Cardo, C., Horner, J. W., 2nd, and DePinho, R. A. (1997) *Genes & Development* 11, 2822-2834

[100] Larue, L., and Beermann, F. (2007) *Pigment Cell Res* 20, 485-497

[101] Lawrence, M. C., and Davis, P. C. (1992) *Proteins* 12, 31-41

[102] Martin, Y. C. (1992) *J Med Chem* 35, 2145-2154

[103] Ewing, T. J. A., and Kuntz, I. D. (1997) *J. Comput. Chem.* 18, 1175-1189

[104] Makino, S., and Kuntz, I. D. (1997) *J. Comp. Chem.* 18, 1812-1825

[105] Taylor, R. D., Jewsbury, P. J., and Essex, J. W. (2002) *J. Comp. Aided Mol. Des.* 16, 151-166

[106] Oprea, T. I., Ho, C. M. W., and Marshall, G. R. (1995) De Novo Design: Ligand construction and prediction of affinity, in computer-aided molecular design: Application

in agrochemicals, materials, and pharmaceuticals. (Reynolds, C. H., Holloway, M. K., and Cox, H. K. eds.), American Chem. Soc., Washington, D.C. pp 64-81

[107] Schneider, G., Lee, M. L., Stahl, M., and Schneider, P. (2000) *J Comput Aided Mol Des* 14, 487-494

[108] Hajduk, P. J., Dinges, J., Miknis, G. F., Merlock, M., Middleton, T., Kempf, D. J., Egan, D. A., Walter, K. A., Robins, T. S., Shuker, S. B., Holzman, T. F., and Fesik, S. W. (1997) *J Med Chem* 40, 3144-3150

[109] Hajduk, P. J., Meadows, R. P., and Fesik, S. W. (1997) *Science* 278, 497-499

[110] Mayer, M., and Meyer, B. (2001) *J Am Chem Soc* 123, 6108-6117

[111] Meinecke, R., and Meyer, B. (2001) *J Med Chem* 44, 3059-3065

Permissions

The contributors of this book come from diverse backgrounds, making this book a truly international effort. This book will bring forth new frontiers with its revolutionizing research information and detailed analysis of the nascent developments around the world.

We would like to thank Guy Huynh Thien Duc, for lending his expertise to make the book truly unique. He has played a crucial role in the development of this book. Without his invaluable contribution this book wouldn't have been possible. He has made vital efforts to compile up to date information on the varied aspects of this subject to make this book a valuable addition to the collection of many professionals and students.

This book was conceptualized with the vision of imparting up-to-date information and advanced data in this field. To ensure the same, a matchless editorial board was set up. Every individual on the board went through rigorous rounds of assessment to prove their worth. After which they invested a large part of their time researching and compiling the most relevant data for our readers. Conferences and sessions were held from time to time between the editorial board and the contributing authors to present the data in the most comprehensible form. The editorial team has worked tirelessly to provide valuable and valid information to help people across the globe.

Every chapter published in this book has been scrutinized by our experts. Their significance has been extensively debated. The topics covered herein carry significant findings which will fuel the growth of the discipline. They may even be implemented as practical applications or may be referred to as a beginning point for another development. Chapters in this book were first published by InTech; hereby published with permission under the Creative Commons Attribution License or equivalent.

The editorial board has been involved in producing this book since its inception. They have spent rigorous hours researching and exploring the diverse topics which have resulted in the successful publishing of this book. They have passed on their knowledge of decades through this book. To expedite this challenging task, the publisher supported the team at every step. A small team of assistant editors was also appointed to further simplify the editing procedure and attain best results for the readers.

Our editorial team has been hand-picked from every corner of the world. Their multi-ethnicity adds dynamic inputs to the discussions which result in innovative outcomes. These outcomes are then further discussed with the researchers and contributors who give their valuable feedback and opinion regarding the same. The feedback is then collaborated with the researches and they are edited in a comprehensive manner to aid the understanding of the subject.

Apart from the editorial board, the designing team has also invested a significant amount of their time in understanding the subject and creating the most relevant covers. They scrutinized every image to scout for the most suitable representation of the subject and create an appropriate cover for the book.

The publishing team has been involved in this book since its early stages. They were actively engaged in every process, be it collecting the data, connecting with the contributors or procuring relevant information. The team has been an ardent support to the editorial, designing and production team. Their endless efforts to recruit the best for this project, has resulted in the accomplishment of this book. They are a veteran in the field of academics and their pool of knowledge is as vast as their experience in printing. Their expertise and guidance has proved useful at every step. Their uncompromising quality standards have made this book an exceptional effort. Their encouragement from time to time has been an inspiration for everyone.

The publisher and the editorial board hope that this book will prove to be a valuable piece of knowledge for researchers, students, practitioners and scholars across the globe.

List of Contributors

Jianli Dong
Molecular Diagnostics Laboratory, University of Texas Medical Branch at Galveston, Galveston, USA

Giuseppe Palmieri, Maria Colombino and Maria Cristina Sini
Unit of Cancer Genetics, Institute of Biomolecular Chemistry (ICB), National Research Council (CNR), Traversa La Crucca, 3 - Baldinca Li Punti, Sassari, Italy

Paolo Antonio Ascierto
Unit of Medical Oncology and Innovative Therapy, Istituto Nazionale Tumori Fondazione "G. Pascale", Via Mariano Semmola, Napoli, Italy

Amelia Lissia and Antonio Cossu
University Hospital Health Unit - Azienda Ospedaliero Universitaria (AOU), Via Matteotti, Sassari, Italy

Guilherme Francisco, Priscila Daniele Ramos Cirilo, Tharcísio Citrângulo Tortelli Junior and Roger Chammas
Department of Radiology and Oncology, School of Medicine, University of São Paulo, Brazil
Center of Translational Research in Oncology, São Paulo State Cancer Institute (ICESP), São Paulo, Brazil

Fernanda Toledo Gonçalves
Department of Ethical and Legal Medicine, School of Medicine, University of São Paulo, Brazil

G. Ribas, M. Ibarrola-Villava and M.C. Peña-Chilet
Health Research Institute-INCLIVA, Av. Blasco Ibañez, Valencia, Spain

L.P. Fernandez
IIB Instituto de Investigaciones Biomédicas "Alberto Sols", Madrid, Spain

C. Martinez-Cadenas
Department of Medicine, University of Castellon Jaume I, Castellon, Spain

Vitali Alexeev, Daria Marley Kemp and Olga Igoucheva
Department of Dermatology and Cutaneous Biology, Jefferson Medical College, Thomas Jefferson University, Philadelphia, Pennsylvania, USA

Alyson Pidich
Temple University School of Medicine, Philadelphia, Pennsylvania, USA

J.G.M. van Beek, N.C. Naus and E. Kilic
Department of Ophthalmology, Erasmus MC, Rotterdam, The Netherlands

A. de Klein
Department of Clinical Genetics, The Netherlands

R.M. Verdijk
Department of Pathology, The Netherlands

A.E. Koopmans
Department of Ophthalmology, Erasmus MC, Rotterdam, The Netherlands
Department of Clinical Genetics, The Netherlands

John O. Mason
Retina Consultants of Alabama, P.C. and the University of Alabama at Birmingham School of Medicine, Department of Ophthalmology, Birmingham, Alabama, USA

Sara Mullins
University of Alabama at Birmingham School of Medicine, Department of Ophthalmology, Birmingham, Alabama, USA

Kavitha Gowrishankar, Matteo S. Carlino and Helen Rizos
Westmead Institute for Cancer Research, University of Sydney at Westmead Millennium Institute and Melanoma Institute Australia, Westmead Hospital, Westmead, Australia

Walter J. Storkus
Dermatology and Immunology, University of Pittsburgh School of Medicine, Pittsburgh, PA, USA
University of Pittsburgh Cancer Institute, Pittsburgh, PA, USA

Devin B. Lowe and Jennifer L. Taylor
Dermatology and Immunology, University of Pittsburgh School of Medicine, Pittsburgh, PA, USA

Konstantinos Arnaoutakis, Dorothy A. Graves, Laura F. Hutchins and Thomas Kieber-Emmons
Division of Hematology/Oncology and Department of Pathology University of Arkansas for Medical Sciences, Little Rock, AR, Winthrop P. Rockefeller Cancer Institute, USA

L.M. Davids and B. Kleemann
Redox Laboratory, Department of Human Biology; Faculty of Health Sciences, University of Cape Town Medical School, Cape Town, South Africa

Hideaki Matsuda, Megumi Masuda and Kazuya Murata
Faculty of Pharmacy, Kinki University, Japan

Yumi Abe and Akemi Uwaya
Research & Development, Morinda Worldwide, Inc., Japan

Kira G. Hartman
Department of Biochemistry and Molecular Biology, University of Maryland School of Medicine, Baltimore, MD, USA

Paul T. Wilder and David J. Weber
Center for Biomolecular Therapeutics, University of Maryland School of Medicine, Baltimore, MD, USA
University of Maryland Marlene and Stewart Greenebaum NCI Cancer Center, Baltimore, MD, USA
Department of Biochemistry and Molecular Biology, University of Maryland School of Medicine, Baltimore, MD, USA

Alexander D. Jr. MacKerell
Center for Biomolecular Therapeutics, University of Maryland School of Medicine, Baltimore, MD, USA
University of Maryland Marlene and Stewart Greenebaum NCI Cancer Center, Baltimore, MD, USA
Department of Pharmaceutical Sciences, University of Maryland School of Pharmacy, Baltimore, MD, USA

Andrew Coop
University of Maryland Marlene and Stewart Greenebaum NCI Cancer Center, Baltimore, MD, USA
Department of Pharmaceutical Sciences, University of Maryland School of Pharmacy, Baltimore, MD, USA

Kristen Varney
Department of Biochemistry and Molecular Biology, University of Maryland School of Medicine, Baltimore, MD, USA
Department of Pharmaceutical Sciences, University of Maryland School of Pharmacy, Baltimore, MD, USA
Center for Biomolecular Therapeutics, University of Maryland School of Medicine, Baltimore, MD, USA

Danna Zimmer
Department of Biochemistry and Molecular Biology, University of Maryland School of Medicine, Baltimore, MD, USA
Center for Biomolecular Therapeutics, University of Maryland School of Medicine, Baltimore, MD, USA

Rena Lapidus
Center for Biomolecular Therapeutics, University of Maryland School of Medicine, Baltimore, MD, USA
University of Maryland Marlene and Stewart Greenebaum NCI Cancer Center, Baltimore, MD, USA